The History of Neuroscience in Autobiography

VOLUME 4

The History of Neuroscience in Autobiography

VOLUME 4

Edited by Larry R. Squire

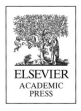

ELSEVIER
ACADEMIC
PRESS

Amsterdam   Boston   Heidelberg   London   New York   Oxford
Paris   San Diego   San Francisco   Singapore   Sydney   Tokyo

Permissions may be sought directly from Elsevier's Science & Technology Rights
Department in Oxford, UK: phone: (+44) 1865 843830, fax: (+44) 1865 853333,
e-mail: permissions@elsevier.com.uk. You may also complete your request on-line
via the Elsevier homepage (http://elsevier.com), by selecting "Customer
Support" and then "Obtaining Permissions."

Academic Press
An imprint of Elsevier
525 B Street, Suite 1900, San Diego, California 92101-4495, USA
http://www.academicpress.com

Academic Press
84 Theobald's Road, London WC1X 8RR, UK
http://www.academicpress.com

Library of Congress Catalog Card Number: 2003 111249

International Standard Book Number: 0-12-660246-8

PRINTED IN THE UNITED STATES OF AMERICA
04   05   06   07   08   9   8   7   6   5   4   3   2   1

Contents

Previous Contributors

Volume 1

Denise Albe-Fessard
Julius Axelrod
Peter O. Bishop
Theodore H. Bullock
Irving T. Diamond
Robert Galambos
Viktor Hamburger
Sir Alan L. Hodgkin
David H. Hubel

Herbert H. Jasper
Sir Bernard Katz
Seymour S. Kety
Benjamin Libet
Louis Sokoloff
James M. Sprague
Curt von Euler
John Z. Young

Volume 2

Lloyd M. Beidler
Arvid Carlsson
Donald R. Griffen
Roger Guillemin
Ray Guillery
Masao Ito
Martin G. Larrabee

Jerome Lettvin
Paul D. MacLean
Brenda Milner
Karl H. Pribram
Eugene Roberts
Gunther Stent

Volume 3

Morris H. Aprison
Brian B. Boycott
Vernon B. Brooks
Pierre Buser
Hsiang-Tung Chang
Augusto Claudio Guillermo Cuello
Robert W. Doty
Bernice Grafstein

Ainsley Iggo
Jennifer S. Lund
Edith Graef McGeer
Patrick L. McGeer
Edward R. Perl
Donald B. Tower
Patrick D. Wall
Wally Welker

Preface to Volume 1

Before the Alfred P. Sloan Foundation series of books began to appear in 1979, the scientific autobiography was a largely unfamiliar genre. One recalls Cajal's extraordinary *Recollections of My Life*, translated into English in 1937, and the little gem of autobiography written by Charles Darwin for his grandchildren in 1876. One supposes that this form of scientific writing is scarce because busy scientists would rather continue to work on scientific problems than to indulge in a retrospective exercise using a writing style that is usually outside their scope of experience. Yet, regardless of the nature of one's own investigative work, the scientific enterprise describes a community of activity and thought in which all scientists share. Indeed, an understanding of the scientific enterprise should in the end be accessible to anyone, because it is essentially a human endeavor, full of intensity, purpose, and drama that are universal to human experience.

While writing a full autobiographical text is a formidable undertaking, preparing an autobiographical chapter, which could appear with others in a volume, is perhaps less daunting work and is a project that senior scientists might even find tempting. Indeed, a venture of this kind within the discipline of psychology began in 1930 and is now in eight volumes (*A History of Psychology in Autobiography*). So it was that during my term as President of the Society for Neuroscience in 1993 to 1994, I developed the idea of collecting autobiographies from senior neuroscientists, who at this period in the history of our discipline are in fact pioneers of neuroscience. Neuroscience is quintessentially interdisciplinary, and careers in neuroscience come from several different cultures including biology, psychology, and medicine. Accounts of scientific lives in neuroscience hold the promise of being informative and interesting, and they could be a source of inspiration to students. Moreover, personal narratives provide for scientists and non-scientists alike an insight into the nature of scientific work that is simply not available in ordinary scientific writing.

This volume does have a forerunner in neuroscience. In 1975, MIT Press published *The Neurosciences: Paths of Discovery*, a collection of 30 chapters in commemoration of F. O. Schmitt's 70th birthday edited by F. Worden, J. Swazey, and G. Adelman. The contributing neuroscientists, all leaders of their discipline, described the paths of discovery that they had followed in carrying on their work. While writing in the style of the conventional review article, some authors did include a good amount of anecdote, opinion, and personal reflection. A second, similar volume, *The Neurosciences: Paths of Discovery II*, edited by F. Samson and G. Adelman, appeared in 1992.

In any case, neuroscience writing that is deliberately and primarily autobiographical has not been collected before. This project, *The History of Neuroscience in Autobiography*, is the first major publishing venture of the Society for Neuroscience after *The Journal of Neuroscience*. The book project was prepared with the active cooperation of the Committee on the History of Neuroscience, which serves as an editorial board for the project. The first chairperson of the committee was Edward (Ted) Jones; its members were Albert Aguayo, Ted Melnechuk, Gordon Shepherd, and Ken Tyler. This group compiled the names and carried out the deliberations that led to the first round of invitations. In 1995 Larry Swanson succeeded Ted Jones as chair of the committee, and as we go to press with Volume 1 the committee members are Albert Aguayo, Bernice Grafstein, Ted Melnechuk, Dale Purves, and Gordon Shepherd.

In the inaugural volume of the series, we are delighted to be able to present together 17 personal narratives by some of the true pioneers of modern neuroscience. The group includes four Nobel Laureates and 11 members or foreign associates of the National Academy of Sciences, USA. The contributors did their scientific work in the United States, Canada, England, Australia, France, and Sweden. It is difficult to imagine a finer group of scientists with which to inaugurate our autobiographical series. The autobiographical chapters that appear here are printed essentially as submitted by the authors, with only light technical editing. Accordingly, the chapters are the personal perspectives and viewpoints of the authors and do not reflect material or opinion from the Society for Neuroscience.

Preparation of this volume depended critically on the staff of the book's publisher, the Society for Neuroscience. The correspondence, technical editing, cover design, printing, and marketing have all been coordinated by the Society's Central Office, under the superb direction of Diane M. Sullenberger. I thank her and her assistants, Stacie M. Lemick (publishing manager) and Danielle L. Gulp (desktop publisher), for their dedicated and skillful work on this project, which was carried out in the midst of the demands brought by the first in-house years of the Society's *Journal of Neuroscience*. I also thank my dear friend Nancy Beang (executive director of the Society for Neuroscience), who from the beginning gave her full enthusiasm to this project.

Larry R. Squire
Del Mar, California
September 1996

Preface to Volume 2

This second volume of *The History of Neuroscience in Autobiography* presents 13 autobiographical chapters by senior neuroscientists. The authors tell about the experiences that shaped their lives, the teachers, colleagues, and students with whom they worked, and the scientific work that has absorbed them during their careers. As with Volume 1, this volume was prepared with the help of the Committee on the History of Neuroscience at the Society for Neuroscience. This group, which serves as editorial board for the project, compiled the names of those who were invited to contribute to the volume, and the committee's chairperson (Larry Swanson) shared in editing the manuscripts.

At the Society for Neuroscience, Holly Seltzer (production director) coordinated the early phases of Volume 2. In 1997, Academic Press joined with the Society for Neuroscience as a partner in this project. Although the volumes continue to be official publications of the Society for Neuroscience, Academic Press has coordinated the technical editing, printing, and marketing for Volume 2 under the very capable direction of Jasna Markovac (Editor-in-Chief, Biomedical Sciences). The collaboration between the Society for Neuroscience and Academic Press has proceeded smoothly, and I hope readers will find Volume 2 as informative and enjoyable as Volume 1.

Larry R. Squire
Del Mar, California
May 1998

Preface to Volume 3

This third volume of *The History of Neuroscience in Autobiography* includes 15 autobiographical chapters by neuroscientists. The authors tell about the experiences that shaped their lives, the teachers, colleagues, and students with whom they worked, and the scientific work that has absorbed them during their careers. Their essays serve as enduring records of a lifetime of discovery and achievement. We are particularly fortunate to be able to include a contribution from Brian B. Boycott, who passed away on April 22, 2000.

As with Volumes 1 and 2, this volume was prepared with the help of the Committee on the History of Neuroscience at the Society for Neuroscience (Lawrence Kruger, chairperson). This group, which serves as editorial board for the project, compiled the names of those who were invited to contribute to the volume.

At the Society for Neuroscience, Allison Pearsall (production director) coordinated the project. Although the volumes are official publications of the Society for Neuroscience, since 1997 Academic Press has been a partner in the project and has coordinated the technical editing, printing, and marketing under the very capable direction of Jasna Markovac (Vice President, Editorial Director). I hope readers will find Volume 3 as interesting and enjoyable as Volumes 1 and 2.

Larry R. Squire
Del Mar, California
October 2000

Preface to Volume 4

This fourth volume of *The History of Neuroscience in Autobiography* includes 14 autobiographical chapters by senior neuroscientists. The authors tell about the experiences that shaped their lives, the teachers, colleagues, and students with whom they worked, and the scientific work that has absorbed them during their careers. Their essays serve as enduring records of a lifetime of discovery and achievement.

We are particularly fortunate to be able to include a contribution from W. Maxwell (Max) Cowan, who passed away on June 30, 2002. Although his chapter was largely completed, we are able to thank his former student Brent Stanfield, Ph.D., who kindly reviewed the chapter and suggested some modest organizational and editorial changes.

As with the first three volumes of this series, Volume 4 was prepared with the help of the Committee on the History of Neuroscience at the Society for Neuroscience. This group, which serves as editorial board for the project, compiled the names of those who were invited to contribute to the volume.

We are especially grateful for the contributions of Louise Marshal, Ph.D., member of the History Committee, who passed away on July 12, 2003 at the age of 94. Her enthusiasm and support for history of Neuroscience projects were widely known and deeply appreciated by the Society for Neuroscience and her colleagues at UCLA.

At the Society for Neuroscience, Charyl Delaney (Chapters and Special Programs Manager) coordinated the project with vigor and efficiency. Although the volumes are official publications of the Society for Neuroscience, since 1997 Academic Press (now part of Elsevier) has been a partner in the project and has coordinated the technical editing, printing, and marketing under the very capable direction of Jasna Markovac (Senior Vice President, Elsevier, Life Science). I hope readers will find Volume 4 as interesting and enjoyable as the earlier volumes.

Larry R. Squire
Del Mar, California
August 2003

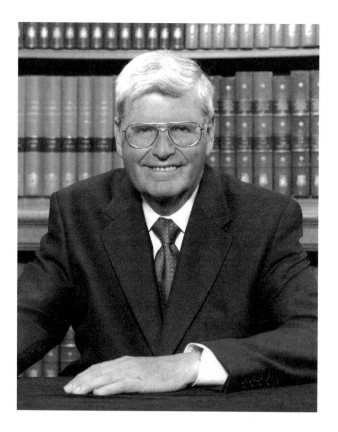

Per Andersen

BORN:

Oslo, Norway
January 12, 1930

EDUCATION:

University of Oslo, M.D. (1954)
University of Oslo, Dr. med., Ph.D. (1960)

APPOINTMENTS:

University of Oslo (1958)

HONORS AND AWARDS (SELECTED):

Fridtjof Nansen Prize, Norwegian Academy of Science (1968)
Norwegian Academy of Science (1980)
Norwegian Research Council (1988)
Honorary Doctorate, Zurich University (1988)
Royal Swedish Academy (1991)
Ipsen Prize (Neuronal Plasticity) (1993)
Foreign Associate, National Academy of Sciences, USA (1994)
Fernström Prize (1995)
Lundbeck Prize (1996)
Honorary Doctorate, Karolinska Instituet (1998)
Foreign Member, Royal Society London (2002)

*Per Andersen pioneered the analysis of the physiology of the hippocampus.
He described the trisynaptic circuit, pioneered the development of the
hippocampal slice, discovered inhibitory neurons in the hippocampus,
and helped establish long-term potentiation as a tool for the study of
neuronal plasticity.*

Per Andersen

Playing with the Seahorse

I thank the Society for Neuroscience and the Editor of *The History of Neuroscience in Autobiography* for the invitation to share with neuroscientific colleagues, younger and older, some of my experiences in our literally exciting field of investigation.

Family and School

Of the many factors of importance for a scientific activity, I think the values you develop through your upbringing may be the most relevant. In both verbal and practical ways, my parents insisted that education was the essential thing. With limited resources, they both made their utmost so that their four children could receive the best education possible. Fortunately, our Scandinavian system allows for public education, up to and including university education. In the suburb of the small, quiet city of Oslo, I enjoyed a happy childhood, living in a favorable position for outdoor life, a Norwegian national pastime.

I enjoyed school, all the way from the early days through high school. I was particularly engaged by physics. However, as the years went by, I was more and more taken to the idea of being a physician. School work was relatively easy, in particular, science and mathematics. Other subjects, particularly essays, called for more maturation than I could muster at the time. However, by concentrating, I got through the numerus clausus barrier and could enter the medical curriculum.

Scientific Introduction

In the medical curriculum, I was fortunate to meet some outstanding neuroanatomists who set me on the scientific path. By their own example, they showed me the importance of well-informed guidance, genuine excitement, and quality standards. The first was Jan Birger Jansen, who in 1930 revived the Norwegian neuroscientific tradition which was started by Fridtjof Nansen through his doctoral thesis from 1887, later to be a famous polar explorer and high commissioner for refugees under the Union of Nations in Geneva. Jansen, supported by the Rockefeller Foundation, created the Brain Laboratory at the Anatomical Institute, which soon attracted a set of young, eager collaborators. Between them, Jansen and Alf Brodal created the so-called Oslo school by concentrating on experimental studies of the cerebellum and its connectivities. Jansen's enthusiastic and instructive lectures on the brain emphasized the magnitude of the controlling and regulating tasks undertaken by the brain and how it influenced virtually all other bodily functions. These thoughts awoke a desire to learn more about this topic and to take part in the search for understanding the brain's control functions. Later, after I obtained a student's assistantship to help in simpler demonstrations, I was fortunate to enjoy Jansens eminent leadership, helping and encouraging his subordinates far more than most scientific leaders. The whole institute felt like a family, with him and his lovely wife Helene as the central figures. Having lost my father when I had just turned 17, Jansen became a sort of father figure for me.

Neuroscientific Apprenticeship

By providence, Birger R. Kaada returned to Oslo from his two-year studies at Yale and McGill. Until this time, about 1950, teaching of neural function at all universities was dominated by clinical syndromes and reflex studies. Kaada, who was trained by John F. Fulton, Wilder Penfield, and Herbert Jasper, was granted laboratory space at the Anatomical Institute by Jansen and told us a series of new and exciting stories, in which electrical recording from brain structures and even individual cells added a new dimension. When he announced that he wanted two student assistants for his research, I eagerly applied and was fortunate to be accepted early in 1951, just as I turned 21 years old. I had started on my neuroscientific career.

Kaada had made an elaborate electrocorticographic study of the so-called rhinencephalon, comprising much of what later has been termed the limbic system. He was interested in examining the physiological roles of specific subdivisions. Thus, he asked Jan Kristian Schøning Jansen, the son of Professor Jansen, and myself to take part in a study with implanted stimulation electrodes in awake cats. We did these experiments in addition to the usual medical curriculum. The way we found time was to drop some of the lectures and theoretical discussions, but not any of the clinical demonstrations. In addition, we got used to long working days.

Stimulation of the amygdala complex in freely moving cats caused licking, chewing, salivation, and retching, but also emotionally colored behaviors, as if the cats were frightened or angry. In contrast, hippocampal stimulation gave much less dramatic responses, but a slowly developing reaction which we called the orienting response. It was as if the animals became aware of something surprising or new in the contralateral environment. The same reaction followed stimulation of the medial frontal cortex and the anterior and middle cingulate gyri. No doubt, the many hours at the microscope during the following histological analysis and the painstaking reconstructions of electrode sites and lesions provided an anatomical insight which has been highly useful later in life. Eventually, Kaada taught us how to plan and write an article on our findings. I still remember the excitement on seeing our names in print as authors of a real scientific article.

Later, I realized how fortunate we were in being introduced to neuroscience by such experienced and dedicated supervisors. Kaada, as well as Jansen and Brodal, emphasized the importance of a sharply formulated problem and then the selection of an appropriate method. Alf Brodal was particularly keen that the chosen problem should not only be clearly defined, but be of biological significance. "Only attack real problems," he used to say. The basic training I received from Kaada, Jansen, and Brodal, supported by their own adherence to sound scientific principles, has been more valuable than is easily measured.

After some years with stimulation of limbic structures in freely moving cats, I got my own project. This time also the inspiration came from a close colleague, Theodor Blackstad, who had just returned from a year studying brain anatomy in Paris. In 1949, Brodal received from Walle Nauta in Zürich a new method for tracing fiber degeneration, even before it was published. This was the famous Nauta 1950 method. Blackstad tried it out on hippocampal pathways and was tremendously rewarded. Fiber degeneration in this structure stood out as a painting of Joan Miró, with black stripes on a yellow background. For example, after an entorhinal lesion, the degenerated perforant path appeared as a black band in the molecular layer of the dentate fascia. So intense was the degeneration that it could easily be seen by the naked eye! In a moment, this slide of Blackstad's set my entire scientific course. Immediately, I saw that this would make a fabulous preparation for a neurophysiologist interested in cortical physiology. By stimulating a proper selection of input fibers, I could engage a set of synapses located to a restricted part of the dendritic tree of the target neurons.

Within a few weeks, I started the first experiments, and with beginner's luck I got some very large and apparently simple signals in the first few experiments. However, after this initial success, things got more complicated, and I had to struggle for several years before I saw light at the end of the tunnel. Here we come to a condition for scientific progress which was not present in Oslo in the early 1950s! Today, a beginner in neurosciences has the advantage to join a number of excellent neuroscience programs and can enjoy instructive textbooks and a large number of review books and articles. Above all, she or he can enjoy the information plethora available on the Internet. In Oslo in 1952, when I started the first hippocampal electrophysiological experiments, very little help was at hand. Although Kaada had recorded gross electrocorticographic signals, he had little experience with evoked potential analysis. Jan K.S. Jansen and myself, Kaada's two first pupils, therefore, had to find out on our own how to proceed. In all Scandinavia, there were few people to ask for help. Nearly all the many outstanding neuroscientists in Sweden had worked on problems related to spinal cord or bulbar (mechanisms. Few, if any, had studied field potentials, the gross signals generated in a central structure after synchronous activation of a major afferent source.

In short, Jan and I had to fend for ourselves. His interest was cerebellar connectivity, linking into the work by his father and Brodal. I was captivated by the elegance, the stringency, and the beauty of the hippocampal histology. Thus, we started with histology. In my case, I cherished the two-volume book by Santiago Ramon y Cajal, translated to French (1911). Here, I may, perhaps, interject a point of satisfaction for European scientists. Because I enjoyed French, the Ramon y Cajal volumes were not too difficult. I devoured them. What a genius! And his countryman, Lorente de Nó, had written a masterpiece on Golgi-stained hippocampal neurons in 1934, also a great source of information. These two masters of the Golgi method gave me tremendous stimulation through the histological details provided and also a number of ideas for physiological thinking.

But, classical anatomy aside, how could I translate the electrical signals I saw into a meaningful picture? Here, I was supported by two giants in the history of neuroscience, Fréderic Bremer and Alan Hodgkin. Bremer was the father of the two important preparations, encephale isolée (a brain isolated from the spinal cord by a section above the C1 segment) and cerveau isolee (the brain isolated from the lower brain stem by a section above the mesencephalon). He wrote a survey of his experiences in *Physiological Reviews* (Bremer 1958), and his logical and clear exposé was a great help. In 1952, Alan Hodgkin and Andrew F. Huxley published their famous set of four papers, which later earned them the Nobel Prize. Hodgkin also wrote a review of this work in *Biological Reviews* in 1951. This became my neuroscientific bible. At first, I found the article extremely difficult because of all the terms and processes I had not met before. I do not know how many times I had to read it before I got the main ideas right. Over and over again, but slowly the major ideas took hold, and I could start to use this information in the interpretation of the hippocampal signals I recorded.

In parallel, I read the 1953 book of John C. Eccles, *The Neurophysiological Basis of Mind*. This book explained in cellular terms many of the results of Sherrington, but for me this book was less important than the Hodgkin review. A different story was, however, the small, red-covered book of his, *The Physiology of Nerve Cells*, in which he summarized the first few years' experience with intracellular studies of motoneurones. At this time, the small red book of Mao was much talked about. For me, and thousands of other neuroscientists, Eccles' small volume would be our Famous Red Book. Given as the Herter Lectures at the Johns Hopkins University in 1955, Eccles managed to give a wonderfully authoritative survey of cellular motoneuronal physiology in a way that could be used as a guideline for studies of most other nerve cells. If Hodgkin's *Biological Review* article was my neurobiological "Old Testament," Eccles little red book became my "New Testament." Feeling I was on my own, however, I developed a certain degree of inferiority. Other neuroscientists had their education from large universities with a proper training in basic topics, not the least biophysics, chemistry, and mathematics. I acutely felt that my medical training, adequate as it probably was for work as a clinical doctor, was inadequate for the basic scientific enterprise.

The reader should not get the impression that I was the only fledgling neuroscientist with difficulty in understanding brain signals. At the time, probably all of us who tried to understand evoked brain signals were uncertain. Probably surprising to many today, we were not that many who worked on the hippocampus. Some pioneering work was done by Richard Jung and Jan F. Tönnies in Alois Kornmüller's laboratory in Berlin. In 1938, they discovered the low threshold for seizure development in the hippocampus. In the same year, Kornmüller, who for years was searching for a physiological correlate to the Brodmann areas, reported with Jung that the hippocampus displayed a large amplitude sinusoidal activity which they coined the theta activity. To my knowledge, in the middle 1950s there were only five scientific groups working with hippocampal field potentials, spontaneous or evoked. These groups counted Brian Cragg and Lionel Hamlyn at University College London, Pierre Gloor and his associates at Montreal Neurological Institute at McGill, John D. Green and Ross Adey with colleagues at the Brain Research Institute at UCLA, Arnaldo Arduini and colleagues in Pisa and, finally me, working by myself in Oslo. Somewhat later, Jim Olds in Ann Arbor made significant additions, and Eric Kandel and Alden Spencer in Karl Frank's laboratory in Bethesda started their remarkable collaboration. To various degrees, we all struggled with interpretation of the extracellular signals recorded from the hippocampus, either after a triggering stimulus, after spontaneous activity, or during an epileptiform seizure activity.

The first unit recording from individual brain cells was, in fact, also made in the hippocampus by Renshaw, Forbes, and Morison in 1940. Green and Arduini rediscovered the theta waves in 1954 and noted that discharges of single hippocampal units were in moderate synchrony with the theta waves. Brian Cragg and Lionel Hamlyn in London were in 1955 the first to record sharp, spike-like signals which were conducted slowly along the apical dendrites after local synaptic excitation. These signals my colleagues and I later named population spikes and proved through recording of a large number of single unit discharges that they were composed of a large number of near synchronously discharging pyramidal or granule cells (Andersen et al., 1971a).

Guided by Bremer, I interpreted the local negative slow waves as signs of excitatory synaptically induced depolarizations of the target neurons. By using the histological evidence from Blackstad's experimental work, I found that commissural activation gave extracellular negative waves exactly in those areas where Blackstad found terminal degeneration. I must admit that I found the thesis work rather tedious. The tradition was that you had to do it all yourself to show your independence and that you were in command of all aspects of the relevant scientific work. An additional element was the fact that I lost the help of Sarah Mørch, the charming artist of the Anatomical Institute. She got cancer, and Jansen would not signal to her that the outlook was bad. Consequently, for more than a year he refused to hire somebody in her place so as not to add to her worries. The result was that I spent nearly every evening in the artist's room, trying to make my own figures from oscilloscope prints and histological micrographs. The artist's room was next to Jansens office. Because he came in every evening for an extra session, undisturbed by the hustle of the day, we came to see each other quite a bit, working as we were in neigboring rooms. Although he concentrated on his work in his own office, he sometimes needed some material from the outer rooms. Quite often, he found me struggling over my figures. He usually came with some encouraging words. I got the impression that he liked to see that I kept at it, but he never commented on the artist's absence. Just as the figure-making took a considerable time, I accept that this training later gave me an upper hand toward people who had not made their own films, prints, line drawings, reversals, enlargements, composites, and lettering.

In those days, we recorded all signals on the oscilloscope face with a camera, initially fully manually operated and later with a semiautomated system that still needed a manual push for every sweep to be saved. A successful experiment could generate about 200 ft or more of 35-mm exposed film. Returning the next day, the first task was to salvage the film containers and develop the films. After fixing and rinsing, the impossibly long films were dried by hanging in one of the tall staircase towers between the basement and the third floor for a few hours. Therefore, everyone in the whole institute could know whether it had been a successful experiment or not. Later, we had to mark each of the several hundreds, or thousands, of traces with India ink by reference to the experimental protocol. In those days, there were no computers and few semiautomatic measuring devices. Nearly all measurements were made by placing the marked films on a light box covered with translucent millimeter paper, and the latencies and amplitudes were measured with an accuracy of a tenth of a millimeter. With experience, it was amazing how good the trained eye can be. For critical measurements, we always used two or more investigators who did not know the results of the others, and in special cases, we used projectors giving enlargements of the original records.

Toward the end of the thesis work, I received a call from Professor Ragnar Granit in Stockholm, whom I met when he was external examiner for Kaada's thesis. He asked me whether I would like to come to his institute to give a seminar of my work. It was like lightning had struck! First, I was excited beyond belief! Second, how could I afford it? Being the first invited seminar in my life, I did not know that people who invite you to give a seminar usually provide both travel and accommodation. I think that Granit understood because he quickly added that I would get a train ticket by post and that I could stay at Hotel Eden "because I have some shares in that hotel." What a wonderful person! Obviously, I was ever so grateful. Coming to, however, I started to worry because the famous Curt von Euler, who had worked on the hippocampus with John Green at UCLA, was Granit's next-in-command. What would he say about my records and interpretations. Maybe I was in for a scientific slaughter?

The Stockholm trip was a revelation. It was the first time I experienced the international brotherhood of science. People were not only friendly, but they treated me as one of their own, as if I really had something to contribute. Obviously, there was opposition, but in a constructive way. In the end, I felt utterly rewarded. Throughout my career, Ragnar Granit and Curt von Euler remained my close friends, two eminent scientists whose memory I honor.

The thesis eventually saw the light of day. At the time, I was happy that the work was done, but I had no idea about its reception and certainly no feeling for its possible future use. In particular, I did not expect to return to it more than very occasionally. Posterity has shown, however, that I have been using all the papers in the thesis quite extensively, a source of quiet satisfaction for a mature neuroscientist. Before the dissertation I was scared stiff, mostly by the reputation of my external examiner, Professor Curt von Euler. I knew he was a gentleman, but how was he as a Ph.D. examiner? Curt used the rule I later heard from my friend Tomas Hökfelt about a similar skirmish: the opponent "showed his claws, but did not use them." A highly civilized behavior!

Throughout the thesis work, I felt a strange, Janus-like effect. Much as I enjoyed finding apparent explanations for synaptic activation of hippocampal neurons, the weakness of my scientific education became all too obvious. My consequent lack of confidence caused an urge to join a first-class laboratory where I could receive top-level training. Once again, my guardian angels Jansen and Brodal came to the rescue. Both belonged to a small group of international neuroscientists, led by the neuroendocrinologist Wolfgang Bargmann, which had yearly meetings in Europe. Eccles was also a member. One sunny day Brodal asked me whether I had thought of going to Australia. I understood immediately what he meant and felt that my heart took a few somersaults. In my very private dreams I had entertained the thought of being trained by Sir John. But in real life? Never! However, this incidence illustrates how important it is to have good supervisors. In Eccles eyes, the Oslo school stood for quality. Brodal wrote and got an immediate positive reply. Later, Eccles told me that this expectation was one of the reasons he said yes to Brodal's inquiry. Here, I can reveal one of Eccles' relatively few mistakes. He believed that I was a trained neuroanatomist, coming from the Oslo group of anatomists. I was, however, not quite without anatomical knowledge. I had been an Instructor at the Brain Dissection Course for the medical students for a few years. Although different from the brains of lower animals, there is still a considerable similarity. A thorough understanding of the three-dimensional relations and some of the gross connectivity turned out to come in very handy later on.

Professor Jansen's excellent relation with the Rockefeller Foundation was probably a major factor behind my stipend, granted in 1961. I was later told that it was one of the last Rockefeller stipends to European scientists because the Foundation had made a strategic change to switch its support to Africa and Asia, in view of the higher prosperity of most European nations. One difficulty was the fact that the Rockefeller Foundation granted travel assistance to my wife and me, but not to our three children. When Professor Jansen heard about that, he immediately said that I should leave that to him. About a week later, he had a solution. Not only had he got hold of money for the children's tickets, but he had arranged so we could go by air. He felt that looking after three children, one only eight months old, for six weeks on a boat would be too strenuous, particularly for my wife. More than anything, this shows what kind of man he was. Obviously, I was more than grateful, but I was anxious to know where the extra money had come from. There were rumors that previous, unexplained financial miracles had been paid by Jansen himself. Thus, I politely said that I hoped that my children's ticket could be reimbursed by a scientific fund. He made as if he was irritated and asked me, "Who is the Boss at this Institute, you or me?" I had to confess that he was the boss. So, he said, with a flicker of a smile, "So leave that one to me, will you?"

Australia and Sir John

My stay in Australia was a fantastic period. From the first to the last day, it was a stay colored by excitement, intense learning, new discoveries, friendship, and a deep satisfaction with the field as such. The main factor was John Eccles himself. The many young international pupils who flocked around his pulpit called him Prof, a term I think he liked a great deal. In addition, there was the excellent working conditions, because the Australian authorities had created one of the few research schools in the world. The superb working and research facilities were thoroughly enjoyed. For us youngsters in the crew, it was like basking in the sun. With the best of equipment, the best of collaborators and technicians, and the best neuroscientist leader in the world, it was a dream. Our setting in the Australian community added to the excitement. Canberra is a garden city with about 20 million fruit trees planted along the boulevard-like streets. The spring flowering has to be seen to be believed! The Aussies, as the indigenous population is called, are a delightful flock, open, honest, and enclosing. All our family came to love them.

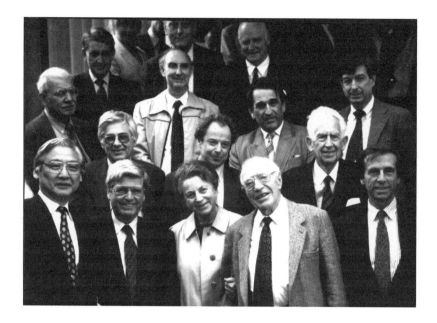

Fig. 1. A group of the many colleagues and friends of Sir John C. Eccles who celebrated his 90th birthday in Frankfurt in May 1993. From left to right, 1st line; Masao Ito, Per Andersen, Helena Eccles, Sir John C. Eccles, Piergiorgio Strata; 2nd row: Mario Wiesendanger, Henri Korn, Janos Szentágothai; 3rd row: Manfred Klee, Jeff Watkins, Joszef Hamori, Roger Nicoll; 4th row: Ian McDonald, Hans Kornhuber, Yngve Løyning.

Among the many findings I was fortunate to be a part of, I would like to mention the description of corticofugal presynaptic inhibition in the spinal cord; analysis of presynaptic and postsynaptic inhibition in the dorsal column nuclei; analysis of rhythmic thalamic responses with recurrent inhibition and postinhibitory rebound as the instrumental mechanism; the finding that hippocampal basket cells are inhibitory; the principle that synapses on soma of pyramidal cells are inhibitory; the finding that cerebellar basket cells are inhibitory; and the discovery of the trisynaptic circuit of the hippocampus.

Spinal and Dorsal Column Nuclei Studies

As a start, Sir John—or Prof—asked me whether I would like to take part in an investigation of a possible corticofugal presynaptic effect on spinal reflexes. Sir John, who knew about the pioneering results of Hagbarth and Kerr (1954) which showed that descending signals from the cerebral cortex could reduce, or even block, spinal signals induced by peripheral activity, wanted to see whether corticofugal impulse volleys could produce presynaptic inhibition in the spinal cord. Having some experience with cerebral cortical stimulation from our work in Oslo, and prodded by Sir John, I suggested that we stimulate the pre- and postcentral gyri. Our immediate success both pleased and impressed Sir John, presumably creating an advantageous position for further collaboration with the young lad from the north. We found that a corticofugal burst of stimuli created the same dorsal root potential and increased the excitability of afferent fibers in the dorsal roots that followed spinal nerve stimulation.

I suggested to Prof that we should try to look for presynaptic inhibition in the dorsal column nuclei because these had a fiber and cell arrangement that allowed recording very close to the fiber terminals. Prof had predicted that the mechanism involved axo-axonic synapses that acted on the terminals themselves. The regular anatomy of this system allowed us to get intra-axonal records from dorsal column fibers as close as 0.5 mm from their terminals. Consequently, the intracellularly recorded depolarization had a large amplitude and was associated with enhanced fiber excitability, just as in the case of spinal afferent fibers.

Thalamic Mechanisms

Following a detailed analysis of the transmission through the cuneate and gracilis nuclei and the associated pre- and postsynaptic inhibition (Andersen et al., 1964b–e), Prof was eager to proceed up to the next station of the somatosensory system, the ventrobasal nucleus of the thalamus. For this approach, we needed some precision of the placement of the recording electrodes. Prof had not used sterotactic procedures before and was genuinely surprised that Tom Sears and I were able to find the ventrolateral nucleus. During a visit to the John Curtin School for Medical Research (JCSMR) by King Bhumipol of Thailand, Eccles showed him around and explained what we were doing. Pointing to Tom and me, he said, "They have to find this little speck of nerve cells in the middle of the brain, and quite amazingly, they hit it every time!" Naturally, we greatly enjoyed these admiring words of his.

While Prof was an accomplished dissector of peripheral nerves and spinal roots, he always left the surgery of the brain to me. We needed to remove the dorsal part of the cortical mantle without getting too much bleeding from the many vessels there, whereafter I sucked away the hippocampus to expose the web of arteries on the dorsal aspect of the thalamus and tried to find an area for penetration of the recording electrodes. Fortunately, it usually worked and reinforced Prof's belief that I was a real neuroanatomist!

When we recorded from thalamic neurons in response to stimulation of an appropriate skin nerve, we were struck by the large size of the excitatory postsynaptic potentials (EPSPs) and that they were composed of a small number of elementary steps. An additional surprise was the large and long-lasting hyperpolarization that followed. It answered to the various tests we had for inhibition, so we concluded it was an IPSP. However, because Prof never had seen such amplitudes and durations in spinal cord neurons, it took some time before he was convinced. Once that occurred, though, he was the most excited of us all and told everyone around how huge the inhibitory processes were in the brain. Still, the most surprising finding in the thalamic cells was the large depolarizing responses, measuring tens of millivolts and lasting for some 20 msec or more, that appeared as unitary events just after the IPSPs. This was an entirely new response type. When we tested whether the IPSP could be elicted by antidromic activation of thalamo-cortical neurons, and thus be part of a recurrent loop, we saw to our further surprise that the recurrent IPSPs also were followed by the depolarizing wave response. Further, a hyperpolarizing current pulse gave a similar reaction as well. Influenced by the enhanced excitability of peripheral nerve fibers after an anodal current, Eccles named the reaction post-inhibitory rebound (Andersen and Eccles, 1962). Later work, notably by Llinas and Jahnsen (1982) and by David McCormick's group (von Krosigk et al., 1993), has shown that the original name was not without foundation. The response is due to calcium influx following resetting of calcium conductance mechanisms by the prominent hyperpolarizing IPSP. Another important factor is the I_h current, of which we were ignorant in 1962. This current is activated by hyperpolarization and provides the depolarizing drive to elicit the rebound response. An additional surprising finding was that there was not one, but a set of repeated IPSPs in ventrobasal thalamic neurons in response to a single stimulus to a peripheral nerve or to the somatosensory cortex. In extracellular recordings, we noted that there was a cluster of cell discharges on top of the rebound response. Many neurons fired nearly synchronously, and each of them emitted a burst of spikes. Such repeated burst discharges were reflected by a set of cortical waves in the appropriate projection area from the thalamic location. I remember how it made me recall the oscillatory responses described by Adrian in 1941, which he interpreted as repeated thalamic activations. In the thalamic work (Andersen et al., 1964 a,f), one of the collaborators was an old friend and colleague of Prof's, Chandler McCuskey Brooks from Downstate University, New York. This real gentleman had been working with Eccles in Dunedin, New Zealand, in 1946. The result was the first description of the focal potential, a field potential resulting from the near simultaneously discharging motoneurones in response to a fiber volley in the relevant peripheral nerve or dorsal root (Brooks and Eccles, 1948). This was the extracellular counterpart of the EPSP which Brock, Coombs, and Eccles discovered in 1951. Chandler was a highly experienced scientist, quiet and reflective and without any high-brow manners. It was a privilege to work with him on these experiments and in the later analysis.

Several of the discoveries led to letters to *Nature*. The two years I spent with Sir John created eight such letters. We were so proud, because it meant that out efforts were appreciated by the rest of the world. Unquestionably, the application of intracellular recording on problems from the central nervous system was an important factor. But equally important was Prof's drive and ambition—he really wanted to discover new land. It was so exciting. Every day was like a birthday party, all the new information and insight were like precious gifts. I woke up every morning eager to get started at work and wondering about what we would find out today. Fortunately, my family also enjoyed the Australian way of life so I could enjoy my work and spend truly long hours in the lab. Weekends were free, though, at least in general.

Hippocampal Synapses

After nearly a year with work on presynaptic inhibition and on the somatosensory system, Sir John came one day and proposed to start investigations on the hippocampal pathways. I was thrilled because some months earlier he had fleetingly suggested that we should concentrate on spinal and brain stem mechanisms during my Canberra time, leaving me as he said "to tackle the hippocampus when you return to Oslo." At the time, I was slightly disappointed, but obviously accepted his proposal. With his changed mind, however, I was thrilled since I knew that our progress would be much faster, and I enjoyed my good luck.

I had used rabbits in my previous work, but Prof preferred cats. Following the routine for spinal cord work, they were anaesthetized by barbiturates. I do not know how wise this choice was because the signals had much lower amplitude than those I was used to. Once we got intracellular records, my apprehension was somewhat allayed. Nevertheless, the use of barbiturate may have had some advantages because barbiturates enhanced inhibition as Eccles later showed in his last experimental paper in a collaboration with Roger Nicoll (Allen et al., 1977). We exploited the experience I had with the field potentials and used a set of afferent sources to the CA1 neurons. With Prof's and Chandler's experience (Brooks and Eccles, 1948), it was now much easier to interpret the field potentials. From the start, Prof was struck by the long duration and smoothness of the field potentials. He suspected something was wrong. I tried to convince him that this was to be expected in the hippocampus. Only slowly did he accept my standpoint, however. The whole situation changed in a wink as soon as we got our intracellular recordings. This turned out to be more difficult than Prof had anticipated. There were several reasons for this situation. Motoneurones are hardy cells. They can be penetrated repeatedly and can withstand impalement by quite coarse electrodes. Therefore, most of the Dunedin and Canberra motoneuronal work was made with microelectrodes with input resistance of a few megohms and a tip of about 1–1.5 μm. A great advantage of spinal cord work was the ease with which one could apply mechanical clamps securing good stability. Finally, most reflex and single cell work was made in the lumbar and sacral spinal cord after it had been separated from the upper segments by a transverse cut in the lower thoracic region. This procedure removed much of the longitudinal movement otherwise conveyed by the respiratory pump. Eccles was fortunate to have excellent mechanical and electronic engineers around him. George Winsbury designed both the fine mechanical clamps and the micromanipulators which probably were the finest in the world at this time. The stimulation and recording unit constructed by Eccles' long-time collaborator, the physicist Jack Coombs, was superb and a major reason for the Canberra success. In the hippocampus, the situation was very different. The cells did not tolerate impalement with coarse electrodes. In addition, mechanical movements from circulation and respiration were quite marked. It took quite some time to learn how to draw and fill higher impedance electrodes and to adjust the amplifier system accordingly. Unfortunately, we had nothing similar to the spinal cord equipment to help us stabilize the hippocampus. We tried to apply a Plexiglas pressure foot with a central hole for the recording electrode, but the pressure could easily be too heavy and damage the hippocampus. We tried several other approaches, pouring liquid agar so as to make a rigid lid to reduce the movements and having a closed system by having only narrow holes drilled in the skull to allow the recording and stimulating electrodes. In addition, we tried fast and small volume respiration volumes and higher respiratory rates, and a pneumothorax system with metal tubes through the thorax wall connected to rubber balloons to reduce the transmission of lung to chest wall movement.

None of these trials was fully successful. However, although the quality and length of the recordings were far from ideal, we got sufficiently many observations to draw some qualitatively valid conclusions. In this regard, it is interesting to recall something Eric Kandel told me some years back. He described how he and Alden Spencer (Kandel, et al., 1961) succeeded in getting excellent records already in their second experiment. If that had not happened, they might well have given in, he told me, because after the glorious start there were only failures for a full year.

A frequent observation was that virtually all inputs produced an IPSP. Excitatory responses were less frequent, but when EPSPs did occur, they always had a few millisecond shorter latency than the IPSPs. As Kandel and Spencer first observed a year before us, antidromic activation of pyramidal cell axons gives rise to IPSPs. We hypothesized that there was an intercalated interneuron in the circuit. Our main reason was the latency difference of about 1–2 msec between the EPSP and IPSP, the widespread distribution of the IPSPs suggesting a distributing mechanism, and finally, the frequent observation of ripples on the initial phase of the inhibitory potentials suggesting its mediation by a high-frequency discharging cell. We searched for such postulated interneurons in areas of the hippocampus where histologists had pointed out the presence of what could be non-pyramidal cells. We found a number of cells that filled the adopted criteria for interneurons: they fired in bursts, but at a lower frequency than pyramidal cell bursts; were often located outside the pyramidal layer; and showed converging effects from different afferent fiber systems.

Identification of Inhibitory Synapses

The identification of these interneurons and their synapses was, arguably, the most dramatic experience I had in Canberra. Impressed by the ubiquity of the IPSPs and their large amplitude, we exploited the special histological arrangement to find their source of origin. We turned to the field potentials and their distribution along the main dendritic axis of the CA1 pyramidal cells. We noted that the onset of IPSPs was associated with a positive extracellular wave when recording from the pyramidal layer. By charting the amplitude distribution of the field potential, the peak was consistently located to the pyramidal layer, irrespective of the afferent fibers used. I remember very well the evening when I showed him the complete set of graphs, all pointing in the same direction. We were disussing our data in his office at the end of an experiment, the famous 11 PM tea break. Since both Kandel and Spencer and we ourselves observed that the IPSPs reversed by chloride injection or diffusion, the hyperpolarization was likely to be mediated by inward movement of chloride ions, in other words an outward current, following classical rules. Consequently, Eccles explained to me that the chloride current generates the outward current and thereby the hyperpolarization of the membrane. Because the field plot had its maximal amplitude in the pyramidal layer, the hyperpolarizing current flows across the soma membrane or a region very closed to it.

> I nearly yelled, because I both saw the light and beamed with delight:
> "Sir, given the conclusion that the inhibitory current flows across the soma membrane, I can tell you which cell type and synapses that do it!"
> He stared at me, but I went on:
> "Cajal has drawn both the cell, its synapses and how it connects to the pyramidal cells."
> "Where?" he said, surprised about my boyish excitement, but clearly starting to think I had a point. He had never heard about such interneurons before.
> "In his volume 2," I nearly shouted. "Let me show you!"
> We ran down the corridor. A super thing about the JCSMR was that the well-equipped library was open round the clock.

We rushed in, and since I had so often searched Ramon y
Cajal's two-volume (1911) masterpiece, I found Figs. 473 and
474 straight away, showing the beautiful basket cells and their
elaborate relation to the many pyramidal cells they innervate.
Prof was elated, starting to laugh, and exclaimed:
"Here it is, here it is!"

I did not quite understand what he alluded to, but later he said that
he saw what he had been chasing so long: the first example of an identified
interneuron in the brain and, above all, the first identification of inhibitory
synapses in central nervous structures. He had himself identified Renshaw
cells as inhibitory interneurones in the spinal cord, but not found their
synapses. Further, E.G. Gray in 1959 described the symmetric and asym-
metric synapses in electron micrographs, although he made clear that the
available evidence did not allow a distinction of their physiological roles.
However, although both types were found in abundance, both in the hippocampus and in the neocortex, we did not know the identity of the parent
neurons nor of the target cells. The closest step to identification came in an
influential paper by Lionel Hamlyn (1963) in which he described the various
bouton types which contacted hippocampal pyramidal cells. However, in the
days before marking substances for a cell or cell type, he could not know the
origin of the fibers attached to the boutons.

But, in November 1962, we succeeded in Canberra. It was difficult to
sleep that night. The next day, Prof came into my little 60-square feet cubicle
and kept on rejoicing. I had a big homemade chart of the hippocampus on
the wall with the key cellular elements depicted. He pointed and pointed,
and soon, as was his habit, he had taken over and explained to me how all
the cells were arranged and how they interacted and told me how we would
proceed. Fantastic!

> After some time, I ventured:
> "Prof, maybe we should check whether the basket cell arrange-
> ment is a general organization or only something peculiar to the
> hippocampus."
> He did not understand at first. I went on:
> "There is an additional structure with basket cells with a very
> similar termination on their target neurons—the cerebellum."
> His answer was very disappointing:
> "Oh no, when Raggen and Charles could not make head and tails
> of it, we will not manage either."

He referred to a paper in the *Journal Physiology (London)* by the Nobel
laureate Ragnar Granit and Charles Phillips, well known for his cortico-
motoneuronal studies (Granit and Phillips, 1956). They intended to exploit

Phillips' long experience with intracellular recording from motor cortex in baboons and record intracellularly from cerebellar Purkinje cells during various reflex situations. For some reason, it proved very difficult. Admittedly, they discovered the burst discharge, which we know today is due to the intense climbing fiber activation, and called it the "inactivation response," but did not acquire good enough records to unravel the underlying mechanism. This had to await the work by Eccles, Llinas, and Sasaki (1966a).

Cerebellar Studies After All

I was very disappointed, but as usual my respect for him prevented any open protest. However, as had happened in our work on hippocampus, a long fortnight later, he came one day into my cubicle and mused: "I wonder whether we should test the basket cell idea in the cerebellum. It is a good idea, you see!" I have to assume that he remembered my proposal on the same issue only some weeks earlier, but he made no remark in that direction. It did happen that he "adopted" ideas from others. Be that as it may, I was excited and told him which option I could see for a suitable experimental approach, an idea he adopted straight away. I had followed Anders Lundberg's work in Lund, Sweden, on the many spinal afferent systems to the cerebellum. In addition, just before I left Oslo, Jan K.S. Jansen and I had made a study of the effects of local stimulation of the surface of the folium, through which I got acquainted with the field potential and its reversal with depth. The fact that it was rejected by the *Journal of Neurophysiology* did not prevent me from acquiring useful experience for our initial cerebellar work in Canberra. We also tested both cerebellar and hippocampal inhibition for possible glycine sensitivity, but found that neither were influenced by strychnine at doses which completely blocked spinal glycine-mediated inhibition. This provided a backdrop for the discovery by Ito and his collaborators (Obata et al., 1967), who found that the Purkinje cell-mediated inhibition on vestibular neurons was mediated by gamma-amino-butyric acid. A few years later, a further Canberra group led by David Curtis discovered that hippocampal inhibition also was GABAergic (Curtis, 1970). Eccles also had a previous engagement in cerebellar neuroscience. His second publication was, in fact, a collaboration with D. Denny-Brown and E.G.T. Liddell (1929) on the effect of cerebellar stimulation on spinal reflexes.

With our previous experience, we quickly found that the field potential profile was very similar to that of the hippocampus and that the Purkinje cells also showed large and long-lasting IPSPs. In addition, we found cells discharging with high-frequency bursts during the rise time of the IPSP. These neurons were found at a depth corresponding to the expected position of basket cells. Consequently, we put forward the hypothesis that recurrent collaterals of Purkinje cells activated basket cells, which in turn disynaptically induced IPSPs in a number of neighboring Purkinje cells. Looking back, it gives some satisfaction to know that I could help in the start of Eccles' glorious last scientific endeavor, which he carried through in a remarkable collaboration with Janos Szentágothai and Masao Ito, namely, the analysis of the properties of cerebellar neurons and the principles behind their interactions (Eccles et al., 1967).

Finally, I received additional training in Canberra by working with David Curtis, the father of the iontophoretic analysis of neuronal activity. In a most efficient collaboration with Jeff Watkins and later with Graham Johnston, he developed this method to give us a new view of the effect of transmitters and their receptors in central nervous synapses. We discovered that thalamic neurons were highly sensitive to iontophoresed acetylcholine (ACh) with a latency approaching that of the Renshaw cells in the spinal cord. This meant that ACh was likely to play an important role in the control of the excitability level of thalamic neurons and thereby of the cortical cells which they bombarded with impulses (Andersen and Curtis, 1964). Today, we know that this system is essential for the general cortical arousal system and an important factor in the manifestation of Alzheimer disease symptoms. Naturally, we also observed the sensitivity of thalamic neurons to application of glutamate and N-methyl-D-aspartic acid (NMDA). In 1962, we did not have the classification of the glutamate-sensitive receptors generally accepted today through the work of Jeff Watkins and his collaborators (Watkins and Evans, 1981), so we had to be content with a description of the effects that we elicited.

I was extremely fortunate to be able to work consistently with Sir John throughout my two years in Canberra, usually two and sometimes three times a week. Altogether, we must have made close to 200 all-day experiments together. This gave me invaluable experience, my main scientific capital, in fact. The usual experiment started at about 8:00 AM and lasted until about 2:00 AM the following night. Our wonderful technicians, Sheila and Carol, had already fetched the cats in the animal house and anaesthetized and shaved them. We, the younger members of the team, put in the tracheal tube for free airways or artificial respiration and venous cannulas for intravenous infusions of fluid or drugs. Then followed the preparation of the peripheral nerves, which we dissected free and provided the end with a cotton tie and loop for good electrode contact. We dissected from 8 to 13 nerves in hindlimb experiments and 3 to 5 nerves when forelimb afferents were asked for, sometimes bilaterally. These dissections usually took us several hours and then came the time for the laminectomy to expose the spinal cord and its attached roots. Eccles was proud to demonstrate his surgical abilities, so he often took part in the dissection. Each time he announced: "It won't take me more than 10 minutes!" His pupils did not protest, but did not quite believe him either. He was particularly proud of being able to split the peroneal nerve in its muscular and skin subdivisions, each only about a third of a millimeter in diameter. These ran together for about 20 mm enclosed in a common sheath. For experimental purposes, it was useful to separate them, however. It was impressive to watch how the famous 60-year-old scientist concentrated on this task of dexterity, a task he solved perfectly every time I saw him do it.

During the recording session, Eccles was the captain, sitting in front of the camera and shooting pictures at a frightening speed since we could not know how long the penetration would last. I was number 2, as they say in the navy, having the responsibility to take notes of stimulated nerves, amplifier settings, and all the other parameters in the complicated operation. With Prof's formidable speed, it was a challenging task. If things went too fast, he used to say: "Don't worry, I remember it all!" Fortunately, we worked so close and often together that I felt I could read his mind to some extent, and I could get the correct settings down in the protocol when he shouted some wrong figure. His memory was truly remarkable, but I am afraid that some information was lost. We were usually three in a team, and the third member was operating the micromanipulator and control instruments, in fact, the all-important fishing part of the enterprise. The day after the experiments was used to mark the films and start the tedious measurement phase. Then followed the analysis and eventually the setting up of graphs. That was the rewarding bit, because we could get some insight in the process under examination. On Friday night Prof came along to collect material from us youngsters. He put graphs and notes and film in a big cardboard box. Quite often, when he returned on Monday morning, he had been able to write all or the best part of another manuscript. The handwritten draft was then typed by the secretary before the control phase came when we all tried to improve on the draft.

Things changed somewhat when we started on experiments on the dorsal column nuclei, where we needed preparation of forelimb nerves, and on thalamic and hippocampal tissues, where no nerve preparation was needed. Here, Prof had no previous experience and he left the forelimb surgery to his younger colleagues. The dorsal column and brain surgery fell to me. For this task, my training as an anatomical lecturer in Oslo came in handy. The exposure of the dorsal column nuclei was relatively simple by ventroflexing the head, allowable because of the tracheal tube, and by gentle removal of parts of the occipital bone. For the hippocampal experiments, we needed to remove the neocortex, a procedure I had carried out time and again in Oslo. I had found a set of small tricks to reduce the bleeding from the skull bones and from the neocortical edges left by the suction. For the thalamic experiments, I needed to remove the overlying hippocampus in order to see the relevant anatomical landmarks. I think some of my colleagues will feel with me when I say that it hurt somewhat to set the suction pipette into this gleaming white structure, so pristine in shape, having given me my vocation and income for years, and just remove it into the bucket. Shameful! The thalamus appears much less glorious. Covered in a dense network of arteries and veins, its dorsal surface looks directly untidy. As one gets to know its inhabitant neurons, however, one recognizes that the rough and red surface is just a camouflage for some of the most interesting and challenging neurons in the brain.

The Trisynaptic Circuit

The last story I will tell from the Canberra period is the discovery of the trisynaptic circuit. Sir John had been the undisputed leader in all the other experimental series in which I took part in Canberra. When it came to the trisynaptic circuit, I was on my own. That is to say, I had two great collaborators with me, Birgitta Holmqvist from Sweden and Paul Voorhoeve from the Netherlands. But this time I was the leader and had the starting idea and the control of the experiments. Once again, the background had been drawn up by neuroanatomists. The big master, my hero Santiago Ramon y Cajal, had made a splendid diagram, summarizing the major points of hippocampal structure in Fig. 479 in Vol. 2 of his *Histologie de Système Nerveux* from 1911. More than anybody else, his rich research findings had inspired and guided me through my initial years. But the diagram contained one error. An arrow indicated that the CA1 neurons were sending their impulses along axons traveling forward to the CA3 neurons and into the fimbria and, thus, out of the hippocampus toward the septum and hypothalamus. My last effort in Canberra was to turn that arrow around. The main target of CA1 neurons is in the exactly opposite direction, namely, the posteriorly lying subiculum.

In the spring of 1963 (Southern Hemisphere version), Prof was away for a grand tour of the world of lectures and symposia. He had asked me whether I knew an interesting problem which could keep Birgitta, Paul, and myself busy in that period, and my answer was a big yes. For a long time, I had wondered where the CA1 neurons sent their impulses, either as the Ramon y Cajal idea went down to hypothalamic nuclei to influence autonomic homeostasis or to other sections of the hippocampal formation for whatever function. Because this was my show, I decided to use rabbits, my own favorite. In urethane-cloralose anesthetized animals, we stimulated the main input to the hippocampal formation, the perforant path, and we recorded simultaneously from three stations: the dentate granule cells, the CA3, and the CA1 pyramidal cells. The initial effect of the perforant volley was the excitation of granule cells as seen by both field potential and intracellular records. The next station was the excitation of CA3 neurons, although their excitability was much lower and only a minor fraction gave discharges. Raising the stimulation rate improved the engagement prominently, however. With a clearly longer latency, the CA1 pyramidal cells were the third group of cells to be recruited, again much better if we used a short train of stimuli. Perhaps the most convincing piece of evidence was the effect of a surgical cut of fibers between the CA3 and CA1 areas. The CA3 activity was not changed, but all CA1 signals vanished altogether. So, the signals traveled from CA3 to CA1 and not in the direction that Ramon y Cajal had drawn. Some years later, my group showed that the main CA1 output is to the subicular neurons, thus finalizing what we called the trisynaptic circuit. We should add, however, that much remains to be learned about the physiological significance of this circuit, and it may well be that much hippocampus-dependent activity is mediated by other pathways.

All fairy tales have a happy end, so also here. My Canberra period ended in November 1963, but not before an incredible occasion occurred. By a night call, Prof was notified by a Melbourne newspaper that he had received the Nobel Prize for Physiology or Medicine, as it is called. He refused to believe it, thinking it was a hoax. The reason was that he twice before had gotten false announcements about the Nobel Prize and had decided to be utterly skeptical. However, when later in the day, his old time friend from the Oxford days "Raggen" Granit called from a meeting in Italy to congratulate him, Prof accepted the fact. What a day! I immediately helped to organize an impromptu lab feast and ran out in town to buy the necessary champagne. John Hubbard, a long-term Kiwi visitor (New Zealander), and Robert Schmidt (an inventive German) made the in-house arrangement and announcement. Then, we invaded Prof's office with an accolade so intense that I felt he had some difficulty in swallowing our overexcitement. Clearly, he was pleased beyond description. Still, I feel that his collaborators and admirers of all ages that day were perhaps even more excited and happy than he was himself. It was as if we had a part in the achievement, even if the prize was given for discoveries made in the early and middle 1950s, partly in Dunedin and partly in Canberra, nearly 10 years before our term in the John Curtin school. Obviously, most of us had expected it to occur. However, the real thing is something else. It was a high point in my life and in those of Eccles' many Canberra colleagues.

On the way home, we traveled across the United States. I had written to many of my American colleagues in the field, most of whom I had not met, and received a most overwhelming response. Every one of them wanted to hear about results from Canberra, and many of the meets gave rise to lifelong friendships. This was a new experience to me. I shall never forget, and stop thanking for, the generosity I met then and later from my U.S. colleagues. I understood that the various aspects of international fraternity that I had experienced in Australia were only a small fraction of the vast brotherhood of similarly thinking people, everyone possessed by the idea to understand more of the nervous system.

Setting Up My Own Laboratory

Coming home from Canberra was quite a transition. On the one hand, the reunion with family and friends was fantastic. While we were in Australia, the Cuban crisis occurred, and for some days there I remember how scared my wife and I were that we might never be able to return to a normal Norway and Europe. During those days, we realized how far from the rest of the world Australia was. Over the last 25 years or so this has changed, but in 1962 the feeling of distance was real. An Adelaide professor has used the term "the evil of distance" for the feeling many Australians have had about their cultural and social isolation from United States and Europe. During the Cuban crisis, we felt that evilness forcefully in our close family.

Our reunion with family and friends in Oslo in 1963 was emotional and reminded me how much our background means. Although the two Canberra years no doubt were the best two years of my scientific life, the homecoming brought back to me other aspects of life, above all the importance of your close family and friends. These feelings, coupled to the intense pleasure of my family in our national peculiarities such as skiing, sailing, and hiking, made up my mind: we would like to stay in Norway.

Nobel Festivities in Stockholm and a Papal Symposium in Rome

Through the kind assistance of Ragnar Granit I was able to secure a ticket for the Nobel festivities in Stockholm when Sir John would receive his Nobel Prize together with Sir Alan Hodgkin and Sir Andrew Fielding Huxley. The Swedes know how to make a festival! With 50,000 red roses from the city of San Remo decorating the Stockholm Concert House, the best scientists in the world received their diplomas, medals, and prizes from the hand of King Gustav Adolf II, himself an accomplished archeological scientist. Prof got his prize for the work on the ionic basis for spinal inhibition. The prize winners were asked to give a set of lectures at other Swedish universities. I was very pleased to hear that examples of central inhibition made up a major theme in his talks that week.

In the winter of 1964, Eccles invited me to a symposium on Brain and Conscious Experience to be held in the Vatican under the auspices of the Pontifical Academy of Science of which Sir John was a prominent member. Created in 1936, the Pontifical Academy arranges a Study Week every year in which a central theme is discussed. Although some of the participants were religious, most were not. Only one demand was made: The group must decide on which points the group could not agree and which experiments had to be conducted to resolve the disagreement. The meeting place was grandiose: the house of Pope Pius IV, Casa Pio Quattro, with an undescribable roof, painted by Michelangelo. Even if we were housed in such clerical surroundings, the discussions were very direct, not least the response to our hosts' proposals for cortical mechanisms where the mind could meet the brain. I was impressed how people could retain their deep respect and friendship in spite of quite strong feelings for or against non-physical explanations for aspects of conscious behavior. It was particularly interesting to hear how

Roger Sperry rejected a simple religious description of willed action, but at the same time had great difficulties with a total rejection of determinism. In his talk he said: "There may be worse 'fates' than causal determinism." The meeting was a glorious lesson in the breadth of scientific knowledge, but also about the willingness to hear each other out, in spite of obvious and at times strong disagreements. Sir John dedicated the book that came out of the meeting to two Pontifical Academicians who had deeply pondered about human nature, Charles S. Sherrington and Ernst Schrödinger.

My Own Laboratory

After the glamour in Stockholm, I returned to Oslo and started to set up my own laboratory. I was well received by my home university with much help, not least from my superiors. A new, albeit small, lab was waiting, and some money for equipment was available. Fortunately, I was successful with an application to the NIH for an initiation grant. Maybe the success of my Rockefeller stipend period helped as well? Tom Sears, who is a master experimenter, came across from the United Kingdom with his family and helped me to set up the new instruments and procedures and get the first experiment going. In 1964, it was supremely rewarding to record nerve and cell activity in my own little laboratory!

Having seen the excellence of the best university groups in the world, I realized that any hope for success of my own neurobiological research had to rest on a strategy which exploited whatever special advantage was available at the University of Oslo or in the not too distant vicinity. One considerable asset was the neuroanatomical group in Oslo and another was the relatively large number of well-educated young people eager to work on problems related to the nervous system.

I count myself fortunate to have been able to assemble around myself a number of Norwegian and foreign scientists, in all more than 80, who have contributed greatly to various hippocampal or thalamic problems. Among the topics we managed to attack with some success, I would like to mention the identification of spine synapses as excitatory (1966); the realization that direct thalamo-cortical connections are the main substrate for the alpha type rhythmic activity in the EEG (1968); the discovery of the lamellar organization (1971); the introduction of the transverse hippocampal slice (1971); the identification of hippocampal output systems (1972); the discovery of long-term potentiation (LTP, 1973); the first intracellular recording from hippocampal slices (1975); the input specificity of LTP (1977); the equipotentiality of excitatory dendritic synapses (1980); two types of GABAergic responses in hippocampal pyramids (1980); linear summation of EPSPs (1983); f/I relations for hippocampal pyramidal cells (1984); dendritic depolarization is essential for LTP induction (1986); behavioral learning promotes new spine synapses (1994); behavioral learning promotes short-lasting synaptic enhancement (STP, 1995); LTP depends on phosphorylation through PKC and CaCaMKII (1988); LTP depends upon the cytosolic tail of NMDA receptors (1996); LTP is absent in mice lacking the A-subtype of AMPA receptors (1999); in such GluR-A$^{-/-}$ mice, LTP is rescued by re-expression of A-subunits (2000); and lamellar orientation of directly recorded CA3 axons (2002).

One of the first tasks we tackled was to identify the functional nature of four afferent hippocampal systems. Here, serendipity occurred. Blackstad, whose Nauta-stained sections set me on the hippocampal path, was working on a method whereby a nerve fiber from a given source could be identified in the electron microscope. With colleagues from the Anatomical Institute, he gave the first description of the electron dense boutons belonging to previously lesioned fibers (Alksne et al., 1966). Using this method, we first stimulated four different fiber systems in isolation and observed monosynaptic excitation of their target cells by intracellular recording or by recording field potentials with cell discharges. We also charted the region of maximal synaptic effects to know where to look for histological evidence. After having lesioned these fiber systems, they were examined by Blackstad a few days later in the electron microscope. All four excitatory fiber systems had degenerating boutons associated with dendritic spines (Andersen et al., 1966). These results gave a functional role to the electron microscope (EM) observation of E.G. Gray (1959) of two synapse types in normal cortical tissue. Gray cautiously stated, "At present there is no evidence to suggest that type 1 and type 2 synapses are functionally different." Only a few years later, Eccles (1964) and Andersen and Eccles (1965) came close, but did not quite make this suggestion, largely because of a lack of evidence for the location of excitatory synapses. With our combination of functional and EM degeneration data from 1966, we could now propose a simple rule: excitatory synapses on two cortical cell types, hippocampal pyramidal cells and dentate granule cells, were located to dendritic spines while inhibitory synapses were located to the somata of these cells. However, the last point had to be modified quickly after Eccles et al. (1966b) found that cerebellar stellate cells, which terminate on dendritic shafts at various distances from the cell body of Purkinje cells, also were inhibitory. Further, while most excitatory boutons are located to spines, there are several exceptions. Hence, the synaptic categorization is not quite so rigid as we proposed in our simple rule in 1966.

Between 1967 and 1970, I deserted my dear hippocampus to take up a challenge derived from our thalamic studies in Canberra. Listening to the loudspeaker, Tom Sears and I, working together in Eccles' laboratory, heard that there often were series of burst discharges without any stimulation. When we recoded these events, they looked remarkably like those we both recognized from our electroencephalographic experience, where the cortical counterparts were called barbiturate spindles. Much charting remained, however, not least at the cortical level to determine the nature of these thalamocortical responses and the location of the rhythmic pacemaker, if any. In this endeavor, I was lucky to be joined by Sven A. Andersson from Gothenburg University who had worked in Vernon Mountcastle's laboratory in Baltimore. We alternated between experiments in Gothenburg and Oslo and became close friends. So much so that Sven, who is an accomplished carpenter, is responsible for a good deal of my mountain cabin in the ranges of central Norway. Our main scientific result was that the spindle waves of various cortical areas were closely controlled by the rhythmic activity of the thalamic projection nuclei and not by the intralaminar or midline nuclei, going against a common opinion at the time. Sven and I wrote a book describing our results, *The Physiological Basis for the Alpha Rhythm* (1968). Until it appeared, the emphasis had been on the so-called unspecific nuclei of the thalamus. We feel that the book introduced another aspect and helped to reorient peoples' ideas about the alpha rhythm.

Long-Term Potentiation

No question, this phenomenon is the single topic which has created the most intense interest among my colleagues. The phenomenon consists of a period of enhanced synaptic transmission after a short session with high-frequency stimulation of a set of afferents to the hippocampal formation. The great interest derives from the many LTP attributes which could support learning and memory. In my thesis work in the late 1950s, I often observed a slow decline of the hippocampal potentials, a sort of fatigue I thought. However, in such cases much could be restored by a few seconds worth of high-frequency stimulation. In my thesis, I noted that a few seconds of 10-Hz stimulation gave a synaptic enhancement which could last from 4 to 6 min (Andersen, 1960). Interesting as they were, I felt it was still not long enough to distinguish it from posttetanic potentiation (PTP). When Terje Lømo joined me in 1964, I showed him this stimulation trick. We compared the effect of raised stimulation frequency on excitation and inhibition. In our intracellular records, we found that the recurrent inhibition remained unchanged for several seconds before a small decline, probably because of a changed internal chloride concentration. Excitatory responses, on the other hand, showed a dramatic increase during the tetanic stimulation and remained enhanced for minutes afterwards. We saw this as a candidate for a learning process. In fact, in 1965 we concluded in a symposium article, not published until 1967, that the posttetanus increased responses were short lasting, they could be seen as "an example of primitive synaptic learning" (Andersen and Lømo, 1967). A major change occurred when Terje gave a series of tetanic stimulations. Now, the enhancement could last for more than 1 hour after the stimulation. This long duration convinced us that we had observed a new phenomenon, different from PTP. The first description of this LTP effect was given by Terje at the Scandinavian Physiological Congress in Åbo in

Finland in 1966 (Lømo, 1966). I talked about the phenomenon at a meeting
in London in 1967. In the audience sat Tim Bliss who had just completed his
thesis on neocortical plasticity. He was highly impressed by our preliminary
results and wanted to come to Oslo for a postdoctoral study. Here, he and
Terje made a set of critical experiments and, with a clever use of an experimental and a control line, found nearly all the important properties: the
long duration, the physiological induction rates, and the synapse specificity.
Hence, the Bliss and Lømo (1973) paper is rightly regarded as the birth
of LTP, although they used the term long-lasting potentiation. Later, my
colleagues and I showed input specificity of LTP because it only occurred
at the tetanized synapses of a given cell while a set of control synapses
remained unchanged (Andersen, 1977). Other highlights were the finding of
McNaughton et al.'s (1978) of the cooperativity phenomenon (many fibers
need to be co-active), the discovery by Collingridge, et al. (1983) that the
NMDA-channel blocker 5-amino-valerate blocks LTP but not synaptic transmission, and Wigström and Gustafsson's (1986) demonstration that pairing
of postsynaptic depolarization and synaptic activation could induce LTP.

The Lamellar Organization

While in Oslo, Bliss took part in an additional investigation with an interesting result. By antidromic and orthodromic activation of four different
excitatory pathways, we found that they all were oriented nearly trans-
versely to the longitudinal axis of the rabbit hippocampus, an arrangement
we coined the lamellar organization (Andersen et al., 1971a). The term suggests that the majority of connections in the trisynaptic pathway are along
one plane, but not exclusively so, since excitation was also found to either
side, only less well developed. Some people misunderstood the term and felt
we had hypothesised an exclusive activation of a thin sliver of tissue, while
some of the fiber systems involved show a much broader distribution. The
lamella should be taken in a statistical sense only, since our original curves
showed a ridge-like structure of activated tissue and not a thin sheet.

  The lamella gave rise more or less directly to a useful preparation,
the transverse hippocampal slice (Fig. 2). For many years, I had tried
to develop an isolated preparation of the whole or part of the hippocampal formation. I had tried various methods, from small chunks kept in
hyperoxygenized saline at low temperature to slabs taken from hibernating
hedgehogs, which in those days crawled in plenitude under the hedges in our
family garden. Nothing was successful. I knew about the pioneering work of
Henry McIlwain with various isolated slice types. The work on the pyriform
cortex was particularly promising (Yamamoto and McIlwain, 1966). However, the tangential sectioning employed by McIlwain would be likely to
lesion the hippocampal neurons. With the lamella idea in hand, a transverse
slice appeared possible. My colleague Knut Skrede went over to London,

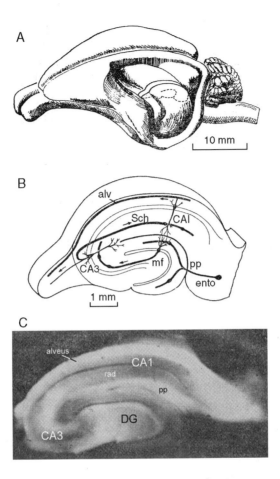

Fig. 2. The transverse hippocampal slice. (A) The lateral part of the neocortex of the rabbit has been removed to expose the large hippocampal formation. (B) The orientation of a lamella is indicated and the main intrahippocampal pathways are seen to lie in the same, lamellar plane. (C) An unstained transverse slice as it appears in the recording chamber, with the three major subdivisions marked (CA1, CA3, DG [dentate gyrus]) and two myelinated fiber bundles labeled (alveus, carrying the axons of the CA1 neurons; pp, perforant path with fibers from the entorhinal area to the dentate gyrus; and CA1 rad, stratum radiatum, a favorite region for study of dendritic synapses. In CA1 the cell body layer is seen here as a black stripe.

where Chris Richards, an associate of Tim Bliss' at Mill Hill and a former pupil of McIlwain, was kind enough to show him how to cut and handle slices from the pyrifom cortex. With a minimal budget, Knut was able to get the first transverse hippocampal slice going in Oslo. Within weeks we knew it was a winner, showing us all the usual field potential properties we knew from intact preparations. Knut and Rolf Westgaard demonstrated the versatility of the preparation in the first report on transverse hippocampal slices (Skrede and Westgaard, 1971).

An Oxford Sojourn

I abstained from the authorship because these two colleagues had worked so hard, in part in my absence, while I spent half a year on sabbatical leave to work with Charles Phillips in Oxford. Charles had arranged for me to be a Visiting Fellow at Trinity College, a most interesting and agreeable stay. The college life was fantastic, a glimpse of a wealth of tradition mixed with people of charm and peculiarities as well. This was my first and only opportunity to work with monkeys. By microstimulation, we studied the origin of cortical neurones that could drive motoneurones monosynaptically as signaled by single units in the electromyogram of small hand muscles. Our results showed that area 4 cortico-motoneuronal cells were not assembled in tight columns as one of the popular hypotheses maintains, but rather were dispersed over a considerable area, although mainly in layer 5, in an arrangement we called a colony of cortico-motoneuronal neurons (Andersen et al., 1975).

Intracellular Experiments in the Hippocampus

Back in Oslo, I was joined by a number of young neuroscientists, in all more than 80, too many to name all. Philip Schwartzkroin was special by being willing to put in a large effort to make sufficiently fine micropipettes to give acceptable intracellular penetrations of hippocampal neurons, whereby he amply demonstrated the advantages of the slice preparation (Schwartzkroin, 1975). The excellent performance of a newly designed amplifier by our electronic engineer Trond Reppen made the job easier. By iontophoretic application of glutamate, Phil Schwartzkroin and I found that minute currents were still effective provided the electrode tip was at certain localized "hot spots" inside a double cone-shaped volume corresponding to the apical and basal dendritic trees. In response to a long application pulse, the initial discharges were assembled in a burst, whereas the remainder consisted of relatively regular low-frequency discharges. Each of these steady state discharges was, however, preceded by a slowly rising depolarization. Thus, glutamate application causes spike discharges through several mechanisms, one depending upon fast depolarization and a different one probably depending upon a slow conductance (Schwartzkroin and Andersen, 1975).

In 1980, we published two papers in the *Journal of Physiology* which created some interest. In the first paper, we described that iontophoretic application of GABA could elicit two completely different responses depending on the application site. Delivery to the soma region gave hyper-polarization, while delivery to certain dendritic regions gave depolarization (Andersen et al., 1980a). In the second paper, we compared the efficiency of various afferent fibers lying at different distances from the cell body of CA1 pyramidal cells in hippocampal slices. Surprisingly, with the exception of the soma and the peripheral fifth of the apical dendritic tree, all other parts of the afferent fibers were equipotent, assuming that the constant stimulation current excited roughly the same number of fibers (Andersen et al., 1980b). Later, Iver Langmoen and I found that stimulation of two such fiber bundles created EPSPs that summed linearly such that the summed input gave an EPSP which was exactly like the algebraic sum of the two subdivisions elicited alone (Langmoen and Andersen, 1983). More recent work has shown that this picture must be modified, in that both cable attenuation and peripheral boosting mechanisms exist.

Over the years, I have been lucky to take part in some interesting discoveries. However, you cannot win all the time. As years go by, the latter seems to become more and more common. In 1985, my colleagues Øivind Hvalby, Massimo Avoli, and I were beaten close to the finishing line. We wanted to study the conditions underlying the induction of LTP. Looking at the field potential distribution during 100-msec-long tetani, we concluded that the dendrites receiving the synaptic input had to be depolarized above a certain amount to observe subsequent LTP. Therefore, we hypothesized that the co-activation threshold discussed by McNaughton et al. (1978) was represented by local dendritic depolarization. If so, we should be able to induce LTP by artificial depolarization and couple that to low-frequency synaptic activation, in itself unable to give LTP. I wanted to avoid spike discharges during the priming such that any effect should not be ascribable to cell discharges as such. This was a mistake. We paired just subthreshold, intracellularly delivered depolarizing current with synaptic activation at the end of the current pulse, but could not detect any clear effect. My former pupil Holger Wigström and his colleague Bengt Gustafsson, both in Gothenburg, did the same type of experiment. Neither of us knew about the other group's activities. Holger and Bengt had arrived at the same idea along a different route. They observed that blocking of GABA-mediated inhibition greatly reduced the threshold for LTP induction. Supported by field potential recordings, they also predicted the importance of dendritic depolarization for LTP. With much stronger depolarization, they observed a positive effect of pairing in the form of long-lasting enhancement of a test synaptic input, exactly as for tetanus-induced LTP.

In our laboratory we tried an alternative procedure. We produced dendritic depolarization by local delivery of glutamate and paired the response with low-frequency synaptic activation. Here, we saw a long-lasting enhanced response to a test stimulus, similar to the Gothenburg results (Hvalby et al., 1987). Again, without knowing of the other group, we both sent a letter to *Nature* and both had our manuscripts rejected. In Oslo, we tried to follow the advice of the referees which meant new experiments and, consequently, more time. In the end, our revised manuscript was rejected as well. Holger and Bengt went about it differently and published their result as a short article in *Acta Physiologica Scandinavica* (Wigström, Gustafsson 1986). Two longer and well-documented reports of theirs appeared later that year and in the next year in *Journal of Neuroscience*. So they deserved to win, but slightly bitter it was.

Molecular Studies of LTP

In 1984, I got a phone call from Torsten Wiesel at the Rockefeller University asking me if I was interested in being a candidate for election to The Neuro- science Institute, run by Gerald M. Edelmann at the same university. What a lovely surprise! Thirty-six associates met twice a year to discuss principles of brain organization and mechanisms, in particular, cortical functions. I had met many oustanding scientists before, but never so many in one and the same room. It was enormously stimulating and enjoyable. Gerald M. Edelman, Gerry among friends, who received the Nobel Prize with Roger Porter for their analysis of the immunoglobulin molecule, was a tremen- dous host with his broad knowledge, from brain mechanisms to music. I am very grateful to have been a member of this Institute for nine eventful years.

Among the many benefits was to meet new colleagues. I made a lasting and warm friendship with many of them, including Paul Greengard. Paul pioneered the discovery of protein phosphorylation as a major mechanism for control of central nervous processes. Because LTP was associated with cal- cium influx, we wondered whether protein kinases could be engaged and, if so, which one. Paul's laboratory provided blockers of various protein kinases which we loaded into microelectrodes and injected into individual CA1 neu- rons. The strategy was to see whether LTP was prevented in the impaled cell, while it appeared as normal in the field potential generated by surround- ing cells. Other laboratories had shown that the calcium-calmodulin protein kinase II (CaMPKII) was involved. We compared the effect of blockers of this kinase with antagonists of cAMP-dependent protein kinase (PKA) and of diacylglycerol-dependent protein kinase (PKC). Blocking the effect of PKA did not change standard LTP, but blockade of the other two did. The effec- tive concentration to produce blockade was considerably lower for the PKC blocker, suggesting an important role for PKC in LTP generation (Hu et al., 1987).

Another branch of our work also involved molecular neuroscience. During the late 1980s, it became increasingly clear that the enhanced synaptic current which is the hallmark of LTP could be explained by a change of the AMPA receptors involved. This could happen either by a changed configuration of the receptor channel itself or by a recruitment, aggregation, or insertion of new receptor molecules. Peter Seeburg at the Max-Planck-Institute for Medical Research in Heidelberg had cloned the genes for AMPA and NMDA receptors, simultaneously and independently of Stephen Heinemann's group at the Salk Institute. Peter was collaborating with Bert Sakmann, of patch clamp fame, to analyze the functional properties of these molecules, with many of the experiments made by recombinant molecules being expressed in frog oocytes or cultured human embryonic kidney cells (HEK). Bert and Peter asked me whether my group would join them in an effort to study the molecular processes underlying induction and expression of LTP. Obviously, my colleagues and I were delighted. This collaboration has now lasted for about 15 years and has been both productive and agreeable. A piece of good luck helped considerably. In 1987, I won a prize from the Norwegian Research Council which gave my group firm support for five years. This prize, supplemented by allotments from Bert's and Peter's own grants, made it possible to acquire adequate instrumentation and to keep together a research group dedicated to this molecular LTP analysis. This collaboration has been a pleasure, and we feel we have made considerable progress. Perhaps the most significant observation was that mice which lack the gene for the A-subunit of the tetrameric AMPA receptor fail to develop LTP, while ordinary low-frequency synaptic transmission remains intact. The pivotal role of AMPA receptors with A-subunits for LTP expression appears as an important observation (Zamanillo et al., 1999). Another exciting result was the dramatic reduction of LTP in mice lacking the cytosolic tail of the 2A-subunit of the NMDA receptor (Sprengel et al., 1998). As is often the case in science, for each new advance more questions are raised. Apparently, there is a complex molecular arrangement in the postsynaptic density of spines, involving both AMPA and NMDA receptors and binding proteins linking these to the cytoskeleton, which influence a variety of mechanisms for receptor changes involved in various stages of the LTP expression. There are enough problems for another life!

Rewards

Many would agree with me that for a scientist, the highest reward is when your own research results have given a glimpse of a new insight into a major problem. The intense pleasure derived from the fact that you have made a useful contribution to human knowledge is hard to explain to other people. That being said, another reason for satisfaction is the acceptance and appreciation received from your colleagues outside those in your own research group. I am particularly grateful for the consistent and strong support I have received from Vernon Mountcastle and Eric Kandel in the United States; from David Curtis and Steve Redman in Australia; from Ragnar Granit, Anders Lundberg, and Sten Grillner in Sweden; and from Tom Sears and Tim Bliss in the United Kingdom.

A highlight of my career was my election to be a Foreign Member of the National Academy of Sciences (NAS) in Washington, D.C. in 1994. Being an European without any extended period of research in the United States, my main knowledge about the NAS was the journal *PNAS*. I did not know enough about the importance of the Academy and its many other activities. Only when I attended the welcome ceremony for inauguration of new members did I understand the high regard in which the fellowship of American scientists holds the distinction of being a member of this honorable institution. After learning how many hurdles there are for a candidate before the final success and how hard and long my proponents must have worked, I was more than grateful and indeed somewhat embarrassed. How could I deserve such a distinction? Equally moving was the large number of kind letters that I received from so many American neuroscientists, even from people I had not heard from for decades.

In March 2002, I learned that I was nominated as a candidate to the Foreign Membership of the Royal Society of London, and in May, I received a letter from Professor Julia Higgins, Foreign Secretary of the Royal Society (RS), that I was elected Foreign Member of the Royal Society of London for Improving Natural Knowledge. It was as wonderful as unexpected. This time I knew a bit more about the institution. Because I had worked both in Canberra and Oxford, I had appreciated the extremely high regard in which my Commonwealth colleagues hold a fellowship in RS and the other activities of this society, notably the professorships and fellowships that the RS offers. Once again, I felt a mixture of pride and embarrassment, knowing the large number of colleagues who clearly deserve such a distinction. Also, I know that my supporters must have been eager and persistent. Because both the National Academy of Sciences and the Royal Society conduct their elections in great secrecy, I am unaware of my proponents and can only thank them indirectly, as in this article.

The election to the Royal Swedish Academy of Science in 1991 was not only a great honor, but has a practical advantage in that I am allowed to nominate candidates to the Nobel Prize in Physics and Chemistry. Because chemistry includes biochemical topics, I have used this opportunity for nomination of outstanding neurochemists. As a Nordic professor in physiology, I have had the priviledge to nominate candidates for the Nobel Prize for Physiology or Medicine, an opportunity I have used every year since I became a professor in 1972.

Looking back, one of the most rewarding aspects of my scientific life has been to make so many international friends. There is something very special about science. The combination of hard and long-lasting work and competition, often fierce, must be set against the collaboration with intelligent, highly motivated individuals. For a really good result, I feel that friendship between the participants is an essential element. An important factor is trust. Because the quality of the results depends so much upon the care invested by the team members, they have to trust each other. The growth of the mutual trust and friendship in the many research groups in which I have taken part is one of the best experiences of my scientific activity. Although the scientific exercise can be quite strenuous, and sometimes directly disappointing, one of the tangible rewards is to be surrounded by persons with deep knowledge and good intellects. To have the opportunity to enjoy considerate arguments or debates, and to be allowed to share information at all levels, is a nearly invaluable aspect of science, a gift I have cherished deeply.

As a small contribution from our side, my wife and I have asked many scientists to come with us to our mountain cabin, well placed for hiking and skiing. Here, we have had the pleasure of greeting a number of visitors from abroad and have also tried to teach them the glorious sport of skiing in between good meals and evenings in front of the open fire.

Although science is competitive, I have often met unselfish friendliness, even magnanimity. Maybe I am easily fooled, but my impression is that generosity is most often shown by people who are of the highest quality, while persons showing more mundane behavior may be less agreeable.

Selected Bibliography

Adrian ED. Afferent discharges to the cerebral cortex from peripheral sense organs. *J Physiol (Lond)* 1941;100:159–191.

Adrian ED. Rhythmic discharges from the thalamus. *J Physiol (Lond)* 1951;113:9–10.

Alksne JF, Blackstad TW, Walberg F, White LE, Jr. Electron microscopy of axon degeneration: A valuable tool in experimental neuroanatomy. *Ergeb Anat Entwicklungsgesch* 1966;39:3–32.

Allen GI, Eccles JC, Nicoll RA, Oshima T, Rubia FJ. The ionic mechanisms concerned in generating i.p.s.ps of hippocampal pyramidal cells. *Proc R Soc Lond Ser B* 1977;198:363–384.

Andersen P. Interhippocampal impulses. II. Apical dendritic activation of CA1 neurons. *Acta Physiol Scand* 1960;48:178–208.

Andersen P, Andersson SA. *Physiological basis of the alpha rhythm.* Neuroscience Series 1. New York; Appleton-Century Crofts, 1968;235.

Andersen P, Blackstad TW, Lømo T. Location and identification of excitatory synapses on hippocampal pyramidal cells. *Exp Brain Res* 1966;1:236–248.

Andersen P, Bliss TVP, Skrede KK. Unit analysis of hippocampal population spikes. *Acta Physiol Scand* 1971a;13:208–221.

Andersen P, Bliss TVP, Skrede KK. Lamellar organization of hippocampal excitatory pathways. *Acta Physiol Scand* 1971b;13:222–238.

Andersen P, Brooks C McC, Eccles JC, Sears TA. The ventro-basal nucleus of the thalamus: Potential fields, synaptic transmission and excitability of both presynaptic and postsynaptic components. *J Physiol (Lond)* 1964a;174:348–369.

Andersen P, Curtis DR. The excitation of thalamic neurones by acetylcholine. *Acta Physiol Scand* 1964;61:85–99.

Andersen P, Dingledine R, Gjerstad L, Langmoen IA, Mosfeldt Laursen A. Two different responses of hippocampal pyramidal cells to application of gamma-amino-butyric acid (GABA). *J Physiol* 1980a;305:279–296.

Andersen P, Eccles J. Inhibitory phasing of neuronal discharge. *Nature* 1962;196: 645–647.

Andersen P, Eccles JC. Locating and identifying postsynaptic inhibitory synapses by the correlation of physiological and histological data. *Symp Biol Hung* 1965;5:219–242.

Andersen P, Eccles JC, Oshima T, Schmidt RF. Mechanisms of synaptic transmission in the cuneate nucleus. *J Neurophysiol* 1964b;27:1096–1116.

Andersen P, Eccles JC, Schmidt RF, Yokota T. Slow potential waves produced in the cuneate nucleus by cutaneous volleys and by cortical stimulation. *J Neurophysiol* 1964c;27:78–91.

Andersen P, Eccles JC, Schmidt RF, Yokota T. Depolarization of presynaptic fibers in the cunate nucleus. *J Neurophysiol* 1964d;27:92–106.

Andersen P, Eccles JC, Schmidt RF, Yokota T. Identification of relay cells and interneurons in the cuneate nucleus. *J Neurophysiol* 1964e;27:1080–1095.

Andersen P, Eccles JC, Sears TA. The ventro-basal complex of the thalamus: Types of cells, their responses and their functional organization. *J Physiol (Lond)* 1964f;174:370–399.

Andersen P, Hagen PJ, Phillips CG, Powell TPS. Mapping by microstimulation of overlapping projections from area 4 to motor units of the baboon's hand. *Proc R Soc Lond Ser B* 1975;188:31–60.

Andersen P, Lømo T. Control of hippocampal output by afferent volley frequency. In Adey WR, Tokizane T, eds. Structure and Function of the Limbic System. *Progr Brain Res* 1967;27:400–412.

Andersen P, Sears TA. The role of inhibition in the phasing of spontaneous thalamo-cortical discharge. *J Physiol (Lond)* 1964;73:459–480.

Andersen P, Silfvenius H, Sundberg SH, Sveen, O. A comparison of distal and prox-imal dendritic synapses on CA1 pyramids in guinea-pig hippocampal slices in vitro. *J Physiol* 1980b;307:273–299.

Andersen P, Sundberg SH, Sveen O, Wigström H. Specific long-lasting potentiation of synaptic transmission in hippocampal slices. *Nature* 1977;266:736–737.

Bliss TVP, Lømo T. Long-lasting potentiation of synaptic transmission in the dentate area of the anaesthetized rabbit following stimulation of the perforant path. *J Physiol (Lond)* 1973;232:331–356.

Bremer, F. Cerebral and cerebellar potentials. *Physiol Rev* 1958;38:357–388.

Brooks CMcC, Eccles JC. Inhibitory action of a motor nucleus and pathway through the spinal cord. *J Neurophysiol* 1948;11:401–416.

Collingridge GL, Kehl SJ, McLennan H. Excitatory amino acids in synaptic transmission in the Schaffer collateral-commissural pathway of the rat hippocampus. *J Physiol (Lond)* 1983;334:33–46.

Cragg BG, Hamlyn LH. Action potentials of the pyramidal neurons in the hippocampus of the rabbit. *J Physiol (Lond)* 1955;129:608–627.

Curtis DR, Felix D, McLellan H. GABA and hippocampal inhibition. *Br J Pharmacol* 1970;40:881–883.

Denny-Brown D, Eccles JC, Liddell EGT. Observations on electrical stimulation of the cerebellar cortex. *Proc R Soc Lond Ser B* 1929;104:518–536.

Eccles JC. *The neurophysiological basis of mind*. Oxford: Oxford University Press,1953; 314 pp.

Eccles JC. *The physiology of nerve cells*. Baltimore: The Johns Hopkins University Press, 1955; 270 pp.

Eccles JC, Ito M, Szenthágothai J. *The cerebellum as a neuronal machine*. New York, Heidelberg: Springer-Verlag, 1967.

Eccles JC, Llinas R, Sasaki K. The excitatory synaptic action of climbing fibres on Purkinje cells of the cerebellum. *J Physiol (Lond)* 1966a;182:268–296.

Eccles JC, Llinas R, Sasaki K. The inhibitory interneurones within the cerebellar cortex. *Exp Brain Res* 1966b;1:1–16.

Granit R, Phillips CG. Excitatory and inhibitory processes acting upon individual Purkinje cells of the cerebellum in cats. *J Physiol (Lond)* 1956;133:520–547.

Gray EG. Axosomatic and axo-dendritic synapses of the cerebral cortex: An electron microscopical study. *J Anat (Lond)* 1959;93:420–433.

Green JD, Arduini AA. Hippocampal electrical activity in arousal. *J Neurophysiol* 1954;17:533–557.

Hagbarth K-E, Kerr DIB. Central influences on spinal afferent conduction. *J Neurophysiol* 1954;17:295–305.

Hamlyn LH. An electron microscope study of pyramidal neurons in the Ammon's Horn of the rabbit. *J Anat (Lond)* 1963;97:189–201.

Hodgkin AL. The ionic basis of electrical activity in nerve and muscle. *Biol Rev* 1951;26:339–409.

Hvalby Ø, Lacaille J-C, Hu G-Y, Andersen P. Postsynaptic long-term potentiation follows coupling of dendritic gutamate application and synaptic activation. *Experientia* 1987;43:599–601.

Hu G-Y, Hvalby Ø, Walaas SI, Albert KA, Skjeflo P, Andersen P, Greengard P. Protein kinase C injection into hippocampal pyramidal cells elicits features of long-term potentiation. *Nature* 1987;328:426–429.

Kandel ER, Spencer WA, Brinley FJ, Jr. Electrophysiology of hippocampal neurons. I. Sequential invasion and synaptic organization. *J Neurophysiol* 1961;24:225–242.

Langmoen IA, Andersen P. Summation of excitatory postsynaptic potentials in hippocampal pyramidal cells. *J Neurophysiol* 1983;50:1320–1329.

Llinas R, Jahnsen H. Electrophysiology of mammalian thalamic neurones in vitro. *Nature* 1982;297:406–408.

Lorente de Nó R. Studies on the structure of the cerebral cortex. II. Continuation of the study of the Ammonic system. *J Psychol Neurol (Lpz)* 1934;46:113–177.

Lømo T. Frequency potentiation of excitatory synaptic activity in the dentate area of the hippocampal formation. *Acta Physiol Scand* 1966; 68(Suppl. 277):128.

McNaughton BL, Douglas RM, Goddard GV. Synaptic enhancement in fascia dentate: Cooperativity among coactive afferents. *Brain Res* 1978;157:277–293.

Obata K, Ito M, Ochi R, Sato N. Pharmacological properties of the postsynaptic inhibition by Purkinje cell axons and the action of γ-aminobutyric acid on Deiter's neurones. *Exp Brain Res* 1967;4:43–57.

Ramon y Cajal, S. *Histologie de Système nerveux chez l'Homme et des Vertébrés*. Paris: A. Maloine, 1911, Vol. II.

Renshaw B, Forbes A, Morison BR. Activity of isocortex and hippocampus: Electrical studies with micro-electrodes. *J Neurophysiol* 1940;3:74–105.

Schwartzkroin PA. Characteristics of CA1 neurons recorded intracellularly in the hippocampal in vitro slice preparation. *Brain Res* 1975;85:423–436.

Schwartzkroin PA, Andersen P. *Glutamic acid sensitivity of dendrites in hippocampal slices in vitro.* In Kreuzberg G. ed. *Advances in neurology, vol. 12*, New York: Raven Press, 1975;45–51.

Skrede KK, Westgaard RH. The transverse hippocampal slice: A well-defined cortical structure maintained in vitro. *Brain Res* 1971;35:589–593.

Sprengel R, Suchanek B, Amico C, Brusa R, Burnashev N, Rozov A, Hvalby Ø, Jensen V, Paulsen O, Andersen P, Kim JJ, Thompson, RF, Sun W, Webster LC, Grant SGN, Eilers J, Konnerth A, Li J, McNamara JO, Seeburg PH. Importance of the intracellular domain of NR2 subunits for NMDA receptor function in vivo. *Cell* 1998;92:279–289.

von Krosigk M, Bal T, McCormick DA. Cellular mechanisms of a synchronized oscillation in the thalamus. *Science* 1993;261:361–364.

Watkins JC, Evans RH. Excitatory amino acid transmitters. *Annu Rev Pharmacol Toxicol* 1981;21:165–204.

Wigstrőm H, Gustafsson B, Huang YY, Abraham WC. Hippocampal long-term potentiation is induced by pairing single afferent volleys with intracellularly injected depolarizing current pulses. *Acta Physiol Scand* 1986;126:317–319.

Yamamoto C, McIlwain H. Potentials evoked in vitro in preparations from the mammalian brain. *Nature* 1966;210:1055–1056.

Zamanillo D, Sprengel R, Hvalby Ø, Jensen V, Burnashev N, Rozov A, Kaiser K, Köster HJ, Borchardt T, Worley P, Lübke J, Frotscher M, Kelley PH, Sommer B, Andersen P, Seeburg PH, Sakmann B. Importance of AMPA receptors for hippocampal synaptic plasticity but not for spatial learning. *Science* 1999;284:1805–1811.

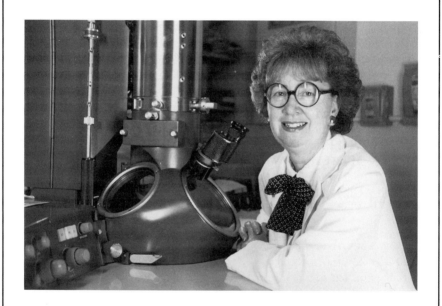

Mary Bartlett Bunge

BORN:

New Haven, Connecticut
April 3, 1931

EDUCATION:

Simmons College, B.S. (1953)
University of Wisconsin Medical School, M.S. (1955)
University of Wisconsin, Ph.D. (1960)

APPOINTMENTS:

Columbia University, College of Physicians and Surgeons,
New York (1963)
Harvard Medical School, Boston (Sabbatical, 1968)
Washington University School of Medicine, St. Louis (1970)
King's College, London (Sabbatical, 1984)
University of Miami School of Medicine, Miami (1989)
Interim Scientific Director, The Miami Project to Cure
Paralysis, University of Miami School of Medicine,
Miami (1996–1997)
Christine E. Lynn, Distinguished Professor of Neuroscience
Member, National Advisory NINDS Council (1987–1991)

HONORS AND AWARDS (SELECTED):

Chair, Development of Women's Careers in Neuroscience
Committee, Society for Neuroscience (1994–2002)
Wakeman Award, Spinal Cord Repair (1996)
Dana Alliance for Brain Initiatives (1999)
Dean's Research Award, University of Miami School of
Medicine (1999)
Vice President, National Neurotrauma Society (2001–2002)
Mika Salpeter Women in Neuroscience Lifetime Achievement
Award (2000)
Christopher Reeve Research Medal for Spinal Cord Repair (2001)
Florida Woman of Achievement (2002)

*Early work by Richard and Mary Bunge demonstrated that demyelination
and remyelination occur in the adult mammalian spinal cord. This and
other work led to a better understanding of myelin formation in the central
and peripheral nervous systems. Mary Bunge has contributed information
on the mechanisms of axonal growth in culture. Both Bunges have been
pioneers in the area of neural cell-extracellular matrix interactions and
spinal cord injury and repair.*

Mary Bartlett Bunge[1]

As an only child growing up in a small Connecticut River harbor town, I was fortunate to have the woods at my back door and, down a long steep incline, a small stream at the front of the house. Spending much time alone, the woods and the stream provided hours of exploration and enjoyment. Steering my rowboat slowly near the banks overhung with elderberry bushes, the tadpoles and frogs were endlessly intriguing. This led to a developing interest in biology and to borrowing books from the library about Marie Curie. How romantic it seemed to be stirring pitchblende for hours! Beyond the stream was a meadow that, when flooded and frozen in the winter, provided an opportunity to pretend I was Sonja Henie, a three-time Olympic gold medalist who brought beauty and ballet to figure skating. A mile down the road lived my ballet teacher, whose lessons inspired me to dream of being a dancer like Anna Pavlova, one of the greatest ballerinas of all time. Being chosen to represent the Girl Scouts in that area of the Connecticut River valley brought me into contact with my fourth heroine, Mrs. Eleanor Roosevelt. The prowess of my maternal grandmother in sewing led to my ability to create my own clothes and, thus, to dream of being a fashion designer in New York City.

A profession involving artistic expression vied heavily with one in science. Both my parents were artistic. My mother, Margaret Elizabeth Reynolds Bartlett, was descended from the renowned British painter and founder of the Royal Academy, Sir Joshua Reynolds. She herself painted and was a decorator with no college education; her father thought college education was useless for women. My father, George Chapman Bartlett, spurned education after high school to study the violin intensely. Despite having a very gifted student who gave a recital in New York, he tired of teaching and turned to creating new houses and renovating very old ones, such as a 1785 house built by Captain Ebenezer Williams where we lived for a few years.

Being different from my classmates in that I was actually interested in learning, it was a relief to migrate to a more northern area of the Connecticut River valley to the Northfield School for Girls for the last two years of high school. My education was greatly improved and led to matriculation

---

[1]With partial commentary on Richard P. Bunge.

at Simmons College in Boston. This college was chosen because interests in biology had finally surpassed the others. I reasoned that the artistic interests could be pursued as hobbies, but it would be impossible to do laboratory work without training. My goal was to be a laboratory technician, and Simmons offered a course in laboratory technology. It was the vision of businessman John Simmons that women should be given both a liberal arts and a practical education. Upon graduating from college, I would be prepared for a job. This goal was to change, however.

At the end of my junior year in college, I was accepted into the well-known college program at the Jackson Memorial Laboratory in Bar Harbor, ME. For the first time I was in a community of 18 highly motivated students pursuing medical and/or research professions. Not only did we attend classes and participate in research, but we also were responsible for preparing our meals and ate in a common dining room. It was a dream summer socially and scientifically, including socializing with the senior scientists. Though renowned for cancer research in animals, I was placed with Dr. Philip R. White, who, in order to study crown gall tumors, had devised plant tissue culture techniques, including the formulation of a completely synthetic medium for plant cells. After being there for a week, he informed me that he was going on a trip and requested that I change the medium of his 20-year-old tomato root cultures. Because prepared culture medium was not available at that time, I nervously weighed each component to prepare the medium from scratch and was enormously relieved to find that the cultures survived uninfected. Dr. White occasionally grew animal tissue in culture, and after viewing contracting heart muscle one day, I was hooked on research. This extraordinary summer experience changed the course of my life and attending graduate school suddenly became compelling.

To Madison, Wisconsin: Fall of 1953

Though scheduled to start a teaching career and a Master's program at Vassar, a telegram arrived from Dr. Robert F. Schilling offering me a Research Assistantship that would be funded by the Wisconsin Alumni Research Foundation while I became a graduate student in the Department of Medical Physiology at the University of Wisconsin Medical School. Dr. Schilling had become renowned for developing a diagnostic test for pernicious anemia. He was studying a substance called intrinsic factor, which is lacking in this condition. Would I be interested in working in his laboratory for my thesis work? The Vassar plan was dumped forthwith, and my parents started to plan the car trip that would take me to Madison in the autumn of 1953.

Intrinsic factor in normal human gastric juice enhances the absorption of vitamin B_{12} from the gut. In the mid-1950s, the mechanism by which this occurs had not yet been elucidated, but it was known that binding of the vitamin to the factor was necessary, although not sufficient. Pseudovitamin

B_{12}, in which the 5,6-dimethylbenzimidazole (DMBI) moiety is replaced by adenine, was considered not to substitute for vitamin B_{12}. We investigated whether the pseudovitamin or the DMBI moiety alone competed with vitamin B_{12} for the process that leads to intestinal absorption of the vitamin and found that the two compounds were not effective competitors *in vivo* and did not bind to gastric juice *in vitro*. Thus, we determined that the binding of B_{12} by normal gastric juice is a highly selective process. This was the subject of my first publication in 1956. A second publication in 1957 reported the results of testing the effect of ten vitamin B_{12} analogs on vitamin B_{12} binding in gastric juice compared with certain other biologic substances (serum, saliva, colostrum). Gastric juice exhibited the greatest preference for vitamin B_{12} in the presence of excess analog. Occurrence of a sulfate, nitrate, or chloride ion in lieu of the cyanide ion of the vitamin did not diminish competition for vitamin B_{12} binding sites by gastric juice. This work also was the basis of a thesis, enabling receipt of an M.S. degree in medical physiology in 1955. Following this, during the first year of marriage, I worked full time in Dr. Schilling's laboratory while deciding about Ph.D. work.

Thus, this was a productive time and an exciting introduction to basic research with clinical relevance, an introduction that was to influence future research decisions. Dr. Schilling was an outstanding mentor who set high standards and viewed data very critically. His input into my first manuscript writing established a valuable foundation for years to come. As a beginning graduate student enjoying some of the many benefits of Madison and Lake Mendota and the unique and wonderful Student Union, a slight hint from him over lunch to work harder, including evenings, was sufficient to change my work habits to this day.

But the research experience was only part of the gain from being in Dr. Schilling's laboratory. Every summer Dr. Schilling took on medical students, and in the summer of 1954, one of those medical students was Richard P. Bunge. Although Dick spent most of the summer in the cold room working on a Raynaud's disease project, and though he vanished at 5:00 PM to wash dishes in the hospital cafeteria to help fund medical school, we became acquainted in a sailboat. Because I thought that he needed some fresh air, I invited him to go sailing and the wind often died down when we were in the middle of Lake Mendota. I had found a gem. In time I was to realize how much he personified midwestern values: no airs, no nonsense, plain speaking, integrity, modesty, and consideration that every person has value. These traits undoubtedly also resulted from having grown up in a home with a strong Christian influence.

Just three years earlier, the tall, lanky young man with a crewcut had arrived in Madison to enter the University of Wisconsin as an undergraduate. This was a big change from the rural Midwest settings where the Bunge home was often situated in an expanse of corn fields and next to a Lutheran church where his father was pastor. He had attended a one-room schoolhouse in early years; a short period at a high school in Albany, MN, where he was a basketball star, awakened his intellect. This intellect flourished in the presence of great minds he encountered at the University and led to entry into medical school.

To pay for his education, in addition to the cafeteria job, he decided to split a year, working half of the time in research and attending medical school part time. A faculty member in the Department of Anatomy, Dr. Paul Settlage, was studying the administration of anaesthesia via the cisterna magna in adult cats. The cerebrospinal fluid was drawn into a syringe, the anaesthetic was added, and the fluid was returned; this was repeated several times. Because these animals exhibited a temporary paralysis, he considered it important to test this procedure of cerebrospinal fluid exchange without the anaesthetic. The person he chose to study this was Dick, who prepared the spinal cord tissue, stained it for myelin, and observed a non-staining rim around the lower medulla and upper spinal cord periphery. Then, one month later, he observed thin circles of new myelin in the area earlier bereft of myelin, at a time when the animals showed neurological improvement. Though the mechanism was not understood, this was the first sighting of demyelination and remyelination in the adult mammalian spinal cord, at that time a revolutionary finding. This led to a lifelong career dedicated to research, preferring that to the practice of medicine. Following medical school, he chose to enter a postdoctoral fellowship rather than to proceed to further medical training.

During my coursework for my M.S., I took a cytology course from a noted cell biologist, Dr. Hans Ris. Known for his work on the configuration of DNA in chromosomes, he was an electron microscopist. His course was fascinating, starting with descriptions of early cytologists Schleiden, Schwann, Boveri, Brown, etc. and providing captivating laboratory periods that included preparations of chromosome squashes and cell fractions and tissue sections. But, most importantly for me, he introduced us to the electron microscope. Even using the first electron microscope at the University of Wisconsin (in the Biochemistry Department), when we often had to hammer the lenses into appropriate positions and the resolution was inferior by today's standards, the images were enthralling, and I saw the opportunity to combine the acquisition of scientific data with artistic expression. The decision to work with Dr. Ris for my Ph.D. in the Zoology Department came easily.

What project to pursue? Several questions had arisen from Dick's discovery. Was demyelination partial or complete? What cells reformed the myelin? How was the myelin laid down? The spiraling mechanism for peripheral myelination had been reported in 1954. Was the same mechanism utilized by central glia? Why was the central myelinating cell not obvious as it was in the periphery? Clearly, what was needed was an electron microscopic characterization of the lesion that Dick had studied at the light microscope level. Despite Dr. Ris' lack of experience with nervous tissue, he took me on. He was an outstanding mentor, committed to the highest standards of excellence and willing not only to mentor a now committed developing neuroscientist but also a young woman. The availability of these two mentors most certainly helped shape my future in a beneficial way. Both, to their credit, were gender blind, and I never thought of myself as a female graduate student, but as a graduate student period. He was an effective teacher as well, and I learned the preparative techniques from Dr. Ris, including thin sectioning, very quickly. He was a master of interpretation of electron micrographs.

And so Dick and I set out on our new research journey. But first I had to meet my teaching requirement for my Ph.D., teaching Zoology I laboratory at 7:30 AM. We had found an apartment close to the University, not far from the bottom of the steep hill that led to some of the main campus buildings, including the zoology building. On bitter cold, dark mornings in the heart of winter, Dick pushed me up the hill. When the teaching commitment was finished months later, we started the work in earnest. We were to have our own laboratory for a time in a brand new medical school research building due to the unfortunate death of Dr. Settlage in a drowning incident. A substitute for teaching Gross Anatomy was needed, and, when this opportunity was offered to Dick, he decided to take a year off from medical school to teach as well as do research. Thus began a love for teaching this subject (exceptionally well) for many, many years, which provided valuable background for leading The Miami Project some 30 years later. This one-year instructorship also enabled us to stay out of debt for our remaining graduate education.

Adequate preservation of central nervous tissue was difficult to achieve. Glutaraldehyde had not yet been discovered as an effective preservative. We heard tales of enormous quantities of expensive osmium tetroxide being used for whole animal perfusion in a Boston laboratory. But we were lucky because the area to be studied was at the rim of the spinal cord. Consequently, we simply withdrew the cerebrospinal fluid from the cisterna magna and replaced it with buffered osmium tetroxide. This was repeated twice to facilitate circulation throughout the intrathecal space. Only a very shallow area of tissue was preserved, but it was within this subpial circumference that the lesion was located. Small wedges of tissue were cut from the rim for dehydration and embedding. We were among the first in the United States to find that araldite was far superior to methacrylate for embedment for electron microscopy.

We studied tissue changes from 29 hr to 460 days after cerebrospinal fluid exchange in a total of 19 cats. Dick's brother, Walter, also a student at the University of Wisconsin, procured the cats for us from local farmers. Twenty-nine hours after lesioning, most myelin sheaths were deteriorating and typical macroglia (fibrous astrocytes and oligodendrocytes) were no longer visible. Myelin breakdown presented as layers of varying thickness split apart, with the edges of these layers yielding subsequently to a honeycomb- or alveolar-like pattern of dispersion. These configurations were clearly different from inadequate preservation. Phagocytosis of the myelin debris had begun. The phagocytes typically displayed long, sheet-like processes that embraced the axon and its myelin sheath or invaded the deteriorating sheath itself. In three-day lesions, despite the extensive myelin breakdown, axons were intact. Axons, completely demyelinated by six days, were ensconced in expanses of greatly swollen debris-laden macrophages. They were denuded only very briefly, however, for by six days macroglia appeared in the lesion area and started to invest some of the axons. These glial processes resembled neither fibrous astrocytes nor oligodendrocytes; their cytoplasm was dense with closely packed organelles and numerous filaments that were not observed in normal astrocytes.

An occasional myelin sheath was first seen at 19 days; by 64 days all axons were at least thinly myelinated. The cytoplasm of the myelin-forming cells was, as above, unlike that of either the oligodendrocyte or fibrous astrocyte that is observed in normal cord. These macroglia were large, and one cell dispatched many processes that embraced many axons. A spectrum of intermediate types between these reactive macroglia and highly filament-laden glia (fibrous astrocytes) became evident after remyelination had begun. Many of the myelinating cells became scarring astrocytes. We proposed that these macroglia were identical to the hypertrophic or swollen astrocytes common to many neuropathological processes and were considered to be progenitors of the scarring fibrous astrocytes. Consequently, we raised the possibility that the presence of hypertrophic astrocytes in multiple sclerosis plaques may be responsible for remyelinating fibers that could then lead to the characteristic clinical remissions.

Recognizable oligodendrocytes appeared in the lesion at 45 days, well after remyelination had begun. Phagocytes disappeared gradually; seen only rarely at 220 days, they were not found in the lesion thereafter. At 460 days, slender processes filled with large compact bundles of filaments dominated the tissue. Oligodendrocytes were more numerous at this time.

We observed that the myelin sheath was formed by spiral wrapping of a sheet-like glial process around the axon. When the first turn of the spiral was completed, a mesaxon was formed. As cytoplasm was lost from this process, the plasma membrane came together along its outer and cytoplasmic surfaces to form compact myelin. Only a small amount of cytoplasm was retained, confined to the paramesaxonal region inside the sheath and, on the sheath exterior, to an external mesaxon or a longitudinal ridge which appeared in cross-section as a small loop. This outer ridge or loop resulted from the loss of glial cytoplasm on one side of the external mesaxon. The orientation of the outer loop compared with that of the inner mesaxon implied a spiral. These vestiges of spiral membrane wrapping were also found in normal adult spinal cord. This mechanism was basically similar to that proposed for the peripheral nerve. It did not agree with the current view on the mechanism of central myelination. In fact, even the electron microscopic identification of central glia was very controversial at that time. In our exceptionally well-preserved control cord, fibrous astrocytes and oligodendrocytes could be identified and distinguished easily.

An obvious question was whether this spiraling mechanism of a glial cell process that we observed during remyelination was the same as the mechanism of first myelination during development. This led us to studies of kitten spinal cord, first in Madison and later in New York. Initially, we observed the same inner mesaxonal and outer loop configurations, suggestive of a similar mechanism. The five-day kitten spinal cord was the best time to observe the continuity between the glial cell perikaryon and its extended processes, at the ends of which myelination occurred. My first glimpse in the electron microscope of an area from the five-day cord was one of my most exciting research moments. As I increased the electron beam to view the tissue, there in the center of the field was a configuration not unlike oldfashioned ice tongs: an oligodendrocyte nucleus and surrounding cytoplasm (lacking the filaments seen during remyelination), from which extended two processes tipped by axons being myelinated. This configuration appears in the 1962 reference. It must be admitted that the rather poor preservation, which led to substantial space in this immature tissue, eased the detection of such configurations. In this way, we discovered that in the central nervous system myelination occurred at some distance from the glial perikaryon, in contrast to Schwann cell myelination in the peripheral nervous system. With maturation, these processes lose much of the cytoplasm, and the resulting thin process is not detectable in the thicket of myelinated axons. This explained why we and others had not yet observed the cytoplasmic life lines to myelin in the remyelinated or normal adult cord. Our observations were incorporated into a cartoon showing the relationship between an oligodendrocyte and the myelin sheaths it formed; this figure continues to appear in textbooks.

It was an intense and exciting time, arriving home between 1:00 and 2:00 AM and then rising a few hours later to resume our work. We worked together extremely well, each bringing different strengths to the project. The electron microscopic images were not only revelatory, but also satisfied my artistic bent as anticipated; I loved creating the most handsome micrographs possible. I have to the present remained intrigued with the developments in electron microscopy in the 1950s and 1960s. One moment of panic occurred when our longest term animal, 460 days following lesioning, escaped from his cage and was seen heading for remote parts of the campus. With a stroke of luck, we somehow managed to catch him. Madison was an idyllic location for graduate students, not only for sailing in the summer, but for swimming at lunch breaks as well. The observations made in Madison led to our first European trip to present at the IVth International Congress of Neuropathology in 1961. We did not realize at the time that this was a harbinger of much travel to come. We managed to be awarded our M.D. and Ph.D. degrees, respectively, at the same graduation ceremony in 1960.

To New York City: Summer of 1960

We set out for Columbia University College of Physicians and Surgeons where we were to be postdoctoral fellows with Drs. Margaret R. Murray (Laboratory of Cell Physiology, Department of Surgery) and George D. Pappas (Department of Anatomy). Dr. Pappas, an electron microscopist, had trained at the Rockefeller Institute with Dr. Keith R. Porter, who along with Drs. George Palade and Albert Claude had pioneered the development of a new body of knowledge that could only have arisen by using the electron microscope. Dr. Margaret R. Murray was herself a pioneer in developing the organotypic explant culture system for both peripheral and central nervous tissues. Dick was to learn these nerve tissue culture techniques so as to be able to ask biological questions without the complexity of performing studies in the whole animal. I was to serve as a bridge between the Pappas and Murray laboratories to initiate electron microscopic characterization of the sensory ganglion and spinal cord culture systems. We were funded by fellowships from the NIH (MBB) and from the National Multiple Sclerosis Society (RPB). We set up a household in the shadow of the medical school on 163rd Street, so that we could walk to work. This northern area of Manhattan was at that time an old and stable neighborhood beside the Hudson River.

Margaret Murray and I had much in common: she, too, was an only child who spent time near the water in a family home on Put-in Creek off Chesapeake Bay; both our precedent families had arrived in the 1600s; she was visually oriented; and she had spent time at Washington University in St. Louis. Her career started in 1929 when she was invited to Columbia University College of Physicians and Surgeons to help establish a research program in surgical pathology, the aim of which was to study human tumors grown *in vitro*, in part to reveal their cellular origins. The nomenclature that she and Dr. Arthur Purdy Stout developed for tumors stands today. She received more notoriety when in 1939 she reported that peripheral nerve sheath tumors originated from Schwann cells. She and her long-term and gifted collaborator, Mrs. Edith Peterson, reported another milestone in 1955: that myelination occurred in culture, proof that a remarkable degree of differentiation could be obtained in the organotypic explant culture system. Her efforts led to the formation of the Tissue Culture Association, which helped devise standardized nerve tissue culture techniques that, among other developments, led to the production of commercial culture media. She opened her laboratory to trainees and investigators from all over the world to learn the techniques that she had developed; in 1970 it could be said that about 75% of the worldwide research effort in nerve tissue culture was carried out by scientists (and their students) trained in her laboratory.

In contrast to what would be future directions in nerve tissue culture techniques, the goal was to try to mimic the *in vivo* environment as closely as possible. Consequently, the culture medium was complex due to inclusion of human placental serum and embryo extract, and the pieces of tissue were cultured intact in the complex Maximow double coverslip assembly. The tissue culture room was basically a surgical suite, whose walls were scrubbed down once a week and in which full surgical regalia was worn. The talents of Mrs. Peterson enabled the cultures to be grown for months or more, during which differentiation of the initially embryonic tissue occurred. The nests of healthy sensory ganglion somata were particularly beautiful and easily seen. Because myelin also was visible in living cultures, the somata and sheaths could be followed continuously for weeks or months to better understand neuronal reactions and causes of myelin breakdown after various treatments. The gradual replacement of culture medium with fixative and the lack of mechanical handling of the tissue enabled outstanding preservation for electron microscopy.

Long-term cultures (up to 76 days) of 17- to 18-day fetal rat spinal cord were characterized electron microscopically. It was known that myelination occurred and that the cultures were capable of complex bioelectric activity, due to the efforts of Dr. Stanley Crain and Mrs. Peterson. Neurons were positioned in several strata beneath a region of neuropil. The general ultrastructural characteristics of *in vivo* mammalian central nervous system (CNS) tissue were found in culture, including well-developed Nissl bodies and an extensive system of microtubules and filaments in the neuronal cytoplasm; close packing of cells and processes with little intercellular space; typical oligodendrocytes and fibrous astrocytes as well as glia intermediate in morphology, the characteristic pattern of CNS myelin, including nodes of Ranvier and typical axosomatic and axodendritic synapses (including Type 1 and Type 2 synapses of Gray). A basis for the complex synaptic networks detected by electrophysiology had been found by electron microscopy.

When the fetal tissue was examined at the time of explantation, it was observed to be very immature, indicating that most of the differentiated features had developed *in vitro*. For example, whereas in the mature cultures synapses were found in nearly every field, a recognizable synapse was extremely rare in the new explant. This offered an opportunity to study for the first time the morphological development of mammalian synapses *in vitro* and to see if there was a close correlation between the initiation of synapse formation and the onset of functional synaptic networks.

Synapses first appeared consistently in 70-hr cultures of 14-day fetal rat cord. These initial profiles covered only a small area, displayed only small clusters of vesicles, contained little cleft material, lacked mitochondria, and were exclusively axodendritic. The time at which these immature synapses were first seen was the time that bioelectric evidence of functioning synaptic networks was found. As the synapses increased dramatically at 78–100 hr, the response of the explant to electrical stimuli became more easily elicited and more complex. Some synapses displayed more associated vesicles and covered a larger area, although mitochondria were still seldom seen. The gradual accumulation of vesicles and, later, mitochondria mirrored results from *in vivo* studies. Synapses on dendritic spines and axosomatic terminals were now observed. It was at this time, after 93–100 hr, that strychnine sensitivity was first detectable, suggesting that inhibitory networks were starting to function. The close correlation of morphology and activity was thus observed despite isolation of the tissue from normal afferent and efferent connections.

Long-term organotypic cultures (up to three months) of fetal ($16\frac{1}{2}$–19 days) rat dorsal root ganglia were characterized as well. The neurons resembled their *in vivo* counterparts in nuclear and cytoplasmic content and organization. The larger neuronal somata exhibited "cytoplasmic roads" composed of neurofilaments and microtubules. Nissl bodies were prominent in the larger perikarya. Satellite cells formed a complete investment around the neuronal perikarya, and their exterior was covered by basal lamina. From the central cluster of neuronal cell bodies, neurites emerged to form a rich network of organized fascicles that often reached the edge of the coverslip (10 mm). This outgrowth, of course, was formed completely in culture. Unmyelinated and myelinated fibers were in the typical relationship with Schwann cells, with only one Schwann cell being related to one myelinated axon, but one Schwann cell being related to multiple unmyelinated fibers. The abaxonal Schwann cell surface was covered by basal lamina. Collagen fibrils and *in situ*-like perineurial ensheathment were also components of the fascicles. The myelin sheaths exhibited their *in vivo* attributes: mesaxons, Schmidt-Lanterman clefts, and nodes of Ranvier. Despite the overall cytological fidelity to similar tissue *in vivo*, perikaryal size, myelinated fiber diameter, and myelin internode length did not reach the larger dimensions observed *in situ*. Ganglion cultures, in which neuronal perikarya and Schwann cells and their myelin sheaths could be well visualized in the living state, were to be the objects of many future studies in numerous laboratories.

When Dick became an Assistant Professor in the Anatomy Department at Columbia in 1962, he set up a tissue culture laboratory. Once again, training in the Murray laboratory had led to the birth of a new nerve tissue culture facility and more third generation culturists began to be trained. Dick was successful in acquiring grants from both the NIH and the National Multiple Sclerosis Society. I became a Research Associate to be supported by the grants that Dick obtained, spurning the goal to be a tenure-track faculty member. By that time our first son, Jonathan Bartlett Bunge, had joined our family. I could not envision lecture preparation, teaching, grant writing, and committee membership added to my research schedule and new motherhood responsibilities. I worked part-time for the ensuing eight years (with the exception of a sabbatical period). A second son, Peter Taeuber Bunge, was born in 1964. I felt more and more like a symphony conductor, trying to keep all the instruments playing in harmony.

Among the studies that we started in our own laboratory was a project investigating the cytological outcome of X-irradiation of the organotypic rat dorsal root ganglion cultures over a two-week period. Investigators continued to ask whether degenerative changes observed after ionizing radiation to the animal were primarily the result of direct radiation injury to the neural elements, and thus independent of secondary effects from a radiation-damaged vascular supply, or whether they resulted from other host-associated humoral or inflammatory responses. The well differentiated, two- to three-month-old organotypic ganglion cultures would be an appropriate tool to address this question. A trainee, Dr. Edmund B. Masurovsky, who worked with us to correlate light and electron microscopic images, saw a striking spectrum of neuronal changes that started as a chromatolytic pattern and evolved into vacuolar or granular degeneration over a two-week period. Interestingly, degenerative changes were not observed in the occasional binucleate neuron. The neurons were more radiation resistant than the satellite cells, which were decimated acutely; this satellite cell loss left only basal lamina coverage of the neuronal cell body. When this occurred, the small evaginations that normally arose from the perikarya and were surrounded by satellite cell cytoplasm were abnormally deeply invaginated into the neuronal perikaryon. A corresponding wave of acute degeneration also was evident in Schwann cells ensheathing unmyelinated fibers; breakdown of myelin (beginning at the node) and their associated Schwann cells followed a few days later. This selective radiation sensitivity of nonmyelinating Schwann cells had not been noted before. Axonal changes were not apparent until 14 days. The demise of the cellular elements took place within the basal lamina tubes. Our observations demonstrated that X-irradiation produced striking cytopathological changes in nervous tissue that was isolated from the host and that many of these changes resembled the effects of radiation *in vivo*.

Dick pursued additional studies utilizing the organotypic ganglion culture system with new trainees. Also, he and Dr. Masurovsky determined that fluoroplastic (Aclar) coverslips could replace glass for long-term culture; differentiation of the cultures was the same as on glass, and the plastic was highly inert, unbreakable, and easily separated from polymerized epoxy resin when cultures were embedded for electron microscopy. The plastic was to be important in devising new culture strategies later in St. Louis. I collaborated with Dr. Murray and one of her trainees, Dr. Celia F. Brosnan, to study the effect of adding chlorpromazine to sensory ganglion cultures. Its mode of action was unknown, and, because it is a fluorochrome, its destination could be followed in the highly visible neurons. The initial diffuse fluorescence seen within a few minutes in the cell soma became abnormally granular, starting at 4 hr. These chlorpromazine-induced granules were enlarged lysosomes, as determined by electron microscopy and by the Gomori technique for detecting acid phosphatase. Cultures recovered within a few days. This reaction to the tranquilizer was considered to be a general cytological reaction by which the cytoplasm is cleared of an abnormal substance. There was the possibility, however, also suggested in the work of others, that the lysosomal response was the primary mechanism by which chlorpromazine exerts its pharmacological action. Work in our Columbia laboratory was to be interrupted by a sabbatical period, and, upon our return for our last year at Columbia, much time was taken to update the 16th edition of Bailey's *Textbook of Histology*, a venerated textbook started in 1904. Dr. Copenhaver, Chairman of the Anatomy Department who was involved in more recent editions, requested our participation. An exciting artistic-related endeavor in the mid-1960s was working with the Director of Photography at the Museum of Modern Art in Manhattan to choose electron micrographs for an exhibit.

To Boston for a Sabbatical: 1968–1969

An opportunity arose for Dick to initiate culture of lobster ganglia with Dr. Edward Kravitz and for me to explore the motile leading tips of lengthening nerve fibers in the laboratories of Drs. Edwin Furshpan and David Potter, all in the Department of Neurobiology in the quadrangle at Harvard Medical School. We moved children and cats to a wonderful town-house on Griggs Park in Brookline. It was an exciting year, in part due to the discussions and frequent seminars at lunchtime when so many of the faculty and trainees convened, often to listen to a visitor. It was a neurobiological feast! Dick grew impatient with the slower development of lobster ganglia compared with those from the mammal, but, nevertheless, he developed the culture system that remains an important part of current research in the Kravitz laboratory (Ganter et al., 1999).

Working with Drs. Furshpan and Potter was a trainee named Dr. Dennis Bray. He had begun novel studies on dissociated sympathetic neurons. Their growth cones were remarkably visible in the culture dish and enticing enough that I began a study of their fine structure. Also, it was our aim to have recorded the recent history (in life and during fixation) of the growth cone that was subjected to electron microscopy. Because the growth cones were flattened on the dish, they were serially thin sectioned in a plane parallel to the dish, not for the faint-hearted because their thickness occupied only a few thin sections at the surface of the dish. The moving parts of the cone, the leading flange and/or filopodia, contained only a filamentous network and occasional membranous structures. Additional organelles, agranular endoplasmic reticulum, vacuoles, vesicles (including dense-cored and coated), mitochondria, microtubules, some neurofilaments, polysomes, and lysosomes, were clustered in the central core of the cone. We were particularly interested in the structural basis for the movement of the growth cone and for the addition of surface membrane. The feltwork of microfilaments (actin) appeared to provide the structure for movement. Dennis had already acquired data to support the idea that the growth cone was the site of surface membrane addition. The plethora of agranular membranous components in the cone and their occasional continuity with the plasma membrane that we observed was consistent with this idea. Our evidence for autophagic vacuole formation in the cone suggested recycling of membrane. A detailed investigation of membrane uptake would be accomplished later.

To St. Louis: Summer of 1970

We received an invitation from Dr. W. Maxwell Cowan to consider faculty positions in the Department of Anatomy (and later, also Neurobiology) at Washington University School of Medicine. He was building an outstanding department that would be among the best in neurobiology in the country. It was a great honor to be asked to join his department, and I will be forever grateful for the exceptional quality of the environment that I greatly valued and benefitted from for the next 19 years. Again, I chose to be a Research Assistant Professor rather than be on the tenure track for reasons given earlier, but was on a full-time schedule. By 1974, I had started to teach and was promoted to Associate Professor with tenure; I became Professor in 1978. We purchased a home in University City, close to the Washington University campus and Forest Park, still preferring to live close to work; the medical center was at the other end of the park.

We were sitting on unpacked boxes, awaiting completion of our new laboratory, when Dr. Patrick M. Wood sauntered in to inquire about job opportunities. An Assistant Professor of Botany, he had been informed that the Botany Department was to be abolished. Fortunately, we said yes to his query, one of the very best decisions that we ever made, because in time he would become one of the most gifted nerve tissue culturists in the world.

The spinal cord, cerebellum, and ganglion culture systems were soon replicated in St. Louis, with laminar flow hoods instead of a designated Columbia-type culture room. Another holdover from Columbia was the Maximow double coverslip assembly, which was too cumbersome and too time-consuming for the feeding regimen and was inadequate to support pieces of tissue large enough for the transplantation work that Dick envisioned. Pat took on the task of modifying the culture chamber. He prepared a mold that could be heated to shape the Aclar coverslip into a bottle cap configuration which could hold more tissue and culture medium. Three of these could simply be placed in a petri dish for long-term culture. One of the first experiments with myelinated sensory ganglion cultures in these Aclar "hats" was conducted with Dr. William Blank, Jr., who found that the Schwann cell-axolemmal junction at the paranode was sensitive to lowered calcium levels in the medium; fluid accumulated between the axon and the myelin sheath due to loss of adhesion of the cytoplasmic loops to the axolemma.

When Dr. Karl Pfenninger came to our laboratory to initiate freeze-fracture studies of axonal growth cones in culture, he introduced the use of fluorodeoxyuridine to create an outgrowth free of non-neuronal cells. This anti-mitotic agent was next used by an M.D./Ph.D. student, Mitchael Estridge, to remove non-neuronal cells from sympathetic and sensory ganglion cultures in order to compare the surface membrane content of those two types of neurons. About that time, James Salzer, in the laboratory for a rotation, treated sensory ganglion cultures with this agent. He could remove Schwann cells temporarily, but they kept coming back (without fibroblasts). When Dick inspected Jim's cultures, he immediately grasped the potential to obtain purified populations of Schwann cells for transplantation. He mentioned this insight in print in 1975. Simply by cutting out the explant, where the neuronal somata were located, the axons quickly degenerated and left only Schwann cells behind. This was the preparative method for Schwann cells for many years. With additional anti-mitotic treatment, the sensory neurons could be rid of Schwann cells. The ability to prepare these purified populations and then add them in different combinations gave us the opportunity to study interactions between neurons, Schwann cells, and fibroblasts *in vitro*. This became a major focus of work in our laboratory.

Pat observed that the purified populations of Schwann cells did not divide after neurons were removed. He then added ganglion neurons (bereft of Schwann cells) to beds of Schwann cells and found that where the outgrowing axons contacted Schwann cells, they started to divide. There was a mitogenic signal from the axon that caused Schwann cells to proliferate. This was the first interaction discovered using the new ganglion culture system and led to a series of experiments to define the signal; this effort was headed by Dick and, as I was not involved, will not be further detailed here.

While these culture systems were being perfected, I continued studying growth cones, again taking advantage of their superior visibility in culture. Rosemary Rees, Dick, and I characterized morphological changes in the pre- and postsynaptic elements during their initial contact and maturation in sympathetic neuron/spinal cord explant cultures. Upon contact, the growth cone filopodia of the cord neuron became extensively applied to the sympathetic neuron plasmalemma, and numerous punctate regions developed in which the membranes were closer together than normal. The Golgi apparatus of the target neuron exhibited increased numbers of coated vesicles, which also were seen in continuity with the close contacts; it appeared that they contributed undercoated postsynaptic membrane, the first definitive sign of synapse formation. Tracer work confirmed that the coated vesicle traffic was from Golgi to surface. Following the appearance of postsynaptic densities, filopodia disappeared, synaptic vesicles gradually accumulated, cleft width and content increased, presynaptic density appeared, and membranous structures and lysosomal structures vanished.

In a solo study I found that protein tracer uptake occurred within minutes, not at the base of the cone, but at the leading edge into a variety of membranous structures, some of which became related to the lysosomal system. More endocytosis occurred at the neurite tip than along the shaft. Vincent Argiro, Dr. Mary Johnson, and I observed that neurites of sympathetic neurons from embryonic, perinatal, and adult rats extended at different rates in culture. We made the novel finding that this resulted from variations in individual growth cone behavior, i.e., differences in growth cone form and pattern of translocation. Growth cones of younger neuronal origin moved at high peak rates of advance and exhibited filopodial and lamellipodial excrescences in contrast to those from adult neurons, which exhbited scant cytoplasm, short filopodia, lack of lamellipodia, and more stationary phases. When the younger cones advanced at their fastest rates, the conformation was predominantly lamellipodial rather than filopodial. Filopodia of growth cones arising from embryonic neurons exhibited higher initial extension rates than did those of postnatal neurons.

Growth cone activity will determine the final geometry of the nerve cell; those that migrate more rapidly and branch with a higher frequency lead to the formation of a larger and more complex geometry. Dr. Dennis Bray, Kevin Chapman, and I (while on sabbatical; see below) found that differences in this neuronal geometry depended upon both extrinsic (the culture substratum) and intrinsic (stage of development of the neuron) factors. Other studies, showing that neurite outgrowth patterns on varying substrata reflect not only differences in neuronal age, but also variation in the behavior of accompanying non-neuronal cells, will not be described here. Dr. March Ard, working with Dick and me, observed in culture that either the Schwann cell surface or the extracellular matrix produced and assembled by Schwann cells (the bands of Bungner) promoted and guided neurite outgrowth from several types of peripheral and CNS neurons.

My major focus, however, was on characterizing the culture requirements for Schwann cell function. One of my favorite experiments was to demonstrate that Schwann cells required contact with matrix in order to differentiate. Dick and I had noticed that when Schwann cells in differentiation-supporting medium did not contact the collagen substratum, but were present on guy-roping fascicles of sensory neurites that extended from the explant to a distance beyond in the outgrowth, they lacked basal lamina and also were abnormally clumped and rounded rather than regularly spaced and aligned on the neurites. We placed small pieces of plastic coated with collagen onto regions of the cellular clumps. Only those Schwann cells that were able to contact this collagen rapidly began to align along the neurites and then to ensheathe and form myelin, a very striking result.

This demonstration of a requirement for connective tissue contact for normal Schwann cell function led us to question whether an extracellular matrix deficiency explained the abnormalities that were observed in nerve roots and peripheral nerves in the dystrophic (*dy*) mouse. The Schwann cells perched on unensheathed axons in the *dy* root were reminiscent of the clumped cells we observed on the suspended fascicles in culture. Working with Dr. Eiko Okada, we were able to mimic in cultures of *dy* sensory ganglion the abnormalities found in *dy* nerves *in situ*: deficient Schwann cell basal lamina, elongated nodes of Ranvier, short myelin internodes, abnormal positioning of the Schwann cell nucleus, and occasional incomplete ensheathment of unmyelinated axons. Co-cultures of *dy* Schwann cells and normal axons showed these abnormalities, whereas normal Schwann cells combined with *dy* axons did not. When fibroblasts were omitted from the cultures, the Schwann cell basal lamina defect was more pronounced than when they were present. Also, when fibroblasts from a normal mouse were added to *dy* neuron and Schwann cell cultures, the basal lamina and ensheathment defects were corrected. We speculated that fibroblasts had contributed matrix because more matrix was in evidence in the corrected cultures. We concluded that an abnormality of contact between Schwann cells and a matrix component could underlie the abnormal Schwann cell behavior in the *dy* mouse nerve.

The possibility that fibroblasts and extracellular matrix components promote Schwann cell differentiation was further investigated in later experiments conducted by a graduate student, Valerie Obremski, working with Dr. Mary Johnson, Pat, and myself. It was learned from work done by Dr. Dikla Roufa in our laboratory that when Schwann cells were cultured with *sympathetic* neurons (without fibroblasts), and in medium that promoted differentiation of Schwann cells associated with *sensory* neurons, ensheathment and basal lamina and collagen assembly were all deficient. Valerie found that adding fibroblasts to the sympathetic neuron/Schwann cell cultures corrected these deficiencies. The addition of purified basal lamina components (laminin, Type IV collagen, and heparan sulfate proteoglycan) partially mimicked the effect of adding fibroblasts. We speculated that superior cervical ganglion neurons were unable to stimulate full Schwann cell extracellular matrix expression and that this led to a basal lamina deficiency which prevents ensheathment from occurring. It will be mentioned later that Schwann cells require neurons to generate basal lamina. Valerie discovered that Schwann cells organized basal lamina in the presence of fibroblasts or in fibroblast-conditioned medium without neurons. Even without neurons, the generation of matrix led to dramatic changes in Schwann cell morphology: the cells elongated and aligned with each other.

The availability of purified populations of sensory neurons and Schwann cells lacking fibroblasts provided an opportunity to determine the endoneurial and perineurial constituents that are contributed by Schwann cells. Axons of neurons cultured alone were unensheathed and devoid of basal lamina and extracellular banded collagen fibrils. When Schwann cells were added to cultures of neurons, Type IV collagen-containing basal lamina and fibrils were formed. Two matrix experts, Drs. J. Uitto and J. Jeffrey in the Division of Dermatology, aided Pat Wood, Ann Williams, and me in also detecting Types I, III, and A-B collagens in the cultures. That Schwann cells produced this variety of matrix components had not been hitherto recognized. When fibroblasts were added to neuron/Schwann cell cultures, the collagen fibrils were larger in diameter, and typical perineurium formed. We laid to rest a long-standing question: Is perineurium formed from Schwann cells or fibroblasts? With the help of Dr. Joshua Sanes in our department, we infected Schwann cells or fibroblasts with a retrovirus carrying the gene for β-galactosidase. We discovered that the perineurium formed in culture expressed this enzyme when fibroblasts were lac-Z positive, but not when Schwann cells were lac-Z positive. Pat, Ann, and I found that neurons were required for the generation of basal lamina (but not its persistence) on the Schwann cell. Further work with Dr. M. Blair Clark revealed that substantial contact between axon and Schwann cell was necessary for the assembly of normal-appearing basal lamina; neither released diffusible neuronal factors nor products released from adjacent basal lamina-assembling Schwann cells were sufficient. The outstanding quality of electron micrographs of these and other cultures was due, in large part, to Ann Williams and later to Margaret Bates, both long-term assistants in our laboratory.

The finding by Dr. Fernando Moya working with Dick and me that a defined medium (N2) supported Schwann cell proliferation but not differentiation enabled us to further explore Schwann cell–neuron interactions, specifically ensheathment and myelination. In N2 medium only, Schwann cells neither ensheathed and myelinated axons nor formed basal lamina and collagen fibrils, even after many weeks in culture. When serum and embryo extract were added to N2, however, within a few days ensheathment, myelination, and basal lamina and collagen formation were evident. This contrast was particularly striking in electron micrographs; in N2, the Schwann cell processes were long and meandering and only adjacent to axons rather than in an encircling mode. Charles Eldridge, a Ph.D. candidate, determined that when embryo extract was eliminated from serum-containing culture medium, Schwann cell differentiation was arrested; the substitution of ascorbic acid was sufficient to promote myelination and basal lamina assembly. Further work demonstrated that in a number of culture conditions it was the level of ascorbic acid in the medium that was critical for myelination and that myelination and Schwann cell basal lamina assembly were paired. Our thinking was that the ascorbic acid in embryo extract was required for Type IV collagen assembly, which is an important component of basal lamina formation, and that this assembly was required for myelination and ensheathment to proceed. The hypothesis that this assembly was required was supported by finding that provision of exogenous basal lamina matrix to cultures grown in defined medium without ascorbic acid promoted these Schwann cell functions. In this way (in part), we discovered that acquisition of basal lamina (or binding to laminin receptors) was a critical prefatory step for Schwann cell differentiation. We developed the concept that Schwann cell surface molecules required polarization (as in epithelia) prior to undergoing the shape changes involved in ensheathment and myelination. The importance of the collagen substratum as well has been noted earlier.

Our laboratory in St. Louis had been not only a productive, but also a happy place. Dick and I were guided by the golden rule: treat others as we would want to be treated. We also allowed ourselves to be "vulnerable" in the sense that we welcomed criticism and would act on it. In the early years in St. Louis, when the group was smaller, all birthdays were celebrated in the laboratory at a sit-down lunch with candles, tablecloth, casserole, and salad brought from home and a birthday cake. A weekly tea, at which the focus was on the goodies brought by everyone to accompany the tea, enabled all to be informed of latest developments, be they scientific advances or personal milestones. Telling jokes was as important as the pastries, and Dick liked nothing better than to embellish them for greatest impact. The laboratory had a "family" feel. Many of our trainees reflected happily on this atmosphere and carried it with them to their new destinations. A glass sculpture by Dale Chihuly, commissioned by me to remember a graduate student, remains in the foyer of the medical school.

To London for a Sabbatical: 1984

We chose to spend nearly half a year in Dr. Dennis Bray's laboratory in the MRC Cell Biophysics Unit, King's College, on Drury Lane in London. A site of historical significance, the seminar room still held some of Wilkin's DNA models. We had always admired Dennis's ability to devise simple and direct experiments to answer basic questions about axonal growth. He had worked in our laboratory in 1978–1979 when he did seminal, often cited work on the avoidance of retinal and sympathetic fibers when they confronted one another in culture and other work on the sorting out of nerve fibers to form fascicles that contained only one type of fiber. He was a conscientious host and a valued discussant. The sabbatical was a time not only of scientific gain, but also of cultural enrichment, because the laboratory was ensconced in the heart of the Covent Garden district. Influences on the formation of outgrowth from a single neuron were studied, as described above. Here we started one of my favorite experiments as well.

We pursued a project to better understand the mechanism by which peripheral myelin is formed. Because it had been known for many years that the Schwann cell nucleus shifted during this process, we asked if following this movement and then coordinating it with the orientation of the Schwann

cell membranes (as detected electron microscopically) could contribute useful insight into the mechanism. In particularly thin areas of dorsal root
ganglion neurites and Schwann cells in culture, we could identify potential
sites of myelination because both the region of the axon and the relating and
elongating Schwann cell tellingly increased in size. Dick and I took turns,
every 4 hr, to map the position of the Schwann cell nucleus as myelination
began and proceeded for one to three days. We spurned time lapse photography because we had to be there to focus the microscope to determine
the exact position of the nucleus. Our histories of nuclear circumnavigation
and carefully preserved and mapped cultures returned with us to St. Louis,
where the samples were put into the hands of Margaret Bates, our electron
microscopy assistant who possessed a special talent for finding a specific area
in a culture and preparing it successfully for electron microscopic scrutiny.
It was critical that, through all the preparation stages, the same orientation
be maintained. We found eight consistent cases in which the direction of
nuclear circumnavigation corresponded to that for the inner, not the outer,
lip of Schwann cell cytoplasm, suggesting that myelin was laid down by progression of the innermost leading edge of the Schwann cell around the axon.
Consistent with this finding was that the observation of basal lamina and
macular adhering junctions on the outer lip of cytoplasm implied anchorage
rather than movement.

To Miami: Summer of 1989

As superior as the Washington University milieu was, we nonetheless
decided to take new faculty positions in The Miami Project to Cure Paralysis
at the University of Miami School of Medicine. Dick was selected to be Scientific Director. With his medical education, extensive knowledge of gross
anatomy as well as cell biology, breadth of understanding, and now a new
and total commitment to spinal cord injury, this was an inspired decision.
Whereas Dick had envisioned transplantation of tissue, particularly purified populations of Schwann cells, into injured spinal cord for over 20 years
and had actually performed a number of transplantation studies, we saw
this as a chance to tackle spinal cord repair anew. A part of the vision was
the promise of using Schwann cells from a piece of peripheral nerve from
a spinal cord-injured person for autologous transplantation. (To generate
large numbers of human Schwann cells in culture was a goal sought and
accomplished by Dick and his collaborators in Miami.) Schwann cells could
also provide myelin for demyelinated or regenerated fibers. Going to Miami
provided an opportunity to bring to the challenge of spinal cord repair our
cumulative knowledge of the biology of the cell of Schwann, Dick's preferred
terminology.

From work with Dr. Carlos Paino, we knew that axons would grow into
a Schwann cell graft placed in lesioned spinal cord. Cultures of Schwann

cells in association with neurites were prepared to create bands of Bungner upon neurite demise by removal of neuronal somata. Transplants were prepared by loosening the supporting collagen substratum from the dish and rolling it and the bands of Bungner (or dissociated Schwann cells) into a jelly roll configuration. Twenty-eight days after positioning the transplant in a photochemically induced lesion, abundant axonal growth was observed within the roll of surviving collagen. After moving to Miami, I initiated a detailed characterization of the photochemically induced lesion up to a year and a half after induction, employing the 1 μm thick plastic sections of tissue prepared for electron microscopy for superior light microscopic histology. Despite this study and the promise of the rolled Schwann cell/collagen implants, we decided to develop a new complete transection/Schwann cell bridge model to obtain unambiguous results; complete transection would eliminate the complication of spared and sprouted fibers and enable detection of regenerated fibers with certainty. Dick termed these implants "the bridges of Dade County."

It was fortunate that a new postdoctoral fellow, Dr. Xiao Ming Xu, came to our laboratory, for it was he who was most responsible for developing this new model. Also, Dr. Veronique Guénard, with us at the time, had gained experience in using the polymer tubes when she was a Ph.D. student with Dr. Patrick Aebischer. Dr. Naomi Kleitman, in our St. Louis laboratory as a Fellow starting in 1985 and then in The Miami Project as faculty, was an important contributor to initial and subsequent bridging studies. Help from Anna Gomez was key in beginning to generate the very large numbers of rat Schwann cells that we needed for transplantation, six million per bridge. By placing a cable of Schwann cells inside a polymer (polyacrylonitrile/polyvinylchloride) channel and then inserting stumps of the transected cord into the channel, nerve fibers were coaxed to regenerate into the cable from both stumps. Careful tracing revealed that the fibers, originating from spinal cord and sensory ganglion neurons, did not exit the grafts in this complete transection paradigm. This was probably due, at least in part, to the presence of proteoglycans at the Schwann cell/host spinal cord interface. Dr. Giles Plant, a Fellow in our laboratory, was to observe their presence later in a detailed immunostaining study.

Because of the eventual possibility of autotransplantation, we desired to determine if human Schwann cells derived from adult tissue and generated in culture would support axonal regeneration as did the rat Schwann cells. Dr. James Guest, working toward a Ph.D. in our laboratory in the middle of a neurosurgery residency in Vancouver, transplanted human Schwann cell bridges into the transected spinal cord of the adult nude rat. The human cells were found to be as effective as the rat cells. Dr. Martin Oudega, a former Fellow in our laboratory and later a collaborating faculty member, began to explore another polymer, polylactic/polyglycolic acid, as a substitute for the channels we usually used. Also, Dr. Xu began to develop a lateral hemi-section/Schwann cell/hemi-channel transplantation paradigm before leaving our laboratory. In this case, some regenerated axons exited the hemi-bridge, possibly because the spinal cord was more stable than in the complete transection model.

Studies of Schwann cell biology in cultures of purified sensory neurons had not been abandoned. Dr. Cristina Fernandez-Valle, a Fellow in our laboratory, made numerous observations. In her first investigation, she demonstrated that the addition of ascorbate, which promotes basal lamina assembly, induced expression of the protein zero gene that encodes the major structural protein of myelin. Expression of protein zero mRNA and protein occurred only in the subset of Schwann cells contacting myelin-inducing axons; Schwann cells in contact with axons that did not induce myelin did not express protein zero mRNA, although they generated basal lamina components. Because the ascorbate requirement could be bypassed by adding a purified basal lamina component, laminin, she next explored receptors for laminin, the β1 subfamily of integrins. Undifferentiated Schwann cells were observed to express large amounts of α1β1 and α1β6, whereas, when myelinating, the predominant integrin was α6β4. Function-blocking antibody to β1 inhibited attachment to laminin, and myelin formation and basal lamina assembly were deficient. This work showed that a β1 integrin bound the laminin present in the basal lamina to the Schwann cell surface and transduced signals critical for differentiation into a myelinating cell. In a third study, actin polymerization disruption was found to inhibit myelin formation and to prevent expression of mRNA encoding the myelin-specific proteins, cyclic nucleotide phosphodiesterase, myelin associated glycoprotein, and protein zero. F-actin, therefore, influenced myelin-specific gene expression in Schwann cells. The combination of purified populations of sensory neurons and Schwann cells without macrophages enabled us to address the long-standing question of the participation of Schwann cells in myelin degradation and their ability to proliferate in Wallerian degeneration. Cristina demonstrated that rat Schwann cells were capable of both substantial myelin degradation and proliferation without the assistance of macrophages.

Studies of Schwann cell bridges continued, but in combination with additional strategies. Clearly, a thoracically positioned Schwann cell bridge was an encouraging start, but the complete transection paradigm was inadequate to promote growth of regenerated fibers off the bridge or to promote regeneration of fibers from brain stem neurons. Drs. Aqing Chen and Xu tested the addition of the corticoid methylprednisolone to the bridge paradigm because this compound was in routine use after human spinal cord injury to curb secondary damage. We found that the cord stump tissue placed into the polymer channel did not break down, the interface between bridge and cord exhibited far less scar tissue, two times as many cord neurons extended axons into the bridge, three times more myelinated axons were in the bridge, fibers from brain stem neurons grew into the bridge as well, and a modest number of regenerated fibers exited the bridge when methylprednisolone treatment was combined with bridging. The combination strategy was, thus, a substantial improvement. Because methylprednisolone has numerous effects, it is not possible to know how it acted to improve outcome in our paradigm. In a separate strategy, Dr. Martin Oudega observed that when methylprednisolone was administered at the time of transection (without a bridge in this case), at a number of time points up to eight weeks, the number of microglia/macrophages was substantially diminished in both stumps, tissue loss was lessened, and dieback of vestibulospinal fibers was reduced.

Neurotrophin administration was combined with Schwann cell bridging. Dr. Xu delivered brain-derived neurotrophic factor (BDNF) and neurotrophin-3 (NT-3) for 14 days into the channel around the Schwann cell cable and found, after an additional 14 days, that the number of myelinated axons in the bridge and the number of cord neurons growing axons into the bridge were significantly increased. Importantly, brain stem neurons responded by extending axons into the bridge, even though the bridge was far from the brain stem. Thus, regeneration of some neuronal populations distant from the injury and the transplant could be elicited by combining trophic factors with a favorable substrate. In another study, Drs. Philippe Menei and Claudia Montero-Menei came from France to initiate an investigation to transplant Schwann cells infected with a retroviral vector carrying the human gene for BDNF/cDNA. Dr. Scott Whittemore, a faculty member in The Miami Project, added his molecular expertise to the project. The Schwann cells were deposited in a 5-mm-long trail extending into the distal cord stump from the complete transection site and also injected into the transection site itself. The trails were largely intact for the month-long experiment. In a comparison of engineered versus untreated Schwann cells, more fibers from brain stem neurons were present in the trail. When no Schwann cells were transplanted, no such fibers were found beyond the transection site. Thus, the increased levels of BDNF improved the regenerative response across the transection and into the thoracic spinal cord. More recently, Dr. Bas Blits from Dr. Jost Verhaagen's laboratory and Dr. Oudega injected adeno-associated viral vectors encoding for BDNF and NT-3 directly into the cord beyond the Schwann cell bridge to transduce the cells in that area. Transgene expression was observed predominantly in neurons for at least 16 weeks. A modest but significant improvement in hindlimb function was observed, and twice as many lumbar neurons extended processes toward the thoracically positioned Schwann cell bridge with vector injection. The lack of evidence for improved growth of regenerated axons from the bridge into the cord was possibly related to inadequate diffusion of the neurotrophins to the region next to the bridge.

Another combination strategy was to inject olfactory ensheathing glia into the stumps beside a Schwann cell bridge. Earlier reports suggested their efficacy. Also, they are positioned *in situ* to escort growing fibers from the periphery into the CNS. We reasoned that these glia might promote the exit of fibers from the bridge. This they did; regenerating fibers left the graft in contrast to lack of such growth with the Schwann cell bridge alone. There was also evidence for the long-distance axonal regeneration (at least 2.5 cm) of ascending fibers that crossed both interfaces. Fibers from a brain stem nucleus, the raphe, were able to reach the distal stump and extend at least 1.5 cm into it. With the prospect of continuing olfactory ensheathing glia transplantation, Drs. Henglin Yan and Plant tested a number of mitogens in culture to find a more effective means of obtaining sufficient numbers from adult rat olfactory bulbs. Combinations of factors, such as heregulin plus fibroblast growth factor-2, were more effective than each factor tested alone in stimulating the glia to divide; forskolin potentiated their activity. In considering Schwann cell versus olfactory ensheathing glia transplantation, one important issue is the development of myelin for the newly regenerated fibers. In a number of studies by others, transplantation of the olfactory glia has appeared to lead to myelination of regenerated or demyelinated fibers. We performed a very carefully controlled study to eliminate contaminating Schwann cells from sensory neuron-ensheathing glia cultures. Under culture conditions that enabled Schwann cells to form myelin around sensory neurites, ensheathing glia did not. Also, in electron micrographs, the typical ensheathing pattern of Schwann cells was not seen in the olfactory glia-sensory neuron cultures; the olfactory glial processes only meandered through fascicles. The cells we employed, immunopanned from adult rat olfactory bulbs, may not be as plastic as those from younger animals. More work needs to be done.

Recently, we have initiated studies of transplantation into contusion injuries, due to their clinical relevance. Drs. Giles Plant and Oudega determined that transplantation of olfactory glia was preferable (based on tissue sparing and hindlimb performance) in medium rather than in fibrin and at seven days rather than at the time of injury. Drs. Toshihiro Takami and Oudega then compared transplantation of olfactory ensheathing glia with Schwann cells into contused spinal cord; some animals received both cell types. Significantly more tissue was spared in all grafted animals. All three types of grafts contained axons, but Schwann cell grafts contained the highest number. Significantly higher numbers of propriospinal and brain stem axons extended 5–6 mm beyond the Schwann cell or Schwann cell/olfactory glia graft than the olfactory glia graft. A modest but statistically significant improvement in hindlimb locomotor performance in the Schwann cell-transplanted animals was detected by two months. Thus, in this first comparison, a Schwann cell graft appeared more effective than the others, but more remains to be learned about olfactory glia survival in the moderately contused adult rat thoracic spinal cord.

I am committed to continue investigating strategies in combination with Schwann cell bridges, not only to improve the regenerative capability of the injured spinal cord, but also to devise neuroprotective interventions to lessen secondary tissue loss. New findings in our laboratory make this even more compelling than before. Dr. Giselda Casella, a Ph.D. candidate working with Pat and me, found that even though blood vessels were destroyed in the contusion lesion epicenter by two days, at seven days new vessels had appeared to form a seemingly continuous cordon through the lesion. By 14 days, however, the number of vessels had decreased. If this demise of the new vascular bridge could be prevented, the bridge could serve as an early scaffold to hasten axonal regeneration across the injury site. A study by Drs. Takami and Oudega combined methylprednisolone and interleukin-10 (IL-10) as a potentially more effective strategy than the use of either one alone; even with the combination, gray but not white matter damage was reduced and hindlimb locomotion was not improved. We are currently testing two new neuroprotective strategies: the administration of substances to modify the inflammatory response and provision of anti-sense oligonucleotides to interfere with the production of tumor necrosis factor-α following injury. These may be more effective than methylprednisolone and IL-10 as neuroprotective agents.

Other current projects continue to test regeneration strategies and to ask what combination of strategies will lead to successful treatment of spinal cord injury. We are testing, for example, the application of chondroitinase to the Schwann cell bridge–host spinal cord interface to interfere with the accumulation of proteoglycan molecules that may inhibit, at least in part, the exit of regenerated fibers from the bridge. A multifaceted approach will be key. Possibilities for a combination strategy could include neuroprotection, bridging with genetically altered cells that secrete appropriate neurotrophic factors, treatment to overcome inhibitory molecules, and training/rehabilitation. The development of appropriate biomaterials and application of new knowledge about guidance molecules are on the horizon. I think that I shall be as busy and as challenged in the next few years as I have been in the past. I love it! It has been a great and rewarding trip, but it is not quite over yet.

Acknowledgments

This chapter is dedicated to Richard P. Bunge, M.D. (Fig. 1). Not only my husband, best friend, and collaborator for 40 years, he served as my most valued mentor for all that time. I believe that I also mentored him. We completed each other. Among Dick's most impressive traits were his generosity of spirit and the ability to think broadly; to synthesize information from varying disciplines; to envision many novel testable ideas; and to make

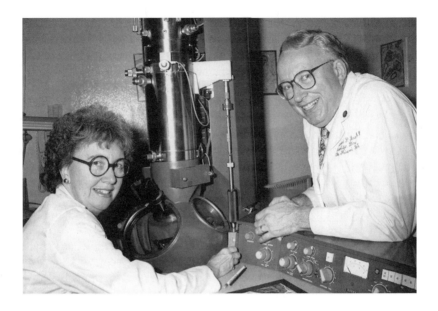

Fig. 1. Mary Bartlett Bunge and Richard P. Bunge.

cogent, insightful, and witty comments in public places. He could wander into the culture room, take a glance at a culture, and make an observation, missed by others, that might spawn a new project. The work reviewed herein includes projects in which we collaborated; to also review his manifold discoveries in which I was not involved is beyond the scope of this effort. Some information is available elsewhere (Salzer and Colman, 1996; Zu Rhein and Duncan, 1997; Vikhanski, 2001). A glass sculpture by Jon Kuhn, commissioned by me to honor Dick, now resides in our new building.

I also dedicate this chapter to sons Jonathan and Peter, two highly exceptional persons. They have enriched and broadened my life experience immeasurably and have taught me much that I otherwise would not have learned. Their support in recent years has been most caring and generous and is greatly appreciated.

Enormous gratitude is due Patrick M. Wood, by far our most important collaborator. Dick and I were honored to be associated with such a clear and logical thinker, gifted experimentalist, and keen observer. In Miami, Dr. Naomi Kleitman added important strengths to our team due to her prowess in culturing Schwann cells, planning experiments, and critically evaluating (including statistically) experimental data.

To all the talented students and fellows and loyal assistants who cast their lot in the Bunge/Wood laboratory, a most appreciative thank you!

Since Dick died of esophageal cancer in 1996, I have greatly appreciated and benefitted from being in the company of outstanding scientists as a member of the Christopher Reeve Paralysis Foundation Research Consortium.

The NINDS deserves loud accolades for continued funding of our work, starting with my postdoctoral fellowship in 1960. When we assumed positions at the Washington University School of Medicine in 1970, we applied for a grant which continues to the present; throughout its course, our work has received three Javits Neuroscience Investigator awards, most recently from 1998 to 2005. Program Project grants from NINDS have been key to certain projects. The National Multiple Sclerosis Society was very generous in their long-term support. From 1989 on, the generosity of The Miami Project and Buoniconti Fund, and the Christopher Reeve Paralysis, Hollfelder and Heumann Foundations is most gratefully acknowledged.

Provision of information about Dr. Margaret R. Murray from Dr. Betty G. Uzman is hereby gratefully acknowledged.

Selected Bibliography

Ard MD, Bunge RP, Bunge MB. A comparison of the Schwann cell surface and Schwann cell extracellular matrix as promoters of neurite growth. *J Neurocytol* 1987;16:539–555.

Argiro V, Bunge MB, Johnson MI. Correlation between growth cone form and movement and their dependence on neuronal age. *J Neurosci* 1984;4:3051–3062.

Argiro V, Bunge MB, Johnson MI. A quantitative study of growth cone filopodial extension. *J Neurosci Res* 1985;13:149–162.

Blank WF Jr, Bunge MB, Bunge RP. The sensitivity of the myelin sheath, particularly the Schwann cell-axolemmal junction, to lowered calcium levels in cultured sensory ganglia. *Brain Res* 1974;67:503–518.

Blits B, Oudega M, Boer GJ, Bunge MB, Verhaagen J. Adeno-associated viral vector-mediated neurotrophin gene transfer in the injured adult rat spinal cord improves hindlimb function. *Neuroscience* 2003;118:271–281.

Bray D, Bunge MB. The growth cone in neurite extension. In *Locomotion of tissue cells*, CIBA Foundation Symposium 14. New York: Associated Scientific Publishers, 1973;195–209.

Bray D, Bunge MB, Chapman K. Geometry of isolated sensory neurons in culture: Effects of embryonic age and culture substratum. *Exp Cell Res* 1987;168:127–137.

Bray D, Wood P, Bunge RP. Selective fasiciculation of nerve fibres in culture. *Exp Cell Res* 1980;130:241–250.

Brosnan CF, Bunge MB, Murray MR. The response of lysosomes in cultured neurons to chlorpromazine. *J Neuropathol Exp Neurol* 1970;29:337–353.

Bunge MB. Fine structure of nerve fibers and growth cones of isolated sympathetic neurons in culture. *J Cell Biol* 1973;56:713–735.

Bunge MB. Initial endocytosis of peroxidase or ferritin by growth cones of cultured nerve cells. *J Neurocytol* 1977;6:407–439.

Bunge MB. The axonal cytoskeleton: Its role in generating and maintaining cell form. *TINS* 1986;9:477–482. (Invited review for special issue.)

Bunge MB. Bridging areas of injury in the spinal cord. *Neuroscientist* 2001;7:325–339.

Bunge MB, Bunge RP, Pappas GD. Electron microscopic demonstration of connections between glia and myelin sheaths in the developing mammalian central nervous system. *J Cell Biol* 1962;12:448–453.

Bunge MB, Bunge RP, Peterson ER. The onset of synapse formation in spinal cord cultures as studied by electron microscopy. *Brain Res* 1967;6:728–749.

Bunge MB, Bunge RP, Peterson ER, Murray MR. A light and electron microscope study of long-term organized cultures of rat dorsal root ganglia. *J Cell Biol* 1967;32:439–446.

Bunge MB, Bunge RP, Ris H. Ultrastructural study of remyelination in an experimental lesion in adult cat spinal cord. *J Biophys Biochem Cytol* 1961;10:67–94.

Bunge MB, Clark MB, Dean AC, Eldridge CF, Bunge RP. Schwann cell function depends upon axonal signals and basal lamina components. *Ann NY Acad Sci* 1990;580:281–287. (Invited paper.)

Bunge MB, Holets VR, Bates ML, Clarke TS, Watson BD. Characterization of photochemically induced spinal cord injury in the rat by light and electron microscopy. *Exp Neurol* 1994;127:76–93.

Bunge MB, Johnson MI, Ard MD, Kleitman N. Factors influencing the growth of regenerating nerve fibers in culture. In Seil FJ, Herbert E, Carlson BM, eds. Amsterdam/New York: Elsevier, *Progress in brain research.* 1987;71: 61–74.

Bunge MB, Schilling RF. Intrinsic factor studies. VI. Competition for the vit. B_{12} binding sites offered by analogues of the vitamin. *Proc Soc Exp Biol Med* 1956;96:587–592.

Bunge MB, Schloesser LL, Schilling RF. Intrinsic factor studies. IV. Selective absorption and binding of cyanocobalamin by gastric juice in the presence of excess pseudovitamin B_{12} or 5-6-dimethylbenzamidazole. *J Lab Clin Med* 1957;48:735–744.

Bunge MB, Williams AK, Wood PM. Neuron-Schwann cell interaction in basal lamina formation. *Dev Biol* 1982;92:449–460.

Bunge MB, Williams AK, Wood PM, Uitto J, Jeffrey JJ. Comparison of nerve cell and nerve cell plus Schwann cell cultures, with particular emphasis on basal lamina and collagen formation. *J Cell Biol* 1980;84:184–202.

Bunge MB, Wood PM, Tynan LB, Bates ML, Sanes JR. Perineurium originates from fibroblasts: Demonstration *in vitro* with a retroviral marker. *Science* 1989;243:229–231.

Bunge RP, Bunge MB. Evidence that contact with connective tissue matrix is required for normal interaction between Schwann cells and nerve fibers. *J Cell Biol* 1978;78:943–950. "Rapid Communication."

Bunge RP, Bunge MB. Cues and constraints in Schwann cell development. In *Studies in developmental neurobiology*. Cowan WM, ed. New York: Oxford University Press, 1981;322–353.

Bunge RP, Bunge MB. Interrelationship between Schwann cell function and extracellular matrix production. *TINS* 1983;6:499–505.

Bunge RP, Bunge MB, Bates M. Movements of the Schwann cell nucleus implicate progression of the inner (axon-related) Schwann cell process during myelination. *J Cell Biol* 1989;109:273–284.

Bunge RP, Bunge MB, Eldridge CF. Linkage between axonal ensheathment and basal lamina production by Schwann cells. *Annu Rev Neurosci* 1986;9:305–328.

Bunge RP, Bunge MB, Peterson ER. An electron microscope study of cultured rat spinal cord. *J Cell Biol* 1965;24:161–191.

Bunge RP, Bunge MB, Ris H. Electron microscopic study of demyelination in an experimentally induced lesion in adult cat spinal cord. *J Biophys Biochem Cytol* 1960;7:685–696.

Bunge RP, Bunge MB, Ris H. Electron microscopic observations on normal, demyelinating, and remyelinating white matter. In Jacob H, ed. *Proc. IV International Congress of Neuropathology*, Sept. 1 4–8, 1961, Munich, Vol. II. Stuttgart, Germany: George Thieme Verlag, 1962;136–142.

Bunge RP, Bunge MB, Williams AK, Wartels LK. Does the dystrophic mouse nerve lesion result from an extracellular matrix abnormality? In Schotland D, ed. *Disorders of the motor unit*. New York: Wiley, 1982;23–34.

Bunge RP, Settlage PH. Neurological lesions in cats following cerebrospinal fluid manipulation. *J Neuropathol Exp Neurol* 1957;16:471–491.

Casella GT, Marcillo A, Bunge MB, Wood PM. New vascular tissue rapidly replaces neural parenchyma and vessels destroyed by a contusion injury to the rat spinal cord. *Exp Neurol* 2002;173:63–76.

Chen A, Xu XM, Kleitman N, Bunge MB. Methylprednisolone administration improves axonal regeneration into Schwann cell grafts in transected adult rat thoracic spinal cord. *Exp Neurol* 1996;138:261–276.

Clark MB, Bunge MB. Cultured Schwann cells assemble normal-appearing basal lamina only when they ensheathe axons. *Dev Biol* 1989;133:393–404.

Copenhaver WM, Bunge RP, Bunge MB. *Bailey's Textbook of Histology*, 16th edition. Baltimore, Md: Williams & Wilkins, 1971.

Eldridge CF, Bunge RP, Bunge MB. Effects of cis-4-hydroxy-L-proline, an inhibitor of Schwann cell differentiation, on the secretion of collagenous and non-collagenous proteins by Schwann cells. *Exp Cell Res* 1988;174:491–501.

Eldridge CF, Bunge MB, Bunge RP. Differentiation of axon-related Schwann cells *in vitro*: II. Control of myelin formation by basal lamina. *J Neurosci* 1989;9:625–638.

Eldridge CF, Bunge MB, Bunge RP, Wood PM. Differentiation of axon-related Schwann cells *in vitro*. I. Ascorbic acid regulates basal lamina assembly and myelin formation. *J Cell Biol* 1987;105:1023–1034.

Fernandez-Valle C, Bunge RP, Bunge MB. Schwann cells degrade myelin and proliferate in the absence of macrophages: evidence from *in vitro* studies of Wallerian degeneration. *J Neurocytol* 1995;24:667–679.

Fernandez-Valle C, Fregien N, Wood PM, Bunge MB. Expression of the protein zero myelin gene in axon-related Schwann cells is linked to basal lamina formation. *Development* 1993;119:867–880.

Fernandez-Valle C, Gorman D, Gomez AM, Bunge MB. Actin plays a role in both changes in cell shape and gene expression associated with Schwann cell myelination. *J Neurosc* 1997;17:241–250.

Fernandez-Valle C, Gwynn L, Wood P, Carbonetto S, Bunge MB. Anti-β1 integrin antibody inhibits Schwann cell myelination. *J Neurobiol* 1994;25:1207–1226.

Fernandez-Valle C, Wood PM, Bunge MB. Localization of focal adhesion kinase in differentiating Schwann cell/neuron cultures. In Martini R, ed. Microsc Res Tech Special issue: *Myelin formation and maintenance*. New York: Wiley-Liss, 1998;41:416–430 (original data).

Ganter GK, Heinrich R, Bunge RP, Kravitz EA. Long-term culture of lobster central ganglia: Expression of foreign genes in identified neurons. *Biol Bull* 1999;197:40–48.

Guénard V, Xu XM, Bunge MB. The use of Schwann cell transplantation to foster central nervous system repair. *Sem Neurosci* 1993;5:401–411.

Guest JD, Hesse D, Schnell L, Schwab ME, Bunge MB, Bunge RP. The influence of IN-1 antibody and acidic FGF-fibrin glue on the response of injured corticospinal tract axons to human Schwann cell grafts. *J Neurosci Res* 1997;50:888–905.

Guest JD, Rao A, Bunge MB, Bunge RP. The ability of human Schwann cell grafts to promote regeneration in the transected nude rat spinal cord. *Exp Neurol* 1997;48:502–522.

Kleitman N, Bunge MB. Olfactory ensheathing glia: Their application to spinal cord regeneration and remyelination strategies. *Topics Spinal Cord Inj Rehab* 2000;6:65–81.

Masurovsky EB, Bunge MB, Bunge RP. Cytological studies of organotypic cultures of rat dorsal root ganglia following X-irradiation *in vitro*. I. Changes in neurons and satellite cells. *J Cell Biol* 1967a;32:467–496.

Masurovsky EB, Bunge MB, Bunge RP. Cytological studies of organotypic cultures of rat dorsal root ganglia following X-irradiation *in vitro*. II. Changes in Schwann cells, myelin sheaths, and nerve fibers. *J Cell Biol* 1967b;32:497–518.

McDonald JW and the Research Consortium of the Christopher Reeve Paralysis Foundation. Repairing the damaged spinal cord. *Sci Am* 1999;281:64–73.

Menei P, Montero-Menei C, Whittemore SR, Bunge RP, Bunge MB. Schwann cells genetically modified to secrete human BDNF promote enhanced axonal regrowth across transected adult rat spinal cord. *Eur J Neurosci* 1998;10:607–621.

Moya F, Bunge MB, Bunge RP. Schwann cells proliferate but fail to differentiate in defined medium. *Proc Natl Acad Sci USA* 1980;77:6902–6906.

Obremski VJ, Bunge MB. Addition of purified basal lamina molecules enables Schwann cell ensheathment of sympathetic neurites in culture. *Dev Biol* 1995;168:124–137.

Obremski VJ, Johnson MI, Bunge MB. Fibroblasts are required for Schwann cell basal lamina deposition and ensheathment of unmyelinated sympathetic neurites in culture. *J Neurocytol* 1993;22:102–117.

Obremski VJ, Wood PM, Bunge MB. Fibroblasts promote Schwann cell basal lamina deposition in the absence of neurons in culture. *Dev Biol* 1993;26:119–134.

Okada E, Bunge RP, Bunge MB. Abnormalities expressed in long term cultures of dorsal root ganglia from the dystrophic mouse. *Brain Res* 1980;194:455–470.

Oudega M, Gautier SE, Chapon P, Fragoso M, Bates ML, Parel J-M, Bunge MB. Axonal regeneration into Schwann cell grafts within resorbable poly(α-hydroxyacid) guidance channels in the adult rat spinal cord. *Biomaterials* 2001;22:1125–1136.

Oudega M, Vargas CG, Weber AB, Kleitman N, Bunge MB. Long-term effects of methylprednisolone following transection of adult rat spinal cord. *Eur J Neurosci* 1999;11:2453–2464.

Oudega M, Xu XM, Guénard V, Kleitman N, Bunge MB. A combination of insulin-like growth factor-I and platelet-derived growth factor enhances myelination but diminishes axonal regeneration into Schwann cell grafts in the adult rat spinal cord. *Glia* 1997;19:247–258.

Paino CL, Fernandez-Valle C, Bates ML, Bunge MB. Regrowth of axons in lesioned adult rat spinal cord: Promotion by implants of cultured Schwann cells. *J Neurocytol* 1994;23:433–452.

Plant GW, Bates ML, Bunge MB. Inhibitory proteoglycan immunoreactivity is higher at the caudal than the rostral Schwann cell graft-transected spinal cord interface. *Mol Cell Neurosci* 2001;17:471–487.

Plant GW, Christensen CL, Oudega M, Bunge MB. Delayed transplantation of olfactory ensheathing glia promotes sparing/regeneration of supraspinal axons in the contused adult rat spinal cord. *J Neurotrauma* 2003;20:1–16.

Plant GW, Currier PF, Cuervo EP, Bates ML, Pressman Y, Bunge MB, Wood PM. Purified adult ensheathing glia fail to myelinate axons under culture conditions that enable Schwann cells to form myelin. *J Neurosci* 2002;22: 6083–6091.

Plant GW, Ramón-Cueto A, Bunge MB. Transplantation of Schwann cells and ensheathing glia to improve regeneration in adult spinal cord. In Ingoglia NA, Murray M, eds. *Axonal regeneration in the central nervous system*. New York: Marcel Dekker, 2001;529–561.

Ramón-Cueto A, Plant GW, Avila J, Bunge MB. Long-distance axonal regeneration in the transected adult rat spinal cord is promoted by olfactory ensheathing glia transplants. *J Neurosci* 1998;18:3803–3815.

Rees RP, Bunge MB, Bunge RP. Morphological changes in the neuritic growth cone and target neuron during synaptic junction development in culture. *J Cell Biol* 1976;68:240–263.

Roufa D, Bunge MB, Johnson MI, Cornbrooks CJ. Variation in content and function of non-neuronal cells in the outgrowth of sympathetic ganglia from embryos of differing age. *J Neurosci* 1986;6:790–802.

Roufa DG, Johnson MI, Bunge MB. Influence of ganglion age, non-neuronal cells and substratum on neurite outgrowth in culture. *Dev Biol* 1983;99:225–239.

Salzer JL, Colman DR. In Memoriam: Richard Paul Bunge. *Neuron* 1996;17:811–812.

Takami T, Oudega M, Bates ML, Wood PM, Kleitman N, Bunge MB. Schwann cell but not olfactory ensheathing glia transplants improve hindlimb locomotor performance in the moderately contused adult rat thoracic spinal cord. *J Neurosci* 2002;22:6670–6681.

Takami T, Oudega M, Bethea JR, Wood PM, Kleitman N, Bunge MB. Methylprednisolone and interleukin-10 reduce gray matter damage in the contused Fischer rat thoracic spinal cord but do not improve functional outcome. *J Neurotrauma* 2002;19:653–666.

Vikhanski L. A Schwann cell chauvinist. In *In search of the lost cord. Solving the mystery of spinal cord regeneration*. Washington, D.C.: Joseph Henry Press, 2001;73–82.

Xu XM, Chen A, Guénard V, Kleitman N, Bunge MB. Bridging Schwann cell transplants promote axonal regeneration from both the rostral and caudal stumps of transected adult rat spinal cord. *J Neurocytol* 1997;26:1–16.

Xu XM, Guénard V, Kleitman N, Aebischer P, Bunge MB. A combination of BDNF and NT-3 promotes supraspinal axonal regeneration into Schwann cell grafts in adult rat thoracic spinal cord. *Exp Neurol* 1995;134:261–272.

Xu XM, Guénard V, Kleitman N, Bunge MB. Axonal regeneration into Schwann cell-seeded guidance channels grafted into transected adult rat spinal cord. *J Comp Neurol* 1995;351:145–160.

Xu XM, Zhang S-X, Li H, Aebischer P, Bunge MB. Regrowth of axons into the distal spinal cord through a Schwann-cell-seeded mini-channel implanted into hemisected adult rat spinal cord. *Eur J Neurosci* 1999;11:1723–1740.

Yan HL, Bunge MB, Wood PM, Plant GW. Mitogenic response of adult rat olfactory ensheathing glia to four growth factors. *Glia* 2001;33:334–342.

Zu Rhein GM, Duncan ID. In Memoriam: Richard Paul Bunge, MD. *J Neuropathol Exp Neurol* 1997;56:319–320.

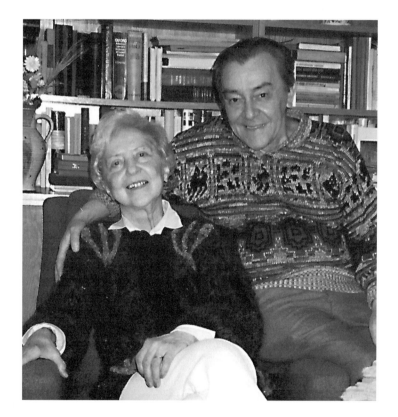

Jan Bures

BORN:

Ctyri Dvory, Ceske Budejovice, Czech Republic
June 13, 1926

EDUCATION:

Faculty of Medicine, Charles University, Prague,
M.D. (1950)
Czechoslovak Academy of Sciences, Prague, Ph.D. (1955)
Czechoslovak Academy of Sciences, Prague, D.Sc. (1963)

APPOINTMENTS:

Institute of Physiology, Czechoslovak Academy of
Sciences (1952–present)

HONORS AND AWARDS (SELECTED):

Central Council of the International Brain Research
Organization (1964–1979)
Governing Council of the International Brain Research
Organization (1992–1998)
Council of the European Neuroscience Association
(1992–1996)
Member of Academia Europea (1992)
Honorary Doctorate, University of Lethbridge,
Canada (1992)
Foreign Associate, National Academy of Sciences,
USA (1995)
Foreign Member of the Polish Academy of Sciences (2000)
Honorary Member of European Brain and Behavior
Society (2000)
Honorary J. E. Purkynje Medal, Czech Academy of
Sciences (2001)

*Jan Bures pioneered the reversible ablation technique by programmatic
analysis of the morphological, physiological, and behavioral effects of
spreading depression. He further studied the neurophysiology of vertebrate
learning, adopting an integrative and systems-level approach to the
analysis of animal cognition.*

Jan Bures

T he aim of an autobiographic chapter is to assess the significance of various factors which may have oriented the subject to science. The two main factors usually considered are genetic endowment and environmental influences. In my case, there is no evidence of intellectual activities in my remote paternal and maternal ancestries. Not much clearer are the environmental factors arousing my early interest in science. But environmental factors in the politically hot climate of Central Europe created situations that tested the resilience of my decision to pursue science and demonstrated the support offered by the international scientific community to the individual scientist.

My father, Rudolf Bures, was born in 1874 at a small farm in central Bohemia. As a younger son he had no chance to stay at the farm and decided, therefore, after termination of his military service in the Austrian army to join police work in gendarmerie. He learned German, passed a number of examinations, mastered good knowledge of the Austrian Law, and became a junior police officer in Trhove Sviny, a small town in South Bohemia. Here in 1904 he met my mother, Marie Pislova, a 20-year-old daughter of a local wheelwright. She had just returned from Vienna and Prague, where she had been working for a year as a maid. Her father, who died before I was born, was a known artisan. Unfortunately, his plans to modernize the workshop were frustrated by the premature death of his eldest son who died as a prisoner of war in a Russian camp during World War I. His two younger sons, Peter and Josef Pisl, were the first members of the family to receive a high school and university education: Peter as a lawyer, working later as a small town notary, and Josef as geodetic engineer, who graduated at the Prague Technical University and was working there as an Assistant Professor until 1934, when he retired because of health problems and returned to his home. He was a true scholar with encyclopedic knowledge and vast files of excerpts from all fields of science, spoke four foreign languages (German, French, English, and Russian), and was always prepared to help children in the neighborhood to master difficult problems in mathematics, physics, and foreign languages. On the other hand, he was a very impractical person, unable to manage the small fields he owned and the old house in which he was living. He never married and was until his death dependent on the help of his older sisters, Cecilia and later of my mother. This was probably the reason why I admired him, but did not find him an attractive example.

My brothers Rudolf and Charles were born in 1906 and 1910 when my father's gendarmerie unit was stationed in Borovany, a small village close to Trhove Sviny. After the end of World War I, which led to collapse of the Austrian empire and the birth of independent Czechoslovakia, he advanced to a more senior position in the Czech gendarmerie and was moved to Ctyri Dvory, now a suburb of the large town Ceske Budejovice, better known to Americans under the German name Budweis, from which the name Budweiser beer is derived. Famous beer has been produced in this locality since the 15th century. The closeness of the city and the many high schools simplified access for my brothers to education. They both attended Jirsik's gymnasium in Ceske Budejovice and after graduation went to study medicine at the Medical Faculty of the Charles University in Prague, the oldest university in Central Europe, which had been founded by the Czech king and Roman emperor Charles the IVth in 1348. When I was born in 1926, Rudolf was already a medical student and Charles was in the last years of high school. The history of my family illustrates rapid transition from a farmer-artisan status to intellectually active middle class, characteristic for the Czech population in the first half of the 20th century.

What could be the important environmental factors attracting me to science in my childhood? Although infantile amnesia seems to block reliable recollection of episodic memories from the first four years of my life, some information can be obtained from my relatives. I was born to old parents, but this did not put me at a disadvantage, because my mother exposed me as much as possible to the company of other children in the neighborhood and spent a lot of time reading me books, which were probably intended for considerably older boys, but which surprisingly aroused my interest and motivated me to hear more. My brothers advised my mother not to read me the standard fairy tales, but something they considered more interesting— adventure stories, geographical discoveries, and science fiction. Taking into account what was available at the time in the Czech language, my mother's choice was Jules Verne. In my preschool years, I was exposed to at least 20 books by this wonderful author, some of them repeatedly, because I insisted that the particularly interesting passages be read to me again and again. The admirable patience of my mother was soon rewarded by my motivation to be independent of her reading. As soon as I learned to read, I attempted to use this new skill for rereading the already known books and for exploring the content of other promising volumes. In fact, this early experience, akin to imprinting, made me addicted to books. I still remember how deeply impressed I was during my first year in the high school in Ceske Budejovice by visiting the municipal library which allowed the juniors like myself to visit the shelves with thousands of books and select those they wanted to borrow for home reading. I learned that books in a public library can be appreciated, not only according to their content, but also according to the traces left on them by their readers. Impact factors and citation rates of the electronic era were reflected in the worn down look of the most popular books.

Another less apparent consequence of the early reading was that I accepted and identified myself with the Jules Verne's philosophy. Some of his books were an impressive glorification of knowledge and of creativity supported by knowledge. Cyrus Smith, the hero of his book *Mystery Island*, is an engineer whose balloon carrying four other passengers wrecked on a deserted island. Although they have nothing more than the content of their pockets, engineer Smith finds a solution for all their problems. He shows his friends how to make fire, what to eat, and where to find safe dwelling. He shows his friends how to make fire, to find safe dwelling, to prepare bricks from baked clay, to produce iron by melting iron in a blast furnace, to domesticate wild animals, to start a plantation from a seed found in a pocket, to synthesize nitroglycerine and use it for construction purposes, to estimate the geographical location of the island and find ways to leave it. Cyrus Smith demonstrates that man can do something from nothing, provided that he has the necessary knowledge. It seems that the possibility of applying knowledge to solving problems of vital importance impressed me already at this age and that I accepted that changing the world for the benefit of mankind was the ultimate purpose of knowledge and science.

In 1931 my father retired from the gendarmerie and our family moved from Ctyri Dvory to Trhove Sviny to live in the house of my aunt Cecilia, who had recently died. Beginning in the autumn of 1932, I attended here the first four classes of primary school. I was good in reading and counting, but had problems with calligraphy and drawing, which has persisted throughout my life. At the age of 10, I prepared for the entrance examination to the Jirsik's gymnasium in Ceske Budejovice, the high school attended by my brothers. I passed the exam and in September 1936 started to study there. I was living in a rented room within walking distance of the school and returned on Sundays by train and bus to my parents in Trhove Sviny. This was a very dramatic time in international politics: Hitler occupied Austria and insisted on annexing the Sudeten, regions of Czechoslovakia at the border of Germany and Austria with majority of German population. Our government, relying on French and British support, invested enormous effort into fortifications and weapons for defense of the Czechoslovak territory, but in the critical negotiations between Germany, Italy, France, and Great Britain taking place in September 1938 in Munich, the Western powers agreed with the German demand and recommended to the Czechoslovak government to yield all territories with German majority to Germany. Because all the fortifications were close to the German border, this made the remnants of Czechoslovakia not defensible. Within several weeks, the Czech population was forced to leave the to-be-occupied regions and find resettlement in the central parts of the country. It was obvious that this was only a temporary solution. On March 15, 1939, the German troops occupied the rest of Czechoslovakia and split it into the Protectorate of Bohemia and Moravia and into independent Slovakia. The democratic Czechoslovakia was destroyed, and the legal basis of personal security, equality, free speech, and foreign travel suddenly disappeared. Most students in my class were affected by the takeover in some personal way. My older brother Rudolf, who ran a medical practice in Ctyri Dvory, was imprisoned by Gestapo on the first day of occupation because he was the chairman of the local organization of Friendship with the Soviet Union. He spent several months in Czech prisons before being finally transported to the German concentration camp Buchenwald. He had the good luck to be released two years later, shortly before the German invasion of the USSR. There were other more sad fates. A number of Jewish students were at first forced to leave schools and start working at menial jobs. Later they disappeared when their families were shipped to concentration camps. Gestapo had a large network of confidants who reported all forms of anti-German attitudes, which were punished in the most severe way (death penalty for listening to the Czech transmission of the BBC). The pervasive atmosphere of terror made even 13-year-old boys and girls very reticent in the company of unknown people.

In spite of the stressful conditions, school followed the traditional curriculum. There were more hours of German language, other disciplines (Czech history, literature, and art) were purged of topics unacceptable for the occupants, and some books were removed from the school and public libraries. But mathematics, physics, chemistry, geography, and languages (Latin and French) remained untouched. I became most interested in mathematics and physics, and in anticipation of future development, I attempted to improve my language education by learning English and Russian. I passed the final examination (which had to be done in the German language) in June 1944. There was no opportunity to continue study because the Czech universities had been closed since 1939 after students' protests against occupation. We had to work in factories or in agriculture, constructing runways at the military airport and repairing damage caused by Allied bombers. I acquired a number of useful skills during this period (working on a turning lathe and using tools for fine mechanics) and came to know different people, all hating the war and hoping that they would be lucky enough to survive and to do something to prevent a relapse of this nightmare.

The war ended in South Bohemia, the southern part of which was taken by the American army and the northern part by the Soviet army. Many lives were lost in the last days of war because the retreating German troops, particularly the SS divisions, fought desperately to escape the Russians and to surrender to the Americans.

With the end of war, the University opened and started to compensate the losses. The priorities were to allow students whose study was interrupted in 1939 to finish their education as fast as possible and to prepare the University for accepting into the first years of undergraduate studies all students accumulated over the six years of university closure. I arrived in Prague already in June to study mathematics in the extraordinary summer semester. This proved to be a wrong decision, because the introductory lectures I attended in the overcrowded lecture halls of the Faculty of Mathematics and Physics were explaining the philosophy of basic mathematical operations and appeared to me trivial and uninteresting. I believed (probably correctly) that my failure to appreciate mathematics was due to a lack of talent and decided to try my luck in a field that was successfully mastered by my brothers, i.e., medicine.

Medical Faculty of the Charles University in Prague

In September 1945, I became a student of the Faculty of Medicine. The first-year lectures were attended by several thousand students and were given in the big entertainment center Lucerna, seating more than 1000 people. The textbooks were another difficulty that could be only partly overcome by the use of German books. The first two years of medical study were devoted to preclinical disciplines, including physics, chemistry, biology, embryology, histology, anatomy, and physiology. In spite of the overcrowded lectures, the teaching done by the best professors we had was interesting and sometimes exciting. Thus, the fact that liquids are incompressible was demonstrated in the course of medical physics by a pistol shot into a cardboard box filled with water. Whereas the totally filled closed box exploded upon the impact of the bullet, a partially filled box was only penetrated by two small openings. It is regrettable that this demonstration was later removed from the course program as too dangerous for the audience, although it could be nowadays included in the psychology course to demonstrate facilitation of memory acquisition by emotional experience.

I was particularly impressed by lectures in biology, delivered by Professor J. Belehradek (who later emigrated to Great Britain, and lectures in physiology, delivered by Professor V. Laufberger. The two courses were very different in style. While Belehradek based his teaching on his textbook published before the war, which contained an excellent survey of pertinent international literature, Laufberger offered students improvised mimeographed texts prepared by his assistant professors and concentrated his attention on creating a practical course in physiology, giving a detailed step-by-step description of the theoretical principles, technical tools, practical procedures, and expected results of the experiments the students had to perform. Similarly different was the content of their lectures. Whereas Belehradek described systematically the theoretical and philosophical issues and the current trends of world research, he did not speak much about the work done in his laboratory. Laufberger's lectures did not attempt to explain physiology, but to describe what he found interesting and on what research problems he was currently working. In the first years after the war, he was interested in neurophysiology; in the work of Norbert Wiener; in recording electrical activity of nerves, brain, and heart; and in the design of simple robots. His lectures were often difficult to understand, but they conveyed clearly his enthusiasm, explained his hypotheses, and described the experiments by which he wanted to confirm them or to falsify them.

During the second year I participated with a group of students in a two-month-long public health service operation aimed at the inoculation of children in North Moravia against tuberculosis and other contagious diseases. Here I met an attractive and pleasant girl, Olga Komoradova, an optimistic and energetic colleague, interested not only in clinical medicine, but also in science. We were both members of the Communist party and participated actively in the political life of university students. We rapidly found that we shared many important views and that we would like to live together. Three years later we married, and on December 23, 1949, our daughter Olga was born while we both were in the last year of medical study.

When studying the preclinical disciplines, I paid attention not only to the lectures, but also to the possibility of joining some ongoing research. This was most common in anatomy, which needed demonstrators for practical courses in osteology, for dissections, and for preparation of schematic illustrations for teaching. Several years of such student work in anatomy was an excellent recommendation for surgery or pathology and was popular among students with clear ideas about their future medical career. This was not my case, because the first two years of medicine had increased my interest in biomedical research and reduced my motivation to become a physician. I wanted to join a field offering the possibility of independent experimental work under the guidance of an experienced colleague, but I knew that the choice of the field would be determined by the available opportunities. Thus, my decision for neuroscience was a result of rational assessment of the advantages and disadvantages offered by the various laboratories I explored.

The most attractive opportunity was the Laboratory of Experimental Neurophysiology, organized in the newly established Central Institute of Biology. Its head, Assistant Professor Zdenek Servit, was a young neurologist who believed that advances in diagnosis, prevention, and therapy of diseases can only be achieved by strong basic research. His primary target was epilepsy, a common neurological disease due to disturbed interaction of excitatory and inhibitory mechanisms, which he wanted to study by using an evolutionary approach, comparing epileptic seizures at different levels of phylogenetic and ontogenetic development. He was a pleasant, eloquent man with limited experimental experience, but with excellent knowledge of pertinent literature and with the skill to prepare and write research reports. He was offered two large rooms on the second floor of the Institute of Physiology of the Medical Faculty, salaries for two technicians, and the possibility of recruiting students who would like to stay as employees after graduation. In early spring 1948 I became, as a third-year medical student, a member of his group.

First Steps in Science

The laboratory was not yet equipped for experimental work, but because Servit considered it important to announce its existence by some published paper, he suggested that I help him prepare a statistical study evaluating medical records of almost 4000 epileptic patients treated during the previous 15 years by the Neurological Clinic. The vast material was collected by students who transcribed the relevant information from the case sheets into prepared questionnaires. My task was to organize the collection of data and to perform statistical analysis of the results. The first part of the study was published two years later (Servit and Bures, 1950), and the second part was published in 1952. Animal experiments, started in 1949, were aimed at testing the hypothesis that the grand mal epileptic seizure is similar in various representatives of vertebrates. The seizure was elicited by transcranial electroconvulsive shock applied to mice (*Mus musculus*), lizards (*Lacerta viridis*), and frogs (*Rana temporaria*). The similar size of these animals simplified the question of whether differences in threshold current eliciting clonic-tonic convulsions of the limbs could be explained by brain volume or should be ascribed to evolutionary factors. I addressed this problem together with Mojmir Petran, another medical student who preferred basic research to medical practice and joined Servit's laboratory. Mojmir, who was an expert in physics (he contributed later to the invention of the confocal microscope), introduced me to the use of measuring instruments and cathode ray oscilloscopes. After several months of preliminary experiments, we proposed the density of the quantity of electricity passed between an intraoral electrode on the palate and a cranial electrode on the occiput as the best estimate of threshold, which was 92 uAsec/mm^2 in mice, was 3 times higher in lizards, and was 15 times higher in frogs. Still more important was the fact that mice and rats had the same threshold, 92 uAsec/mm^2, although rats were 10 times heavier than mice (Bures and Petran, 1952). Several other papers studied the effect of hypothermia, the effect on seizure threshold of hydration of the brain, and the effect of positive or negative DC current, which was applied on the head against a large indifferent electrode on the belly.

Ph.D. Dissertation

Simultaneously with the examination of the phylogenetic development of epilepsy, directed by Professor Servit, I was working on an independent project that was the subject of my Ph.D. thesis. In fact, this degree was called at that time "candidate of science" (CSc.) because Czechoslovakia and other countries of the East Block modified the system of academic degrees according to the Soviet model. After consultations with Professor Servit, who was my supervisor, I decided to study an interesting form of epilepsy, the so-called audiogenic seizures, which can be elicited in rats and mice by strong acoustic stimuli, e.g., by jingling a bunch of keys or by exposing the animal to a 120-dB bell. The advantage of this model was that unlike spontaneous epilepsy, the acoustic reflex epilepsy could be elicited by a defined stimulus that made it possible to trace the spread of excitation from the acoustic projection to mesencephalic and prosencephalic structures mediating the generalization of the seizure, manifested by convulsions and by high amplitude spikes and waves in the EEG. This seemed to be a feasible task, but difficulties soon emerged. The incidence of audiogenic epilepsy in the Wistar rats available in Prague was rather low and not reliably reproducible. The first thing was to introduce a sensitizing procedure, increasing the susceptibility of the animals to the acoustic stimulus. This was easy, because a subconvulsive dosage of pentamethylentetrazol (50 mg/kg) increased the percentage of susceptible animals to 50%. A more serious difficulty was the EEG recording. The only EEG apparatus in Prague was an eight-channel Grass device donated to Czechoslovakia by the United Nations Relief and Rehabilitation Administration (UNRRA). It was used for the examination of patients at the Neurological Clinic of the Medical Faculty. Its use for animal experiment was an almost clandestine operation made possible by cooperation with staff employees of the clinic.

In spite of the above technical and organizational problems, I succeeded in finishing in three years (1950–1952) six experimental studies related to the theme of my dissertation, which was completed and submitted in December 1952. The individual papers were published in 1953 in Russian or English in *Physiologia Bohemoslovaca*, and their English summary appeared 10 years later (Bures, 1963). The main results illuminated behavioral, integrative, and electrophysiological aspects of reflex epilepsy.

Since the electrophysiological experiments had to be done on restrained animals, it was necessary to examine the effect of restraint on seizure susceptibility. It was found that gentle fixation of the forelimbs and one hindlimb reduced the incidence of audiogenic seizures in sensitized rats or mice from 70 to 10%, but that longer lasting restraint (10 min) lost its inhibitory effect and rather increased seizure susceptibility. If the animal exposed to the auditory stimulus, made ineffective by restraint, was re-exposed to the auditory stimulus when free, no seizure was elicited. This blockade was not due to the duration of the preceding restraint, but to the duration of the preceding acoustic stimulus, which probably left some persisting inhibition in the auditory system. The subsequent study compared the effect of restraint and of other strong stimuli on the blocking of audiogenic seizures. Similar inhibition elicited by electric shock to the lower part of the body started 30 sec after the shock and disappeared 3 min later. Audiogenic seizures were also blocked by forced swimming. It was also demonstrated that repeated presentations (six to eight) of the inhibitory stimulus decreased its efficiency to control level.

Attempts to identify the anatomical substrate of audiogenic epilepsy showed that the first seizures in rats coincided with the maturation of cerebral cortex, i.e., with the appearance of cortical postural reactions and of acoustic evoked responses in auditory cortex. Another study indicated that elimination of the major sensory modalities (vision, olfaction, audition) as well as blockade of most somatosensory and visceral sensations by myelotomy decreased seizure susceptibility. Finally, analysis of the effects of hypothermia on seizure susceptibility indicated that while susceptibility to electroconvulsive shock is not changed by reduction of body temperature to 20°C, audiogenic seizures cannot be elicited at temperatures below 27°C. This is not due to blockade of auditory responses in the cortical projection area where evoked potentials remain preserved at 21°C, but rather at some subcortical level.

Postdoctoral Period

I found the work on the dissertation very stimulating—I could ask questions that I considered interesting, find the best way to solve them, and decide how to interpret the results. Although Professor Servit was a very liberal boss who liked to discuss research with his co-workers, he usually prepared an outline of the project and took responsibility for the formulation of the final version of the manuscript. I believed that the dissertation had qualified me for a more independent position. We discussed the problem in detail and although Professor Servit was not quite enthusiastic about it, he agreed to give me more freedom. This was not too painful for him, however, because this was a period of rapid growth of our science. The Central Institute of Biology became one of the institutes of the newly organized Academy of Sciences, and it was expected that it would rapidly grow by training dozens of new scientists. Ernest Gutmann, the most qualified neuroscientist in the country, was asked to form a Department of Muscle Physiology. He emigrated before the war to England, studied biology in Oxford, and got a British Ph.D. with J.Z. Young as supervisor. He had extensive experimental experience and understood how modern science should be done. It was very fortunate that he was around when *Physiologia Bohemoslovaca*, the foreign language output for Czech research, was started and when the institute library was organized. Another mature scientist who appeared in Servit's group was Friedrich Eckert, a specialist in comparative physiology of invertebrates. He was a former Assistant Professor at the German University in Prague, who married before the war a Jewess and after German occupation of Czechoslovakia refused to divorce her. His moral integrity saved her life for which he paid several years of imprisonment in a concentration camp.

Servit had a number of new graduate students, some of them (Josef Zachar, Daria Zacharova, and Domin Svorad) coming from Slovakia and others from Bohemia (Olga Hudlicka, Vera Novakova, Zdenek Martinek, Libuse Chocholova, Jaroslav Sterc, and Zdenek Lodin). He allowed me to find, investigate, and publish my own research projects; to collaborate with my wife Olga, who left the position of Lecturer at the Physiological Institute of the Medical Faculty and was concluding her Ph.D. dissertation under Servit's supervision; to use the help of two technicians for our experiments; and to find additional postgraduate students whose Ph.D. dissertations would be related to our program.

While the above negotiations were proceeding, we started to look for an interesting, promising, and feasible theme that could serve as a reliable basis for team research. The possibility appeared in one of the joint papers (Servit et al., 1953) that examined the effect of DC current on the duration of anesthesia. Later analysis (Bures, 1954a) of EEC changes, observed in the polarized hemisphere, indicated that the current onset is accompanied in the cortex adjacent to the polarizing electrode by a striking decrease of EEG amplitude which spreads during several minutes over the entire neocortex. The properties of this phenomenon closely resembled spreading EEG depression (SD), described 10 years earlier by Leao (1944). To identify it as SD required recording the negative slow potential wave accompanying the wavefront of the EEG depression and determining the velocity of propagation (3 mm/min), the two characteristic markers of SD. Convenient DC recording was achieved by the chopper technique (Goldring and O'leary, 1951), which made it possible to record the slow potential directly in one EEG channel, the input of which was short-circuited and only once per second briefly connected to a 1 μF condenser placed between the nonpolarizable calomel cell electrodes that were applied to the points where the potential difference was measured. This was demonstrated in a subsequent paper (Bures, 1954b), which also reported that SD can be elicited in non-anesthetized rats and that its properties are not different from those seen under anesthesia. These findings seemed to us sufficient for considering SD as a suitable theme for collective multidisciplinary research. In fact, I am still surprised that our plan to study the very abstract, academic problem of SD did not meet opposition, but was well accepted. The reason was probably the atmosphere of intellectual preparedness for phenomena mediated by non-synaptic interaction of neurons. SD fitted well into the vague, but plausible concept that besides nerve impulses the brain employs other means to integrate its activity. While most examples of ephaptic transmission, propagation of nerve signals across cuts and field-mediated synchronization of activity of large neuronal populations, were poorly reproducible, SD remained the only robust and reliable example of phenomena of this class. This was true not only for Western science, but perhaps still more for Soviet neurophysiology, paying much respect to the mysterious concepts of dominant state, parabiosis, and perielectrotonus. Particularly the dominant state, wherein activation of a nerve center increased its responsiveness to a wide range of nonspecific stimuli, seemed to be related to the problems of neural plasticity. Although skepticism prevailed, the underlying beliefs, expectations, and doubts kept the idea of non-synaptic integration alive and gained support for projects offering reasonable chances to address the above questions.

Laboratory of Physiology of the Central Nervous System

Ten years after the discovery of SD, the field was well surveyable, and it was not difficult to accumulate in a couple of years reprints of pertinent papers and to establish contact with the most active research groups. On the basis of such a survey, we tried to formulate the list of the principal research directions connected with SD.

1. Manifestations and concomitants of SD
2. SD eliciting stimuli and conditions blocking SD development
3. Morphological substrate of SD; SD-prone and SD-resistant structures of the vertebrate brain; and phylogenetic and ontogenetic aspects
4. Metabolic nature of SD and SD-related phenomena
5. Electrophysiological consequences of SD in remote brain structures
6. Behavioral manifestations of SD and its effect on innate reactions and on acquisition, consolidation, and retrieval of conditioned reactions

We have split our effort and attempted with Olga to cover in the next two years the above six directions and to explore the possibility of their detailed investigation. Olga took responsibility for point 6, in particular, for developing her idea to use SD as a functional ablation procedure allowing examination of the role of the depressed cortex in different stages of memory trace formation and retrieval. I concentrated on electrophysiological and other technical problems, and we both participated in individual papers according to the time we had spent on them.

The start of the SD project was made possible by another technique of SD initiation: application of DC current to exposed cerebral cortex was replaced by chemical stimuli applied on filter papers to the dura-covered bottom of trephine openings (4 mm in diameter) prepared in the parietal bones. While 1% KCl solution elicited usually a single SD wave, 25% KCl evoked a train of SD waves accompanied by continuous EEG depression lasting 2–3 hr (Bures and Buresova, 1956b). Such prolonged depression was well suited for examination of long-lasting consequences of functional decortication, e.g., for demonstration of reduced excretion of a 5% water load (Buresova, 1957a), of reduced metabolic thermoregulation (Buresova, 1957b), and of blockade of unconditioned reflexes and natural conditioned reflexes (Buresova, 1956). The latter studies were included in Olga's Ph.D. dissertation entitled "Physiological Consequences of Stimulation of the Central Nervous System by Direct Current and by Potassium Ions." Application of chemical substances to the cerebral cortex could also be used for estimation of the threshold concentrations of SD-eliciting compounds or of drugs blocking SD initiation or SD propagation (Bures, 1956; Bures and Buresova, 1956a). Important contributions to the SD-related phenomena were the papers describing the terminal anoxic depolarization of the cerebral cortex and its modification by local treatment of the cortex (Bures and Buresova, 1957) or by systemic application of drugs (Benesova, Buresova, and Bures, 1957). The metabolic aspects of SD were addressed in a study comparing the metabolic effects of 0.1 M KCl on brain slices with the mechanism of the metabolic processes leading to SD initiation by the same KCl concentrations (Bures, 1956). Similarly, the dependence of SD on the body temperature of rats indicated that between colonic temperatures 20° and 40°C the amplitude of the negative slow potential changes with $Q10 = 1$, and the SD propagation rate and the duration of the slow potential change with $Q10 = 1.7$ to 2.0 (Bures et al., 1957). Finally, the morphological aspects of SD were addressed in a study describing the development of SD and of terminal anoxic depolarization during the first 20 days of postnatal life in rats (Bures, 1957).

The results obtained in the three years 1953–1956 confirmed the expectation that the SD project can support meaningful research into the mechanisms of cerebral functions and is closely related to investigations performed in a number of international neuroscience centers. In addition, five papers were published in refereed international journals and thus proved their capability to compete with international production. On the basis of these results, we were given three positions for graduate students who would cover the most promising areas of our SD research: metabolism (biochemist Jiri Krivanek), morphology (anatomist Eva Fifkova), and functional organization of the brain (Tomas Weis). We were also given the positions of an electronic engineer and of three technicians specialized in biochemistry, histology, and electrophysiolgy. In 1958, our team was officially declared the Laboratory of Physiology of the Central Nervous System, and I was nominated its head.

The new employees were coming between 1956 and 1958. The first was Jiri Krivanek, who started immediately with a demanding biochemical program. His main task was to support the electrophysiological analysis of SD by finding the chemical concomitants of the slow potential shift and of the EEC depression. Already during his first year he found that the depolarization of cerebral cortex during SD and anoxia is accompanied by a dramatic decrease of phosphocreatine in the depolarized cortex (Krivanek, Bures, and Buresova, 1958). Soon followed papers describing the decrease of glycogene and glucosis and the increase of lactate in the SD-affected tissue (Krivanek, 1958). His not less important task was to verify Grafstein's (1956) hypothesis that the SD spread is mediated by diffusion of potassium ions liberated from depolarized neurons. This was studied by washing the exposed cortical surface with isotonic NaCl and by comparing the leakage of potassium ions from the normal cortex and from the depolarized cortex into the washing fluid. Although it took at least 2 min to accumulate sufficient volume of the superfusion fluid for measuring the K^+ concentration in the sample with a flame photometer, the method was sensitive enough to show that SD presence is accompanied by a fivefold increase of potassium in the washing fluid (Krivanek and Bures, 1960). This indicated at least a fivefold increase of potassium concentration in the extracellular space during the negative slow potential. The assumption that the real increase can be several times higher was confirmed only 15 years later after ion-sensitive electrodes became available.

Eva Fifkova, an assistant in the Institute of Anatomy of the Medical Faculty, started to work with our group as an externist. She prepared with J. Marsala from the same Institute the first version of a Czech stereotaxic atlas and later performed histological controls for individual electrophysiological studies. She joined our department in 1958, and her main task was to study the morphological substrate of SD, particularly the boundaries of SD propagation in the neocortex, hippocampus, caudate nucleus, thalamus, and cerebellum of rats and in the striatum of pigeons. The above studies formed the basis of her later Ph.D. dissertation.

Tomas Weis started to work in our laboratory as a medical student and returned to us several years later after completion of his medical training as a graduate student. Since he was not technically specialized, he concentrated on electrophysiological analysis of remote effects of cortical or hippocampal SD on subcortical structures and on integrative functions, e.g., sleep.

First International Contacts

The Academy of Sciences was aware of the necessity to establish direct contacts with scientific institutions abroad and between individual scientists, but foreign travel was extremely limited in the first postwar decade. In autumn of 1954, the Academy arranged for me and Jiri Krecek, our colleague working in developmental physiology, a two-month visit to Soviet research centers in Moscow and Leningrad. I wanted to visit laboratories performing electrophysiological experiments in animals, and my hosts did their best to show me all they had. In Moscow I visited the Institute of Higher Nervous Activity and saw the laboratories of Academician V.S. Rusinov, met his co-workers G. Kuznetsova and I. Kozlovskaya, and thoroughly studied his recording equipment that was even according to the Czechoslovak standards desperately obsolete. In spite of the technical shortcomings, experiments showing that the dominant focus produced by polarization of motor cortex attracts acoustically elicited responses were interesting and impressed me as a useful model of plasticity. On various occasions I was asked to give seminar talks describing our current research. The seminars were well attended, but the discussion indicated that most participants were not aware of the existence of SD and were surprised that I did not use Pavlovian terminology to interpret it. I had to explain that there were no reasons to consider the decrease of EEC as a sign of some form of Pavlovian inhibition and that reliable electrophysiological markers of behavioral inhibition were yet to be found. My attitude was not understandable to an audience accustomed to accepting explanations based on old concepts that had never been sufficiently proven, but whose authority should not be questioned. Poor knowledge of non-Russian literature was due to the low percentage of scientists able to use foreign languages and by the absence of English journals in the libraries of the institutes. However, even access to Russian literature was limited by ideological considerations. During one month in Leningrad I was hosted by the Institute of Physiology of the Academy of Sciences. I spent a lot of time in the library of the Institute trying to look up Russian journals not available in Prague and was deeply shocked to find that many volumes had been obviously censored in a very crude way, by removing whole pages or by gluing them together so that they could not be read or by blackening names or whole lines or paragraphs that mentioned scientists who were prosecuted in some political process. Attempts to find an explanation were not answered.

I was later advised by the Russian colleague responsible for my scientific program not to ask questions that cannot be answered or that could expose the questioner to unpleasant interrogation later. The main conclusion drawn from the two months spent in Russia was that in the coming years our field could expect from this country neither technical innovations nor theoretical advances. On the other hand, I found among the people I met in the Russian institutes a number of talented, enthusiastic researchers who wanted to work in Prague and who later succeeded to visit us for shorter or longer periods.

An important consequence of my visit was increased visibility of our group in Russia. We were put on the list of potential foreign partners for collaborative projects, which could not be implemented in the Soviet Union alone. This was illustrated by collaboration with Kh. S. Koshtoyants, an Armenian scientist and Professor of the Moscow State University, who learned about our experiments demonstrating that the SD-eliciting potency of KCl can be counteracted when adding to the KCl solution a definite concentration of $CaCl_2$. He wanted to find some way to test the detoxicating effect of glutathion on the toxicity of $HgCl_2$ and suggested he perform a simple experiment during his several months-long stay in Prague which could (1) test the possibility of eliciting SD by local application of the thiol group poison $HgCl_2$ on the exposed cerebral cortex and (2) test the possibility of blocking the $HgCl_2$-elicited SD by supplying reactive SH groups with an appropriately concentrated solution of glutathione. The experiments performed in a few weeks showed that 5% $HgCl_2$ elicits a train of six SD waves when applied on intact neocortex, but that it remains ineffective when applied on cortex pretreated for 5 min with 10% glutathione. This effect of glutathione was limited to $HgCl_2$ and left the SD waves elicited by KCl unchanged. The results were published in *Proceedings of the Soviet Academy of Sciences* (Bures and Koshtoyants, 1955).

International Congress of Physiology

Perhaps the most important international contact in this period was my participation in the XXth International Congress of Physiology in Brussels. The Czechoslovak Physiological Society sent an official delegation including 17 scientists from the universities and Academy of Sciences and helped the delegates with the language editing of their papers. Our English journal, *Physiologia Bohemoslovaca*, prepared a supplement containing extended versions (3–7 pages) of the 17 contributions of the Czechoslovak delegates. Our abstract in the Congress proceedings (Bures and Buresova, 1956b) and its three-page version in the supplement (Bures and Buresova, 1956c) were the first English reports describing the use of SD as a functional ablation procedure.

Entering Big Science

In autumn of 1957, I was invited by the Georgian Academy of Sciences to participate in the Third Gagra Conference on the Mechanism of Conditioned Reflexes. The conference took place from January 13 to 24, 1958, in a recreation center of Soviet VIPs in the Black Sea resort of Gagra. These conferences organized by Academician I. S. Beritashvili were the most influential meetings of Soviet specialists dedicated to open discussion of controversial problems in the ideologically sensitive field of higher nervous activity. The first conference on bioelectrical phenomena in 1948 was followed by a longer interval due to administrative persecution of Beritashvili by the Stalinist leaders of the Academy who accused him of not being loyal to the materialistic interpretation of Pavlov's ideas. Beritashvili refused to denounce his belief that the behavior of animals is determined not only by conditioned reflexes but also by so-called images, complex representations of the world surrounding the animal, and of corresponding expectations of possible consequences of specific behaviors. After Stalin's death in 1953, Beritashvili's situation gradually improved, and this was manifested in the second Gagra conference on excitation and inhibition in 1955 and in the third conference that should have included also several scientists from Poland, Hungary, and Czechoslovakia. Since the other invited guests were not able to come, I remained the only foreign participant at the conference. Because I had a very junior position in the Czechoslovak Academy of Sciences, the invitation was a surprise not only for me, but also for my superiors. The mystery was solved only during the conference.

The most talented co-worker of Beritashvili, A. I. Roytbak, had written in 1955 a book, *Bioelectric Phenomena in Cerebral Hemispheres*, with a pertinent review of relevant literature. A chapter of this book was devoted to the SD phenomenon, and its properties attracted scientists studying mechanisms of nervous integration. Among the papers quoted by Roytbak were also my two articles on SD published in *Physiologia Bohemoslovaca* in 1954. The paper describing the possibility of eliciting SD in the cortex of non-anaesthetized intact rats was considered particularly important because it opposed the assertion of Professor Gedevani, a Georgian rival of Beritashvili, that the slowly spreading inhibition in the cerebral cortex can only be observed in deep barbiturate anesthesia. In this way I became, without knowing about it, an ally of the Beritashvili clan and a person whose invitation seemed desirable. In addition, Roytbak's assessment of my qualification was wrong. Roytbak had sent in September 1955 a copy of his book "to professor Jan Bures." This dedication suggested that he believed me to be a rather senior person and prepared Beritashvili and the conference organizers for receiving an important representative of the Czechoslovak Academy. I realized all this suddenly in the first minutes after landing at the airport in Adler, the closest airport to Gagra. Although there were only a few passengers disembarking from the plane, it took almost 30 min before the members of the welcome committee who came in two cars to take me to the conference place in Gagra decided that the young boy not at all corresponding to their expectations was the person they should take to the conference. It seemed, however, that as soon as the disappointment was overcome, they were quite happy that I was not a stuffy professor but somebody prepared to answer all their questions and to learn about their problems and plans.

I learned only during the conference about still another reason for my invitation to Gagra. Representatives of the Soviet Academy of Sciences were negotiating with a group of Western scientists about the possibility of organizing an international scientific forum that could help governments find peaceful solutions to the problems of the Cold War period. Study of the brain, psychology, and education seemed to be the fields best suited for this purpose, and the plan was to start this venture with an international conference to be held in October 1958 in Moscow. A Soviet scientist entrusted with the organization of the Soviet block participation in this conference was G. D. Smirnov, whom I had briefly met during my visit to Moscow in 1954 and who was also a participant at the Gagra conference. He explained to me that Gagra was one of the last preparations for the Moscow meeting and that the Soviet speakers would be selected from the Gagra speakers. It seemed that I was invited to Gagra to demonstrate what I could present in Moscow and to discover how I would manage the stresses of the lecture and subsequent discussion.

The first days of the conference were devoted to study of the 16 papers to be presented. The actual lectures and discussions took place from 11:00 AM to 6:00 PM so that the participants had plenty of time to prepare their discussion and edit their contributions that had been prepared by the organizers for later publication. Presentation of the paper (not more than 1 hr) was followed by questions, which were immediately answered by the speaker, and by general comments, summarily answered in the concluding statement of the speaker. The discussion was sometimes very critical, but was always motivated by a sincere effort to find the proper solution to controversial problems. Our paper, "Application of Spreading EEG Depression in Research into the Mechanisms of Conditioned Reflexes," elicited a number of technical questions and critical comments by the representatives of the Vvedenski's school (N.V. Golikov) who wanted me to use Vvedenski's terminology when describing and explaining SD. To this request I replied in a rather harsh way: "I appreciate the historical significance of Vvedenski's contribution to electrophysiology, but I am also aware of the fact that his main discoveries were made 70 years ago. I believe that dogmatic acceptance of his ideas and hypotheses hinders the development of contemporary methodological approaches, which make it possible to understand the nature of the studied phenomenon. This is why we refused to explain SD using Vvedenski's terminology and concentrated our effort on metabolic, physicochemical, physiological and morphological analysis of this phenomenon." I was glad to see that this position was shared by most participants at the conference, who refused the tendency to reduce research problems to a terminological level.

After the conference I was invited to visit Beritashvili's institute in Tbilisi to learn more about his current research, which was concerned mainly with the problems of spatial orientation of animals and humans. He was interested in our plans to concentrate on the physiology of memory and to use SD as a research tool for this purpose. Although he was already quite old at that time, he was very well informed about the recent development of the field and advised me how to do various experiments of a cognitive character. During the conference I met not only the present, but also the future leaders of Soviet neurophysiology, among them P. G. Kostyuk, who became my good friend.

The Gagra conference showed me some weak points in our research. One of them was the absence of unit activity recording required for assessment of remote effects of cortical or hippocampal SD on subcortical structures. To fill this gap, I obtained an Academy fellowship for a three-week visit to the Institute of Physiology of the University in Pisa, where Professor G. Moruzzi had established one of the best microeloectrophysiological laboratories in Europe. I arrived in June 1958 and was accepted in a friendly way. After detailed discussion of my plans with Professor Moruzzi, I was offered an equipped laboratory with a stereotaxic apparatus and microdrive, a two channel preamplifier, and an oscilloscope. I was shown how to prepare tungsten microelectrodes and how to introduce them into the reticular formation of rats and record activity of reticular neurons. In two weeks I was able to obtain reliable recordings and to demonstrate to Professor Moruzzi a marked increase in the firing rate of reticular neurons shortly after elicitation of cortical SD.

While unit activity recording was the main goal of my stay in Pisa, I was less impressed by the organization of the research. The Institute had only three staff employees: Professor Moruzzi and two assistant professors, Arduini and Mollica. Research was mainly done by foreign or Italian students who worked in the Institute for one to three years. During my stay there were four foreign students from Canada, Japan, West Germany, and Chile, as well as five Italian students. Research was organized around the three staff employees. In the autumn, groups consisting of one to two foreigners and one to two Italian students were formed around the three oldest employees. They started to work on agreed projects and tried to complete parts of them in a way that would allow preparation of manuscripts in July. The project continued the following autumn with a partly changed team and somewhat updated goals. I was impressed by the excellent results produced by this simple informal system, based on the prestige of Professor Moruzzi and on the motivation of the visiting scientists, who worked very hard to obtain in the short time available results that would give them the opportunity to become co-authors of publications and confirm their affiliation with a leading research center. I hoped that our laboratory in Prague would one day be able to follow this wonderful example and become similarly attractive for visitors who would come to learn something interesting while contributing to an exciting research project.

After returning to Prague, I spent all summer recording reticular units in our laboratory. The amplified spikes were detected by a Schmitt trigger circuit and converted to standard rectangular pulses which were passed through a diode to a condenser. After 30 sec the condenser was discharged by a relay and started to be charged again. This simple integrator made it possible to record slow changes in unit activity produced by spreading depression waves in the ipsilateral cerebral cortex. Shortly before the Moscow colloquium, our Institute was visited by two American participants at the meeting, M. A. Brazier and H. W. Magoun, who wanted to see our laboratories and speak with people doing this research. They spent almost the whole day in our laboratory, seeing the experiments with SD in freely moving animals, slow potentials in cerebral cortex, and accompanying unit activity changes in remote brain structures. They asked many pertinent questions, offered much useful advice, and seemed to be impressed by what they saw.

The Moscow Colloquium

The meeting in the House of Science from October 6 to October 11, 1958, was attended by 26 scientists from the USSR, 7 scientists from the Central and Eastern Europe, and 1 scientist from China. The Western participants were from the United States (4), France (3), and one each from Belgium, Netherlands, Italy, England, India, Japan, Mexico, and Canada. The Eastern participants presented 16 lectures coinciding in 11 cases with the talks given at the previous Gagra conference. The Western participants presented 13 talks. The proceedings of the conference, including also the discussion following individual talks, were published in 1960 as a supplement of the journal *Electroencephalography and Clinical Neurophysiology* and are rather well known. The main theme of the conference was the dispute about the locus of the plastic changes underlying the formation of conditioned reflexes. While the representatives of the Pavlovian school (Livanov, Trofimov, Anokhin, and Voronin) insisted that the CS-US association proceeds in the cortex, Gastaut suggested that the closure takes place in subcortical structures, especially in the reticular formation and in the non-specific thalamic nuclei. The attempts to find support for either position by electrophysiological evidence did not yield convincing results. Our lecture was well accepted because it approached the same problem in a different way, i.e., by using an easily identifiable electrophysiological phenomenon precisely located in space and time as a functional ablation procedure, testing the brain regions that are in a definite time window indispensable for elicitation of the conditioned reaction. I received flattering commentaries from Professors Magoun, Chang, and Bremer. When Professor Voronin wondered why blockade of the preferred forepaw by SD does not lead to an immediate switch of the habit to the contralateral limb, Professor Jasper mentioned his earlier experiments showing by other functional ablation procedures (local cooling or Novocain anaesthesia) similar effects on handedness. Professor Sarkisov considered rats unsuitable for research of this kind, because their cortex is insufficiently differentiated, and suggested that we pay more attention to the role of subcortical structures in the organization of conditioned reflex activity.

An important result of the Moscow colloquium was the unanimous resolution of its participants to form a permanent international organization for the study of brain, facilitating contacts between scientists interested in brain research. Owing to the efforts of Professors A. Fessard and H. Jasper, this goal was included in the UNESCO program and soon led to the birth of the International Brain Research Organization (IBRO). One immediate consequence for myself was an invitation to visit the United States and to participate in a conference in some respects analogous to the Gagra meetings.

Conference on Central Nervous System and Behavior

I was invited by the Josiah Macy Jr. Foundation to take part in the second conference of the Central Nervous System and Behavior series. This series of 5 yearly conferences was attended by a stable group of about 20 prominent scientists who were each year joined by an additional 10 visitors invited to report on topics relevant to the program. I had to speak about reversible decortication and behavior, V. S. Rusinov spoke about manifestations of conditioning in the human EEG, and E. Grastyan spoke about hippocampus and conditioning. An unusual feature of the Macy conferences was the stress placed on the discussion between the participants. The organizers believed that formal talks taking 90% of the time at standard conferences gave the speakers too much influence on the course of the conference. To give the audience a better opportunity to influence the conference program, it was recommended that the main talk be interrupted by questions, objections, and comments. It was hoped that in this way it would be possible to direct the attention of the conference to problems more important than those covered by the speaker. Although this expectation was not always confirmed, the approach led to rapid clarification of controversial points and increased attention by the audience. In fact, the lecture sometimes resembled a cross-examination in a courtroom rather than a scientific discourse, but the moderator usually succeeded in giving the speaker enough time for presentation of the main points of his talk. This can be quantitatively documented by my talk that was interrupted 94 times by 13 discussants, among whom the most active ones were Jim Olds, Paul MacLean, Frank Fremont-Smith, Dominick Purpura, and Karl Pribram. I learned from this form of discussion how many inaccuracies and ambiguities were present in my presentation and how important it was to try to reduce their frequency. I also found how superficial my preparation was for entering new areas of research (e.g., the anatomical and functional relations of neocortex and the hippocampal formation) and how important it was to lay firm ground to study the morphological boundaries of SD.

After the conference I was given an extremely well selected and efficiently organized tour through neuroscience centers related to my research interests. During four weeks I had the opportunity to visit the following places: the laboratories of H. C. Magoun and J. D. Green at the University of California, Los Angeles; the laboratories of R. W. Sperry and A. van Harreveld at the California Institute of Technology, Pasadena; the laboratory of J. L. O'Leary at Washington University, St. Louis; the laboratory of Jim Olds at the University of Michigan, Ann Arbor; Xavier University,

Cincinnati; the laboratory of R. E. Myers, Walter Reed Army Institute, Washington, DC; the laboratory of W. H. Marshall at the National Institutes of Health, Bethesda; and the laboratories of H. Jasper and D. L. Burns at McGill University, Montreal. Particularly important for me was the opportunity to meet the leaders of contemporary SD research, Marshall and Van Harreveld, as well as other scientists who had made important contributions to the field (Burns and O'Leary). This formed a safe basis for future contacts based on personal friendship. Not less important was the opportunity to establish contacts with Sperry and his former student Myers, whose split brain work we tried to replicate and to expand in our reversible split brain studies. The one-week visit to Jim Olds started an intercontinental collaboration examining the influence of cortical SD on self-stimulation of various subcortical motivation centers. The resulting paper (Bures et al., 1961), the electrophysiological part of which was done in Prague and the behavioral part in Ann Arbor, led to the conclusion that cortical operant mechanisms are greatly suppressed during SD and that this effect blocks all approach behavior and the operant components of aversive behavior.

My trip to America had not only scientific, but also political aspects. The possibility of meeting a large sample of American scientists and discussing with them not only science but also everyday social and economical problems of the world convinced me that political confrontation of East and West is counterproductive and that it is necessary to seek goals on which the two systems can agree. A similar attitude was shared by many American colleagues. Perhaps this was best expressed in a joke often told by Frank Fremont Smith, who suggested that when seeking a slogan which would be acceptable to all races, religions, and political factions, it is best to start with a moral that is understandable even to animals. According to his opinion, the best slogan corresponding to such criteria is "Kids are O.K." He believed that exchange visits of large samples of the young population between countries may considerably improve international relationships. Something confirming this view happened during my short visit to Xavier University, the purpose of which was not quite clear to me, because no SD-related research was conducted there. I was asked, however, to explain to the biology students, assembled in a large lecture hall, what research I was doing, what its purpose was, and what benefits it may bring to people. I did my best, stressing the importance of biomedical research and the hope it brings to patients and to their families. In a subsequent discussion I answered a dozen questions concerning university education, medical care, social conditions, financing of research, etc. After the lecture, the professor who had introduced me explained how happy he was to have me as a living example of the fact that people on the other side of the Iron Curtain are much the same as here, have similar problems, and try to use the same means to solve them. Since Xavier University is one of the Jesuit Universities in the United States and he was a priest, his statement impressed me as a sincere expression of a feeling of the need to overcome the antagonisms of a bipolar world by belief in the force of common human values.

Second International Meeting of Neurobiologists, Amsterdam, 1959

The series of meetings started in Gagra in 1958 was concluded in the autumn of 1959 in Amsterdam by a conference on Structure and Function of the Cerebral Cortex to which I was invited to deliver a talk about metabolic aspects of SD. The paper summarized the chemical substances, the local application of which elicited SD, and the metabolic interventions (anoxia, hypoglycemia) facilitating subthreshold SD-evoking stimuli and described biochemical changes occurring in the cortical regions invaded by SD. Among the discussants were B. Grafstein, A. Van Harreveld, and McIllwain.

The First Book

The first years of electrophysiological research performed with limited access to expert instruction forced all students working in Servit's department to read very carefully the technique sections of the articles they used as the basis for their planned experiments. Of course, quite often we were not able to get some important detail and then had to go to other papers of the same author or had to try a different approach that was described in a more accurate and reliable way. Sometimes it was easier to substitute the missing information by trying a tentative solution that mostly did not work as expected, but helped us understand the theoretical principles involved. All these efforts were informally discussed among three technically minded investigators, M. Petran, J. Zachar, and myself. Petran was an expert in physics and electronics, Zachar was an expert in the muscle and peripheral nerve electrophysiology, and I specialized in electrochemistry and electrophysiology of the central nervous system. After five years of collaboration, we came to the conclusion that the experience we had accumulated in the course of our work could be described in a book, which might serve as an introduction to electrophysiology for graduate students and biomedical researchers. The idea was to write a book that would combine the necessary technical information with detailed description of individual experiments to be performed, covering the principles involved, apparatus and material, animal preparation, procedure, results, and their interpretation. Muralt's *Practical Physiology* for medical students served as an example of a similar book. It was required that the simple experiments be described at a level guaranteeing reproducible results.

After we decided to write and agreed on the general plan of the book, we started to explore the possibility of its publication. Our first choice was Academia, the publishing house of the Academy of Sciences, which was supposed to publish scientific monographs coming from the institutes of the Academy. A preliminary assessment of the proposed manuscript was done by the publication committee, which was chaired by the Vice President of the Academy, Professor V. Laufberger. He rejected the original plan to write the book in Czech because according to his opinion "nobody will read such a book written in Czech" and suggested to Academia that they offer an English version to foreign publishers interested in possible co-editions of attractive titles. He probably liked our cookbook idea of recipes for specific experiments, because he used Muralt's book as a model for his *Practical Physiology*, but I was never sure whether he believed that our book could succeed in international competition or whether he wanted to show three obviously immodest youngsters that they had overestimated their creativity. Surprisingly, Academic Press was interested in a co-edition; we found an English-speaking physiologist, our colleague Peter Hahn, to serve as translator and language editor and two anatomists from the Medical Faculty of the Charles University in Prague, Eva Fifkova and Josef Marsala, to serve as authors of sterotaxic atlases of the brains of rat, rabbit, and cat, which would form a part of the book. The book was ready for publication in 1959 and appeared simultaneously in Prague and in New York in 1960.

In the last year before publication, we wanted to obtain preliminary reviews of various chapters of the book from experts familiar with the subject. While in most cases we got very positive comments and constructive recommendations, some of our invited advisors tried to dissuade us from writing the book. One of them was Professor H. Grundfest, who read during a short stay in Prague several chapters and told us in subsequent discussion that he appreciated very much our effort, but believed that the experiments could be described much better by more experienced scientists who were sensitive to possible pitfalls and who could provide wider interpretation of the results. Needless to say, we were rather worried by such outspoken skepticism. We tried to explain that it was not our intention to write a fundamental treatise, but a practical handbook which would summarize the minimum information necessary for running typical experiments. We hoped that the readers would decide whether this form was what they wanted. And the readers did. The book was sold out in a year. A new printing was published in 1962, and an extended new edition was published in 1967. A Russian translation appeared in 1962 in a huge number of copies. A year later the book was translated into Chinese and published 3200 copies.

Countless discussions with the readers revealed the most probable reasons for the popularity of the book. The students usually stressed the fact that the book contained the information sufficient for simple experiments that are easy to do and that correspond well to their interests. The teachers using the book in practical courses asked the students to follow the book and to contact their instructors only when something does not work as expected. They believed that the book not only saved their time, but that independent attempts of the students to find the correct solution considerably improved their understanding of the problem.

Research Orientation in the 1960s

The series of conferences was followed by a more quiet period in 1960. Contacts with French colleagues led to invitations to two interesting symposia in 1961. One was concerned with audiogenic epilepsy, a field I had left almost 10 years ago, but for me it was the first opportunity to discuss my results with colleagues who could give me useful advice. The second Conference on the Physiology of Hippocampus, organized in August 1961 in Montpellier, corresponded more to my current interests. It was attended by a number of leading specialists I had met earlier (Albe-Fessard, Fessard, Gastaut, Grastyan, Jasper, Lissak, MacLean, and Marshall). I appreciated the talks by Per Andersen, Brenda Milner, and Eric Kandel and the informal discussions with them. Since I knew Kandel's paper (Brinley, Kandel, and Marshall, 1960) on the role of potassium ions in the mechanism of SD, I asked about his further plans and was surprised by his decision to leave not only the SD research but also the promising electrophysiology of hippocampus described in his contribution to the conference and to start investigations of the plastic changes underlying learning in the simple nervous system of the *Aplysia.*

In January 1962, I participated in the Fourth Gagra Conference with a talk describing the use of cortical SD in rats for the study of the tonic influences of the neocortex on the subcortical centers. Further results of this research were reported in September 1962 on the XXII International Physiological Congress in Leyden, Netherlands, where our group contributed three papers (delivered by Bures, Buresova, and Weiss) describing the effect of cortical SD on spontaneous unit activity and evoked responses in thalamic and hypothalamic centers. In March 1963, I was invited by the British Biological Council to the symposium Animal Behavior and Drug Action, taking place in London. In my talk I reviewed results of our experiments describing the effect of atropine and physostigmine on EEC activity and on the acquisition and retrieval of the passive avoidance reaction. After the end of the symposium, most of the participants were invited to continue the discussion in a Ciba symposium that, among other things, paid attention to the possible use of SD as a functional ablation procedure in pharmacological experiments. From late August to early October, due to an invitation of the American Psychological Association, I spent almost seven weeks in the United States, where I attended the XVIIth International Congress of Psychology in Washington, the 71st Annual Meeting of the American Psychological Association in Philadelphia, and the First Conference on Learning, Remembering, and Forgetting in Princeton. At the International Congress, I gave in the symposium Neurophysiology of Learning, organized by R. Galambos, a lecture "Functional Dissection of the Mechanisms of Learning," which was discussed in detail by Larry Weiskrantz. In the intervals between the above meetings I visited, according to a plan carefully prepared by my hosts, a number of neuroscience laboratories in Bethesda, Boston, Cambridge, Providence, New Haven, New York, Rochester, and Houston. The most important new contacts established were with Professor H.-L. Teuber and his group (Chorover, Schiller, and Altman); Dr. Gerstein at MIT; David Hubel and Torsten Wiesel at the Harvard Medical School in Boston; Pfaffman at the Brown University, Providence; Neal Miller at Yale University; and Professor Roy John at Rochester.

The international conference Reflexes of the Brain organized by the Soviet Academy of Sciences and by the IBRO to celebrate the 100-year anniversary of the publication of Sechenov's book of the same name was the last important meeting of the year. Our contribution described the progress made by applying SD to the analysis of the mechanisms of conditioning. I paid special attention to the boundaries of SD propagation, to the duration of unit inactivity during an SD episode, and to the possibility of disrupting conditioned responses seen in the activity of subcortical neurons by cortical SD. Unlike the case of the Moscow colloquium, SD was discussed in two other papers by Meshcherski and Narikashvili, who worked on rabbits and cats, respectively. This led to disagreement about results concerning the effect of cortical SD on evoked responses in specific thalamic nuclei, probably due to incomplete invasion of different cortical layers in cats and rabbits. International recognition of our group was manifested in 1962 by my election to the Central Council of the IBRO. The fact that I was elected as a member at large by postal ballot of the IBRO membership probably reflected publications in journals and participation in international conferences attended by the IBRO members.

The next year, 1965, was very busy. It started with the symposium "Cortico-Subcortical Relationships in Sensory Regulation" organized in February in Havana by the Academy of Sciences of Cuba for 30 participants from 13 countries. We contributed two papers, one describing the use of thalamic SD as a tool for differentiation of cerebral cortex by thalamic spreading depression and the other describing the modulation of reactions of colliculus inferior neurons to acoustic stimuli by changes in their spontaneous firing rate by polarization or by microelectrophoretic application of glutamate. After the conference, I was asked by the local organizers to come next year to deliver a practical course in electrophysiology to a group of graduate students. We made a plan for the course and agreed on technical requirements (apparatus, laboratory space) for it. On September 1 the 23rd International Congress of Physiological Sciences in Tokyo began, and in the symposium "Neural Mechanisms of Conditioned Reflex and Behavior," I delivered a paper on conditioning of isolated neurons by using direct stimulation of the recorded cell as the unconditioned stimulus (Bures and Buresova, 1965).

I also participated as a discussant in the symposium "Structure and Function of the Limbic System" which took place in Hakone from September 10 to September 20. An unexpected bonus to the trip to Japan was an unplanned week-long stay in Cambodia: due to the war between India and Pakistan we had to wait one week for a connecting flight to Europe in Phnom Penh, and this gave us a marvelous opportunity to visit Angkor Vat and other jewels of Indochina architecture.

In 1966, after participation in the Fifth Meeting of the Collegium Internationale Neuro-Psychopharmacologicum in Washington and after a series of lectures in the United States and a brief visit to Mexico, I arrived in Havana to organize the electrophysiology course for graduate students. During 2 weeks we collected the necessary equipment, formed teams of instructors, and arranged demonstration stations for the eight themes of the course. With Dr. Aquino-Cias, who worked for a year in our laboratory in Prague, we first trained two instructors for each of the following themes: electromyography and electrocardiography, normal and epileptic EEC activity, evoked responses to sensory stimuli and event-related potentials, stimulation of cortex and callosal responses, slow potentials— spreading depression, slow potentials—anoxic depolarization, unit activity in reticular formation, and hippocampal population spike elicited by perforant path stimulation. After everything was prepared, the 20 course participants were divided into 8 groups with 2 to 3 students each and rotated during 8 days through the 8 themes. This arrangement gave each student enough time to perform the whole experiment, to understand its biological and technical aspects, as well as to evaluate the results obtained. After conclusion of the experiments, the students were asked to identify the most difficult aspects of the individual methods, and various alternatives were discussed and, if necessary, demonstrated. The course showed that even with simple equipment it is possible to demonstrate almost all basic methods of contemporary electrophysiology to a relatively large audience. I have used this experience when participating in similar courses in Yugoslavia (1969), Chile (1971), and Poland (1984).

The busy contacts with the United States continued also in 1967 and in 1968, when I was invited by Jim McGaugh to attend one of his first Irvine conferences. Everything looked optimistic. In the introduction of my talk entitled "The Reunified Split Brain" (Bures and Buresova, 1970a) about communication between the two halves of the vertebrate brain, I compared the world divided by political, economical, and ideological barriers to a split brain preparation and expressed the hope that the reversible split brain technique, which can be used to restore coordinated activity between the two temporarily separated halves of the brain, will inspire politicians, economists, and philosophers to seek an analogous solution for our planet. Unfortunately, my incurable optimism proved to be wrong. Shortly after my return from the United States, in the first hours of August 21, we received a phone call from a co-worker of our Institute informing us that the Soviet army had begun the invasion of Czechoslovakia. We turned on the television and radio, trying to understand what had happened and how we could cope with the situation. Our 19-year-old daughter Olga, a student of mathematics, was an au pair girl and safe in London and thus was far from any local dangers. We had two foreign guests with small children in the laboratory: Lynn Nadel with Melissa (4 years) and Kenny (3 years) and Takanori Ookawa with his wife and 1-year-old Makiko. We advised them to leave the country as soon as possible and to wait in Western Europe until the situation clarified. While Lynn packed his family in a big van and drove to the German border over highways crowded by Soviet tanks, two days later Takanori joined a transport to Germany organized by the American Embassy for the many foreigners stranded in Prague. The streets were full of protesting people and Russian soldiers, tanks, and armored cars. Fighting started around some strategic buildings, and the Soviet army showed its resolve to use all force available to suppress the protests. The leaders of the Czechoslovak Communist Party were arrested by the Russian army and imprisoned in the Soviet Union. The Czechoslovak parliament was in session, passing resolutions protesting against the Soviet occupation, but could contact the population only through illegal radio transmission because it had no access to the official media. The situation in the Institute was desperate. Many scientists contemplated the possibility of leaving the country and staying abroad. I was, as was Olga, a member of the Communist Party since the first months after the war. We were not happy with all that had happened in our country under the communist regime, but we hoped that a more liberal policy would finally bring our part of the world the so much expected freedom we craved for during the war. The development in the 1960s that culminated in the Prague spring of 1968 seemed to indicate that such a process was underway, but the intervention of the Soviet Union showed us clearly that the liberal intellectuals had no hope to realize their dreams. However, going abroad did not appear to be correct. After the war, we wanted to do something positive for our country. To leave it now, in its time of need, seemed to be treason. We decided to stay as long as we had an opportunity to continue our research. This was a naive decision, because we did not take into account that the possibility of leaving the country, which would have been very easy in 1968, would become very difficult a year later. But in the long run, we feel that it was the correct decision. It gave us the opportunity to see life from a different point of view and to test the assumption that our position in science does not depend on political mafias and on our servile attitude toward them, but only on the output of our brains and hands.

Of course, the consequences of the Soviet invasion for our science did not develop abruptly. Foreign travel was free in 1968 and almost free in 1969. During this time I could still visit Cuba; lecture in Switzerland, Netherlands, Belgium, and Germany; teach together with Olga in an IBRO course in

Kotor, Yugoslavia; give a talk (Bures and Buresova, 1970b) at the symposium "Short-Term Processes in Neural Activity and Behavior," organized by Gabriel Horn in Cambridge; and attend the XlXth Psychological Congress in London where I organized with Olga the symposium "Split-Brain Function." However, the latter Congress marked for us the last opportunity to give an invited talk in the West for a period of 18 years, i.e., up to 1987. I was still allowed to visit Great Britain in 1970 on a commercial trip, the purpose of which was to demonstrate an invention (apparatus for early identification of fertilized eggs) and to accept an invitation from the University of Valparaiso, Chile, to organize a course of electrophysiology for graduate students in 1971. After this trip, the door to the West was completely locked. We were ousted from the Communist Party, because we did not agree with the Soviet occupation of our country. We were considered hostile elements who could perhaps be allowed to do some research provided that we were carefully watched by loyal superiors. This was clearly demonstrated in the case of Olga, who was at the time Associate Professor of Physiological Psychology at the Philosophical Faculty of the Charles University. She was removed from all teaching activities at the University, but was allowed to continue her research in the Academy.

Strategy of Isolated Scientists

We anticipated the reduction of foreign travel from the moment of the Soviet invasion and considered various strategies for maintaining our output in spite of the marked reduction in our contacts with international research. The classical defense plan was to maintain the flow of publications coming from the laboratory and to replace our visits abroad by maintaining a stable flux of visitors coming to work in Prague. Fortunately, we were not fired. I even remained head of the laboratory until 1981, when the pressure on the non-loyal scientists paradoxically increased and this position was given to a younger member of our group, our good friend Gustav Brozek. Worse was the situation of Olga, who in 1982 reached the retirement age of 58 years. Although scientists could postpone retirement until 65, the new director of the Institute insisted on her immediate retirement and formal appeals to the President of the Academy, Academician Riman, pointing out the discriminative nature of this decision, were ignored. Olga continued to work as before, but was paid only for a part-time job, although she remained one of the most productive scientists in the Institute.

Aside from the above demonstrations of administrative arrogance, there were no attempts to change the orientation of our research, the funding of which remained stable. This was advantageous for us, because in the yearly reviews of the productivity of individual departments we could report the low cost of a primary publication. The Academy started to explore the possibility of quantitative evaluation of the output of different laboratories and individual scientists using Garfield's scientometric criteria. Each published paper was multiplied by the impact factor (IF) of the journal, expressing the expected citation rate of the article in the future. The IF values were about 0.5 for *Physiologia Bohemoslovaca*, 3.0 for *Brain Research*, and 15.0 for *Nature*. The sum of the IF weighted values of papers published in different laboratories was proportional not only to the number of articles, but mainly to their IF ranking. This increased considerably the rating of laboratories publishing their results in good foreign journals. Finally, we could retain foreign funding obtained from Western countries in support of specific projects. This was quite important in this period, because in 1969 we obtained from Foundations' Fund for Research in Psychiatry a grant of $28,000 for a laboratory computer LINC 8 which made us independent from the classical LINC owned by the Institute.

Visiting Scientists

It was less clear how the Soviet invasion would influence the number of visiting scientists who formed the main work force of the laboratory. We could only extrapolate from the experience we had so far. While the first paper resulting from collaboration with a visiting scientist was published in 1955 (Bures and Koshtoyants, 1955), next collaborative studies appearing in 1961 were produced by scientists coming from the Soviet Union who were joined in 1962 by visitors from East Germany and later from other East Block countries in Central Europe. Some of them were coming for long-term stays equivalent to Ph.D. training or to a comparable university degree in their countries. Dr. W. Ruediger from the Humboldt University in East Berlin spent 2 years in Prague to prepare his Habilitation based on analysis of the effect of cortical SD in conscious rats on unit activity, excitability, and functional state of the hypothalamic and mesencephalic motivation centers. Visitors from other socialist countries were coming for shorter stays (usually two to three months), depending on the funds reserved for exchange fellowships to Czechoslovakia in their home countries. During their stay in Prague, they concentrated on the experiments that were eventually finished by other members of the team after their departure. In some cases, they could come the following year to prolong a continuing project. In this way, we gradually established tight working contacts with a group in Rusinov's laboratory in the Institute of Higher Nervous Activity and Neurophysiology in Moscow, working on SD (G.D. Kuznetsova and V.I. Koroleva). This collaboration generated almost 20 papers over the years. Similar close contacts with Konorski's group in Warsaw (I. Lukaszewska, A. Markowska, and M. Wesierska) led to experiments using SD-induced functional decortication and other forms of reversible ablation in behavioral research.

Another opportunity for financial support of visiting scientists opened in the UNESCO-sponsored fellowships for potential applicants from developing countries. The Biological institutes of the Academy offered 10 such fellowships each year and our laboratory was among those advertised. We got one applicant from Japan in 1962/1963 (I. Shima), one from Mexico in 1963/1964 (E. Roldan), and another from Cuba in 1965/1966 (J. Aquino-Cias). Shima studied SD in pigeons—the boundaries of spread and effects on unit activity (the affected parts of the striatum and remote brain structures, behavioral consequences of striatal SD). Roldan examined electrophysiology of sleep in rats (sleep cycle, neocortical and hipocampal EEG, REM sleep manifestations). Aquino-Cias explored the effects of thalamic spreading depression on the spread of epileptic afterdischarge, on caudate spindles, and on other integrative phenomena.

Visitors from developed Western countries (United States, Canada, and Australia) started to come in late 1960s, some for regular postdoctoral stays with fellowships paid for by the NIH and others for the shorter periods covered by various foundations. The first was Chuck Woody from W.H. Marshall's laboratory' who came to Prague in 1967/1968 to study the effect of SD on the conditioned eye blink elicited in cats by the glabella tap and introduced us to the use of computers for processing the electrophysiological data. At the same time, Lynn Nadel arrived with his family. He worked on interocular and interhemispheric transfer in rats and published a series of papers on the subject.

As expected, the number of papers co-authored annually by visitors from the Soviet Union and from other East Block countries dropped from 6.1 in the preinvasion period (1963–1967) to 0.25 in 1968–1971, it rose to 1.25 in 1972–1975 and to 3.25 in 1976–1979, and attained the preinvasion level by reaching the value 6.5 in 1980–1983. On the other hand, papers co-authored annually by visiting scientists from other parts of the world rose from 3.1 in the preinvasion period to 11.0 in 1968–1971, decreased to 5.25 in 1972–1975, and stabilized at the level of 3–4 in the 1980s. It was obvious that the reduced number of visitors from Eastern Block countries was due to administrative restrictions limiting travel to the dissident country in order to limit the possible spread of the dissent. It took the Soviet authorities almost 10 years to abandon this inadequate strategy and to start a kind of reform. Gorbachev's "perestroika" came too late, however, to prevent the avalanche collapse of the Eastern Block and of the Soviet Union. From the point of view of our laboratory, the Soviet decision not to allow their scientists to work in Prague was regrettable, but did not interfere with our work. The total number of visitors was not reduced, but the output was substantially increased. Among the guests were first-class researchers (Chuck Woody, Lynn Nadel, Joe Huston, Dave Megirian, Joel Davis, Ian Steele Russell, Bert Siegfried, Hans Welzl, Masaaki Shibata, Takashi Amemori, Nelson Freedman, Bruno de Luca, S. J. Dimond, Andy Greenshaw, George Gerstein, Mitchell Glickstein, Walter Freeman, and many others) who accelerated the progress of our work and continued to collaborate with us afterwards. However, the most important result was the moral boost given to us by the international neuroscience community whose delegates came to be with us in a difficult time. The fact that all the foreign guests from the United States, Canada, Great Britain, Australia, Japan, Switzerland, Italy, and other countries got visas indicates that the government tried to avoid the impression that it blocked international collaboration in science. The practical result was that those of us who could not travel to the West were not completely cut off from contacts with Western science whose delegates were permanently present in Prague.

While the above considerations indicated that our work could go on as earlier, we decided to concentrate our effort on behavior. The name of the laboratory was changed to the Laboratory of Neurophysiology of Memory. SD research continued as a prototype of the functional ablation technique, but was supplemented by other reversible inactivations induced by pharmacological and physical factors. We decided to add conditioned taste aversion (CTA), motor learning, and spatial memory to the behavioral models studied. We finished the search for the role of potassium ions in the mechanisms of SD and anoxic depolarization by demonstrating with potassium-selective microelectrodes an increase of extracellular potassium to 70–90 mM. In 1989, this paper (Vyskocil, Kriz, and Bures, 1972), made possible by our colleague Pavel Hnik, who brought from Salt Lake City to Prague the first specimens of the potassium electrodes based on the Corning ion exchanger, was identified by Current Contents as a citation classic. My visit to the laboratory of Aristides Leao in Rio de Janeiro on my return from Chile gave me the opportunity to see SD in the *in vitro* preparation of the chicken retina (H. Martins-Ferreira) and to use it for the visualization of the circulating SD demonstrated earlier in the cerebral cortex of rats (Shibata and Bures, 1972). The circling retinal SD (Gorelova and Bures, 1983) entered SD into the list of synergetic phenomena.

During the IBRO course in Kotor, Olga and I met Professor John Garcia, the discoverer of CTA. After hearing his lecture, we were immediately impressed by the exceptional properties of the phenomenon: separation of the gustatory CS and of the visceral US by an interval of up to several hours did not disrupt CTA learning, although standard CS–US associations do not survive CS–US delays exceeding a few seconds. Still more puzzling was the fact that CTA was acquired even when the US (administration of the toxin), but not the CS, was applied under deep anesthesia. It seemed that the above CTA properties were ideally suited for examination with the functional ablation methods. We started with the CTA experiments in 1971, and soon found out that CTA learning is prevented by bilateral cortical SD elicited before the CS but not before the US administration. This suggested participation of neocortex in CS processing, but not in CS storage or in the formation of the CS–US association (Buresova and Bures, 1973, 1974). Further analysis indicated the parabrachial nucleus (PBN) of the brain stem as the locus of the CS trace–US association (Ivanova and Bures, 1990). Combination of unilateral functional decortication and unilateral TTX blockade of PBN prevents CTA learning when applied to different halves of the brain, but not when applied to the same side of the brain (Gallo and Bures, 1991). This result suggests that CTA acquisition requires interaction of the cerebral cortex with PBN through ipsilateral pathways. Our CTA research was summarized in a review chapter (Bures and Buresova, 1977) and in two books (Bures, Buresova and Krivanek, 1988; Bures, Bermudez-Rattoni, and Yamamoto, 1998).

Another field we wanted to extend was motor learning. Our behavioral experiments were mostly based on active or passive avoidance tasks and on aversively or appetitively motivated discrimination learning. We hoped that training rats to master motor skills controlled by specific motor centers might simplify electrophysiological and morphological analysis of the neural networks supporting this behavior. We started by forcing the rat to reach deep into a narrow horizontal tube at the end of which was a small food pellet or by releasing the pellet only when the photoelectrically recorded forelimb extension exceeded the preset criterion time (Zhuravin and Bures, 1986). Later, we were attracted by licking, another small movement that occurs during the consumption of liquids and that is generated by rats at a very constant frequency of about 6 Hz. We attempted to slow it down to about 4 Hz using a retractable spout that was removed after each lick beyond the reach of the animal's tongue and returned back only at an interval corresponding to the 4 Hz frequency of licking (Hernandez-Mesa et al., 1985). Rats eventually learned to lick slower, but it took several weeks of training and tedious elimination of various faked solutions (e.g., 3-Hz licking produced by alternation of large amplitude licks detected by the photoelectric lick sensor and short licks that remained unrecognized). Finally, we trained rats more complex skilled movements requiring development of a new synergy between functionally unrelated effectors, e.g., between the tongue and forepaw (Brozek and Bures, 1991). After each lick, the retractable spout was removed by the computer and was returned to the accessible position when the rat pressed and released a bar located under the spout. After several weeks of training, the rats learned to produce this complex movement in a way supporting uninterrupted licking, i.e., with a phase shift of about 180 dg between licking and bar pressing. This indicated that the generator of licking in the reticular formation triggers not only the movements of the tongue, but that training connected it also to the centers controlling the bar pressing forepaw.

In the late 1970s we were deeply influenced by the renaissance of animal cognition, both at the theoretical level (O'Keefe and Nadel, 1978) and at the experimental level (radial maze—Olton and Samuelson, 1976; water maze—Morris, 1981). We were excited by the new experimental possibilities and started immediately experimenting with the homemade versions of the devices. Our first paper on the radial maze technique (Magni, Krekule, and

Bures, 1979) used a two-level apparatus in which an animal exiting from the visited arm had to descend to the floor, return below the 5-cm-elevated central platform, and climb through a central hole to start a new choice. The obligatory return to the same starting point precluded response chaining. Our first paper on the Morris water maze (Buresova et al., 1985) already used an interactive computer tracking system that raised the submerged escape platform only after the rat had spent a continuous criterion interval (1–5 sec) in the goal area. Use of this "on demand platform" eliminated the possibility of accidental detection of the hidden goal during randomly oriented swims. Later experiments concentrated on the capacity and persistence of working memory and on the physiological and pharmacological interventions disrupting the navigation performance.

Some of the above behavioral tasks were used for electrophysiological analysis. Particularly well suited for this purpose were the handedness experiments when the almost immobile rat reaching into the feeder allowed recording of units from motor cortex, basal ganglia, and cerebellum and off-line analysis of the records. Periresponse histograms of unit activity, in the motor cortex and cerebellar dentate nucleus ipsilateral to the reaching forepaw, showed clear peaks starting 100–150 msec before reach detection, but culminating in the dentate nucleus about 60 msec earlier than in the motor cortex. Perireach histograms in the contralateral caudate nucleus were characterized by an earlier and more prolonged excitation (Dolbakyan et al., 1977; Hernandez-Mesa and Bures, 1978; Moroz and Bures, 1982). A similar approach used in the analysis of unit responses of CTA-trained rats to presentation of the drinking spout containing the aversive taste stimulus revealed inhibition starting 100–150 msec after stimulus onset in the gustatory cortex, amygdala, and ventromedial hypothalamus and an excitatory response appearing about 100 msec later in the lateral hypothalamus (Buresova et al., 1979).

Finally, one activity that could be expected to be possible even under the most difficult conditions was writing books. We had hoped to write manuals for behavioral research and for the use of computers in neuroscience similar to the successful "Electrophysiological Methods." At the same time, we wanted to write a monograph about SD and another one about our approach to the neural mechanisms of behavior. The book *The Mechanism and Applications of Leao's Spreading Depression of EEG Activity* by J. Bures, O. Buresova, and J. Krivanek was almost prepared already in 1972, but its publication was delayed by the fact that one of the potential co-authors, Eva Fifkova, stayed illegally in the United States and we were not allowed to have her name among the authors. It was published by Academia in coedition with Academic Press in 1974. The manual *Techniques and Basic Experiments for the Study of Brain and Behavior* by J. Bures, O. Buresova, and J. P. Huston was published in 1976 by Elsevier. It was rapidly sold out, and the second revised and enlarged edition appeared in 1983. Its Russian translation, published in 1991 by the publishing house Vysshaya shkola, had 13,000 copies. The second manual, *Practical Guide to Computer Applications in Neuroscience*, was published in 1982 by Academia in co-edition with Wiley. It was based on a two-week workshop organized by our Institute in 1973 for researchers interested in biomedical applications of computers. The workshop included 40 hr of programming at the computer console, and the participants appreciated the opportunity to learn basic programming skills and to understand simple programs. This book was also translated into Russian and published in 1984 by the publishing house Nauka. The last book appearing in this period was *Brain and Behavior: Paradigms for Research in Neural Mechanisms* by J. Bures, O. Buresova, and J. Krivanek, published again by Academia in co-edition with Wiley. It was an attempt to describe our experience in several areas of experimental research in the context of contemporary science and to call attention to potentially significant solutions of new problems. This book did not cover our spatial memory research.

Back to Freedom

Fifteen years after the Soviet occupation of Czechoslovakia, the situation started to change. Foreign travel became easier even for the unreliable elements; a number of known dissidents were asked to leave the country or were allowed to go abroad with the hope that they would not return or that it would be possible to refuse them a reentry permit. Because I reached retirement age in 1986, restrictions on my exit permits were considerably alleviated. It was believed that a retired citizen who decides to stay illegally abroad will do a positive service to the country, because he will draw no pension.

In 1987 my eligibility for foreign travel was tested by Jim McGaugh's invitation to his "Third Conference on the Neurobiology of Learning and Memory" held in UCI Irvine on October 14–17, 1987. I obtained a permit to leave Czechoslovakia and stay for a month in the United States. I opened the meeting with a keynote address entitled "Neurobiology of Memory: Significance of Anomalous Findings." When Lynn Nadel, who was introducing me to the audience, asked how many people present in the room had been in our laboratory in Prague, more than a dozen hands went up. I was deeply moved by the feeling of being at home with people whom I knew and who knew me. I was reassured that the worst part of the postwar troubles was over for our science and that we would be able to continue from the point where our development was interrupted in 1968. Other invitations followed: in 1987 from Joe Huston to Duesseldorf; in 1988 from Mitchell Glickstein to University College London, from Richard Morris to Edinburgh, from Hans Welzl to Zurich and to the Neuropharmacological Congress in Athens, and from Professor Gispen to Rotterdam; in 1989 from Steve Rose to the European Science Foundation meeting in Sicily, and from Professor Cioffi for teaching at the University of Naples and lecturing at the Italian Congress of Physiology in Firenze. Note that all these trips took place before the Prague Velvet Revolution in November 1989. In 1990, the first free year, I was invited to a short conference in London, to an SD symposium in Brazil, and for a two-month stay in the laboratory of Professor Taketoshi Ono in Toyama University, Toyama, Japan. The frequency of invitations remained stable in the following years. The particularly memorable ones were to the University of Lethbridge, where I received an honorary doctorate in 1992; to the National Academy of Sciences (NAS) annual meeting in 1996 for inauguration as a foreign associate; participation in several meetings of the governing council of the IBRO to which I had been reelected by postal ballot in 1992; meetings of the Central Council of the European Neuroscience Association (ENA), which I was a member of in the years 1992–1999; and a meeting of the Brazilian Academy of Sciences, where I delivered a speech in honor of A. A. P. Leao, commemorating a year since his death.

There were other memorable moments that I remember well. One of them was a completely unexpected wire received on April 25, 1995, from the members of the NAS section 52 congratulating me on my election to NAS. I could not believe it, and only a phone call from Jim McGaugh (chairman of section 52) convinced me that this really happened. I felt deeply honored, but also embarrassed by knowing many colleagues who I believed deserved this distinction more than myself.

The political changes in our country did not influence my position in the Institute. I was 64 years old during the Velvet Revolution and thus too old for an administrative position. Jiri Krivanek became the head of the department, and I continued to work as a research scientist and principal investigator on several grant projects. The Institute agreed to employ me as long as I could get adequate funding and demonstrate corresponding productivity. The present head of the Department of Neurophysiology of Memory is my former student, Andre Fenton, who came as a B.Sc. from McGill University in 1991 to our laboratory to gain some experience in behavioral research. He joined our spatial memory research program and in two years completed four experimental studies dealing with the problem of interhemispheric transfer of lateralized place navigation in rats. He went from Prague to SUNY Brooklyn to become a graduate student of Bob Muller and to learn how to examine place cells. In 1998 he joined our laboratory as a postdoctoral fellow, took full responsibility for the technical and computational development of our place cell research, and significantly extended our behavioral experiments. Two years later, he was appointed head of the Laboratory of Neurophysiology of Memory and in this position became principal investigator of the European Community grant "Network Analysis of Hippocampal Memory Processing" and of a grant of the Grant Agency of the Czech Republic (GACR) "Development of Spatial Memory Tests Suitable for Early Detection of Mnestic Disorders in Neurological and

Psychiatric Disorders." Andre has a unique ability to clearly formulate ideas, rapidly establish personal contacts with colleagues, openly discuss controversial points, and find acceptable solutions. His excellent organizational talent, enabling him to simultaneously supervise a number of independent projects, is best demonstrated by his capacity to head at the same time not only the laboratory in Prague, but also a new laboratory in the Department of Physiology and Pharmacology of the SUNY Downstate Medical Center in Brooklyn. I believe that Andre's example shows that the Czech Academy of Sciences is prepared to open its facilities to foreign scientists who want to continue their research in Prague. Low salaries do not make a scientific career in the Czech Republic financially attractive, but this can be compensated by research traditions, equipped laboratories, trained personnel, and a creative environment. With more foreign scientists working in our institutes, it will be possible to change the somewhat provincial Czech science, pursued almost exclusively by Czechs, into Prague science, represented by the multinational community of scientists working in this part of Europe. I hope that this form of "reversed brain drain" may contribute to the rapid growth of strong international research in Central Europe.

In Conclusion

This chapter should probably help young people and their teachers better understand how to become scientists. I am afraid that my contribution is not much helpful in this respect. In fact, I do not believe that scientists can be educated. Somebody who is not curious, who does not feel the challenge of an interesting problem, who is not excited by the possibility of finding ways to solve it, will not become a scientist even when taught by the best teachers. The problem is not to educate scientists, but to find them and to recruit them for research. I considered each of the 100 graduate students and postdoctoral fellows I have supervised during 50 years of research not pupils but co-workers, who are fully entitled to influence the project with their ideas, technical innovations, and unorthodox interpretations. I hate the deprecatory comments that refuse the opinions of young, inexperienced people because they are "immature." This probably reflects long-term memories of my youth, when an entire generation of young scientists in Prague was clearly immature but nevertheless had entered science quite successfully. Perhaps the reason was the absence of authorities and the lack of hierarchical organization in the ruins of science that survived the war. The fact that the immature people were nevertheless able to build the new Czech science and that many of them who emigrated to West Europe and North America attained professorial positions in the Western academic system suggests that immaturity may be not a drawback but an advantage—open-minded views, less stereotyped thinking, imaginative plans. An excellent teacher, who always knows the best answer to any question, may exert an inhibitory influence on the creativity of his or her students.

Although I had few formal teachers who influenced the development of my scientific views, there were probably hundreds of scientists who helped me understand science. The anonymous reviewers of my first papers written in terrible English who deciphered the content of the message and found it suitable for publication, the unknown poster presenters eager to explain to me the critical tricks of their techniques, the authors of articles who addressed problems of interest to our group in a way that opened new perspectives for our research—these people were and are my teachers to whom I feel greatly indebted. I am trying to pay my debt back by doing the same services for other people who expect them: I am reviewing about 50 papers per year, visitors of our lab can see any technical details they are interested in, and I speak and write openly about all plans and ideas currently used in our research.

Of course there are people who are directly responsible for some important features of my personality—my mother who introduced me to the magic world of books; my brother, Charles, who supported me during my high school studies; my wife Olga who has been for more than 50 years my spouse and my closest partner in science; our daughter Olga who realized my mathematical ambitions by becoming a professor of technical cybernetics in the Czech Technical University in Prague; and our granddaughters Catherine, a neurologist, and Barbara, a lawyer. A bad case of autoimmune polymyositis prevented Olga from continuing experimental research, but she follows closely the activities of the laboratory, translates Dana Foundation documents for the Brain Awareness Week lectures, and firmly directs the activities of our household. We believe that a couple sharing one intact immune and motor system (mine) and one system with superb organizational capacities (her) can live an interesting and happy life, and we are doing our best to demonstrate it.

Selected Bibliography

Benesova O, Buresova O, Bures J. Die Wirkung des Chlorpromazins und der Glykaemie auf das elektrophysiologisch kontrollierte Ueberleben der Hirnrinde bei verschiedenen Koerpertemperaturen. *Arch Exp Pathol Pharmakol* 1957;231:550–561.

Brinley FJ, Kandel ER, Marshall WH. Potassium outflux from rabbit cortex during spreading depression. *J Neurophysiol* 1960;23:246–256.

Brozek G, Bures J. Synchronisation of tongue and forepaw movements in the rat: A model of instrumental muscle synergy. *Behav Brain Res* 1991;43:29–34.

Bures J. On the question of electrotonic mechanisms in the activity of the central nervous system. The production of spreading depression of EEG activity by electrotonus. *Physiol Bohemosl* 1954a;3:272–287.

Bures J. Direct potential difference between the cerebral hemispheres during the depression of EEG activity in anaesthetized and non-anaesthetized rats. *Physiol Bohemosl* 1954b;3:288–295.

Bures J. Some metabolic aspects of Leao's spreading depression. *J Neurochem* 1956;1:153–158.

Bures J. Ontogenetic development of steady potential differences in cerebral cortex of animals. *EEG Clin Neurophysiol* 1957;9:121–130.

Bures J. Electrophysiological and functional analysis of the audiogenic seizure. In *Psychophysiologie, Neuropharmacologie et Biochimie de la crise audiogene.* Paris: Coll. Int. CNRS No. 112. Edition CNRS, 1963;165–179.

Bures J, Bermudez-Rattoni F, Yamamoto T. *Conditioned taste aversion: Memory of a special kind.* Oxford: Oxford University Press, 1998;178.

Bures J, Buresova O. The question of ionic antagonism in spreading depression. *Physiol Bohemosl* 1956a;5:195–205.

Bures J, Buresova O. A study on the metabolic nature and physiological manifestations of Leao's spreading depression. XXth International Physiology Congress, Abstracts of communications, 1956b;143.

Bures J, Buresova O. Metabolic nature and physiological manifestations of the spreading EEG depression of Leao. *Physiol Bohemosl* 1956c;5(suppl):4–6.

Bures J, Buresova O. Die anoxische Terminal depolarisation als Indicator der Vulnerabilitaet der Grosshirnrinde bei Anoxie und Ischaemie. *Pfluegers Archiv* 1957;264:325–334.

Bures J, Buresova O. Plasticity at the single neurone level. XXIII International Congress of Physiological Sciences, Lectures and Symposia, *Excerpta Medica,* Amsterdam 1965;359–364.

Bures J, Buresova O. The reunified split brain. In Whalen RE, Thompson RF, Verzeano M, Weinberger NM, eds. *The neural control of behavior.* New York: Academic Press, 1970a;211–238.

Bures J, Buresova O. Plasticity in single neurones and neural populations. In Horn G, Hinde RA, eds. *Short-term changes in neural activity and behavior.* Cambridge: Cambridge University Press, 1970b;363–403.

Bures J, Buresova O. Physiological mechanisms of conditioned food aversion. In Milgram NW, Krames L, Alloway TM, eds. *Food aversion learning.* New York: Plenum Press, 1977;219–255.

Bures J, Buresova O, Fifkova E, Olds J, Olds ME, Travis RP. Spreading depression and subcortical drive centers. *Physiol Bohemosl* 1961;10:321–331.

Bures J, Buresova O, Huston JP. *Techniques and basic experiments for the study of brain and behavior.* Amsterdam: Elsevier, 1976;277. Second, revised and enlarged edition, 1983;326. Russian translation, Leningrad: Vysshaya shkola, 1991.

Bures J, Buresova O, Krivanek J. Some metabolic aspects of Leao's spreading cortical depression. In Tower DB, Schade JP, eds. *Structure and function of the cerebral cortex.* Proc. Second Int. Meeting of Neurobiologists. Amsterdam: Elsevier, 1960;257–265.

Bures J, Buresova O, Krivanek, J. *The mechanism and applications of Leao's spreading depression of EEC Activity.* Prague: Academia, and New York: Academic Press, 1974;410.

Bures J, Buresova O, Krivanek J. *Brain and behavior: Paradigms for research in neural mechanisms.* Prague: Academia, and Chichester: Wiley, 1988;304.

Bures J, Buresova O, Zacharova D. The effect of changes in body temperature on spreading EEG depression. *Physiol Bohemosl* 1957;6:454–461.

Bures J, Koshtoyants KhS. The role of the tissue SH-bonds in the initiation of spreading depression of the electrical activity of the cerebral cortex (in Russian). *DAN SSSR* 1955;105:1118–1120.

Bures J, Krekule I, Brozek G. *Practical guide to computer applications in neurosciences.* Prague: Academia, and London: Wiley, 1982;399. Russian translation (*Application of computers in neurophysiological research*), Leningrad: Nauka, 1984;240.

Bures J, Petran M. Estimation of seizure susceptibility by the method of electroconvulsive shock (in Russian). *Physiol Bohemosl* 1952;1:24–37.

Bures J, Petran M, Zachar J. *Electrophysiological methods in biological research.* Prague: Publishing House of the Czechoslovak Academy of Sciences, and New York: Academic Press, 1960;512. Second printing 1962. Third revised edition 1967;824. Russian translation (*Electrophysiological methods of investigation*), Moscow: Izdatelstvo Inostrannoy Literatury, 1962;456. Chinese translation, Shanghai: Scientific Publishers, 1963;398.

Buresova O. The influence of spreading cortical depression on unconditioned and conditioned alimentary reflexes (in Russian). *Physiol Bohemosl* 1956;5:350–358.

Buresova O. Influencing water metabolism by spreading depression. *Physiol Bohemosl* 1957a;6:12–20.

Buresova O. Disturbances in thermoregulation and metabolism as a result of prolonged EEG depression. *Physiol Bohemosl* 1957b;6:369–375.

Buresova O, Aleksanyan ZA, Bures J. Electrophysiological analysis of retrieval of conditioned taste aversion in rats. Unit activity changes in critical brain regions. *Physiol Bohemosl*, 1979;28:525–536.

Buresova O, Bures J. Cortical and subcortical components of the conditioned saccharin aversion. *Physiol Behav* 1973;11:435–439.

Buresova O, Bures J. Functional decortication in the CS-US interval decreases efficiency of taste aversive learning. *Behav Neural Biol* 1974;12:357–364.

Buresova O, Krekule I, Zahalka A, Bures J. On-demand platform improves accuracy of the Morris water maze procedure. *J Neurosci Methods* 1985;15:63–72.

Dolbakyan E, Hernandez-Mesa N, Bures J. Skilled forelimb movements and unit activity in motor cortex and caudate nucleus in rats. *Neuroscience* 1977;2:73–80.

Gallo M, Bures J. Acquisition of conditioned taste aversion in rats is mediated by ipsilateral interaction of cortical and mesencephalic mechanisms. *Neurosci Lett* 1991;133:187–190.

Goldring S, O'Leary JL. Experimentally derived correlates between EEG and steady cortical potentials. *J Neurophysiol* 1951;4:275–288.

Gorelova NA, Bures J. Spiral waves of spreading depression in the isolated chicken retina. *J Neurobiol* 1983;14:353–363.

Grafstein B. Mechanism of spreading cortical depression. *J Neurophysiol* 1956;19: 154–171.

Hernandez-Mesa N, Bures J. Skilled forelimb movements and unit activity of cerebellar cortex and dentate nucleus in rats. *Physiol Bohemosl* 1978;27:199–208.

Hernandez-Mesa N, Mamedov Z, Bures J. Operant control of the pattern of licking in rats. *Exp Brain Res* 1985;58:117–124.

Ivanova SF, Bures J. Acquisition of conditioned taste aversion in rats is prevented by tetrodotoxin blockade of a small midbrain region centered around the parabrachial nuclei. *Physiol Behav* 1990;48:543–549.

Krivanek J. Changes of brain glycogen in the spreading EEG depression of Leao. *J Neurochem* 1958;2:337–343.

Krivanek J, Bures J. Ion shifts during Leao's spreading cortical depression. *Physiol Bohemosl* 1960;9:494–503.

Krivanek J, Bures J, Buresova O. Evidence for a relationship between creatin phosphate level and polarity of cerebral cortex. *Nature* 1958;182:1799.

Leao AAP. Spreading depression of activity in the cerebral cortex. *J Nerophysiol* 1944;7:359–390.

Magni S, Krekule I, Bures J. Radial maze type as a determinant of the choice behavior of rats. *J Neurosci Methods* 1979;1:343–352.

Moroz VM, Bures J. Cerebellar unit activity and the movement disruption induced by caudate stimulation in rats. *Gen Physiol Biophys* 1982;1:71–84.

Morris RGM. Spatial localization does not require the presence of local cues. *Learning Motiv* 1981;12:239–261.

O'Keefe J, Nadel L. *The hippocampus as a cognitive map.* Oxford: Clarendon Press, 1978.

Olton DS, Samuelson RJ. Remembrance of places passed: Spatial memory in rats. *J Exp Psychol: Anim Behav Processes* 1976;2:97–116.

Roytbak AI. Bioelectric phenomena in cerebral hemispheres (in Russian). Tbilisi: Publishing House of the Georgian Academy of Sciences, 1955.

Servit Z, Bures J. Epilepsy in the light of a large statistics (in Czech). *Thomayerova sbirka* 1950;10:1–4.

Servit Z, Bures J, Buresova O, Petran M. On the nature of electroanesthesia (in Russian). *Physiol Bohemosl* 1953;2:337–346.

Shibata M, Bures J. Reverberation of cortical spreading depression along closed-loop pathways in rat cerebral cortex. *J Neurophysiol* 1972;35:381–388.

Vyskocil F, Kriz N, Bures J. Potassium-selective microelectrodes used for measuring the extracellular brain potassium during spreading depression and anoxic depolarization in rats. *Brain Res* 1972;39:255–259.

Zhuravin IA, Bures J. Operant slowing of the extension phase of the reaching movement in rats. *Physiol Behav* 1986;36:611–617.

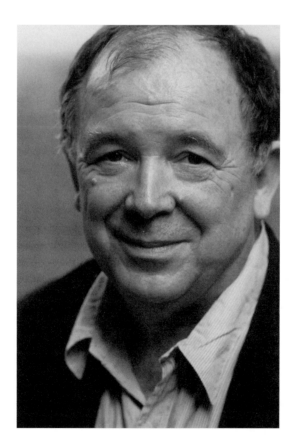

Jean-Pierre G. Changeux

BORN:
Domont (95), France
April 6, 1936

EDUCATION:
Ecole Normale Supérieure, Paris (1955)
Paris University (1957)
Institut Pasteur, Ph.D. (1964)

APPOINTMENTS:
Agrégé-Préparateur of Zoology, Ecole Normale Supérieure,
Paris (1958)
Sous-Directeur, Collège de France, Paris (1967)
Professor, Collège de France (1975)
Professor, Institut Pasteur (1975)

HONORS AND AWARDS (SELECTED):
Gairdner Foundation Award, Canada (1978)
Richard Lounsbery Prize, National Academy of Sciences,
USA (1983)
Wolf Prize, Israel (1983)
Foreign Associate, National Academy of Sciences, USA (1983)
Foreign Member, Royal Academy of Sciences, Stockholm
(1985)
Académie des Sciences, Paris (1988)
Bristol-Myers-Squibb Award in Neuroscience (1990)
Carl-Gustaf Bernhard Medal, Swedish Royal Academy of
Sciences (1991)
Foreign Member, Academy of Arts and Sciences (1994)
Eli Lilly Award, European College of Neuropsycho-
pharmacology (1999)
Balzan Prize for Cognitive Neuroscience, Berne (2001)
Karl Spencer Lashley Award, American Philosophical
Society (2002)

*Jean-Pierre Changeux identified and characterized the acetylcholine
receptor, demonstrated its allosteric transitions, and described its ion
channel. He also helped formalize the concept of synapse selection and
competition during development. In addition, building on his broad
interests in neuroscience and higher function, he has developed theory,
constructed models, and written successfully for the general audience.*

Jean-Pierre G. Changeux

utobiographical accounts are always partial and, therefore, invariably biased. This retrospective examination does not aim at a historical and comparative reconstruction of the development of concepts as general as those of allosteric proteins, the epigenesis of neuronal networks by selection, cognitive learning by reward, or even a faithful description of specific discoveries such as the identification of the acetylcholine receptor. The extraordinary exuberance of scientific research, and the ever-increasing number of scientists throughout the world who contribute either directly or indirectly to the progress of knowledge, and specifically to biological research, are such that, as Carl Popper wrote, "the objectivity of science is not a matter of individuals but a social matter." This objectivity is reached through extensive debates and critics between scientists, through their collaboration as well as through their rivalry. I will therefore limit myself to sketch, in this panoramic synthesis, a personal scientific itinerary that is all but linear, with its successes and failures, its joys and sorrows. Being aware of the collective character of this research and of its multiple dimensions, I would like to start by paying tribute to all those collaborators and colleagues, but also insightful competitors, who have made it possible for this work to exist.

Allosteric Proteins

I owe it to my first mentors, particularly to Jean Bathellier, my Natural Sciences Professor at the Lycée Montaigne, and to Claude Delamare-Deboutteville, who opened to me the doors of the Arago Laboratory of Marine Biology at Banyuls-sur-Mer, for encouraging my adolescent's fascination in life sciences and for converting it to a research vocation. By their teaching and by the example they set, they offered me the demonstration that biology is a branch of knowledge by itself, like mathematics, chemistry or physics, and literature, with the added richness of its multidisciplinary dimension.

From the taxonomy of parasitic marine copepods to the study of the fundamental molecular mechanisms of the living cell, the transition is not as abrupt as it seems. My juvenile philosophy, inspired by the work of Jean Brachet and Christian de Duve, whom I met during a training course in Brussels in 1959, was that the great problems of biology, such as those arising from the evolution of parasites and their unusual embryonic development, were to find their solution at the level of elementary biochemical properties of the egg cell and in the chemistry of its activation by the fertilizing sperm cell thereby eliciting its cleavage and segmentation. My arrival in Jacques Monod's laboratory, at the beginning of 1960, enabled me to put these rather ambitious ideas to the test with the added light shed by structured theoretical reflection and the contribution of rigorous experimentation. Among the several research projects which Jacques Monod and François Jacob proposed for my doctorate thesis, one particularly held my attention. Umbarger and Pardee had shown that in certain bacterial biosynthetic pathways the first enzyme is inhibited, apparently in a competitive manner, by the end product of the pathway. The issue was to understand the molecular mechanism of this elementary regulatory operation, which involved two chemical agents, a substrate and a regulatory signal with very different structures. This topic fitted directly with the spirit of my first theoretical enthusiasms as a biological student. I therefore selected it as my thesis subject. The experimentation was difficult for a beginner. I felt rather isolated. I tried hard, with L-threonine desaminase, to find a method to dissociate regulatory interaction and catalytic activity *in vitro*. Reagents of thiol groups, thermal treatment, and mutations uncoupled the inhibitory effect caused by isoleucine, while conserving this enzyme's catalytic activity on its substrate. In contrast with the hypothesis of a competitive inhibition, the substrate and the regulatory effector were to bind topographically distinct sites (Changeux, 1961). In the sketch I drew in the paper I presented at the 1961 prestigious Cold Spring Harbor Symposium on Quantitative Biology, the model of "non-overlapping" sites was clearly distinguished from the standard scheme of "overlapping" sites, i.e., mutual inhibition by steric hindrance. The interaction between these two sites was postulated to be indirect, or *allosteric* (a word coined by Monod and Jacob in the Concluding Remarks at the same meeting), and transmitted by a conformational change of the protein molecule (Monod, Changeux, and Jacob, 1963). At this stage of the inquiry, the change was viewed as analogous to the "induced-fit" mechanism suggested long before by Daniel Koshland for the catalytic action of enzymes. In passing, I observed that the sigmoid, cooperative, curve of saturation by the substrate was also uncoupled by the chemical treatment which dissociated regulatory and active sites.

At the end of my first public presentation of these results at the Cold Spring Harbor meeting, Bernard Davis stood up and noted the analogy between the cooperative binding properties of L-threonine desaminase and oxygen binding to hemoglobin. This was the beginning of an exciting epic. My research on the properties of L-threonine desaminase progressed. Later (early 1964), I handed Jacques Monod the first version of my thesis work. Max Perutz's results on hemoglobin's tridimensionnal structure as well as Jeffries Wyman's enlightened comments gave rise to vivid reflection and daily debates with my thesis advisor Jacques Monod. The model that emerged from it (Monod, Wyman, and Changeux, 1965) was based on the general principle that the molecular structure of allosteric proteins is organized in a cooperative manner forming "closed microcrystals," or *oligomers*. Furthermore, a mechanism was suggested which links cooperative binding and cooperative structure. It postulated a molecular switch according to which the regulatory protein may exist spontaneously under a small number of discrete conformational states that possess different biological properties. The regulatory signal, under these conditions, *selects* the conformation to which it preferentially binds and shifts the conformational equilibrium, thereby triggering signal transduction. A "Darwinian" selection, rather than a "Lamarckian"-induced-fit-instruction, of conformational states would take place.

In the conclusion of my thesis (1964), I considered the possibility of extending this model to the mechanisms of signal transmission in the nervous system and, more specifically, to the recognition of communication signals at the level of the chemical synapse. The theory was further elaborated together with the solid state physicist Charles Kittel during a first postdoctoral period at the University of California, Berkerley (1966–1967). The possibility was considered that, in membranes, receptors may form highly cooperative assemblies (Changeux et al., 1967). Only recently, Dennis Bray and his colleagues from Cambridge discovered that this mechanism actually takes place in the case of bacterial chemotactic receptors. In any case, these reflexions on membrane receptors were the starting point of investigations that still go on today.

Identification of the Acetylcholine Receptor

At the beginning of the last century, John Newport Langley (1905) postulated the existence of *receptors* engaged in the recognition, and transduction into a physiological response, of drugs or physiological chemical signals, since then called neurotransmitters. The test of the suggested hypothesis that allosteric mechanisms mediate synaptic transmission required the isolation of such a receptor, which since Langley had remained a mysterious entity. I decided to extend my postdoctoral studies in David Nachmansohn's laboratory at Columbia University in New York (1967). During his stay in France at the end of the 1930s, after having fled Nazi Germany, David Nachmansohn discovered the exceptional wealth in biochemical components of the cholinergic synapse of the electric organ from certain fish such as *Torpedo* or *Electrophorus*. He had also set up a preparation of individual cells isolated from the electric organ—or electroplaque—which enables one to investigate electrophysiology, pharmacology, and biochemistry on the same biological system (Nachmansohn, 1959). In his laboratory, I learned to dissect the electroplaque and to record its electrophysiological response to the neurotransmitter acetylcholine and its derivatives, such as nicotine and curare. Jon Singer, whom I had visited a few months earlier at the University of California, San Diego, had generously offered me a sample of an affinity probe, TDF, which he had previously used with antibodies. This molecule presents a trimethylammonium group, like acetylcholine, as well as a reactive diazonium group. The postulated mechanism was that TDF would bind and irreversibly link itself to the receptor site by a covalent bond. TDF behaved with the electroplaque as expected (Changeux, Podleski, and Wofsy, 1967). This was a significant step in the characterization of the receptor. The receptor was amenable to protein chemistry. This method was soon adopted by Arthur Karlin (1968), who was also a postdoctoral fellow in David Nachmansohn's laboratory. Inspired by earlier work on allosteric enzymes, he had initially observed that the electroplaque response to acetylcholine was sensitive to thiol reagents. On this basis, he improved the method of affinity labeling. However, this specificity soon appeared to be insufficient to allow isolation, from crude electric organ extracts, of the receptor in its active form.

Two singular discoveries allowed this obstacle to be overcome. The first one was the demonstration by Michiki Kasai and myself (1970) that membrane fragments purified from the electric organ have the tendency to reseal and form closed vesicles, or "microsacs." Inspired by the method used by George Cohen and Jacques Monod with bacterial permeases, we were able to measure radioactive Na^+ (or K^+) ion fluxes with the microsacs using a simple filtration method. Even better, the microsacs responded *in vitro* by an increase in ion flux to "nicotinic" cholinergic effectors with a specificity very close to that recorded by electrophysiological methods on the electroplaque and the neuromuscular junction. It thus became possible to study *in vitro* the "chemistry" of the physiological ionic response to acetylcholine. The receptor molecule was present in the purified membranes and I immediately started to try to solubilize it by detergents. A second discovery was as decisive. One spring afternoon in 1970, Chen-Yuan Lee, a Taiwanese pharmacologist, unexpectedly came into my laboratory. He informed me of his work on a snake venom toxin, α-bungarotoxin, which he had isolated and purified and which, according to him, almost irreversibly blocks the neuromuscular junction of higher vertebrates at the postsynaptic level. Aware of the Claude Bernard and Louis Pasteur tradition to use toxic compounds as "chemical lancets" to "dissect" physiological mechanisms, I immediately asked him for a sample of this toxin. He accepted, and I tried it as soon as I received it a few days later. The result was remarkable: α-bungarotoxin blocked both the electroplaque's electrical response *in vivo* and the microsacs' ion flux response to nicotinic agonists *in vitro*. It also blocked the *binding* of a nicotinic agonist, decamethonium, to a macromolecule that I had previously solubilized, using a weak detergent, from the microsac preparation. A protein which binds nicotinic agonists and the snake venom toxin in a mutually exclusive manner could then be identified under a detergent-soluble form that still reversibly binds the neurotransmitter (Changeux, Kasai, and Lee, 1970). In a footnote of the original article, I also mentioned that it could be physically separated from an enzyme long studied in David Nachmansohn's laboratory: acetylcholinesterase. For a while, I thought that acetylcholinesterase might form a supramolecular aggregate with the receptor protein: but this did not happen to be the case. The paper was communicated by Jacques Monod to the Proceedings of the National Academy of Sciences. After its publication, the finding was praised by David Nachmansohn, who for decades had tried to identify the receptor, and by the distinguished Swedish pharmacologist Ulf von Euler. The molecule was shown to be a high molecular weight, hydrophobic protein, strikingly different from acetylcholine esterase and which could be purified in my laboratory (Olsen, Meunier, and Changeux, 1972; Meunier et al., 1974). Examined by electronic microscopy (Cartaud et al., 1973), the receptor molecule resembled some kind of transmembrane "rivet" made up of several subunits organized into a compact bundle and whose synaptic side has the aspect of a rosette with a hydrophilic core. The emotion was immense. For the first time, a neurotransmitter receptor could be "seen."

Molecular Organization of the Acetylcholine Receptor

From then on it became possible to display the intimate organization of the receptor molecule. Was it really an allosteric protein? Was it an oligomer as suggested by the theory? An initial study performed in the laboratory with Ferdinand Hucho (1973) on the purified *Electrophorus electricus* receptor revealed a pentameric organization. I hesitated. The theoretical reflections I had with Jacques Monod stressed the importance of twofold symmetry axes. Indeed, these ideas provided a simple explanation for the evolution of a protein monomer into an oligomer. Nevertheless, these early findings were correct. The teams of Raftery and Karlin, who had no preconceived idea on this particular issue, established the pentameric organization, but also discovered that the structure was more "baroque" than we had expected, raising an additional difficulty for the theory. The receptor molecule resulted from the assembly of four apparently quite different types of subunits organized into a $[2\alpha\beta\gamma\delta]$ pentameric oligomer (see Weill, McNamee, and Karlin, 1974). These subunits had been distinguished by their molecular mass. Nothing was known about their chemistry. Anne Devillers-Thiéry, Dony Strosberg, and myself (1979) then established, using a microsequencing technique, the 20 amino acid sequence of the α-subunit N-terminal domain. It was quickly confirmed by Raftery's team. Today, this result may appear to be rather modest. However, at the time, it had a quite significant impact. A "chemical identity card" of the receptor was henceforth available, the first one ever to be established with a neurotransmitter receptor. It was quickly confirmed by Raftery's team which, with the help of Leroy Hood's high technology, determined the *four* subunits N-terminal sequence of the Californian *Torpedo* receptor and revealed important sequence identities between the subunits (Raftery et al., 1980). It was a comeback from baroque to classicism. As expected from the Monod, Wyman, and Changeux theory, the receptor protein was indeed an authentic oligomer, but it was *pseudo-symmetrical*, with an unusual fivefold rotation axis perpendicular to the plane of the synaptic membrane.

Basing themselves on these initial sequence data, the groups of Numa, Heinemann, and Barnard, as well as Anne Devillers-Thiéry and Jérôme Giraudat in my laboratory, cloned the complementary DNAs of the different electric organ subunits, and then those of the muscle, and established their complete sequence (Noda et al., 1982; Ballivet et al., 1982; Giraudat et al., 1982; Devillers-Thiéry et al., 1983). The reading of the sequence revealed several functional domains along the subunits sequences: a long hydrophilic N-terminal segment, four hydrophobic segments, and a short cytoplasmic hydrophilic segment, supposedly organized into extracellular (synaptic), transmembrane, and cytoplasmic domains, respectively.

In order to test the hypothesis of an "allosteric" interaction between distinct sites, this time at the *submolecular* level, the respective locations of the acetylcholine binding site and of the ion channel had to be determined. In this second step, the affinity labeling, which had not enabled the isolation of the receptor, proved to be very useful. A first result was obtained by Karlin's group using an affinity labeling reagent of the acetylcholine binding site, which led to the identification of a pair of adjacent cysteins (192–193), located in the N-terminal domain of the α-subunit (1984) (Kao et al., 1984). However, this result did not reveal the site's pharmacological specificity. The use of DDF, an affinity probe very close to Singer's TDF, which I had used during my stay at Columbia University, brought novel information. The dimethyl ammonium group of DDF creates a resonant molecule that can now be photoactivated by energy transfer from the protein. Indeed, our team, in collaboration with that of Hirth and Goeldner from Strasbourg, identified close to eight amino acids labeled by DDF, six of them with an aromatic side chain and all located in the long hydrophilic NH_2 terminal domain. These amino acids are distributed into three main loops (A, B, C), thus forming a sort of electronegative aromatic basket in which acetylcholine quaternary ammonium is capable of lodging itself (Dennis et al., 1988; Galzi et al., 1990). Another important observation shed a new light on the organization of the binding site. It was that the α-toxin, like DDF, labeled the γ- and δ-subunits, in addition to the α-subunit. From this came the idea that the acetylcholine binding site was located at the *interface* between subunits (Oswald and Changeux, 1982). The groups of Cohen, Taylor, and Karlin quickly confirmed this notion by identifying new loops, D, E, and F, located on the "complementary" side of the γ- and δ-subunits. A first validation of these biochemical results was obtained by directed mutagenesis of the labeled amino acids (see Galzi et al., 1990). However, the most spectacular evidence was recently provided by the Dutch group of Smit and Sixma using crystallographic analysis of a soluble snail protein that binds acetylcholine and happens to be homologous to the receptor's synaptic domain. Most of the amino acids identified by affinity labeling are very precisely found at the acetylcholine binding site level and at the interface between subunits (compare Corringer et al., 2000 and Brecj et al., 2001).

Identification of the Ion Channel

The most difficult task remained: the identification of the ion channel. How would it be possible, using the biochemical methods available, to chemically identify a pore within a protein through which the ions flow? The quest proved to be long and difficult (1974–1999). Relatively old pharmacological observations, made mainly in David Nachmansohn's laboratory and about which I became aware of in 1967 during my stay in his laboratory, inspired the search. Some agents, referred to as local anesthetics, were, in fact, known to block ion currents activated by nicotinic agonists, but in an indirect non-competitive manner and with no significant effect on the receptor binding site. These channel blockers acted, as it were, as a "cork" and offered out-standing tools for channel "labeling." The first step (1974), performed by my student, Michel Weber, and an American postdoctoral fellow, Jonathan Cohen, was to demonstrate, *in vitro*, that the local anesthetics do not directly displace acetylcholine from its site, but bind to a different site (Weber and Changeux, 1974; Cohen, Weber, and Changeux, 1974). The first attempts of reversible binding with a local anesthetic, quinacrine, pointed toward a protein with a molecular mass of 43,000 Da present in the subsynaptic membrane (Sobel, Weber, and Changeux, 1977). However, soon afterward, Jonathan Cohen, who had returned to Harvard University, showed that it was possible to get rid of this protein while conserving the binding of local anesthetics. I then decided to tackle the problem using again the affinity labeling method that was dear to me, but this time with a covalent local anesthetic synthesized in Bernard Roques' laboratory. When we explored the covalent labeling by this photoaffinity probe, Robert Oswald and I (1981) noted that the ultraviolet (UV) irradiation of the control molecule, *without reactive group*, was sufficient to covalently link the molecule to the recep-tor to the δ-subunit. This unanticipated observation, in fact, enabled us to quickly explore the properties of a large number of potential channel blockers which, because of their aromatic structure, could serve as photo-labeling reagents by simple UV irradiation of their complex with the receptor protein. Some among them labeled essentially the δ-subunit, while others labeled several subunits. One of them, chlorpromazine, displayed excep-tional properties (1981, 1983). Chlorpromazine labeled the four types of subunits of the receptor, and this covalent binding was strongly increased by nicotinic agonists and for all subunits at the same time. In addition, the effect of acetylcholine was blocked by d-tubocurarine and α-bungarotoxin. Moreover, my student, Thierry Heidmann, demonstrated that chlorpromazine binds itself to just one high affinity site per [2αβγδ] oligomer (1982, 1983). Furthermore, the kinetics of access to this site increased 100-fold when chlorpromazine was rapidly mixed with acetylcholine, i.e., conditions under which the ion channel opens (Heidmann and Changeux, 1984, 1986). It was then hypothesized that the chlorpromazine binding site is located within the *ion channel*, in the molecule's *pseudo*-symmetry axis (1983, 1984), and becomes accessible to chlorpromazine when the ion channel opens. The conditions under which the channel could be specifically labeled were thus established. The hardest task remained: to identify the amino acid(s) labeled by chlorpromazine.

It took my student, Jérôme Giraudat, more than a year of relentless efforts to demonstrate that, in the δ-subunit, chlorpromazine specifically labels one amino acid *serine* 262 located within the MII transmembrane segment (Giraudat et al., 1986). We were in a state of great tension. No one had, until then, suggested that the MII segment could eventually belong to the ion channel. The result was nevertheless made public at the fall meeting of the American Neuroscience Association (1962). We were reassured when, a few months later, Ferdinand Hucho using exactly the same protocol published the same result, but with a different probe. Jérôme Giraudat (1987) and then Frédéric Révah (1989, 1990) (Révah et al., 1990) continued with shrewdness the identification of the chlorpromazine-labeled amino acids on the other subunits. They confirmed, in agreement with Hucho's work, the contribution of a ring of serines but, in addition, discovered the specific labeling of other amino acids: leucines and threonines located at a distance of three to four amino acids on both sides of the ring of serines. The interpretation we made of these results was (1) that the MII segments contribute to the channel walls, (2) that these segments are folded into an α-helix, and (3) that the chlorpromazine binding site is located at a near equatorial position in the channel's pseudo-symmetry axis. The contribution of MII was quickly confirmed and further documented by the teams of Numa and Sakmann (1986, 1988) and Lester and Davidson (1986, 1988) using site-directed mutagenesis and electrophysiological recording techniques after reconstitution in *Xenopus* oocytes, following the method developed by Barnard and Miledi (1982) (cited in Changeux, 1990).

More recent studies, performed in my team by two postdoctoral fellows, Jean-Luc Galzi followed by Pierre-Jean Corringer, in collaboration with Daniel Bertrand from the University of Geneva, have enabled us to progress further. We identified a group of three amino acids that drive, in a critical way, the conversion of the ion channel cationic selectivity into an anionic one. One of them, which is particularly critical, is located in a loop situated at the cytoplasmic end of the MII segment (Galzi et al., 1992; Corringer et al., 1999). It thus became possible to transform an excitatory acetylcholine receptor into an inhibitory one. The finding has been reproduced by another group with the 5HT$_3$ receptor. The converse result—from anionic to cationic—has recently been achieved by other teams, using the same method, with the inhibitory glycine and GABA receptors.

All the data obtained clearly indicate that the receptor sites and the ion channel belong to topographically distinct proteic domains. Their interaction is therefore *allosteric*. Better, Jean-Luc Eiselé, a Swiss researcher working in my laboratory, successfully constructed a functional chimera joining the nicotinic receptor synaptic domain and the 5HT$_3$ serotonin receptor transmembrane domain (Eiselé et al., 1993). Therefore, the structural data obtained with the nicotinic receptor could be generalized to other receptors of the "nicotinic family."

Allosteric Transitions of the Acetylcholine Receptor

Additional biochemical results, but of a different nature, brought about additional arguments in favor of the allosteric model. First, at equilibrium, acetylcholine binds in a cooperative manner to its two binding sites that are present in each receptor protein molecule (Weber and Changeux, 1974). Furthermore, application of fast mixing methods derived from Manfred Eigen pioneering studies revealed amazing conformational changes. From Langley's (1905) and Katz and Thesleff's (1957) studies, it was known that when acetylcholine is applied onto a muscle cell *in vivo*, a fast (micro- to millisecond) opening of the ion channel, or *activation*, first occurs, followed by the slow closing (0.01 to several seconds) of the channel, or *desensitization*. Electrical recording methods did not allow a direct measurement of acetylcholine binding to the receptor and therefore rapidly appeared insufficient to investigate the molecular mechanisms of the activation and desensitization transistors. The isolation of a novel generation of microsacs, now extremely rich in receptors (20–40%), from the *Torpedo* electric organ, carried out earlier by Jonathan Cohen, Michel Weber, and myself (1972), opened the door to chemical methods. The extensive kinetic analysis of the fast binding of a fluorescent analog of acetylcholine dansylcholine to these membranes rich in receptors, performed by Thierry Heidmann for his thesis, taught us very much (Heidmann and Changeux, 1979, 1980). It revealed several conformational states of the receptor molecule: the kinetics of interconversion to a state of low affinity corresponded to activation, and several states of high affinity corresponded to desensitization upon rapid mixing with a nicotinic agonist. In contrast to a widespread opinion among pharmacologists, the highest affinity states did not correspond to the active states, but the opposite was true. Moreover, consistent with the allosteric scheme, a non-negligible fraction (about 20%) of the receptor was spontaneously found in the high affinity, desensitized state. In separate studies of considerable interest, Meyer Jackson (1984) had observed the spontaneous opening of the muscle receptor in the *absence* of acetylcholine. In agreement with the allosteric model, these two series of observations demonstrated that the transition between low and high affinity states of the receptor protein could therefore occur in the *absence* of acetylcholine. However, the situation appeared more complex than for regulatory enzymes. Regarding the receptor, there was not only one, but a cascade of transitions between discrete conformational states. I took the opportunity to generalize the conclusion to possible mechanisms of synaptic plasticity. In a short theoretical model, I suggested together with Thierry Heidmann (1982) that the characteristic property by which neurotransmitter receptors undergo multiple allosteric transitions with different time scales could be involved in the regulation of synaptic strength, particularly in elementary learning mechanisms. The idea deserves, in my opinion, some consideration as an alternative to the NMDA receptor-Mg^{2+} plug device. Indeed, it could apply to all the other receptors, including the non-NMDA glutamate receptors that display desensitization.

Gain of Function Mutations and Receptor Diseases

These thoughts opened the door, as will be described later, to the idea of a possible contribution of allosteric receptors to higher brain functions. An unanticipated discovery brought an additional dimension: that of neurological pathologies. Marc Ballivet and Daniel Bertrand at the University of Geneva, continuing the studies carried out in the laboratories of Patrick, Heinemann, and Lindstrom on the nicotinic brain receptors, had identified in the chick a new subunit type, which they named $\alpha 7$ (Couturier et al., 1990). Like the other neuronal receptor subunits, it presented important sequence identities with the muscle receptor, but appeared to be more archaic. It possessed the remarkable ability to associate with itself into a homomeric functional receptor, after expression in *Xenopus* oocytes. At last, the demonstration of a nicotinic receptor with perfect symmetry could be established, as expected from the original allosteric model. I immediately recognized that this system was the most appropriate to investigate the functional role of the amino acids homologous to those chemically identified by affinity labeling in *Torpedo*. Marc Ballivet agreed to give us an $\alpha 7$ cDNA. I asked my student, Frédéric Révah, to specifically mutate the chlorpromazine-labeled amino acids in $\alpha 7$ (Revah et al., 1991). The first recordings performed by Daniel Bertrand surprised us. Indeed, the mutation of leucine 247 into threonine did not cause an expected loss of channel function, but, on the contrary, resulted in a "gain of function": a dramatic decrease in the desensitization rate and, in addition, a near to 100-fold increase in apparent affinity. How strange! While discussing these results at a laboratory meeting, an interpretation suddenly came to my mind. The simplest explanation for these effects could originate from the allosteric model, assuming, for instance, that the high affinity desensitized state becomes permeable to ions. If this were the case, any molecule stabilizing the desensitized state should potentiate the response. I then recalled pioneering studies performed in my laboratory by Hans Grünhagen, one of Manfred Eigen's former students, and the discovery that antagonists, such as curare, could stabilize the desensitized state (Grünhagen and Changeux, 1976). If this happened to be the case, we would predict that α7 receptor antagonists, such as dihydro-β-erythroidine, could act like agonists. I called Daniel Bertrand to share this idea with him. He called me back a few days later. Effectively, dihydro-β-erythroidine behaved as an agonist on the L247T receptor (Bertrand et al., 1992). According to me, these results provided additional evidence in favor of a mechanism of allosteric transition between "rigid" states, which would preexist before the interaction with the ligand.

We were even more happily surprised when, in a totally independent way, Andrew Engel, Steven Sine, and their colleagues at the Mayo Clinic in the United States (see Engel and Ohno, 2002) subsequently reported that in some (not all) of the patients suffering from congenital myasthenia paralysis, the disorder observed was caused by dominant mutations of the muscle nicotinic receptor that led to a gain of function. Among the 13 mutations associated with this phenotype, 7 were located in MII, 1 of which was precisely at the homologous position of leucine 247. Stuart Edelstein, Professor at the University of Geneva, whom I had met in Berkeley in 1966, came to visit me at the Pasteur Institute in order to reexamine the application and the generalization of the allosteric model to the known neurotransmitter receptors and ion channels (Edelstein et al., 1996). The quantitative examination of the properties of mutant receptors from myasthenic patients revealed that their properties were exquisitely fitted by the allosteric model (1996, 1997) (Edelstein et al., 1997). The phenomenon can be extended to other receptors. A whole class of "receptor diseases" which include G-protein-linked receptors and tyrosine kinase receptors may be directly caused by the perturbation of the allosteric properties of these receptors (Changeux and Edelstein, 1998).

Epigenesis by Selective Synaptic Stabilization

Parallel to my molecular biology studies on regulatory enzymes and, later, on the acetylcholine receptor, I could not avoid returning to my youth "dreams" on the chemistry of embryonic development. We were in 1970. Jacques Monod had finished writing *Chance and Necessity*. I read the book with great interest, but also with the critical distance of a student who had become somewhat "parricidal," as Jacques Monod wrote in the affectionate dedication of the copy he gave me. Although I greatly shared the philosophy, I found his position on the development of the central nervous system too much based on innate influences. Well informed admirer of Wiesel and Hubel's work on the effects of experience on the postnatal development of the visual cortex (1965), I did not share their views on the "functional validation" by experience of preformed innate patterns of nerve connections. At a meeting organized by Edgar Morin on "l'Evénement," I suggested instead that exuberant and variable distribution of connections would become established through some kind of trial-and-error process and that at "critical" or sensitive periods a *synaptic* selection would occur according to a Darwinian epigenetic mode under the control of network activity (Changeux, 1972). The idea that regressive processes co-occur with mechanisms of synaptic competition during development had already been mentioned on several occasions since Ramón y Cajal (1899). However, this concept had neither been mathematically formalized nor generalized. Philippe Courrège, Antoine Danchin, and myself tried hard to accomplish this (Changeux, Courrège, and Danchin, 1973; Changeux and Danchin, 1976), and this attempt yielded two major consequences. First, the demonstration that a particular spatial and temporal distribution of electrical and chemical activity in a developing network is liable to be inscribed under the form of a particular and stable topology of connections within what I called a "genetic envelope." Second, the proposition, presented as a theorem of "variability," that the selection of networks having different connective topologies can lead to the same input–output behavioral relationship.

This theoretical project according to which an "epigenetic" evolution by synaptic selection could take over from the "genetic" evolution of biological species, both at the level of the individual and of the social group, was, and still is, a major source of debate. Even if the Darwinian metaphor raises discussions, its application to higher levels of organization, known as cognitive, enriched debates with Gerald Edelman, Terrence Sejnowski, Jeff Lichtman, and Dale Purves. Among its benefits, it gave rise to new models, both experimental and theoretical: "top-down" as well as "bottom-up."

An example of the bottom-up model was the junction between the motor nerve and the skeletal muscle, the simplest experimental model of chemical synapse whose anatomy (Couteaux, 1978), physiology (Katz, 1966), and biochemistry (Nachmansohn, 1959), particularly that of its principal component, the acetylcholine receptor (Changeux et al., 1970), were now known.

At the presynaptic level, Redfern (1970) had shown that, during the development of the motor endplate, a multiple innervation with three to five nerve endings occurs at birth and disappears later, since only one motor axon per muscle fiber remains in the adult. During his postdoctoral studies in my laboratory, Pierre Benoit (Benoit and Changeux 1975, 1978) demonstrated, for the first time, that in the newborn rat the state of activity of the junction controls the elimination of supernumerary terminals. Following my suggestion, Francis Crépel and Jean Mariani (1976, 1981) extended this observation to the development of the innervation of cerebellar Purkinje cells by climbing fibers. Later, other groups produced important experimental data in favor of the selectionist model (Lichtman, Constantine-Paton, Stryker, Shatz, etc.). The eventual contribution of instructive Lamarckian processes to the postnatal development of brain networks, yet, is still debated (Sejnowski, Purves).

The studies on the cerebellar mutants led to a casual observation which unexpectedly opened a new area of research. Looking at the protein compositions of the cerebellum of mutant mice deprived of Purkinje cells (Mallet et al., 1974), a freshly arrived postdoctoral fellow, Jacques Mallet, found that a high molecular weight band (called P400) was missing. Katsuhiko Mikoshiba, a very dynamic postdoctoral fellow, confirmed the observation (Mikoshiba, Huchet, and Changeux, 1979) and back in Japan built from it the splendid story of the IP3 receptor (Nikoshiba, 2003).

Molecular Morphogenesis of the Synapse

The model of epigenesis by selection aroused, in parallel, new investigations on the differentiation of the *postsynaptic* domain using the significant contribution of knowledge acquired about the molecular biology of the acetylcholine receptor. In particular, α-bungarotoxin allowed (in an electronic microscopy study performed by my student Jean-Pierre Bourgeois in collaboration with Antoinette Ryter) the evaluation of the number of receptor molecules per unit of postsynaptic membrane surface, showing that their density is extremely high (around $15,000/\mu m^2$) and persists several weeks after denervation (Bourgeois et al., 1972, 1978). The α-toxin was also an exceptional tool in the hands of John Merlie [an American postdoctoral fellow who I converted from bacteriology to neurobiology and collaborated with in François Gros' laboratory (Merlie et al., 1975; Merlie, Changeux, and Gros, 1978)] and also in the hands of Heinrich Betz (my second German postdoctoral fellow) to study the biosynthesis of the muscle receptor. Its repression by electrical activity was demonstrated during muscle development (Betz, Bourgeois, and Changeux, 1977; Bourgeois et al., 1978).

A new conceptual stage was reached with the analysis, using molecular genetics methods, of the genetic determinants that control the regulation of the acetylcholine receptor gene transcription into messenger RNA during the formation of the motor endplate. René Couteaux (1978) had noticed that the muscle nuclei lying directly under the motor nerve terminal presented a very unusual anatomy and, therefore, named them "fundamental nuclei." John Merlie and Josh Sanes (1984) had also noticed that innervated muscle regions were richer in messenger RNAs coding for the receptor subunits than the non-junctional regions. My interest was reinforced by the discovery, made by my medical student Bertrand Fontaine using an *in situ* hybridization method (developed together with Margaret Buckingham's laboratory) (Fontaine et al., 1988; Fontaine and Changeux, 1989), that these messenger RNAs are strictly located at the level of the fundamental nuclei. There is a "compartmentalization" of the expression of the receptor genes at the level of the subneural domain. Several groups (Goldman, Brenner, Sakmann, Burden) confirmed this observation. It enabled the analysis, conducted in my laboratory throughout the years by several students and postdoctoral fellows (André Klarsfeld, 1987; Jacques Piette, 1989, 1990; Jean-Louis Bessereau, 1994; Satoshi Koike, 1996; and Laurent Schaeffer, 1998), of the genetic mechanisms (DNA elements and transcription factors) that regulate this elementary morphogenesis. For instance, we discovered that distinct genetic determinants and signaling systems control the targeting of transcription under the synapse (*N Box*) via trophic factors of neural origin and the repression by electrical activity outside the synapse (*E Box*) (Schaeffer et al., 2001). It lead to the identification of an Ets transcription factor as a crucial element for the normal formation of the neuromuscular junction (De Kerchove d'Exaerde et al., 2002).

The posttranscription stages, studied by Jean Cartaud and colleagues in collaboration with my group, i.e., the transit through a specialized Golgi apparatus (1989), a particular secretory pathway (1990, 1995), and the assembly, by the 43K-Rapsyn protein (discovered in my laboratory by André Sobel in 1977), into sub-synaptic aggregates, confirmed and extended the model of a progressive compartmentalization of gene expression in the course of the formation of the neuro-muscular synapse.

Michel Kerszberg and I (1993) then had sufficient data in hand to describe this process as a cybernetic mathematical model that accounts for the formation of a sharp boundary of gene transcription, during the development of the motor endplate. Further development of the model accounts for the positioning of this boundary in a morphogenesis gradient during embryonic development (Kerszberg and Changeux, 1994, 1998). The mechanism was soon extended to the basic issue of the formation and parcellization of the neural plate in the course of embryonic development, which potentially plays a crucial role in the phylogenesis of vertebrate brain (Kerszberg and Changeux, 1998).

Nicotinic Receptors in the Brain

Naturally, the strategy of understanding neural development at the level of networks of transcription factors linking dispersed populations of promoter elements was to be applied to the expression of neuronal nicotinic receptor genes in the brain. Clarke, Patrick, Heinemann, and others had described the distinct topological distribution of the various types of neuronal nicotinic receptors and of the messenger RNAs of their subunits in the brain. Michele Zoli, a postdoctoral fellow from Italy, carefully examined during development the expression of the $\alpha3$, $\alpha4$, $\beta2$, $\beta4$ genes which starts very early at day 10 of embryonic development and can be synchronous in certain regions (spinal cord), but not in others (cerebral cortex) (Zoli et al., 1995). This required a particularly sophisticated transcriptional regulation. Indeed, my student Alain Bessis (Bessis et al., 1993, 1997) showed, in the case of the genes for the $\alpha2$ and $\beta2$ subunits, that the regulation of their transcription is submitted to a complex interplay between activatory regulatory sequences and inhibitory ones. Moreover, the fine analysis of nicotinic receptor distribution at the neuronal level using electrophysiological methods, performed by my collaborators Christophe Mulle (Mulle and Changeux, 1990; Mulle et al., 1991) and Clément Léna (Léna, Changeux, and Mulle, 1993; Léna and Changeux, 1997), indicated that the receptor protein is not only distributed on the neuronal soma and dendrites, but also on the axonal terminals and on the segments located close to the terminal referred to as preterminal (Léna, Changeux, and Mulle, 1993). A critical question arose: what are the functions of the various brain nicotinic receptor forms associated with such a complex organization? Further theoretical reflection was needed.

Neuronal Man and Cognitive Learning by Reward

In 1983 I published *Neuronal Man: The Biology of Mind*. This book covered the contents of the first seven years of lectures I gave at the Collège de France and was enriched by the laboratory's current research. I ventured to collect and critically synthesize the data which had been gathered thanks to extraordinary progress in neuroscience since the 1970s, from the molecular and cellular levels to cognitive functions, even consciousness. In it, I substantiated and documented the thesis of epigenesis by synaptic selection. In the chapter on "Mental Objects," I extended it to higher brain functions. I developed Hebb's old proposal according to which the representations formed by our brain can be identified with activity states of "cooperative" neuron assemblies. I integrated it with the selectionist model, proposing that acquisition of knowledge, in other words the neuronal inscription of meaning, is carried out in at least two steps: the genesis of multiple and transitory "prerepresentations" followed by the selection of the "adequate" representation(s) of the outside world. The first selection mechanism that was retained was that of "resonance" between prerepresentations of internal origin and the percept evoked by an interaction with external reality (1983).

While realizing the need for deeper analysis, particularly at the cognitive level, I decided to discuss the issue in the mid-1980s with my close friend Jacques Mehler, whose experience with psycholinguistics could be a great source of enrichment. He put me in contact with one of his students, Stanislas Dehaene, who had been trained in mathematics at the Ecole Normale Supérieure but was doing experimental psychology under his supervision. It was the starting point of an exceptionally fruitful collaboration which still continues actively today. Stanislas and I agreed about two major issues from the start: (1) a theoretical model had meaning only if it concerned a defined behavioral task, accessible to experimentation; and (2) the formal model should be based on plausible neuronal data. It should be as "neuro-realistic" as possible. The swamp sparrow's song-learning, as studied by Peter Marler and his group, was first used as basic material for a network of formal neurons capable of learning *sequences* of notes through resonance (Dehaene, Changeux, and Nadal, 1987).

We then decided to extend the modeling to more elaborate cognitive functions and, in particular, to tasks with which I became acquainted during my teaching at the Collège de France. We selected the well-known delayed-response tasks which, in mammals, mobilize the frontal cortex. New modes of selection had to be found at the cognitive level. The involvement of "reward" processes, suggested by Thorndike, Pavlov, and Skinner, in an "empirical" context seemed plausible and adaptable to the selectionist scheme. In addition, this idea enriched the modeling work with a new biochemical dimension. Neuronal systems specialized in reward and punishment had been identified for years. They engaged specific neurotransmitters such as dopamine and serotonin, as well as acetylcholine. Hence, we developed and formalized the idea (Dehaene and Changeux, 1989, 1991) that the prerepresentations produced by a neuronal "generator of diversity" could be selected by the release of a reward signal evoked by a successful interaction with the outside world. Conversely, a punishment would destabilize the system and start again the production of prerepresentations. The model included an elementary mechanism of modulation of synaptic strength by the reward signal. This still hypothetical mechanism was derived from the extension of the allosteric scheme that I proposed with Thierry Heidmann in 1982 of a coincidence reading of two synaptic signals—including a neurotransmitter of reward—by a common allosteric state of the synaptic receptors. In computer experiments, the virtual organisms, constructed on this basis, passed the task. Others were designed for the Wisconsin Card Sorting test (1991) or even the Tower of London task (1997). The models accounted for the expected cognitive behaviors, but also offered many new experimental predictions.

The *in vivo* techniques of gene invalidation in mice provided original experimental avenues to put to the test our hypotheses and computer models that covered intricate organization levels from molecules to cognitive functions. This approach in fact enabled us to approach the role of the various neuronal nicotinic receptor subunits. I entrusted to Marina Picciotto, an American postdoctoral fellow, the task of constructing a mouse invalidated for the β2 subunit, the most largely distributed subunit in the brain. After several difficult years, with the help from several colleagues at the Pasteur Institute and with great courage, she succeeded (Picciotto et al., 1995). The mutant mouse displayed quite peculiar behavioral traits. It no longer responded to nicotine in a passive avoidance learning task, and also showed alterations in reward processes. For instance, nicotine self-administration as well as the effect of nicotine on dopamine release were abolished (Picciotto et al., 1998). The anti-nociceptive effect of nicotine was also lost in the β2 mutant mouse, as well as in the α4 mutant mouse (also constructed by Lisa Marubio, another American postdoctoral fellow). These mice possessed somewhat altered punishment mechanisms. These results are still far from giving a fair evaluation of the suggested models. Yet, they open fruitful experimental perspectives regarding nicotine addiction, analgesia, and cognitive functions.

Conscious Space and Nicotinic Receptors

In *Neuronal Man*, I tackled the issue of consciousness and the neuronal bases of "becoming conscious" and stated that the relevant explanation had to be found at the level of a system of neuronal regulations functioning as a global entity. In my 1992 course at the Collège de France, I suggested that the formal neuronal network that Stanislas Dehaene and myself had proposed for the Wisconsin Card Sorting task could serve as a starting point for the development of a more general model that would include a "conscious workspace." Two events prompted us to tackle this modeling in a direct way. On the one hand, Stanislas Dehaene had created a very active independent research group dedicated to brain imaging and started to apply this technique to investigate conscious versus nonconscious tasks. On the other hand, Antonio Coutiño gave us the opportunity to present our ideas in Portugal to a group of experts brought together by the Gulbenkian Foundation in the monastery of Arrabida in the summer of 1998. Our position differed from Francis Crick's 40-Hz reductionism, from Gerald Edelman's complexity dialectic, and from Rodolfo Llinás' thalamocortical oscillations. Rather, our intention was to imagine a neuronal architecture that would explain altogether the global and unitary character of the conscious workspace, as suggested by the psychologist Baars (1989) *and* the diversity of the underlying processes. It was elaborated as a computer model. Dehaene, Kerszberg, and myself (1998) proposed that neurons with long axons connecting distinct cortical areas, even different hemispheres, play an essential role in the genesis of the conscious space. In effortful tasks, such as the Stroop test, "global" representations would differentially mobilize these neurons together with components from specialized processes through mechanisms of evaluation from the outside world, but also through mechanisms of *self-evaluation* toward the subjective *inner world*. The proposed computer model is able to successfully simulate the Stroop task. The model also accounts for the top-down control of these global representations upon the activity states of the underlying processes by a simple neuronal mechanism. A tentative answer was brought, in neuronal terms, to the paradox raised by Sperry of the mysterious top-down control of consciousness over lower neuronal processes.

Von Economo's (1929) studies on the microarchitecture of the cerebral cortex underlined the abundance of pyramidal neurons with long axons in layers II and III of the cerebral cortex. Interestingly, these layers are specially dense in the so-called association areas which include the prefrontal cortex. Moreover, brain imaging studies, particularly those performed by Stanislas Dehaene and his group, revealed a strong activation of the prefrontal areas during the accomplishment of conscious tasks requiring an effort. Finally, everyone knows about nicotine's effects on wakefulness and on attention.

Was it reasonable to link these theoretical thoughts and the experimental studies carried out with the neuronal receptor? A first link was established by a discovery made by the Australian neurologist Bercovic and the German molecular biologist Steinlein (Steinlein et al., 1995). Bercovic had recognized that several members of the same Australian family suffered from a rare form of autosomal dominant nocturnal frontal lobe epilepsy, which causes loss of consciousness and convulsions. This was the first genetic epilepsy to be identified at the amino acid level; moreover, it resulted from a mutation of the gene coding for the α4 subunit of the acetylcholine nicotinic receptor. My surprise and delight was even greater when I read in the paper that the particular amino acid whose mutation resulted in seizures was homologous to serine 261 in the MII segment that we had initially labeled with chlorpromazine in the *Torpedo* receptor! Spontaneous mutations revealed, independently of any preconceived idea, the *same amino acid* as the one we had labeled in a deliberate way to identify the ion channel. Can a more "objective" validation of these results be conceived?

The subject of the neural bases of consciousness and of its chemistry is henceforth opened to scientific research. The nicotinic receptor may again play a role. Is it a new start for the chemistry of consciousness and cognitive functions? It will require, in order to progress, a multidisciplinary approach that unites life sciences and human sciences at multiple levels of organization, together with human sciences. It is our duty and that of the younger generations to make it work. We are far from the end … .

Bibliographic references of the team can be found on the laboratory's Web site: http://www.pasteur.fr/recherche/unites/neubiomol/bibliography. html. Additional references on the history of the acetylcholine receptors can be found in Changeux references (1981, 1990). This paper is inspired by the document delivered for the Balzan prize ceremony (2000).

Selected Bibliography

Baars BJ. *A cognitive theory of consciousness.* Cambridge, UK: Cambridge University Press, 1989.

Ballivet M, et al. Molecular cloning of cDNA coding for the gamma-Subunit of Torpedo acetylcholine receptor. *Proc Natl Acad Sci USA* 1982;79:4466–4470.

Barnard EA, Miledi R, Sumikawa K. Translation of exogenous messenger RNA coding for nicotinic acetylcholine receptors produces functional receptors in *Xenopus oocytes. Proc R Soc (Lond)* 1982;215:241–246.

Benoit P, Changeux JP. Consequences of tenotomy on the evolution of multiinnervation in developing rat soleus muscle. *Brain Res* 1975;99:354–358.

Benoit P, Changeux JP. Consequences of blocking nerve activity on the evolution of multi-innervation at the regenerating neuromuscular junction of the rat. *Brain Res* 1978;149:89–96.

Bertrand D, Devillers-Thiéry A, Revah F, Galzi JL, Hussy N, Mulle C, Bertrand S, Ballivet M, Changeux JP. Unconventional pharmacology of a neuronal nicotinic receptor mutated in the channel domain. *Proc Natl Acad Sci USA* 1992; 89:1261–1265.

Bessereau JL, Stratford-Perricaudet L, Piette J, Le Poupon C, Changeux JP. In vivo and in vitro analysis of electrical activity-dependent expression of muscle acetylcholine receptor genes using adenovirus. *Proc Natl Acad Sci USA* 1994;91:1304–1308.

Bessis A, et al. Negative regulatory elements upstream of a novel exon of the neuronal nicotinic acetylcholine receptor alpha2 subunit gene. *Nuclei Acid Res* 1993;21:2185–2192.

Bessis A, et al. The neuron-restrictive silencer element (NRSE): A dual enhancer/silencer crucial for patterned expression of a nicotinic receptor gene in the brain. *Proc Natl Acad Sci USA* 1997;94:5906–5911.

Betz H, Bourgeois JP, Changeux JP. Evidence for degradation of the acetylcholine (nicotinic) receptor in skeletal muscle during the development of the chick embryo. *FEBS Lett* 1977;77:219–224.

Bourgeois JP, et al. Localization of the cholinergic receptor protein in Electrophorus electroplax by high resolution autoradiography. *FEBS Lett* 1972;25:127–133.

Bourgeois JP, et al. Quantitative studies on the localization of the cholinergic receptor protein in the normal and denervated electroplaque from Electrophorus electricus. *J Cell Biol* 1978;79:200–216.

Brejc K, Van Dijk WJ, Klaassen RV, Schuurmans M, Van Der Oost J, Smit AB, Sixman TK. Crystal structure of an ACh-binding protein reveals the ligand binding domain of nicotinic receptors. *Nature* 2001;411:269–276.

Brejc K, Van Dijk WJ, Klaassen R, Schuurmans M, van der Oost J, Smit AB, and Sixman TK. Crystal structure of AchBP reveals the ligand-binding domain of nicotinic receptors. *Nature* 2001;411:269–276.

Brodmann K. *Vergleichende Lokalisationslehre des Groshirnrinde in ihren Preinzipien dargestellt auf Grund des Zellenbaues.* Leipzig: Barth, 1909.

Cartaud J, et al. Presence of a lattice structure in membrane fragments rich in nicotinic receptor protein from the electric organ of Torpedo marmorata. *FEBS Lett* 1973;33:109–113.

Changeux JP. The feedback control mechanism of biosynthetic L-threonine deaminase by L-isoleucine. *Cold Spring Harbor Symp Quant Biol* 1961;26:313–318.

Changeux JP. Le cerveau et l'événement. *Communications* 1972;18:37–47.

Changeux JP. The acetylcholine receptor: An allosteric membrane protein. *The Harvey Lectures* 1981;75:85–254.

Changeux JP. *L'Homme neuronal*. Paris: Fayard, 1983;419.

Changeux JP. Functional architecture and dynamics of the nicotinic acetylcholine receptor: An allosteric ligand-gated ion channel. Fidia Research Foundation Neuroscience Award Lectures, Volume 4, 1990;21–168.

Changeux JP, Courrège P, Danchin A. A theory of the epigenesis of neural networks by selective stabilization of synapses. *Proc Natl Acad Sci USA* 1973;70:2974–2978.

Changeux JP, Danchin A. Selective stabilization of developing synapses as a mechanism for the specificication of neuronal networks. *Nature* 1976;264:705–712.

Changeux JP, Kasai M, Lee CY. The use of snake venom toxin to characterize the cholinergic receptor protein. *Proc Natl Acad Sci USA* 1970;67:1241–1247.

Changeux JP, Dehaene S. Hierarchical neuronal modeling of cognitive functions: From synaptic transmission to the Tower of London. *CR Adad Sci Paris* 1998;321:241–247.

Changeux JP, Edelstein S. Allosteric receptor after 30 years. *Neuron* 1998;21: 959–980.

Changeux JP, Podleski T, Wofsy L. Affinity labeling of the acetylcholine receptor. *Proc Natl Acad Sci USA* 1967;58:2063–2070.

Changeux JP, Thiéry J, Tung Y and Kittel C. On the cooperativity of biological membranes. *Proc. Natl. Acad. Sci. Wash.* 1967;57:335–341.

Cohen JB, Weber M, Changeux JP. Effects of local anesthetics and calcium on the interaction of cholinergic ligands with the nicotinic receptor protein from Torpedo marmorata. *Mol Pharmacol* 1974;10:904–932.

Corringer PJ, Bertrand S, Galzi JL, Devillers-Thiéry A, Changeux JP, Bertrand D. Mutational analysis of the charge selectivity filter of the alpha 7 nicotinic acetylcholine receptor. *Neuron* 1999;22:831–843.

Corringer PJ, Le Novère N, Changeux JP. Nicotinic receptors at the amino acid level. *Annu Rev Pharmacol* 2000;40:431–458.

Couteaux R. *Recherches morphologiques et cytochimiques sur l'organisation des tissus excitables*. Paris: Robin et Marenge, 1978;225.

Couturier S, Bertrand D, Matter JM, Hernandez MC, Bertrand S, Millar N, Valera S, Barkas T, Ballivert M. A neuronal nicotinic acetylcholine receptor subunit (alpha7). Is developmentally regulated and forms a homo-oligomeric channel blocked by alpha-BTX. *Neuron* 1990;5:847–856.

Crépel F, Mariani J, Delhaye-Bouchaud N. Evidence for a multiple innervation of Purkinje cells by climbing fibers in immature rat cerebellum. *J Neurobiol* 1976;7:567–578.

De Kerchove d'Exaerde A. Cartaud J, Ravel-Chapuis A, Seroz T, Pasteau F, Angus LM, Jasmin B, Changeux JP and Schaeffer L. Expression of mutant Ets protein at the neuromuscular synapse causes alterations in morphology and gene expression. *EMBO Reports* 2002;3:2201–2207.

Dehaene S, Changeux JP. A simple model of prefrontal cortex function in delayed-response tasks. *J Cognitive Neurosci* 1989;1:244–261.

Dehaene S, Changeux JP. The Wisconsin card sorting test: Theoretical analysis and simulation of a reasoning task in a model neuronal network. *Cerebral Cortex* 1991;1:62–79.

Dehaene S, Changeux JP. A hierarchical neuronal network for planning behavior. *Proc Natl Acad Sci USA* 1997;94:13293–13298.

Dehaene S, Changeux JP, Nadal JP. Neural networks that learn temporal sequences by selection. *Proc Natl Acad Sci USA* 1987;84:2727–2731.

Dehaene S, Kerszberg M, Changeux JP. A neuronal model of a global workspace in effortful cognitive tasks. *Proc Natl Acad Sci USA* 1998;95:14529–14534.

Dennis M, Giraudat J, Kotzyba-Hibert F, Goeldner M, Hirth C, Chang JY, Lazure C, Chrétien M, Changeux JP. Amino acids of the Torpedo marmorata acetylcholine receptor subunit labeled by a photoaffinity ligand for the acetylcholine binding site. *Biochemistry* 1988;27:2346–2357.

Devillers-Thiéry A, et al. The amino-terminal sequence of the 40K subunit of the acetylcholine receptor protein from Torpedo marmorata. *FEBS Lett* 1979;104:99–105.

Devillers-Thiéry A, et al. Complete mRNA coding sequence of the acetylcholine binding alpha subunit of Torpedo marmorata acetylcholine receptor: A model for the transmembrane organization of the polypeptide chain. *Proc Natl Acad Sci USA* 1983;80:2067–2071.

Edelman G. *Neural Darwinism: The theory of neuronal group selection.* New York: Basic Books, 1987.

Edelstein S, Changeux JP. Allosteric proteins after 30 years: The binding and state functions of the neuronal alpha 7 nicotinic acetylcholine receptor. *Experientia* 1996;52:1083–1090.

Edelstein S, Schaad O, Changeux JP. Single binding versus single channel recordings: A new approach to study ionotropic receptors. *Biochemistry* 1997;36:13755–13760.

Edelstein S, Schaad O, Henry E, Bertrand D, Changeux, JP. A kinetic mechanism for nicotinic acetylcholine receptors based on multiple allosteric transitions. *Biol Cybern* 1996;75:361–379.

Eiselé JL, Bertrand S, Galzi JL, Devillers-Thiéry A, Changeux, JP, Bertrand D. Chimaeric nicotinic-serotonergic receptor combines distinct ligand binding and channel specificities. *Nature* 1993;366:479–483.

Engel AG, Ohno K. Congenital myasthenic syndromes. *Adv Neurol* 2002;88:203–215.

Fontaine B, Changeux JP. Localization of nicotinic acetylcholine receptor alpha-subunit transcripts during myogenesis and motor endplate development in the chick. *J Cell Biol* 1989;108:1025–1037.

Fontaine B, et al. Detection of the nicotinic acetylcholine receptor alpha-subunit mRNA by in situ hybridization at neuromuscular junctions of 15-day old chick striated muscles. *EMBO J* 1988;7:603–609.

Galzi JL, Revah F, Black D, Goeldner M, Hirth C, Changeux JP. Identification of a novel amino acid alpha-Tyr 93 within the active site of the acetylcholine receptor by photoaffinity labeling: Additional evidence for a three-loop model of the acetylcholine binding site. *J Biol Chem* 1990;265:10430–10437.

Giraudat J, Dennis M, Heidmann T, Chang JY, Changeux JP. Structure of the high affinity site for noncompetitive blockers of the acetylcholine receptor: Serine-262 of the delta subunit is labeled by [^{3}H]-chlorpromazine. *Proc Natl Acad Sci USA* 1986;83:2719–2723.

Giraudat J, Devillers-Thiéry A, Auffray C, Rougeon F, Changeux JP. Identification of a cDNA clone coding for the acetylcholine binding subunit of Torpedo marmorata acetylcholine receptor. *EMBO J* 1982;1:713–717.

Galzi JL, Devillers-Thiery A, Hussy N, Bertrand S, Changeux JP, Bertrand D. Mutations in the ion channel domain of a neuronal nicotinic receptor convert ion selectivity from cationic to anionic. *Nature* 1992;359:500–505.

Galzi JL, et al. Functional significance of aromatic amino acids from three peptide loops of the alpha 7 neuronal nicotinic receptor site investigated by site-directed mutagenesis. *FEBS Lett* 1991;294:198–202.

Goldman D, Brenner HR, Heinemann S. Acetylcholine receptor alpha-, beta-, gamma-, and delta-subunit mRNA levels are regulated by muscle activity. *Neuron* 1988;1:329–335.

Goldman D, et al. Muscle denervation increases the levels of two mRNAs coding for the acetylcholine receptor alpha-subunit. *J Neurosci* 1985;5:2553–2558.

Grünhagen HH, Changeux JP. Studies on the electrogenic action of acetylcholine with Torpedo marmorata electric organ. Quinacrine: A fluorescent probe for the conformational transitions of the cholinergic receptor protein in its membrane bound state. *J Mol Biol* 1976;106:497–516.

Heidmann O, et al. Chromosomal localization of muscle nicotinic acetylcholine receptor genes in the mouse. *Science* 1986;234:866–868.

Heidmann T, Bernhardt J, Neumann E, Changeux JP. Rapid kinetics of agonist binding and permeability response analyzed in parallel on acetylcholine receptor-rich membranes from Torpedo marmorata. *Biochemistry* 1983;22:5452–5459.

Heidmann T, Changeux JP. Fast kinetic studies on the interaction of a fluorescent agonist with the membrane-bound acetylcholine receptor from T. marmorata. *Eur J Biochem* 1979a;94:255–279.

Heidmann T, Changeux JP. Fast kinetic studies on the allosteric interactions between acetylcholine receptor and local anesthetic binding sites. *Eur J Biochem* 1979b;94:281–296.

Heidman T, Changeux JP. Interaction of a fluorescent agonist with the membrane-bound acetylcholine receptor from Torpedo marmorata in the millisecond time range: Resolution of an intermediate conformational transition and evidence for positive cooperative effects. *Biochem Biophys Res Commun* 1980;97:889–896.

Heidmann T, Changeux JP. Un modèle moléculaire de régulation d'efficacité d'un synapse chimique au niveau postsynaptique. *CR Acad Sci Paris* 1982;3,295: 665–670.

Heidmann T, Changeux JP. Time-resolved photolabeling by the noncompetitive blocker chlorpromazine of the acetylcholine receptor in its transiently open and closed ion channel conformations. *Proc Natl Acad Sci USA* 1984;81:1897–1901.

Heidmann T, Changeux JP. Characterization of the transient agonist-triggered state of the acetylcholine receptor rapidly labeled by the noncompetitive blocker [^{3}H]chlorpromazine: Additional evidence for the open channel conformation. *Biochemistry* 1986;25:6109–6113.

Heidmann T, Oswald RE, Changeux JP. Le site de liaison de haute affinité de la chlorpromazine n'est présent qu'à un seul exemplaire par molécule de récepteur cholinergique et est commun aux quatre chaînes polypeptidiques. *CR Acad Sci Paris* 1982;295:345–349.

Imoto K, Busch C, Sackmann B, Mishina M, Konno, T, Nakai J, Bujo H, Mori Y, Fukuda K, Numa, S. Rings of negatively charged amino acids determine the acetylcholine receptor channel conductance. *Nature* 1988;335:645–648.

Jackson MB. Spontaneous openings of the acetylcholine receptor channel. *Proc Natl Acad Sci USA* 1984;81:3901–3904.

Jasmin BJ, Cartaud J, Bornens M, Changeux JP. Golgi apparatus in chick skeletal muscle: Changes in its distribution during endplate development and after denervation. *Proc Natl Acad Sci USA* 1989;86:7218–7222.

Karlin A, Cowburn DA. The affinity labelling of partially purified acetylcholine receptor from electric tissue of Electrophorus. *Proc Natl Acad Sci USA* 1973;70:3636–3640.

Karlin A, Winnick M. Reduction and specific alkylation of the receptor for acetylcholine. *Proc Natl Acad Sci USA* 1968;60:668–674.

Kao P, Dwork A, Kaldany R, Silver M, Wideman J, Stein S, Karlin A. Identification of the alpha-subunit half-cystine specifically labeled by an affinity reagent for the acetylcholine receptor binding site. *J Biol Chem* 1984;259:11662–11665.

Kasai M, Changeux JP. Demonstration de l'excitation par des agonistes cholinergiques à partir de fractions de menbranes purifiées *in vitro*. *CR Acad Sci Paris* 1970;270D:1400–1403.

Katz B. *Nerve muscle and synapse*. New York: McGraw Hill, 1966.

Katz B, Thesleff S. A study of the desensitization produced by acetylcholine at the motor end-plate. *J Physiol* 1957;138:63–80.

Kerszberg M, Changeux JP. A model for motor endplate morphogenesis: Diffusible morphogens, transmembrane signalling and compartmentalized gene expression. *Neural Computation* 1993;5:341–358.

Kerszberg M, Changeux JP. A model for reading morphogenetic gradients: Autocatalysis and competition at the gene level. *Proc Natl Acad Sci USA* 1994;91:5823–5827.

Kerszberg M, Changeux JP. A simple molecular model of neurulation. *BioEssay* 1998;20:758–770.

Klarsfeld A, et al. A 5' flanking region of the chicken acetylcholine receptor alpha-subunit gene confers tissue-specificity and developmental control of expression in transfected cells. *Mol Cell Biol* 1985;7:951–955.

Koike S, Schaeffer L, Changeux JP. Identification of a DNA element determining synaptic expression of the mouse acetylcholine receptor delta-subunit gene. *Proc Natl Acad Sci USA* 1995;92:10624–10628.

Langley JN. On the reaction of cells and nerve-endings to certain poisons, chiefly as regards on the reaction of striated muscle to nicotine and to curare. *J Physiol* 1905;33:374–413.

Léna C, Changeux JP, Mulle C. Evidence for "Preterminal" nicotinic receptors on GABAergic axons in the rat interpeduncular nucleus. *J Neurosci* 1993;13:2680–2688.

Léna C, Changeux JP. Role of Ca^{2+} ions in nicotinic facilitation of GABA release in mouse thalamus. *J Neurosci* 1997a;17:576–585.

Léna C, Changeux JP. Pathological mutations of nicotinic receptors and nicotine-based therapies for brain disorders. *Curr Op Neurobiol* 1997b;7:674–682.

Marler P, Terrace H. *The biology of learning.* Berlin: Springer-Verlag, 1984.

Mallet J, Huchet M, Shelanski M, Changeux JP. Protein differences associated with the absence of granule cells in the cerebella from the mutant weaver mouse and from X-irradiated rat. *FEBS Lett* 1974;46:243–246.

Merlie JP, Changeux JP, Gros F. Skeletal muscle acetylcholine receptor. Purification, characterization, and turnover in muscle cell cultures. *J Biol Chem* 1978;253:2882–2891.

Merlie, JP, et al. Synthesis of acetylcholine receptor during differentiation of cultures embryonic muscle cells. *Proc Natl Acad Sci USA* 1975;72:4028–4032.

Merlie J, Sanes JR. Concentration of acetylcholine receptor mRNA in synaptic regions of adult muscle fibers. *Nature* 1985;317:66–68.

Meunier JC, Sealock R, Olsen R, Changeux JP. Purification and properties of the cholinergic receptor from Electrophorus electricus electric tissue. *Eur J Biochem* 1974;45:371–394.

Mikoshiba K. Inositol 1,4,5 triphosphate (IP3) receptor. *Nippon Yakurigaki Zasshi* 2003;121:241–253.

Mikoshiba K, Huchet M, Changeux JP. Biochemical and immunological studies on the P 400 protein, a protein characteristic of the Purkinje cell from mouse and rat cerebellum. *Dev Neurosci* 1979;2(6):254–275.

Monod J, Changeux JP, Jacob F. Allosteric proteins and cellular control systems. *J Mol Biol* 1963;6:306.

Monod J, Wyman J, Changeux JP. On the nature of allosteric transitions: A plausible model. *J Mol Biol* 1965;12:88–118.

Mulle C, Changeux JP. A Novel type of nicotinic receptor in the rat central nervous system characterized by patch-clamp techniques. *J Neurosci* 1990;10:169–175.

Mulle C, et al. Existence of different subtypes of nicotinic acetylcholine receptors in the rat habenulo interpeduncular system. *J Neurosci* 1991;11:2588–2597.

Nachmansohn D. *Chemical and molecular basis of nerve activity.* New York: Academic Press, 1959;235.

Nikoshiba K. Inositol 1,4,5 triphosphate (IP$_3$) receptor. *Nippon Yakurigaki Zasshi* 2003;241–253.

Noda et al. Primary structure of alpha-subunit precursor of Torpedo californica acetylcholine receptor deduced from cDNA sequence. *Nature* 1982;299:793–797.

Numa S. A molecular view of neurotransmitter receptors and ionic channels. *Havey Lecture Series* 1989;83:121–165.

Olsen R, Meunier JC, Changeux JP. Progress in purification of the cholinergic receptor protein from Electrophorus electricus by affinity chromatography. *FEBS Lett* 1972;28:96–100.

Oswald RE, Changeux JP. Ultraviolet light induced labeling by non competitive blockers of the acetylcholine receptor from *Torpedo marmorata*. *Proc Natl Acad Sci USA* 1981;78:4430–4434.

Oswald RE, Changeux JP. Crosslinking of alpha-bungarotoxin to the acetylcholine receptor from Torpedo marmorata by ultraviolet light irradiation. *FEBS Lett* 1982;139:225–229.

Patrick J, et al. Molecular cloning of the acetylcholine receptor. *Cold Spring Harbor Symp Quant Biol* 1983;48:71–78.

Piette J, Bessereau JL, Huchet M, Changeux JP. Two adjacent MyoD1-binding sites regulate the expression of the acetylcholine receptor delta-subunit gene. *Nature* 1990;345:353–355.

Piette J, Klarsfeld A, Changeux JP. Interaction of nuclear factors with the upstream region of the alpha-subunit gene of chicken muscle acetylcholine receptor: Variations with muscle differentiation and denervation. *EMBO J* 1989;8:687–694.

Picciotto M, Zoli M, Léna C, Bessis A, Lallemand Y, Le Novère N, Vincent P, Merlo Pich E, Brûlet P, Changeux JP. Abnormal avoidance learning in mice lacking functional high-affinity nicotine receptor in the brain. *Nature* 1995;374:65–67.

Picciotto M, Zoli M, Rimondini R, Léna C, Marubio L, Merlo Pich E, Fuxe K, Changeux JP. Acetylcholine receptors containing 2-subunit are involved in the reinforcing properties of nicotine. *Nature* 1998;391:173–177.

Raftery MA, Hunkapiller M, Strader CD, Hood LE. Acetylcholine receptor: Complex of homologous subunits. *Science* 1980;208:1454–1457.

Ramon y Cajal. *Histologie du système nerveux de l'homme et des vertébrés*. Paris: Maloine, 1909–1911.

Redfern PA. Neuromuscular transmission in newborn rats. *J Physiol (Lond)* 1970;209:701–709.

Revah F, Bertrand D, Galzi JL, Devillers-Thiéry A, Mulle C, Hussy N, Bertrand S, Ballivet M, Changeux JP. Mutations in the channel domain alter desensitization of a neuronal nicotinic receptor. *Nature* 1991;353:846–849.

Revah F, Galzi JL, Giraudat J, Haumont PY, Lederer F, Changeux JP. The noncompetitive blocker ^{3}H chlorpromazine labels three amino acids of the acetylcholine receptor delta-subunit: Implications for the alpha helical organization of the MII segments and the structure of the ion channel. *Proc Natl Acad Sci USA* 1990;87:4675–4679.

Schaeffer L, de Kerchove A. and Changeux JP. Targeting transcription to the neuromuscular synapse. *Neuron* 2001;31:15–22.

Schaeffer L, et al. Implication of an Ets and Notch related transcription factor in synaptic expression of the nicotinic acetylcholine receptor. *EMBO J* 1998;17:3078–3090.

Sobel A, Weber M, Changeux JP. Large scale purification of the acetylcholine receptor protein in its membrane-bound and detergent extracted forms from Torpedo marmorata electric organ. *Eur J Biochem* 1977;80:215–224.

Steinlein O, et al. A missense mutation in the neuronal nicotinic acetylcholine receptor alpha 4 subunit is associated with autosomal dominant nocturnal frontal lobe epilepsy. *Nature Genet* 1995;11:201–203.

Von Economo C. *The cytoarchitectonics of the human cerebral cortex*. London: Oxford University Press, 1929.

Weber M, Changeux JP. Binding of Naja nigricollis ^{3}H-alpha-toxin to membrane fragments from Electrophorus and Torpedo electric organs. 1. Binding of the triatiated alpha-neurotoxin in the absence of effector. *Mol Pharmacol* 1974a;10: 1–14.

Weber M, Changeux JP. Binding of Naja nigricollis ^{3}H-alpha-toxin to membrane fragments from Electrophorus and Torpedo electric organs. 2. Effect of the cholinergic agonists and antagonists on the binding of the tritiated alpha-neurotoxin. *Mol Pharmacol* 1974b;10:15–34.

Weber M, Changeux JP. Binding of Naja nigricollis ^{3}H-alpha-toxin to membrane fragments from Electrophorus and Torpedo electric organs. 3. Effects of local anaesthetics on the binding of the tritiated alpha-neurotoxin. *Mol Pharmacol* 1974c;10:35–40.

Weill CL, McNamee MG, Karlin A. Affinity labeling of purified acetylcholine receptor from Torpedo californica. *Biochem Biophys Res Commun* 1974;61:997–1003.

Wiesel TN, Hubel DH. Single-cell responses in striate cortex of kittens deprived of vision in one eye. *J Neurophysiol* 1965;28:1060.

Zoli M, Le Novère N, Hill J, and Changeux JP. Developmental regulation of nicotinic receptor subunit mRNAs in the rat central and peripheral nervous system. *J. Neurosci.* 1995;15:1912–1939.

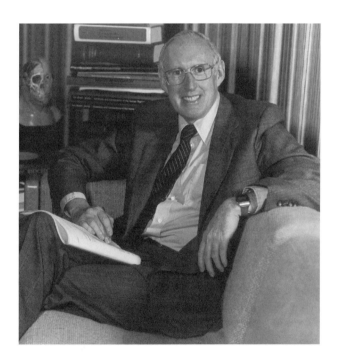

William Maxwell (Max) Cowan

BORN:

Johannesburg, South Africa
September 27, 1931

EDUCATION:

Witwatersrand University, B.Sc. (1951)
Oxford University, D. Phil. (1956)
Oxford University, B.M., B.Ch. (1958)

APPOINTMENTS:

Oxford University (1953)
Washington University School of Medicine (1965)
University of Wisconsin School of Medicine (1966)
Washington University School of Medicine (1968)
The Salk Institute for Biological Studies (1980)
Washington University (1986)
Howard Hughes Medical Institute (1988)

HONORS AND AWARDS (SELECTED):

Institute of Medicine (1977)
Society for Neuroscience, President (1977–1978)
American Academy of Arts and Sciences (1979)
Foreign Associate, National Academy of Sciences, USA (1981)
Fellow, Royal Society of London (1982)
Karl Spencer Lashley Award, American Philosophical Society
(1984)
Foreign Member, Norwegian Academy of Sciences (1984)
Foreign Member, Royal Society of South Africa (1987)
American Philosophical Society (1987)
Honorary DSc., Emory University (1995)
Honorary DSc., Northwestern University (1995)

Max Cowan was a neuroanatomist who specialized in the developing nervous system and pioneered the application of modern neuroanatomical tracing techniques. A gifted scholar and administrator, he was the founding Editor of the Journal of Neuroscience, Editor of the Annual Review of Neuroscience for its first 25 volumes, and Chief Scientific Officer of the Howard Hughes Medical Institute for 13 years.

William Maxwell (Max) Cowan

I was born in Johannesburg, South Africa on September 27, 1931. My parents, Adam Cowan and Jessie Sloan Cowan (nee Maxwell), had emigrated from Scotland to South Africa in the early 1920s, together with my maternal grandparents and the rest of their family, just about the time that the full impact of the British government's decision to close many of the shipyards on the Clyde began to be felt. My father, grandfather, and the three eldest of my uncles had all been involved in one way or another in the shipbuilding industry, and by 1920 the prospects for shipbuilding seemed bleak. In a famous essay on *The Economic Consequences of the Peace*, Maynard Keynes had warned that moving too rapidly from a wartime to a peacetime economy could cause widespread unemployment and social upheaval. Unfortunately, his warning fell on deaf ears, and for much of the 1920s and 1930s the United Kingdom experienced an unprecedented depression. Anticipating that the situation was likely to deteriorate even further, my grandfather went to South Africa to explore the possibilities for engineering in the mines that were springing up along the "gold reef" of the Transvaal. Several months later he urged his family to sell everything they had and join him. My parents were engaged to be married at the time, and it took little persuasion for my father to decide to emigrate with my mother's family.

At first their best hopes seemed to be realized, but soon the mine workers went on strike for higher wages, and within weeks almost the entire industry ground to a halt. Refusing to meet the workers' demands, most mines were closed, and it would be almost 18 months before the workers were allowed to return—at a lower weekly wage than they had received before. In retrospect, it is difficult to know how the family survived this period. My younger uncles decided to abandon mining for other careers, but my father returned to working on structural engineering projects for different mining companies and in the mid-1930s for a private engineering firm where he rose from foreman to works manager. In 1940 he was asked by his company to take responsibility for repairs to ships damaged in the Indian Ocean, and for the next six years my family (consisting of my parents, my brother James, who was six years older than me, and I) moved to the post of East London on the East coast. At the end of World War II, we returned to Johannesburg.

The many moves my parents were forced to make meant that my brother and I had to change schools frequently. In one way I benefited from this. I had been taught by my mother to read, write, and do elementary arithmetic before beginning school when I turned six. Three months later I was transferred to a new school that had just opened. This school had too many second graders and resolved the problem by having an examination and passing on to the third grade the 20 or 30 of us who were judged to be able to cope with that grade. This meant that I had, in effect, completed the first three grades in little more than a year. It also meant that for the rest of my schooling I was two years younger than my classmates. The public schools I attended in Johannesburg were at best adequate, but I was fortunate in East London in being enrolled at Selborne College (named in 1907 for the Second Earl of Selborne, the High Commissioner for South Africa) which was one of the better schools in the country. When my family returned to the Johannesburg area, I stayed for about three months with friends to complete the academic year. While building a new house in a Johannesburg suburb, we lived for almost two years in Germiston, a small town outside the city. Here I completed the last two years of high school, "matriculating" with first class honors at the age of 15.

At the time I had given little thought to what I might do after graduating. One possibility was to join the law firm that my parents had used for some years, as an "articled clerk." This would enable me to work as an "apprentice lawyer" while attending the local law school part time. Since no one in my family had ever attended university, this seemed a reasonable route toward a professional career. Fortunately for me, when my parents and I met with the head of the law firm to sign the articles of agreement, he expressed surprise that I was just 15 and urged my parents to allow me to attend the University of the Witwatersrand ("Wits") full-time for at least one year. Having always taken his advice before, my parents agreed to this and I duly enrolled at the University to take a number of prelaw courses, including English, Afrikaans, Latin, History, and Economics.

That year proved to be decisive in my career. I enjoyed some of the work and did especially well in History and Economics, but soon began to have serious doubts about a career that would probably have involved mainly real estate law. And for the first time, I became seriously concerned about the enormous social disparity between white South Africans and the local African community, most of whom were either employed as domestic servants or in the lowliest (and often the most dangerous) positions in industry and in the mines. I was also much influenced by an elderly friend of my family who urged me to think of an alternative life of service to the community and suggested that I consider going to medical school. As the year progressed, this seemed more and more appealing. Although I knew that admission to medical school was extremely competitive, I thought I had probably done well enough in high school and in my courses at Wits to have a reasonable chance. The one serious snag was that this was a six-year course for which my parents had not bargained. As it happened, the tuition was relatively low, and as I would be living at home and could probably earn some money doing various odd jobs at weekends and during the vacations, my parents finally agreed that I should apply.

The letter acknowledging that I had been accepted into the Medical School class for the following year indicated that although 120 students had been accepted, only 80 would be allowed to proceed to the second year because of space constraints. This meant that competition within the class was likely to be very keen. Like most medical schools that followed the British system of admitting students straight from high school, the first year courses consisted of Physics, Chemistry, and Biology. I had had a fairly good grounding in the physical sciences, but had never taken a biology course. Fortunately, the subject matter was inherently so interesting, and as it was given a decidedly "medical slant" by most of the faculty involved, I found myself more excited by biology than anything I had studied before. I also found that there was a ready market for the lecture notes I took, especially among the Afrikaans-speaking students in the class. Copying out and distributing my notes both aided my own studies and also provided a modest amount of pocket money. At the end of the year, I was ranked third in the class and was comfortably assured of a place in the second year.

In the two-month interval between the first and second years, I got a position as a trainee male nurse at a large, semi-private mental hospital on the outskirts of Johannesburg. This was my first exposure to psychiatry and to what seemed, at the time, to be the distressing treatment of patients with mental illness. Most of those suffering from depression were given electric shock therapy, without the benefits of muscle relaxants or tranquilizers. With three other male nurses, my role was to hold the patients down during their convulsions and, when they had regained consciousness, take them back to their wards, where they awaited their next treatment with growing trepidation. Patients suffering from schizophrenia were routinely given insulin shock therapy which, I was assured, was the best available treatment and, in some instances, seemed to benefit the patients. A number of patients who had failed to respond to all previous treatments were subjected to prefrontal lobotomies. This often enabled the families to cope with their previously intractable behavior, but a number I saw at the hospital seemed to be left in a zombie-like state requiring almost continuous care. My initial shock at what I witnessed during those two months gave way in time to a sense of the extraordinary mystery of how our brains must normally function and a feeling for the desperate plight of those whose brain function is impaired.

The second year curriculum consisted of Gross Anatomy, Histology, Physiology, and Biochemistry. Despite the enormous amount of sheer memorization involved and the general unpleasantness of dissection, I quite enjoyed the courses taught by the Anatomy Department. The newly appointed Head of Physiology and Biochemistry, on the other hand, made these subjects almost incomprehensible to most of the students. Instead of traditional instruction, with lectures and laboratory exercises, he felt that the students should be exposed from the beginning to how scientists "think." To do this, the assembled class watched, listened, or tried to follow an ongoing series of discussions and debates in which all of the faculty participated. There was virtually no coherence in the subject matter from day to day. Studying textbooks was discouraged, and lab exercises were regarded as essentially a waste of time. The Professor himself tended to dominate every session, often going off on some wholly unrelated tangent that left the students bewildered and baffled. Sidney Brenner, who was in his final year, early on recognized that this was an absurd way to teach students who knew nothing about the subject and delighted in getting the Professor off the topic at hand and on to a wild intellectual goose chase. One of Sidney's favorite ploys was to interrupt with a question, "But what about the endocrines?" Rising to the bait the Professor would reply, "You're absolutely right, Sidney, one cannot forget the role of the endocrines," and off he would go, leaving the topic of the discussion, whether it was muscular contraction, temperature regulation, cardiac output, or whatever, as he held forth on "the endocrines." This was my first exposure to Sidney's puckish humor for which, as I later discovered, he was notorious and irrepressible.

Sidney Brenner

I had not realized until quite recently that Sidney Brenner and I had attended the same high school in Germiston, South Africa. He was six or seven years ahead of me, so I did not meet him until some years later when I was a second year medical student at the Witwatersrand University. Sidney was in his final year, having interrupted his medical studies to do a degree in genetics. He had had the most brilliant academic career and managed throughout his clinical years to do research and to teach in the Department of Physiology and Biochemistry. (This was to cost him an additional six months training in Internal Medicine, when the Professor of Medicine refused to give him a passing grade in his final examination, on the grounds that he had rarely, if ever, attended ward rounds.)

I mentioned that it was at Wits that I was first exposed to Sidney's sense of humor, but it was also here that I first discovered his innate and quite extraordinary kindness. Sidney recognized that the bizarre teaching approach adopted by the head of the Department of Physiology and Biochemistry was not teaching the students the fundamentals. About two-thirds of the way through the course, he realized that we could not possibly have learned any physiology and were in imminent danger of being failed by the external examiner at the end of the year. Quite on his own initiative, and at considerable personal inconvenience, he organized a series of tutorials in which he tried to cover in a fairly systematic way the rudiments of biochemistry. Without this, I may never have passed the final examination. Almost everything I learned about biochemistry came from Sidney's seminars, and with my laborious reading of Best and Taylor's huge textbook I absorbed the basic physiology material as well.

I lost touch with Sidney about 2 years later, and it was not until after about another 18 months, in the fall of 1953, that I ran into him again. By this time I was at Oxford working on my doctorate and teaching as a junior faculty member in the Department of Human Anatomy. One late afternoon—it was probably in October or November—I was walking along South Parks Road, which marked the boundary between the science departments and the rest of the University. I was preoccupied and it was not until I had almost passed a duffle-coated figure when I suddenly realized it was Sidney Brenner. "Sidney," I said, "What are you doing here?" With characteristic absence of modesty he replied, "I'm teaching Hinshelwood mathematics." Sir Cyril Hinshelwood was Professor and Head of the Department of Physical Chemistry, a Nobel Laureate for his earlier work on the kinetics of chemical reactions, and a past President of the Royal Society and of the Classical Association. By general consent he was also the most brilliant linguist in Oxford, as fluent in Russian and Chinese as he was in French, German, Italian, Latin, and Greek. Also, if that were not enough, he was a painter of some distinction who had had several exhibitions at various galleries in London and elsewhere. Lately, he had become interested in bacterial growth which, to Sidney's chagrin, he insisted on treating as just another form of chemical kinetics. I gather Sidney had many arguments with his mentor, but apparently failed to convince him of the importance of genetics.

Shortly after Watson and Crick's paper on the structure of DNA appeared, Sidney went to Cambridge to view their model for himself and to talk to people who did believe in genetics. Crick was very impressed (as almost anyone would be) after talking to Sidney for an hour or more and tried to persuade him to join the group in molecular biology at the Cavendish. Unfortunately for Sidney, under the terms of his Beit Fellowship that had supported his stay at Oxford, he was obliged to return to South Africa for a year or two. This proved to be frustrating, but not a complete waste of time as he was able to work in a virology laboratory where he familiarized himself with the exciting work on phage genetics that had played such an important role in the creation of the emerging discipline of molecular biology.

As soon as the mandatory period had expired, Sidney returned to the United Kingdom and took up a staff position in what had now become the Medical Research Council Laboratory of Molecular Biology (LMB) at Cambridge. He was to remain at the LMB until he reached statutory retirement age, having served, after Max Perutz's retirement, as Director of the Laboratory. For many years, until Francis Crick left Cambridge for the Salk

Institute in the late 1970s, Sidney and Francis shared an office during what was one of the most productive collaborations in modern biology. As Francis once remarked to me as we talked of that period, "I always felt that any day that I did not spend at least an hour talking to Sidney was a wasted day."

I need hardly summarize the extraordinary series of seminal discoveries that emerged during that period. It is sufficient to simply mention some of the highlights: the elucidation of the general nature of the genetic code; the discovery of messenger RNA and the formulation of the "central dogma" of molecular biology—"DNA makes RNA and RNA makes protein"; and the introduction of the nematode worm *C. elegans* as a model system for the analysis of development. Sidney's role in all these discoveries was critical, and it is a continuing source of surprise to most biologists that his contributions during this period have not been recognized by the award of the Nobel Prize.[1] With the possible exception of Seymour Benzer, there is no one more deserving of such recognition.

When I emigrated to the United States, for a period of time I lost contact with Sidney. But in the mid 1970s, when I was trying to recruit a molecular geneticist to the Department of Anatomy and Neurobiology at Washington University, I wrote to him asking if he could recommend someone for the position. As it happened, Dr. Bob Waterston, an American postdoc working in Sidney's laboratory on a interesting aspect of genetic regulation in *C. elegans*, was planning to return to the United States. Bob had some reservations about joining a department that was so heavily committed to neurobiology, but at Sidney's urging he accepted the position. (Later, when I left Washington University, Bob transferred his appointment to the Department of Genetics. In due course he became Chairman of the Department and Head of Washington University's Genome Sequencing Center which, with the Sanger Center at Cambridge, has been responsible for sequencing the entire *C. elegans* genome and for contributing the major share of the data in the publicly supported human genome sequencing effort.)

After he retired from the LMB, Sidney became a fairly regular visitor to the Salk Institute, where he continued to astonish us all by the breadth of his knowledge of virtually all aspects of biology and to delight us with his humor. I recall his saying on one occasion when he visited the Salk, having stopped off on the way first at Boston and then at Pasadena, that this has been an unusually interesting trip. In Boston, Ben Lewin, then Editor of *Cell*, the most successful new journal in biology, had complained about the large numbers of papers he was receiving each month. He asked Sidney if he thought they should consider publishing a second more or less parallel journal. "If you do," Sidney replied, "I suggest you call one of them

---

[1]Editorial note: Unfortunately, Max Cowan died before it was announced in the fall of 2002 that Brenner had won the Nobel Prize.

'Hard Cell' and the other, 'Soft Cell.'" (Some years later Lewin did put out a second journal, but under the more prosaic title of *Molecular Cell*.) At Pasadena, Sidney had spent some time with a well-known immunogeneticist who had bent his ear for some hours about the future of genetics and new methods and machinery for DNA sequencing. Sidney's report of this visit went something like this: "You know I've always been very skeptical about artificial intelligence, but having spent an afternoon with ____, I am now totally convinced that it exists."

Sidney currently directs a modest research institute near Berkeley. He is still full of new ideas about the future of genomics (and almost anything else one cares to mention), and every other month he has a piece in *Current Biology* that reminds us that his sense of humor is, if anything, even sharper than before. For example, only Sidney could propose that the Nobel Prize Committee in Stockholm revise its policies. As he tells it, on the prescribed day in October the awardee would receive an early morning phone call, "Professor ____, I am honored to tell you that you have been selected to receive this year's Nobel Prize for Physiology or Medicine." Once the excited recipient of the call had calmed down and stopped saying how shocked he was and how flattered and honored, etc., the heavily accented Swedish voice would say: "I must inform you, Professor ____, that the policy regarding the Nobel Prize has been changed. You now have to decide whether you want the honor or the money—you can no longer have both."

For more than 50 years, Sidney has been one of my scientific heroes. I am fortunate to have been his student and I am honored to be his friend.

An Introduction to Neuroscience

The only integrated course taught my second year was in the area we now refer to as neuroscience, although it was some 20 or more years before that name was introduced. The reason for this was that only one person in the brain sciences was competent to teach both neuroanatomy and neurophysiology. This was Dr. Michael Wright, at the time a senior lecturer in the Anatomy Department. Mike, as I soon came to know him, was essentially self-taught. Like Sidney Brenner, he too had interrupted his medical training to do a degree in anatomy, where he had concentrated on the nervous system. On completing his medical degree, he joined the faculty and soon established himself as *the* local authority on the nervous system. He had a slight stammer and was not a particularly fluent lecturer. But among all our teachers he stood out as not only extremely knowledgeable about his subject, but also determined to engage the interest of his students. I can still recall vividly the lecture he gave on synaptic transmission. This was based (as I later learned) on Eccles' recent review and restatement of his electrical hypothesis for both excitation and inhibition. For the first time my interest was piqued: how exciting it must be to understand something about our brains and how they function. At the end of the lecture, when the other students had left the auditorium, I had the temerity to ask "what would one have to do to work in this field?" Mike's response was to say that if I did well enough in my second year courses, I could drop out of Medical School for a year and take a B.Sc. in Anatomy and focus my interest, as he had done, on the nervous system.

When the results of our first exams were posted, I went to see Mike again and was reassured that I would be accepted into the Department's B.Sc. program. My parents were concerned that this would add yet another year to my education, but were somewhat reassured that I would probably be given a teaching assistantship and, with it, tuition remission. Generally, only one or two students took this approach each year, but in my year six of us chose the B.Sc. program and were joined by a seventh student, Godfrey Getz, who had completed the third year before returning to do a degree in Biochemistry. Of the students in my own year, only two of us continued this diversion, taking a second year to take a B.Sc. Honors degree. My colleague, Bill Andrew, later spent several years as a medical missionary in Swaziland before becoming a consultant radiologist in Pretoria. Godfrey Getz went on to have a distinguished academic career in research, teaching, and academic administration at the University of Chicago.

I had not appreciated that the B.Sc. degree would entail majoring in two subjects, Gross Anatomy and Histology, or that Gross Anatomy included human paleontology. So the amount of time I could spend on neurophysiology, which had been my initial interest, was rather limited. In part because of this, and in part because I was awarded the degree with distinction in both majors, which had been achieved only once before—by Sidney Brenner, no less—I stayed on for a second year. During this year I spent a great deal of time with Mike Wright—much of it in building our own equipment—learning from him much more than neuroanatomy and neurophysiology. He encouraged me to read widely in philosophy, in the history of science, in politics, and in literature. In a special sense this year marked the beginning of my real education.

After completing the requirements for the B.Sc. Honors degree, I returned to the third year of Medical School, mainly Pathology and Pharmacology. But I had only spent about four rather boring months on these subjects when, out of the blue, I was summoned to see Professor Dart, the Head of the Anatomy Department. With characteristic shortness Dart began by saying, "How would you like to go to Oxford?" I was too surprised to answer intelligently, so he went on to explain that he had recently received a letter from his friend Professor LeGros Clark at Oxford, asking if there was anyone in his Department interested in the nervous system who might be suitable for a junior faculty position. After discussing this with Mike Wright, Dart had decided to put my name forward, although, as he was quick to point out, I should not let my expectations get out of hand because it was likely that LeGros was interested in someone who already had a medical degree. The vacancy at Oxford had occurred because a former South African, Harold Daitz, who LeGros had recruited three or four years earlier, had died suddenly. But LeGros had been so impressed with him that he thought it just possible that another South African might be suitable. Dart promised to write to LeGros and, to my amazement, received a letter by return of post saying that Cowan sounds fine; he can do a D.Phil (Oxford's Ph.D) while working as a Department Demonstrator (a position roughly equivalent to a non-tenured Assistant Professor at a U.S. institution) at a salary of £500 per year. This time I was ready with my answer, and in little more than a month I set sail from Cape Town, arriving in Oxford on April 17, 1953.

Raymond Dart

It was not until I arrived in Oxford that I discovered that not all professors of Anatomy were like Raymond Dart, the Professor of Anatomy Wits. For generations, Dart had terrorized students by his irascibility and his intolerance of even the most minor error or infraction of the rules he had imposed. His infrequent visits to the dissection room were terrifying to even the bravest student. At any moment he could fasten on a hapless student and launch a verbal attack on his or her appearance, dress, or posture, with his voice rising in real or feigned anger that sent shivers of fear throughout the entire class. His brusque ferocity was legendary throughout the Medical School. One widely repeated story—probably apocryphal—was that on one occasion a rather mousy faculty member had haltingly announced that his wife was pregnant. "Good God, man," Dart was alleged to have responded, "Who do you suspect?" He was only slightly more accessible and a shade less intimidating to the students who dropped out of Medical School for a year or two to take a bachelor's or honors degree in Anatomy and Histology.

It was during the year I was working toward a B.Sc. in his department that I experienced first hand his wrath. The first occasion was when I gave a seminar on cutaneous sensation to the faculty and my fellow students. I had worked hard in preparing for the seminar and thought it had gone well. But no sooner had I ended than Dart, who had been sitting in the front row, jumped to his feet. "My God man," he railed, "If you have something to say, shout it out. Don't just stand there, holding on to the pointer as if for dear life." And with that he leapt onto the podium, his arms flung high as he repeated, "Shout it out. Let the world know what you think."

My second encounter with Dart was even more traumatic. I had not realized when I enrolled for the degree course that the degree in Anatomy included Anthropology. At the time I had little interest in comparative anatomy or physical anthropology and had paid little attention to either the lectures or the practical work. About a third of the way into the course,

I received a summons to meet "the Prof" in his office, together with Philip Tobias who served as course master for the anthropology program. At the appointed time Tobias and I met at Dart's door. Tobias knocked and Dart responded with a gruff "come in." But as we entered his office, he did not look up. Instead, he continued writing for what seemed to me to be half an hour, but was probably only a minute or two, but long enough to be intimidating. Finally, he looked up at Tobias and said "Well, what is it?" With that Tobias began listing how many lectures and labs I had missed and how far back I was falling in anthropology. When he finished, Dart said, "Is that all?" "Yes," I replied. Dart asked, "Then what the hell have you been doing?" I replied, "I've been working with Dr. Wright. You see I had only dropped out of Medical School for this year because I wanted to study the brain and especially neurophysiology. And for the past three months we have been building equipment."

When I stopped, my heart was beating fast and my palms were cold and clammy. Imagine my surprise when Dart suddenly turned on Tobias and asked, "Is that true?" "Yes," said Tobias—he had obviously talked with Mike Wright. "Then why are you bothering me?" Dart asked. He continued, "We get about 80 medical students a year through this Department, and hardly one of them has ever had an idea in his head. At last we find one interested enough to want to study something he's excited about, and you want to kill his interest by turning him into a measurer of bones like yourself." He had a few more choice words for Tobias, and just as I was beginning to feel sorry for him at this unexpected turn of events, Dart turned on me: "As for you young man, if you don't get the top mark in anthropology at the end of this year I will personally see that you are thrown out of this University. Now get the hell out of here!"

Fortunately, with some effort I was able to catch up with my colleagues, and, in time, I even began to find anthropology quite interesting. At the end of the year I was fortunate to get a "double first" (i.e., honors in both my major subjects) which did not escape Dart's attention. I recall walking down the hallway one day and being alarmed at seeing Dart and a visitor approaching. The most alarming thing was Dart's simian gait: head slightly lowered, brow furrowed, arms hanging loosely at his sides, a curious, almost slouching walk. To my surprise, as he reached me he stopped, turned toward the visitor, and said: "Oh, this is Cowan, one of our bright young boys." With that he turned and continued his Australopithecine-like progression.

In the mid-1970s, when I was Chairman of the Anatomy Department at Washington University School of Medicine, I heard that Dart (who was then in his 80s) was visiting Philadelphia. As he had spent almost two years in the 1920s working in the Anatomy Department at Washington University on a Rockefeller Fellowship, I thought it would be nice to invite him to give the Terry Lecture, named for Robert Terry, Washington University's first Professor of Anatomy and someone whom Dart had known and admired for more than 50 years. Dart said he would be pleased to accept the invitation and duly came to St. Louis. While somewhat frail, in conversation he was as lively as ever, but, as I was pleased to see, a good deal more mellow.

In introducing him to the audience who attended the lecture, I commented briefly on his career. After completing his medical education in Sydney, Australia, he had gone to England to work under Sir Grafton Elliot Smith, at that time the doyen of British anatomy. When he returned from his stay in St. Louis, Elliot Smith had urged him to apply for the Chair of Anatomy at the newly formed Medical School at Wits in Johannesburg, South Africa. In due course he was appointed and took up the position in January 1923. The following year he made one of the most important discoveries in human evolution—the finding of the first Austraopithecine fossil. The story of this discovery has been told frequently, so I shall not repeat it here. But what is less well known is that Dart's report of his finding in the journal *Nature* met with considerable skepticism by the leading British anatomists who, for the most part, were so enamored of the Piltdown skull that they found it hard to believe that the adoption of an upright posture preceded expansion of the brain. Moreover, many of them also remembered that before Dart left for South Africa, he had published a number of papers on the evolution and development of the vertebrate nervous system which not only challenged the conventional wisdom, but in at least one instance was demonstrably wrong. It would be more than 30 years before the correctness of Dart's interpretation of the Taungs baby came to be appreciated. But Dart's immediate response was typical; he refused to publish his next several papers in British journals. As I recall he sent his first post-Australopithecus Africanus paper to an obscure Japanese journal!

After saying all this and more, I ended the introduction by recounting my meeting with Dart and Tobias. In responding, Dart began his lecture by saying, "I can't recall the incident that Dr. Cowan has just recounted, but remembering how I used to be in those days, I must confess it sounds authentic!"

I cannot end my reminiscences about Raymond Dart without adding two further remarks. The first is that I am only one of many South Africans who got their start in science by taking advantage of the introduction to research provided by the degree courses for medical students that Dart had initiated. Although he did not personally participate to any significant degree in these courses (at least by the time I took my degree), he realized long before most other medical educators that the best way to excite students' interest in science is to give them an opportunity to be engaged in research as early as possible. The success of so many who took a B.Sc. or B.Sc. Honors degree during their medical training is a lasting tribute to Raymond Dart. The second thing I wish to add is an abiding memory I have of Dart that stands in striking contrast to his brusque and often frightening manner. It happened during a lecture he gave on human evolution. At one point, he lifted onto the desk what looked like a shoe box. From this, with visibly trembling hands, he removed the original Taungs skull. For fully a minute he held it like a tiny infant in his hands, and from near the front of the lecture room I could see his eyes fill with tears. Was it, I wondered, because he continued to be overawed by the wonder of holding in his hands the first real link to our prehuman past? Or was it from the realization that after so many years he had finally been vindicated? Even his most vociferous critic, Sir Arthur Keith, had finally accepted the correctness of his views and had proposed that the Australopithecines should be called the "Dartians," although unlike the "Martians," they really were of this world. Whatever the reason, the moment was a touching one that revealed an aspect of Dart's persona that for the most part seemed to have been carefully concealed. Like so many men who present a remote and tough exterior, at heart he was as sentimental as anyone I have known in science.

I should also say that it is a source of special pleasure to me that it was largely through the efforts of my mentor at Oxford, Wilfrid LeGros Clark, that the Australopithecines came to be recognized as the earliest human ancestors. And for most of my years at Washington University, a plaster cast of the Taungs fossil stared down at me as I sat at my desk, a stern reminder not only of where I had come from (in more ways than one) but also of how I should (or perhaps better, should *not*) behave toward my colleagues and students.

LeGros Clark

It is impossible to express adequately my indebtedness to LeGros Clark. From my first meeting with him on the morning after my arrival in Oxford until his last brief letter to me some months before his death in 1971, he treated me almost like a son; he guided and nurtured my scientific career, advised me generously on every significant decision I made, and set the finest example of scientific excellence and sound judgment that I have known. In sum, I owe almost everything I have been able to achieve to his personal kindness, thoughtfulness, and encouragement. I had known of his many contributions to neuroanatomy before joining his department, but it was only later that I came to appreciate the importance of his contributions to comparative anatomy, to primatology, and especially to human evolution and in a larger sense through his books and lectures to all aspects of anatomy. To say that he was *the* outstanding anatomist of his generation hardly does justice to the range of his scholarship and the example he set for all who were privileged to know him. Two incidents will serve to illustrate how he influenced my own career, beyond the unique opportunity he provided by inviting me, an unknown student, to Oxford to be his colleague and for 20 years his friend.

Unknown to me he had applied, on my behalf, to the Nuffield Foundation for one of their greatly prized Commonwealth Fellowships. When, some time later, he told me that the Foundation had made an exception to their general policy of only awarding fellowships to individuals currently residing in one of the Commonwealth countries, I was both surprised and delighted; the stipend was significantly more than my Oxford salary, and the fellowship carried a number of other fringe benefits. But when he told me that one of the requirements was that fellows had to return to their own country for at least three years, he immediately sensed my disappointment. "How do you feel about returning to South Africa three years from now?" he asked. When I responded by saying that I had hoped that, if I did well enough, I would be able to continue working at Oxford, he said without a moment's hesitation, "That's what I hoped you would say; I'll let the Nuffield people know that you have declined their offer." Despite the trouble he had gone to, he gave not the slightest hint of annoyance; instead, I took his response as the best possible reassurance that he was pleased with my progress and that I could look forward to a continuing position in the department.

The second incident also occurred without my prior knowledge. In the fall of 1955, he attended a meeting in Johannesburg on the role of the Australopithecines in human evolution. While he was there he got hold of my parents' address and arranged to visit them at their home. On returning to Oxford, he came up to my office to say that he had been giving a good deal of thought to my career and felt that it would be important for me to complete my clinical training and take the B.M.B.Ch. degree. He had already consulted with the University authorities and had been assured that I could be admitted to the clinical school at the Radcliffe hospital in the spring and would not have to meet any of the preclinical requirements, except for Pathology and Pharmacology. In addition, I would continue my appointment as a Departmental Demonstrator (at a somewhat reduced salary) and would be promoted to a tenured University Lectureship when I had taken the degree. This was such a surprise that after thanking him for going to all this additional trouble I could not help asking why he was suggesting what seemed to me an entirely new direction. His answer was: "Two things. First, without a medical degree it will be very difficult for you to achieve the success your career deserves, at least in this country. And, second, when I told your parents how well you were doing and would soon have your D.Phil., your mother said to me, 'That's very nice, but we had always hoped he would become a real doctor.' So you owe it both to yourself and to your parents to do this." Needless to say, I took his advice and was able to complete my medical degree in about two and a half years after finishing the D.Phil in April 1956. But perhaps the kindest and most encouraging gift LeGros bestowed was the freedom to work on whatever topic I chose, while always making himself available for advice and guidance whenever I needed it.

Neuroanatomical Studies with Tom Powell

The first person in the Department of Human Anatomy Le Gros introduced me to was Tom Powell. Little did I realize that morning that Tom and I would work together over the next 13 years or that next to Le Gros himself, Tom would have the greatest impact on my work during my years at Oxford.

As we were walking upstairs from Le Gros's office he told me that he especially wanted me to meet a young clinical research fellow who had been in the department for about a year and a half. He told me: "His name is Tom Powell and although he originally came to Oxford to do neurosurgery with Hugh Cairns, I hope he will stay with us in the Department. He won the Hallet prize and we really need people who know Gross Anatomy as he does. He's been working with me on the thalamus and I'm sure you'll find him helpful." I had no idea what the Hallet Prize was or why this would indicate a good gross anatomist, but I was pleased to know that there was someone else working in the brain to whom I could look for help. When Le Gros introduced us, I was immediately impressed by Tom's friendly response. As we left his office he said, "If I can help you in any way, just let me know."

It was not long before I learned that the Hallet Prize was awarded each year to the top candidate in the primary examination for the FRCS (Fellowship of the Royal College of Surgeons) and that its receipt marked one as knowing essentially everything there is to know about gross anatomy. I also learned that in preparation for the "primary," Tom had spent a year as a Demonstrator in Anatomy at Cambridge, where he had not only mastered the minutiae of anatomy, but had seen Geoffrey Harris working out the direction of blood flow in the hypophysial portal circulation that, arguably, marked the real beginning of modern neuroendocrinology. Later, I learned that he had won scholarships to Edinburgh—at the time the leading medical school in the United Kingdom—and that on graduating he had determined to become a surgeon. After completing an internship he had gone to Cambridge, took the primary FRCS, and was then a surgical resident (to use the American title of this position) at the Royal Postgraduate Medical School with Hammersmith Hospitals. On completing the second part of the FRCS, he had essentially become "board certified" in surgery. But he had set his heart on a career in neurosurgery and had applied for an internship in Cairns' unit at Oxford. Cairns had established his service as the very best neurosurgical unit in the country and competition for places in his program was extremely keen. He only admitted people who had already completed the equivalent of a residency in general surgery. His standards, and those of his colleague, the American Joe Pennybacker, were known to be the most rigorous in the profession.

For some reason that I cannot recall (if I ever knew), Cairns was unable to have Tom begin his neurosurgical training right away and suggested that he spend a year or more doing research in the Department of Human

Anatomy under Le Gros Clark. Le Gros had been pleased to have Tom join him and assisted in Tom's obtaining a Medical Research Council Clinical Research Fellowship.

As it happened, Le Gros had received the brain of a patient who had died some 24 days after having almost the entire cerebral hemisphere surgically removed and felt that the analysis of the thalamus would be an excellent project for Tom's first experience in research. While several studies of near complete hemispherectomy in other mammals (including non-human primates) had been reported, this seemed like a unique case to observe the changes in the human thalamus. The analysis of this brain occupied much of Tom's first year in Oxford and resulted in his first publication, *Residual Neurons in the Human Thalamus following Hemidecortication*, that appeared in *Brain* in 1952. It was to be the first of over 160 papers he would publish over the next 42 years—efforts that constituted an extraordinary research contribution.

Tom's first experimental study was done in collaboration with Le Gros. It involved analyzing retrograde degenerative changes seen in the ventral posterior nucleus of the thalamus after more-or-less selective lesions of three of the cytoarchitectonic fields that comprise the somatosensory cortex in monkeys. The resulting paper appeared in 1953 shortly after I joined the Department. Le Gros had been responsible for most of the surgical procedures and Tom had carried out the detailed (and quantitative) analyses on which their primary conclusions were based. He had also written, as he showed me, four drafts of the paper before Le Gros was satisfied and sent it off to the *Proceedings of the Royal Society*.

About the time Tom began working in the Department, Le Gros recruited to the position of Departmental Demonstratorship a young South African who had for a short while been working in the Anatomy Department at Middlesex Hospital. This was H. M. Daitz, known to my colleagues in Johannesburg as Harold, but to everyone at Oxford as Max. Daitz soon made his presence known in the Department. He was thoughtful, smart, hard working, and unusually outgoing. At the Middlesex Hospital he had worked in an intellectual vacuum but surrounded by others doing research; he blossomed in Oxford. Like Le Gros Clark, who near the beginning of his career had carried out an important experimental study using the simplest of tools—a saucepan, scalpel, scissors, and surgical needle—to place lesions in the brains of rats, Daitz set out to study the hippocampus and its connections. Unfortunately, his life was cut short at the age of 29, and the field lost someone who would undoubtedly have become a major figure judging from the material he had collected and the notes he had made during his brief stay at Oxford.

At Le Gros' suggestion, Tom undertook to work up Daitz's unpublished work, and when I first met him he was in the process of putting the finishing touches on a paper that reported Daitz's first original discovery, namely, that the fimbria are not solely a hippocampal efferent pathway as Cajal and others had stated, but contained afferents from the medial septal nucleus and the diagonal band of Broca which we now know to be the source of the cholinergic inputs to the hippocampal formation. The cellular changes in the septal region after fimbrial lesions had puzzled Tom for some time, and for the first few days I was in the Department we discussed them, looked at the slides, and discussed them further, until finally Tom felt satisfied that his initial conclusion was probably correct. This experience presaged the literally hundreds of hours that Tom and I were to spend over the next 13 years looking at slides, debating the significance of our observations (we always examined the experimental material independently), and trying to resolve difficulties in conference before writing up the results with each of us taking turns to "dictate" a section while the other wrote it down. When we had completed the draft, Tom would type it up, hunting and pecking on an old manual typewriter while I prepared the figures and the photomicrographs. We often had lunch and dinner together at the faculty club adjoining the science area. In the evenings we went back to the lab until 10:00 or 10:30 PM. We were both single at the time and work was the center of our lives. When we were not doing experiments or looking at the slides, we would spend hours on end talking, talking, and talking. For me it was wonderful to have such a colleague and friend, and as our work was going well, I could not have wished for a better start to my career (Fig. 1).

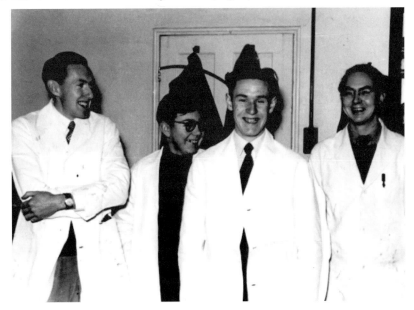

Fig. 1. Max Cowan (far left), Tom Powell (far right), and other lab members at Oxford in the early 1950s.

In many of the brains prepared by Daitz, the anterior thalamic nuclei had been incidentally damaged, and with LeGros' approval, Tom and I used some of these brains to analyze the selective projection of different parts of the medial mamillary nucleus. The large-celled lateral nucleus appeared to be unaffected.[2] Some of the other material Daitz had prepared began what was to be a long-term interest in the organization of the connections of the hippocampus, but apart from enabling us to clearly distinguish the fields that projected into the fimbria and the so-called dorsal fornix, the protargol-stained preparations were of only limited value.

While working up Daitz's material, Tom and I spent a good deal of time thinking about the projection of the midline and intralaminar nuclei. Unlike most of the rest of the thalamic nuclei, which undergo severe retrograde degeneration after lesions of specific cortical fields, the intralaminar nuclei (and especially the centromedian nucleus which is such a striking feature of the primate thalamus) show either no, or only minimal, changes even after virtually complete decortication. In addition, in the 1940s Morison and Dempsey had shown that low-frequency electrical stimulation of the intralaminar system elicited a "diffuse recruiting response" across the cortex. A number of alternative suggestions to account for these findings had been put forward, and most recently, Rose and Woolsey had reported that whereas the nuclei survived large cortical lesions, in rabbits in which the "rhinecephalic" structures were destroyed, the nuclei showed marked degeneration. They had not followed up on this observation, and so Tom and I planned a series of experiments, first in rats and later in rabbits, with lesions directed at the rhinecephalic structures in the basal forebrain, sparing as much as possible the neocortex. The results of these experiments were reported in 1954 and 1955 and seemed to us to establish fairly clearly that, whereas some of the smaller midline nuclei projected to the medio-basal forebrain, the intralaminar nuclei only showed degeneration when the lesions encroached on the striatum (caudate and putamen). There had been earlier findings compatible with the notion that the intralaminar nuclei were part of a thalamo-striate system, but to a large extent this view had been discounted. We were impressed—as was LeGros when we showed him our material—that the severity of the cellular degeneration was as marked as that seen in the principal nuclei after cortical lesions. In retrospect, however, we should have considered the possibility that the changes were

---

[2]I returned to this problem several years later when I was in St. Louis and was asked to examine several cat brains in which F.J. Fry at the University of Illinois, Urbana, had placed lesions at different levels in the mamillothalamic and mamillotegmental tracts either singly or in combination. Following his death, his family asked if I could prepare the work for publication. This was of interest to me because of my prior work on the mamillary connections, but especially because it provided a direct way to test the hypothesis that the existence of proximal collaterals protected neurons against axotomy.

not solely due to damage to the terminals of the axons of the intralaminar nuclei and perhaps given more attention to the much milder changes that from time to time had been reported in the nuclei after large cortical lesions.

At the time, we were excited by an entirely fortuitous observation in the brains of some of our experimental rabbits in which the cingulate cortex had been damaged, without involvement of the striatum or the thalamus itself. This was the finding that, in addition to the expected retrograde degeneration in the three anterior thalamic nuclei, there was marked cell loss in the medial mamillary nucleus. This prompted us to place additional lesions in different parts of the cingulate cortex in young rabbits, following on the lines of Rose and Woolsey's careful analysis of the projection of the anterior nucleus upon the limbic cortex. These experiments confirmed our earlier study that each major part of the medial mamillary nucleus projects upon a different component of the anterior thalamic complex and beyond these to the different cytoarchitectonic fields of the cingulate region. As neither LeGros nor Tom had been aware of such "retrograde transneuronal degeneration," for a few short days I felt I had actually made an original discovery. But, cautious as always, LeGros urged that we look closely at the early German literature in which so much had been reported but largely forgotten. To my chagrin I soon learned that between 1870 and 1884 Gudden had reported atrophy of the medial mamillary nucleus in his young rabbits with extensive cortical lesions. And further reading revealed that there were reports in the ophthalmology literature of primary optic atrophy (due to the death of retinal ganglion cells) in patients with long-standing lesions involving the visual cortex. (Some years later, when I was in Madison, WI, one of my graduate students, Jennifer Hart (later LaVail), and I found that cingulate lesions in neonatal and very young rats could result in degeneration beyond the anterior thalamus and mamillary nucleus, to the ventral tegmental nucleus which was known to project upon the medial mamillary nucleus).

Despite the cost of monkeys for experimental purposes, LeGros Clark felt it was important to obtain funds for Tom and I to place stereotaxic lesions in different parts of the caudate nucleus and putamen in a number of macaques to resolve in particular the long-standing issue of the projection of the centromedian nucleus. Although in some cases the incidental involvement of the internal capsule complicated the findings, it was clear from others that isolated lesions within the putamen resulted in clear-cut retrograde degeneration in the centromedian nucleus and equally convincing changes in the more rostral intralaminar nuclei including the nuclei centralis medialis and lateralis. The resulting paper in *Brain* seemed well received, and it was not until the introduction of new methods that we finally established that, in addition to their primary projection upon the striatum, the intralaminar nuclei have colleratal projections to the cerebral cortex.

During a short trip that Tom and I made to Brussels, at the invitation of Frederic Bremer, one of the outstanding neurphysiologists of his generation, we saw experiments being done on pigeons which seemed among the most tractable of all experimental animals. Since, in avian brains, the striatum comprises almost 90% of the telencephalon, it occurred to us that it might be of interest to examine the projections of the different thalamic nuclei upon the various striatal subdivisions. While the findings in this study proved to be of some interest to comparative neuroanatomists, it had a much longer impact on my own career, again through a wholly unexpected finding.

As we were compiling our study, we were joined for a year by a postdoctoral fellow who wished to learn some neuroanatomical methods. Because he was to be with us for such a short time, we suggested that he might examine the projection of the retina upon the diencephalon and midbrain of the pigeon, using the technique introduced in 1954 by Walle Nauta that clearly showed the course and termination of degenerating axons against a relatively clear background due to the active suppression of staining of normal axons. The findings confirmed what had been known for many years about the retinal projection, but the pattern of degeneration in one component of the visual system, the so-called isthmo-optic tract, seemed quite different in that it began within the isthmic region of the brain and proceeded centrifugally toward the retina. In Nissl preparations made some weeks after unilateral eye removal, the isthmo-optic nucleus (ION) of the opposite side was completely degenerated. What we had stumbled upon was a centrifugal projection within the visual system, that is, a pathway that arises in the brain and projects to the retina. Again, a search of the older literature revealed that this pathway had been described in the late 19th century by the Dutch neuroanatomist Wallenberg, but had been largely ignored. Some time later, one of Tom's students, James McGill, interrupted his medical studies to do a D.Phil. and chose to work on the detailed organization of the projection of the ION upon the retina and of the projection of the retina upon the ION, by way of the optic tectum. The ION and its connections were to play a large role in my subsequent career when in the mid-1960s and later I began working on the development of the nervous system.

But several things were to happen before this. I had begun my clinical training in the fall of 1956 and was able to supplement my demonstrator's salary by tutoring students at Pembroke College in Anatomy.

In the late summer of 1954, I learned that Mike Wright and his wife were coming to London—he to do electroencephalography at the National Hospital for Neurological Diseases in Queen's Square and she to continue her clinical training at the Hammersmith Hospital. Shortly afterwards, with LeGros' approval, Mike and I agreed to pick up on some of the work we had been doing at Wits on the use of "strychnine neuronography," although by this time it was clear that the complex pattern of "suppressor bands" that

Dusser de Barenne, McCulloch, and their colleagues at MIT had claimed to have found using this approach were almost entirely artifactual. We were still interested in the possible relationship of trains of strychnine spikes to the "spike and dome" recordings seen in petit mal epilepsy. And since, by this time, everything I had worked on had been done in collaboration with Tom Powell, it was natural that he should join us in this endeavor.

Michael (Mike) Wright

Apart from a handful of close personal friends, two or three former colleagues, and perhaps a dozen of his students, Mike Wright is essentially unknown. Yet to those whose lives he touched, he will always be remembered as a fine scholar, outstanding teacher, and a wonderfully caring human being. I personally owe as much to Mike Wright as to any of my other mentors, and in an act of quite extraordinary generosity, he changed my entire life.

Mike, like so many of the junior faculty members I encountered in my first year or two at medical school, had interrupted his medical training to do a degree in science (he ended up doing an M.Sc.) and shortly after graduating was offered a faculty position. He had had an excellent academic record as a student, but what was most remarkable was that he had, entirely through his own efforts, become the most knowledgeable neurobiologist in South Africa (although the term neurobiology was not then in vogue). It is true that as a young scientist Raymond Darrt had published papers on the brains of some Australian reptiles and on this basis had arrived at a rather odd view of brain evolution, but there was no one else in Johannesburg at this time who had any first-hand experience of neurophysiology or neuroanatomy. To this degree Mike was a self-taught man.

I don't know what had prompted him to turn his attention to the study of the nervous system. Perhaps it was because as an infant he had suffered some form of neurological injury which left him with a marked foot drop, a somewhat unsteady gait, and a mild stammer. But by the time I met him, he had not only mastered the intricacies of neuroanatomy, including its esoteric and often capricious methods, but was aware of all the latest developments in neurophysiology and had learned enough about electronics to begin building his own equipment to record activity from the brain. It was probably because he was so engaged with the field that he became such an engaging teacher. Unlike most of his colleagues who were content in their lectures to rehash the contents of the prescribed textbooks, Mike made a point of introducing his students to the most recent new work in the field, while in no way trying to snow them with his erudition. Because of his slight speech impediment, he was not considered a good lecturer by those who judged lectures on the forcefulness of their presentation rather than their content; but to those of us who were disappointed by the generally low level of medical school teaching, his lectures stood out as both intellectually exciting and challenging.

I have already recounted my first encounter with Mike (as he later insisted I call him) and how I soon came to work in his lab. Mike was very accommodating and made it possible for me to spend odd hours working with him, mainly constructing electrophysiological equipment. This was in the days before research grants, and most of Mike's work was funded out of his own pocket. I was able to help in a small way by selling the microscope my parents had given me for doing well in my first year of medical school. The proceeds of this sale enabled us to buy a cathode ray oscilloscope tube and some of the other components needed to build a recording set-up.

In a real sense my education began when I started working with Mike. As we sat on opposite sides of a lab bench, Mike would talk to me about science, philosophy, literature, and politics. Most days he would suggest that I read something, usually unrelated to my course work. It was through these "private tutorials" that I first became acquainted with the British empiricists, with Bertrand Russell, Wittengenstein, etc. What little I know about electronics I learned from him in those pretransister days, and I owe essentially all my grounding in neuroanatomy and neurophysiology to his patient yet demanding tutorials. It was because I had learned so much from Mike that year that I decided to spend a second year with him for a B.Sc. degree.

For my honors thesis Mike suggested that I describe the anatomy of the hypothalamus of the common South African baboon. In retrospect, this was a fairly boring exercise since the baboon hypothalamus proved to be no different from that of other primates that had been well described by others. But my real interest was in electrophysiology, and Mike taught me much both in South Africa and later when he was visiting England.

I have already described how I came to be recommended to Le Gros Clark by Raymond Dart, and Mike's role in this was an act of quite exceptional selflessness. As I left Dart's office, after I had learned that he would put my name forward, I began to wonder why Mike had not put his own name forward. He had a medical degree and also an M.Sc.; he had been on the faculty for a few years and had just completed an excellent textbook on the nervous system for medical students. In every respect he seemed ideally suited for the position and obviously much better qualified than I was. Yet the fact remained: he had recommended me. In retrospect, I should have gone directly to ask him why he had chosen not to seek the position. Regrettably, I did not do this and to this day do not know why he put my name forward.

When at Oxford I learned that Mike was coming to England, I contacted him on his arrival and arranged to visit him. This led to the suggestion of our once again working together. Tom Powell was eager to learn some electrophysiology, and this led to my working on a project with both my closest present colleague and my closest prior collaborator.

During their stay in London, Mike's wife Priscilla fell in love with a visiting Australian physician at the Hammersmith and shortly thereafter Mike fell in love with one of the EEG technicians with whom he had been working. Priscilla went to Australia and before long achieved some distinction as a clinical nephrologist. Mike returned to Johannesburg and was later joined by his friend and soon-to-be second wife.

I have always regretted that I did not keep in touch with Mike after his return to South Africa, and it came as a painful surprise, about two years later, to learn that he had died under rather tragic circumstances. I was later told that those last two years were very unhappy ones for Mike professionally. He had been approached by a group of neurologists to be responsible for their EEG service, as it was clear that he was the most experienced and knowledgeable person in Johannesburg. Mike agreed to do this, although he must have realized that it would leave him with little or no time for research. But, I understand that this was not the main source of his unhappiness. He had not been "reading" EEGs very long, when he realized that the neurologists were taking advantage of both their patients and him. There was no justification for ordering an EEG for the great majority of the patients he saw, and while he was being paid a rather modest fee for carrying out the procedure, analyzing the records, and providing a written report, the clinicians were billing the patients at what he considered an exorbitant rate. When he confronted the neurologists with this, they simply terminated the arrangement leaving him without his principal source of income. He became seriously depressed, and in 1961 he sadly passed away at the age of 37.

I have no doubt that had Mike lived in the United States or in the United Kingdom he would have had a substantial impact on the emerging field of neuroscience. He had a fine grasp of neuroanatomy and, although self-taught, was as knowledgeable about neurophysiology as anyone I knew. As it was, his scientific legacy was an excellent short textbook on the fiber systems of the brain and spinal cord, published by Wits and sadly long out of print, and the respect and affection of those few students whose lives he influenced so profoundly.

The Oxford Years

Each Tuesday and Thursday during the fall of 1954 Tom and I caught the first available train from Oxford to Paddington, and the "tube" to Queen's Square, where we spent the day in a partially darkened room observing photically driven strychnine spikes at different frequencies and for different periods of time. Two findings soon emerged. The first was that the maximum frequency the spikes could be driven was about 3.5/sec, and at this rate there was a progressive separation of the photic-evoked response and the strychnine response until after about 10 sec, when the separation was quite distinct, the train of strychnine spikes ceased to follow the evoked responses. The second was that it was possible to record photically driven strychnine spikes well beyond the visual cortex, if reinforced by local strychnine applied at intervals of roughly every 7 min, spreading it seemed within the plane of the cortex, since it continued even when the non-visual cortex was undercut a la B. D. Burns. The first finding correlated well with the tendency of spike and dome seizures to last about 10 sec and then end abruptly. Also, judging from its rate of propagation, the spread of the strychnine activating mechanisms appeared similar to the so-called "deep response" Adrian had reported following direct electrical stimulation of the cortex.

By mid-December we felt we had enough data to work up our findings, and Mike agreed to come to Oxford over the Christmas holiday to work on the paper. This was my first experience of an English winter. It was not so much that the temperature was low, as the dampness of the cold and the absence of central heating that one felt most. The only heating in my rooms was from a small gas fire that one had to keep feeding shillings every hour or so. Unfortunately, we ran out of shillings in the middle of our first afternoon together and were reduced to wearing our overcoats and gloves while trying to analyze our recordings and preparing to write a draft of the paper. As soon as the pubs opened, we lost all interest in writing and made our way to the "local," not so much for liquid refreshment as for warmth and a renewed supply of shillings.

By the end of the holiday, we had completed the drafts of two papers which Mike said he would ask the head of the EEG lab, William Cobb, to look over and perhaps submit to the *Journal of Physiology*. His response was to say he would send them on to the *Journal of Physiology*. To our surprise, when we received the proofs, his name appeared as the first author (which followed the Journal's then policy of listing authors alphabetically), although he had not actually participated in the design or execution of the experiments or in their preparation for publication. In fairness I should add that Cobb suggested that we should present the work at the next meeting of the Physiological Society which was to be held at one of the London medical schools. But, when the time came, he was adamant that either Mike or I should present the paper before what he knew would be a formidable audience of neurophysiologists. Mike and I tossed a coin to determine who would face the music—I lost.

By contrast, LeGros had always insisted that his name *not* appear on any of the papers, even though his guidance had been critical and his careful, line-by-line reviewing of our papers before they were sent off to editors was exemplary. His scientific integrity revealed itself about this time in a very special way. During the years following the introduction of prefrontal leucotomy, there was considerable interest in the connections of the prefrontal cortex and especially those linking it to the hypothalamus. One day LeGros pointed out to Tom and me that some years before Mrs. Margaret Meyer who had worked as a research assistant in his lab had prepared and analyzed the brains of several monkeys with lesions in different parts of the frontal cortex that had been stained by the Glees modification of the Bielschowsky technique. LeGros had alluded to some of the findings from this material in a brief review he had written for a special issue of the *British Medical Bulletin*, but the material, valuable as it was, had never been written up after Mrs. Meyer had moved with her husband to London. At his suggestion, we wrote to her and she enthusiastically endorsed the idea and made available to us all her lab notes and mappings of the changes seen in the hypothalamus and neighboring structures. As we usually did, Tom and I independently examined each brain, made our own sketches of the "degeneration" etc., and a week or two later got together to compare notes. Two things became immediately clear. First, we had confirmed all Mrs. Myers' findings, but, second, it did not seem to matter where the lesion was located, the "sheep's droppings" that were considered indicative of degenerating terminal axons in Glees' preparation were always found in the same locations (and in roughly the same amount). It occurred to us that degeneration of this type had been reported in a number of other papers that had been published over the past few years, after lesions of the fornix and areas as diverse as the temporal neocortex and entorhinal area. Even more puzzling was the fact that in all this material (which had been carefully stored in the Department) we could find no evidence that a normal control brain had been prepared (no doubt because it had been judged too costly to "waste a monkey").

It was with some trepidation that at the first opportunity we showed our findings to LeGros. But as soon as he examined the material and was convinced of the correctness of our findings, he insisted that we prepare a normal monkey brain and also obtain a suitable human brain from the Pathology Department. When these revealed exactly the same findings he insisted that we prepare a note for *Nature* pointing out that in the hypothalamus the Glees method gave rise to an artifact that had been mistakenly reported as evidence for degeneration after various cortical lesions. He had no hesitation about this. A serious mistake had been made, and the scientific community should be alerted to the fact. Our paper in *Nature* evoked a firestorm of criticism from one of those whose work done at Oxford had been called in question; Paul Glees and Mrs. Meyer were equally upset and let LeGros know their feelings in no uncertain terms. We only learned of some of this from LeGros who had adamantly defended us in private letters to those who had complained. Although the reason for this artifactual appearance has never been fully explained, over the years a number of other workers, including Walle Nauta and Janos Szentágothai, using quite different methods, confirmed our basic finding that many of the purported connections do not, in fact, exist. For me, this "vindication" was less important than the lesson I had learned from LeGros about genuine scientific integrity.

Unlike most medical schools I have known, Oxford proved to be extremely flexible. I was allowed to enroll in Howard Florey's remarkable course in General Pathology and the much less inspiring course in Pharmacology while I was completing my D.Phil. thesis. Since the examinations did not have to be taken immediately after the course, I was able to postpone these until I was well into my clinical years. This is not something I would necessarily recommend, but it saved me more than six months and enabled me to complete the requirements for the B.M. B.Ch. degree in just over two years. While I was preoccupied with my clinical studies, in 1957 Tom spent a sabbatical year at Johns Hopkins, where he worked closely with Vernon Mountcastle and Gian Poggio and got to know Philip Bard, Jerzy Rose, Steve Kuffler, David Hubel, and Torsten Wiesel. This year had a profound effect on Tom's career. He published a number of important papers with Vernon on the functional properties of neurons in the postcentral gyrus of the monkey and participated in the earliest experiments on the poorly understood posterior complex of the thalamus with Vernon and Gian. His enthusiasm for the research climate in the United States was such that, on his return, I decided that at the first convenient opportunity I would try to visit it myself. Another consequence of his visit was that Larry Kruger, who had been in the Physiology Department with Jerzy Rose, came to Oxford for a six month postdoctoral fellowship, and when I returned to full-time teaching and research, we shared an office and the beginnings of a lifelong friendship. Visits to Oxford by Clinton Woolsey and Vernon Mountcastle— the latter to put the finishing touches on his papers with Tom—ensured that when I finally made it to the United States, I would find myself among friends.

In the mid-1950s we realized that the time had come to focus our further efforts on the tracing of efferent pathways using Nauta's important new method. We were aided in this by a succession of visitors to the Department, each of whom worked on the connections of different regions of the brain, including John Carman from New Zealand with whom we worked on cortico-striatal and cortico-claustral connections. Our own work focused on the efferents of the piriform lobe and on the relation between the olfactory system and the thalamus.

I was especially fortunate to have had as one of my best students at Pembroke College Geoffrey Raisman, who decided to do a D. Phil. under our supervision. Geoff brought enormous energy to his work, which included a complete reexamination of the afferent connections of the hippocampus which followed, but added extensively to, the work of Ted Blackstad and his colleagues at Aarhus, Denmark. Geoff's later EM work on the reorganization of synapses in the septum following its partial denervation did much to revive interest in the important subject of morphological plasticity in the central nervous system (CNS) and has continued over the years in his work on promoting CNS regeneration. It also provided what was to be one of the continuing foci of my own work when I moved to the United States in the mid-1960s.

The years I spent at Oxford were among the most enjoyable in my life. Shortly after completing my D. Phil., I was married to Margaret Sherlock, whom I had known for the better part of two years. She was teaching in a private orphanage in London and her dedication to the children under her care had convinced me beyond words of her sense of values and her commitment to the needs of others well beyond any self-ambition she may have had. Over the next few years our three children (Margaret Ruth, Stephen Maxwell, and David Maxwell) were born. We had a modest house in a 13th century village on the outskirts of Oxford. More or less concurrent with the completion of my medical degree, I was appointed to a tenured University lectureship (for which, as was the common pattern, I received an honorary MA, making me an official "Don"). I was given a lectureship to teach Anatomy to students at Balliol College, and although this meant that during each of the three eight-week Oxford terms I spent a good deal of time either demonstrating in the dissection room or in hour-long tutorials with one or two students in my rooms at Pembroke, I found that I enjoyed teaching and did not begrudge the time involved in preparing lectures or tutorials or in direct contact with students. This love of teaching has stayed with me, and it has been enormously gratifying to hear from time to time from former students that something I said in a lecture or a modest act of personal kindness had had a lasting influence on their lives.

Sabbatical to St. Louis

Apart from a planned sabbatical to the United States, I had not seriously thought of ever leaving Oxford. But when LeGros Clark reached mandatory retirement age, it soon became clear that life in the Department would no longer bask in the benign ways I had known since 1953. LeGros' successor, Geoffrey Harris, was a brilliant scientist whose work on the hypothalamic regulation of pituitary function is rightly regarded as the cornerstone of neuroendocrinology. But, while greatly admiring of his science, I soon realized that most of the resources of the Department were likely to be funneled into his research group. So when the time came for us to apply for visas for our sabbatical year, we took the precaution of applying for "green cards" that assured us that if we so chose we could return to the United States as resident aliens.

Our decision to spend the year in St. Louis was quite fortuitous. Ed Dempsey, who was Head of the Anatomy Department at Washington University, had just completed a difficult five-year term as Dean of the School of Medicine and had come to Oxford for a "mini-sabbatical" with a long-term friend, Graham Weddell, a Reader in our Department. As it happened, Ed and I had offices across the hall from each other, and in the course of our frequent chats, he persuaded me that with three children it would be virtually impossible to live in the United States on the $7000/year stipend offered to Rockefeller Traveling Fellows. Instead, he offered me a one-year-long appointment in his Department at roughly twice the salary. He also pointed out that his Department was well equipped with electron microscopes—whose use I was anxious to learn—and that he would himself be returning to full-time research for much of the year. I knew a good deal about Washington University Medical School (WUMS) with its long tradition in neuroscience: Erlanger and Gasser had won the Nobel Prize for their work done there on the compound action potential; Lorente de Nó, Cajal's last and greatest student, had spent time in the adjoining Central Institute for the Deaf; and of special interest to me was the fact that Viktor Hamburger and his colleagues Rita Levi-Montalcini and Stanley Cohen in the Biology Department had just discovered the first neuronal growth factor, NGF, and had clarified for the first time the existence of widespread neuronal death during the normal development of the sensory ganglia and certain regions of the spinal cord itself.

I shall leave for another occasion an account of the bizarre process of obtaining the immigrant's visa from the U.S. Embassy in London. Suffice it to say that all was soon set for our departure and on or about September 1, 1964, we arrived in St. Louis. It had been cold and wet when we left Oxford for Heathrow Airport, but when we arrived in St. Louis on a TWA flight at about 4:00 PM the temperature was 98° and the humidity must have been close to 95%! Stepping off the plane, in coats and sweaters, we felt as if we had been immersed in a hot bath. Our situation was not helped by discovering, several minutes later, that our luggage had been unloaded in Cincinnati where we had an hour or two layover.

By the time we arrived and checked into our hotel, the children were exhausted, having been on the go for more than 18 hr. Unfortunately for Margaret and me, their internal clocks caused them to wake up at about 2:00 AM, hungry, asking for breakfast, and generally disoriented by their new environment. Luckily, we had ordered sandwiches before going to bed and these sufficed until the coffee shop opened.

Two memories stand out from that first week in the United States. First, when we went to breakfast and ordered eggs and bacon, the waitress asked: "How do you want your eggs?" I said, innocently, "just fried." "Sunny-side up," she responded. I looked out the window. The sun was already up, the sky was clear, and the day promised to be as hot as it had been the day before. "Yes," I said, "it does look like a sunny day." I also remember on our third day, while I was at the medical school, there was a flood in the bathroom which excited the children, but momentarily alarmed Margaret.

Before we left Oxford, Ed Dempsey had written to say that we should not make arrangements for accommodation or the purchase of a car. I learned why during my first day in the Department. Apparently, Ed had been invited by the Secretary of the Department of Health, Education & Welfare to go to Washington to work on President Johnson's Health Care program and expected to be there for at least a year. So he planned to offer us the use of his house in University City, at a reasonable rent, and to sell us his car, a 1957 Buick sedan for its book value of $100! These arrangements suited us just fine, but I did wonder why he had not told us earlier that his plan to return to research and to work had perforce been set aside.

The Dempsey's house proved to be more than adequate for our needs. It seemed to have every electronic device RCA made for domestic use: a large color TV, several electrical tooth brushes, radios, washing machine, dryer, trash compactor, etc., and a small but good library. (I later learned that Dempsey had a specially close relationship with RCA and had purchased a number of RCA electron microscopes, and I couldn't help wonder if this was somehow related to the number of RCA items in his home.) The 1957 Buick, on the other hand, left much to be desired. Its fuel consumption was excessive, and during the course of the year we had to spend $300–$400 for various repairs, to say nothing of the frustration of frequent breakdowns, usually at the most inconvenient times.

Second only to the surprise of learning that Dempsey was not going to be present was the shock of learning that I was expected to teach Gross Anatomy throughout the first semester of my stay. The Head of the Gross Anatomy program, a wonderful, charming—but very tough—woman named Mildred Trotter (or "Trot" to her colleagues and generations of medical students) upon hearing that I was joining the Department had insisted that I teach in her course, seemingly on the grounds that English anatomists are all expected to teach most aspects of anatomy, including Gross Anatomy. Since, at that time, Gross Anatomy consumed about 400 "contact hours"— most of them in the dissecting room—this meant that I would spend a good deal of the first five months of my sabbatical teaching and would only be able to do research for about 2 or 3 hr per day.

This experience, however, turned out to be one of the more enjoyable during my year in St. Louis. The first-year medical students were, on average, not much smarter than those I had taught at Oxford, but as they had all completed four years of college before entering medical school (as opposed to entering directly from high school) they were generally more mature and more committed to their studies. Spending long hours in the dissecting room, I took the opportunity to get to know many of them and continue to hear from some of them even over 30 years later.

For many of the students the chance to talk to a Professor about their work, their pasts, and their career expectations was unusual. One told me that in the four years he had been at college (one of the larger Midwestern land-grant institutions with a student body in excess of 35,000) he had never actually spoken to a Professor. They lectured, of course, but left more direct contacts to Teaching Assistants. At Oxford, by contrast, each student met with his tutor, usually singly but sometimes with a fellow student, for at least an hour each week.

Gross Anatomy is not a difficult subject, but it requires an unusual amount of rote learning. It has been estimated that a medical student learns about 15,000 new terms in his/her first year. Most of these are anatomical, but in addition to assimilating (and remembering) the names of the hundreds of bones, muscles, joints, tendons, nerves, arteries, veins, and the component tissues of all of the organs of the body (including the brain), they have to know the relationships of each of these to the others—the attachments of muscles to particular parts of bones; the course of arteries, nerves, and veins, from their origin to their terminations; etc. To "enliven" all those dry facts, I tried to relate the material to the clinical experiences the students would encounter in their later years and when they entered clinical practice. We also tried to enliven the otherwise fairly boring process of dissection-based learning in other ways.

I recall one occasion when the students were about to dissect the heart. Two young women in my section, both intelligent and serious students, had become good friends, but were from completely different backgrounds. One was from New York and politically well to the left of center. The other was from Wyoming and characteristically conservative. I'm not sure if they ever discussed politics, but in an election year, politics was very much in most people's minds. Recall that this was 1964: Goldwater, the darling of the extreme right was challenging Johnson (LBJ) for the presidency. Not only were the differences between the two parties more clear-cut than in most elections (Johnson spoke of "not sending American boys to fight a war that Vietnamese boys should fight on their own": Goldwater's reply was that "extremism in defense of liberty is no vice" and his supporters rallied around the slogan: "In your heart you know he's right"), but the issues of war in Southeast Asia versus a war on poverty in America seemed to sum up the alternative courses open to the electorate.

The night before the students were to open the heart, I surreptitiously inserted a small strip of paper in a gelatin capsule of the type we used for preparing material for electron microscopy and placed this into the left ventricle of the cadaver the two women were dissecting. The next morning I took the New Yorker aside to urge her (without telling her why) to stay back and let her Wyoming colleague open up the heart. About 30 min later, the ventricle was opened up and I was called over by the two students who wondered why this strange-looking capsule was lodged inside. I suggested to our western student that she remove it and look inside. By this time several other students and two instructors had gathered around the dissection table. Cautiously, the capsule was opened and the strip of paper removed. "What does it say?" asked the New Yorker, in all innocence. "Well, it says," responded her colleague, "In your heart you know he's *WRONG*." This was greeted with laughter and cheers all around from the largely pro-Johnson students.

A second memory from my hours in the dissecting room stems from meeting one of the more brash students who informed me that he was an authority on the pineal gland. Since so little was known about the pineal at the time, I was prompted to ask what he felt made him an authority on the gland. "Oh, I've published four papers on it," was his smug response. "In that case," I said, "you might well be," since no one I had met had published more than two papers on the subject. As he seemed anxious to convince me of his standing in this field, he promised to let me have reprints of the papers at our next meeting. When he gave these to me I took them home and read them over that weekend. When I saw him the following Monday, I said, "I must be missing something, so correct me if I'm wrong; but, as I read these papers in the order in which they were published, I got the impression that the first paper described the development of an enzyme assay; the second describes the levels of the enzyme in the pineal; the third reports that the assay was not as specific as you first thought; and, finally, the fourth paper concludes that since the assay was not specific, the data in the second paper were inconclusive." "I wouldn't put it quite that way," he responded, "but I guess you could get that impression." "Tell me," I asked, "how long did you work in the lab to be able to publish these four papers?" "Oh, I spent the whole 10 weeks of that summer working on that project," was his reply. Four papers from a ten-week stint as an undergraduate told me all I needed to know about the quality of his "research experience" and what it promised for his future career if he planned to do research.

My other experiences teaching Gross Anatomy were more rewarding, and by the end of the semester I felt I had learned a lot about U.S. medical students, about the folly of having them spend so much time learning the minutiae of the subject (which most would forget within weeks of the final exam), and especially how pleasant this particular group of students were. A few years later, when I returned to Washington University as Head of the Anatomy Department, the class arranged a welcoming party for me, and a number of the students have kept in touch with me over the years and many have gone on to have very successful careers as clinical investigators. In addition, I got to know several of the faculty since we spent so much time together.

The senior person, Mildred Trotter, became an especially good friend and was helpful in instructing both Margaret and me on how to behave like Americans. "Women should not go out to luncheon without white gloves" was the sort of advice she freely dispensed. Her social sense, we learned, came from having been a student of Robert Terry, the first Head of the Department who—as she told us—would not only tell her whether or not she should wear a hat, but exactly which one was appropriate for each occasion. During the later 1940s Trot had spent a good deal of time in Hawaii on behalf of the U.S. Army, trying to identify soldiers killed in action in the Pacific from examination of their skeletal remains. Over the years she had measured, weighed, and determined the ash content of the hundreds of skeletons that Terry had accumulated and on this basis she felt confident that she could identify whether a particular bone (especially the longer limb bones) was from a white or black individual, male, or female. Together with other material, such as clothes, dog tags, etc., this enabled many remains to be returned to their families. About the time I arrived in St. Louis, Trot received an invitation to give a lecture on her anthropological work at University College London. It was some time since she had done much in the way of research, and she was reluctant to accept the invitation. She finally agreed to do this if I would assist her in organizing the material.

This was not easy. Most of her work had been done on the skeletons of the cadavers dissected over the past 40 years by successive generations of medical students. Until about 1950 most of the cadavers came from the local charity hospitals; a majority were black males; there were fewer whites and comparatively few females. Most were poorly nourished, had many untreated illnesses, and, in a word, were hardly representative of the population as a whole. While the race of each cadaver was noted, it was unclear how homogeneous the groups were or if the recorded ages were correct. Despite these limitations, the mass of data she had collected was unique and when presented in an orderly and unpretentious way formed the basis for her lecture, which was well received.

The one faculty member whom I got to know best was Robert (Bob) Laatsch. Bob was a WUMS graduate, who after an internship had been persuaded to join the Department as an Instructor. Before I met him he had done a fair amount of electron microscopy and was technically very good at cutting ultrathin tissue sections. As we both taught in the Gross Anatomy class, I spent a fair amount of time with him and discovered that, while he was interested in research, he was studying no specific project and had no publications from the two years he had been in the Department. So I asked if he would like to join me in looking at the ultrastructual organization of the hippocampus and some of its connections. (At Oxford I had been working on this topic at the light microscopic level for some time with my student, Geoffrey Raisman.) Bob seemed pleased at this suggestion, but soon realized that to do this properly he would need to perfect completely a different approach to tissue fixation than he had used before.

Fortunately, others had described ways to fix brain tissue by perfusion that enabled one to see excellent tissue preservation and to select carefully oriented blocks of tissue for thin sectioning. Once we had gained a good sense of the normal fine structure of the tissue, I did a number of experiments in which the commissural connections (from the opposite side) were interrupted at varying postlesion intervals. In these we were able to clearly identify degenerating axon terminals in the appropriate regions. This work resulted in two papers in the *Journal of Comparative Neurology* that appeared in 1966 and 1967. Although in retrospect I think they were fairly modest contributions, at the time they attracted a fair amount of attention because they were among the earliest studies in which degeneration in identified axon terminals was used to study connections in the CNS.

An incidental observation we made during this work was of an unusual membrane specialization at nodes of Ranvier which we thought might be significant for the flow of current at nodes during impulse conduction. We sent a short note about this finding to *Nature*, which, for some unknown reason, delayed its publication for several months, by which time others reported the same findings.

Once my teaching obligations were over, I was able to visit several other universities around the United States, and at many of these I gave seminars about the work my colleagues at Oxford and I had done over the previous two or three years. Following a visit to Johns Hopkins to give a seminar, John Dowling and I were able to combine our different expertises to identify experimentally, at the EM level, the mode of termination of the centrifugal fibers to the pigeon retina upon a distinct group of amacrine cells. But the most useful experience followed a seminar in the Biology Department at Washington University, during which I pointed out that the isthmo-optic system and other parts of the avian visual system would be wonderful subjects to analyze using the methods that Hamburger and Levi-Montalcini had perfected. I still recall vividly Viktor jumping up and saying in his wonderfully animated way: "You must do those experiments while you are here, and I'll ask one of my research assistants, Eleanor Wenger, to drop what she has been doing, to work with you." Thus began my direct involvement in developmental neurobiology, and for much of the rest of my year in St. Louis, Eleanor and I worked together making partial and complete excisions of the chick optic vesicle and optic cup, preparing the material by the special staining procedures Rita had perfected and the more conventional neuroanatomical methods I was familiar with. It would be a year or more before I could get around to analyzing the material, and in the meantime we had to return to Oxford so I could complete my teaching obligations, prepare to sell our home, and plan for a new life in the United States. We had so greatly enjoyed ourselves during the year, I had come to realize that it would be a great deal easier to support my research through NIH grants (rather than depend on the generosity of the Department Head), and in the relatively short while we had been in the country, we had made so many good friends that our qualms about leaving the United Kingdom (and especially Margaret's extended family) were largely overcome.

The University of Wisconsin

During our stay in St. Louis, I had the opportunity to visit several of the leading medical schools on the two coasts and the universities of Chicago and Wisconsin (Madison) in the Midwest. To my surprise, I was approached about the possibility of faculty positions at several of these institutions and, in retrospect, may have done well in accepting any of them. Washington University pressed me to stay on; the University of Chicago's offer was financially extremely attractive; and because of my contacts at Hopkins, it too was very appealing. In the end I decided to take the offer from Madison, not only because of my past associations with Ray Guillery (with whom Tom Powell and I had published two papers prior to his joining the "brain drain") and with Clinton Woolsey, but also because I was so impressed following my interview with James Crow, who, as I later learned, was acting Dean of the school.

My appointment was to be in the Anatomy Department, and it came as something of a surprise when in the summer of 1966 I quickly learned that with the notable exception of Ray, the Department left much to be desired, and the students were in a very different class from those I had grown used to at Oxford. Nevertheless, our family enjoyed Madison (even its long, cold winters), and I especially enjoyed my interactions with the fine group of scientists that Woolsey and Rose had assembled in the Department of Neurophysiology.

I had only been there a little more than a year when, out of the blue, I was visited by Ollie Lowry from WUMS. Ollie was chairing the search committee that had been appointed to recruit a new Head of Anatomy. In the meantime, Ed Dempsey had returned from Washington and resigned to become Chairman of Anatomy at Columbia. I was impressed by Ollie's candor when he told me that the WUMS' first choice had been Walle Nauta, but they had been unable to lure him away from MIT. I had not given any thought before this of the possibility of taking on the administrative responsibilities of a department chair, but agreed to visit the WUMS and meet with the search committee. It was an open secret that WUMS had just passed through a very difficult period, mainly focused on the one side by the determination of Mr. Queeny, Chairman and President of Monsanto, who was President of the Hospital Board and thought that the hospital should close its "charity wards" and be run like an efficient business corporation and on the other side by the faculty who stood firmly behind the school's traditional academic policies. But things had changed quite rapidly. Mr. James McDonnell (of the McDonnell Douglas Aircraft Company) had replaced Queeny on the Hospital Board; a new administrative structure had been put in place in the Medical School; and, perhaps most importantly, the school had succeeded in recruiting a number of outstanding new department heads, including Roy Vagelos (later CEO of Merck) in Biochemistry, Cuy Hunt in Physiology, and Phil R. Dodge in Pediatrics.

After a good deal of heart searching and equivocation (I was especially concerned that I had been at Wisconsin for such a short time and was not at all sure of my competence to rebuild a department that was reduced to just two associate professors, two instructors, and three graduate students), I finally decided to take the risk, having become convinced from my meetings with the Dean, the Vice-Chancellor (Bill Danforth), and several of the department heads that they were determined to be helpful. It was going to take about eight or nine months before new laboratory space could be constructed for me, so in the end I spent almost two years at Madison before moving to St. Louis in the summer of 1968. Much of the intervening time was spent in the Department of Neurophysiology, where I profited greatly from almost daily discussions and arguments with Jerzy Rose. I was also joined at this time by two graduate students, Jennifer Hart (who as mentioned earlier would become Jennifer LaVail) and Jim Kelly, and later by one of Jim's colleagues in the Zoology Department, David Gottlieb. The three of them formed the nucleus of my new lab at WUMS, with each of them working on a different problem in neural development.

Return to St. Louis

Almost from my arrival in St. Louis, Cuy Hunt and I found that we shared many of the same interests in teaching and neuroscience and agreed to develop our work more or less in parallel. Cuy had begun his research career at Rockefeller; had written two classical papers on the γ-efferent control of muscle; and had already built two excellent departments, first at the University of Utah and later at Yale. He had all the qualities of a fine administrator: soundness of judgment, excellence of taste in the selection of faculty, and an architect's eye for transforming rundown space into first-class research laboratories. I have always remembered fondly his advice and encouragement and the generous way in which he effectively removed all the usual barriers that so commonly divide academic departments.

It took me much longer to rebuild the Anatomy Department (Fig. 2), but with the clear determination that although we would certainly teach the required courses in Gross Anatomy, Histology, and Neuroanatomy as rigorously as before, the research focus of all the initial appointments would be in what was now generally referred to as neurobiology or neuroscience.

Among the first faculty appointments I was able to make were Harold Burton, who had been a postdoctoral fellow at the University of Wisconsin, working on the physiology of the somatosensory system, and Joel Price, who had been a graduate student at Oxford with Powell and for his thesis had completed one of the best fine structural studies of the olfactory bulb with its unusual pattern of reciprocal dendro-dendritic synapses. A major coup was the joint recruitment from Columbia University College of Physicians and Surgeons of Richard and Mary Bunge to independent faculty positions. Richard's work on the structure of central and peripheral myelin had quickly found its way into the standard textbooks. Mary's later work on the structure of growth cones set the standard for years to come. Together, Richard and Mary added immeasurably to the entire life of the Department: their teaching was exemplary; their laboratory a model of creativity and friendliness;

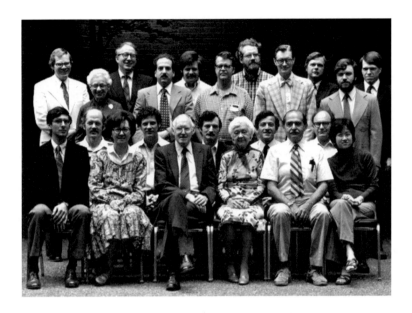

Fig. 2. The faculty of the Department of Anatomy and Neurobiology at WUMS in the late 1970s. Standing (left to right): David Menton, Estelle Brodmann (Departmental Librarian), Richard Bunge, Arthur Lowey, Dave Gottlieb, Tom Thach, Dick Bischoff, Roy Peterson, Tom Woolsey, Joel Price, and Mark Willard. Seated (left to right): Harold Burton, Bob Waterston, Mary Bunge, Larry Swanson, Max Cowan, Ted Jones, Mildred Trotter, Ted Cicero, Adolf Cohen, Len Tolmach, and Charlene Gottlieb.

and their advice and judgment, given freely and generously, was appreciated by all who were fortunate to come in contact with them.

Later we were joined by Edward (Ted) Jones who had been a New Zealand fellow at Oxford with Tom Powell and in his three years there set a research pace as astonishing for its quantity as its quality. After an obligatory period back in Otago, Ted and his family emigrated to the United States, where he has spent the rest of his distinguished career, mastering almost every useful technique and applying them with imagination and astonishing energy to a wide range of scientific problems from the somatosensory and motor systems to the pathology of schizophrenia and other developmental brain disorders. After several years at WUMS, he served as Chair of Anatomy at the University of California, Irvine and more recently as Director of Neuroscience at UC Davis. In 1999 he served with distinction as President of the Society for Neuroscience.

A measure of the breadth of the Department's research activities is its inclusion of Tom Thach, well-known for his contribution to motor learning in the cerebellum; John Chirgwin who, while in Rutter's laboratory at UCSF, had cloned the insulin gene; and Bob Waterston who joined us from Sidney Brenner's lab at the MRC Laboratory for Molecular Biology. With John Sulston, Bob led the U.S./U.K. effort to sequence the genome of the nematode *C. elegans* and later played a major part in generating human and mouse expressed sequence tags (ESTs) and in the human genome effort, which reported its final draft of the genome in the summer of 2000.

My own group grew slowly. In addition to the students who came with me from Wisconsin, about a year later I was joined by Larry Swanson, who for his Ph.D in the Department of Psychiatry had done one of the first immuno-histochemical studies of the nonadrenergic system of the brain and soon became a first-rate neuroanatomist familiar with almost all areas of the CNS. On completing an internship in surgery, Tom Woolsey who, while he was a medical student at Johns Hopkins, with Hendrik van der Loos discovered the exquisite "barrels" in layer IV of the mouse cerebral cortex and had been able to show that each barrel was uniquely associated with one of the mystacial vibrissae arranged in rows and columns across the whisker pad of the animal's snout also joined me. No more elegant demonstration of functional localization in the cortex exists, and over the years Tom, with a succession of students and other colleagues, explored the problems it posed with indomitable persistence and style. As the group expanded, our regular lab meetings began to attract others, including several faculty members, and by the mid-1970s these "Saturday morning seminars" came to be regarded as a central focus for the exchange of ideas where, in the most informal setting (lubricated by free coffee and doughnuts), students, postdocs, and faculty met each week to learn from each other. To see Viktor Hamburger, already well into his 70s, assiduously taking notes from a seminar by a recent postdoctoral fellow is an image deeply burned in the memories of most of us.

Editorial and Other Neuroscience-Related Activities

Shortly after moving from Madison to St. Louis, I was approached by Jerzy Rose, on behalf of the Editorial Committee of the *Journal of Comparative Neurology (JCN)* and the management of the Wistar Press Publications, about the possibility of being Editor-in-Chief of the journal. The *JCN* was the oldest scientific publication devoted to the nervous system, having been founded in 1891 by C. Judson Herrick. Its title reflected Herrick's own interest and to a large extent the principal research interest in the field at that time. Unfortunately, over the years it had not only lost its primary focus, but with only minimal resources was having great difficulty in keeping abreast with the newer journals in the field and even with its own publication schedule. By the mid 1960s it had an extensive backup of papers and was more than a year behind the listed publication date. This led the Wistar Press to seriously consider dropping *JCN* from its list, and it was only at the suggestion of two of the Editorial Board Members that it considered extending the life of the *JCN* for a further two years, provided a new Editor was appointed, the backlog of papers was dealt with, and a new focus was given to the Journal.

I had never seriously considered taking on such a responsibility, but after meeting with the Board and being reassured of their determination to radically change the journal, I agreed to serve for an initial period of two years. Given a free hand to make whatever changes were considered necessary and sufficient resources to carry them out, I made every effort to transform *JCN* into a modern neuroscience publication covering most aspects of the field, with only one concession—the title of the journal was to remained unchanged.

In the end it took about four years to put the changes into effect, and I think it is fair to say that by the mid-1970s *JCN* was successfully competing for many of the most interesting articles in the field. Indeed, the rate of publication more than doubled, and it was soon recognized as the most successful of the Wistar publications. Its success, however, came with a price, in this case an enticing bid from a commercial publication house that Wistar Press felt it could not forgo, even though it was clear that the new publication expected the journal to abandon its not-for-profit status. I was opposed to this change and indicated that if the sale went forward, I would resign as Editor after one year, during which a new Editor could be appointed. By this time I had served for 11 years, and it seemed an appropriate time to step aside and for someone else to take over. In addition, I had been asked to help launch the *Journal of Neuroscience*, which I did, serving for several years as the Editor-in-Chief, and I felt that obligation would preclude me from continuing to give the *JCN* my full attention.

By the early 1970s, the unprecedented growth of the Society for Neuroscience had attracted several publishers as a fruitful field into which to expand their portfolios. One of these was the Annual Reviews Inc. (ARI), a not-for-profit organization that had been started by J. Murray Luck, a Stanford biochemist, to publish authoritative and archival reviews in several areas of science. The Editor-in-Chief and CEO of ARI was encouraged by his Board to look into the possibility of beginning a new series in neuroscience, and at the next annual meeting the Society organized open meetings that were attended by about 250 individuals to discuss this possibility. Despite some reservations that such a series might adversely impact those in psychology and physiology, there seemed to be considerable support for the idea, and, with the Board's approval, the *Annual Review of Neuroscience* was launched in 1978, with an Editorial Committee consisting of Eric Kandel, Zach Hall, Richard Thompson, and myself. I had agreed to serve as Editor for 5 years, but by the simple expedient of ignoring my letter of resignation at the end of the 5th year, Bill Kaufman extended my appointment at 5 yearly intervals, for now well over 25 years!

Developmental Neuroanatomy

Beginning in the interval before I left Oxford and through my years at Wisconsin, my work began to follow two closely related lines. Much of the material prepared by Eleanor Wenger showed that early removal of the developing vesicle and optic cup resulted in death of a significant proportion of the cells in the trochlear nucleus, which in its time course paralleled that seen in normal animals which had been termed "naturally occurring cell death." This parallelism suggested that the causative mechanism, whether spontaneous or induced by the excision of the trochlear mesoderm, was likely to be the same. Also, unexpectedly, we found that the induced ganglion cell degeneration we observed in the ciliary ganglion was followed after the shortest of intervals by secondary degeneration in the accessory oculomotor nucleus which, in birds, provides the preganglionic parasympathetic outflow to the ciliary ganglion. This implied that not only did immature neurons die when they were surgically separated from their natural peripheral targets, but also that the degenerative process could extend even further back, in a manner not unlike the retrograde transneuronal degeneration in the anterior thalamic/mamillary nuclear system we had reported earlier in rabbits and rats.

But my greatest interest lay in the ION. Here we found that very early, partial lesions of the optic vesicle could lead to a small, rounded eye and a correspondingly small, but otherwise normal-looking ION. When the lesions were placed somewhat later (the difference was only a few hours), that part of the nucleus which corresponded to the partial optic cup lesion showed marked cell death in the relevant sector of the ION, but the rest of the nucleus looked normal. By contrast, when the entire optic vesicle or cup was completely ablated, there were no signs of the ION. This type of center/periphery interaction had been pioneered in the motor and sensory systems by the great Ross Harrison and his many students (especially Sam Detwiler) and had served as the basis for Viktor's classic study of the effects of early limb ablation in chicks and for his classic study with Rita on the sensory ganglia. Fortunately, by this time (the mid-1970s) several new methods were becoming available. With Bill Crossland and then Peter Clark, a postdoctoral fellow from the United Kingdom, we were able to extend the story of the ION a good deal further, and in Peter's hands it continued to be a rich source for other work for a decade or more.

Our attempts to study in greater detail many of the events in early neural development were increasingly frustrated by the limitations of the experimental methods available. This was true also of the methods used to trace pathways in the mature nervous system, which depended for the most part on the induction of degenerative changes following the placement of destructive lesions. This caused my colleagues and me to think of alternatives that would take advantage of such physiological properties of neurons as their ability to synthesize proteins in the cell body and then actively transport them along the lengths of their processes. Cajal had recognized that the cell body served as the "trophic center" of the neuron, but it was not until years later that Weiss and Hiscoe showed by constricting nerves at different levels that the contents of axons are in continuous flow, mainly centrifugally from the cell body toward the axon terminals, but also retrogradely back toward the cell body. When isotopes became available for biological studies, Taylor and Weiss showed that proteins formed by introducing a labeled amino acid into the eye could be traced back to the visual centers of the brain. This soon led to a great outpouring of work on axonal transport, much of it led by Bernice Grafstein and her students. Ray Lasek at Denver demonstrated very elegantly that after labeling dorsal root ganglia one could trace the central course of the sensory pathways in the spinal cord, but stopped short of introducing the label directly into the brain itself to analyze intracerebral pathways.

At about this time, I met Anita Hendrickson who was in the Department of Ophthalmology at the University of Washington in Seattle. Anita had injected labeled tracer into the eyes of a group of monkeys and had followed it to the lateral geniculate body. But, most importantly, she had shown that a considerable proportion of the labeled proteins had reached the terminals of the optic nerve fibers and could be clearly seen overlying the retino-geniculate synapses. Joining forces with Anita, Tom Woolsey, David Gottlieb, Joel Price, and I set out to develop an experimental protocol for using this "autoradiographic method" for tracing pathways from the site of the uptake of the label by cell bodies (but, importantly, not by fibers of passage) to their terminal projection fields and for demonstrating its usefulness in a variety of different neuronal systems.

The paper describing the method and discussing frankly both its advantages and its limitations appeared in *Brain Research* in 1972 (Cowan et al., 1972). At the time it attracted considerable interest, and Walle Nauta whose suppressive axonal degeneration method had given such an impetus to neuroanatomy was kind enough to refer to it as the most significant advance in the field in nearly two decades.

Equally important, however, was a report in *Science* by my former student Jennifer LaVail and her husband Matt, who were then postdoctoral scientists in Richard Sidman's lab. Following on an observation by Olson that peripheral axon terminals could take up exogenous proteins and transport them retrogradely to the cell body, the LaVails showed that the enzyme horseradish peroxidase (HRP; for which there was a simple histochemical staining procedure) could be used to determine the sites of origin of central neural pathways. Although it was later found that HRP could be transported bidirectionally, this meant that for the first time axonal pathways could be analyzed without destroying either their origins or terminations. Also, from the point of view of our own interest, it was now possible to study the development of neural systems in ways that only a few years before seemed quite impossible.

It is hardly necessary to list the many topics we now began to study— from the precise time of arrival of optic nerve fibers at their terminations within the tectum, to the identification that early in development some neurons migrated to ectopic sites yet sent their axons to the correct targets, while others that attained their correct locations projected to inappropriate regions. Quantitative analyses of silver grain distributions enabled us to show that axons that project to the same region compete for synaptic space, and at least in one region (the dentate gyrus) the outcome of this competition was determined on a "first come first served" basis.

Shortly thereafter, Bernice Grafstein made the seminal observation that some of the transported label was released or escaped from the axon terminals where it became available for uptake by the second order neurons. LeVay, Hubel, and Wiesel took advantage of this to use the autoradiographic technique to map the distribution of the so-called "eye-dominance columns" in the visual cortex, and later Rakic showed that the initial overlap in the distribution of the inputs from the lateral geniculate nucleus was progressively refined later in development. It was an exciting time for neuroanatomists and several long-standing problems (such as the projection of the intralaminar thalamic nuclei and of the cells of the reticular nucleus itself) were finally laid to rest. Others that had been bedeviled by the "fiber of passage" problem (such as the precise origin of the "hippocampal" projection to the mamillary complex) were at last settled. It was gratifying that several of these studies were done at Washington University, but even more gratifying to see these new methods used by both neuroanatomists and neurophysiologists throughout the United States, Europe, Japan, and elsewhere.

The essentially digital nature of the silver grains seen in autoradiographs had prompted us to use grain counts to define more precisely the borders of projections. But manually counting grains was tedious, and so with the help of colleagues in the Department of Electrical Engineering, especially Donald Wann and one of his students, Mike Dierker, we began to explore the possibility of developing a variety of computer systems for quantifying morphological data. A contract I negotiated with the National Eye Institute provided the funds required to design and build the necessary hardware (this was some years before computer-controlled Z-axis focusing became standard on light microscopes) and to write the operational programs. My colleague in the Anatomy Department, Tom Woolsey, was especially helpful in all this and deserves much of the credit for the ultimate success of the systems that were developed and for a period used by colleagues at Washington University and elsewhere, until a few years later when commercially available instruments were produced. Among the systems we developed were: (1) a fully automated program for the counting of silver grains in autoradiographs; (2) an interactive program for determining the three-dimensional structure of Golgi-impregnated neurons or physiologically identified cells with an appropriate label such as HRP or biocytin, that gave precise measurements of individual dendrites, dendritic branching patterns (primary, secondary, third order, etc.), and, if needed, the location and densities of spines and of axons and collaterals (the reconstructed tree-like images could, of course, be rotated and viewed from any spatial angle); (3) a program for determining the diameters of myelinated axons taken directly from electron micrographs; and (4) a digitized tablet for measuring areas of any displayed image. These various programs were duly published and made readily accessible to other investigators, a number of whom came to Washington University to use our facility.

Two other technical developments engaged our attention during this period. The first, and in terms of its ultimate usefulness, most important was developed by Gary Banker, who in the mid-1970s came to my lab as a postdoctoral fellow from the group at the University of California, Irvine. This was the development of a culture system for growing dissociated hippocampal neurons (from E16-E18 day rat fetuses). Our aim was to produce cells that could survive for long periods in a chemically defined medium to follow the development of their processes; and, if they formed synapses *in vitro*, to study their physiological properties. At the time this seemed a fairly long shot, but Gary's persistence finally paid off, and in due course cultured hippocampal neurons were to become one of the most widely used preparations in cellular neurophysiology and for the study of short- and long-term changes in neurons under different physiological conditions.

The second technical development arose when, in the late 1970s, Jerry Pine, a high energy physicist from Cal Tech, spent a sabbatical year in our lab developing a "chip" on which neurons could be grown and form connections with each other. The chips contained up to 100 sites in which the cells could be electrically stimulated and from which their activity could be recorded. Jerry's original idea was to see if these artificial systems could be "taught" to conduct information in specific patterns. By the end of the year, several such chips had been made, and their ability to stimulate cells grown on them were tested (by concurrent intracellular recordings) and found to be surprisingly successful. Unfortunately, because of other demands on his time when he returned to Pasadena, Jerry did not pursue the problem. But some years later, the basic idea was adapted for studying the activity of fairly large populations of retinal ganglion cells, and out of this emerged the important work done in Carla Shatz's lab at UC Berkeley on the key role of propagated waves of spontaneous activity in the early refinement of retino-geniculate connectivity.

In 1972 I was asked by Jim Watson to participate in the first neuroscience course to be taught at Cold Spring Harbor (CSH). Most of the other participants were from the Harvard Neurobiology Department, and I was mainly involved in lectures and demonstrations on neuroanatomy and neural development. This was my first exposure to such high intensity teaching and to the outstanding students who are attracted to CSH. Among those in the first course were George Zweig, co-discoverer of quarks, Seymour Benzer, and three young molecular biologists who were to form the core of the molecular neuroscience group at the Salk Institute. This proved to be a wonderful three weeks, and I was pleased to return again and again over the next decade. In addition to attracting Mark Willard, who joined my lab later that year as a postdoctoral fellow (having been trained at UC Berkeley as a phage geneticist), my short stay at CSH was to have an unexpectedly long-lasting effect on my life.

One of the hitherto unaddressed problems in the study of axonal transport was that very few of transported proteins were known. Mark seemed to be in a good position, given his past experience, to do something about this, although at the time my lab was ill-equipped for such work. Fortunately, in a conversation with Roy Vagelos, I had mentioned this, and Roy responded by saying that one of his postdoctoral fellows was leaving unexpectedly and he would be glad to let Mark have the use of the vacated lab space. The fact that Roy was always looking for tennis partners and Mark happened to be an unusually good player sealed the arrangement. Within about two years Mark had identified more than 60 different proteins in the optic nerves of rabbits that were transported in at least four different phases as judged by their rate of movement along the length of the axons. Later, with one of his graduate students, he identified a protein, GAP 43, whose expression was significantly increased in regenerating amphibian optic nerves and regenerating peripheral nerve fibers and was one of the first to be associated with axonal growth.

My First and Only Experience with Parapsychology

Washington University has been singularly fortunate in the support it has received from the leaders of St. Louis business and society, and during the 1960s and 1970s no one was more supportive than James McDonnell, founder of the McDonnell aircraft company and later Chairman of McDonnell Douglas, one of the nation's leading aerospace companies. In the early 1960s, "Mr. Mac," as he was generally referred to in St. Louis, had played a critical role in maintaining the traditional relationship between the School of Medicine and Barnes Hospital; he had generously endowed the University's planetary science program and had provided funds for the creation of the new Medical Sciences building and endowed its Department of Genetics. Not surprisingly, the University was always quick to respond to any new proposal he suggested. It was in response to one such suggestion in 1978 that I first got to know Mr. Mac personally. This is how it came about.

Out of the blue, one afternoon I received a phone call from the Chancellor of the University, Dr. William (Bill) Danforth. "Max," he began, "what do you think about parapsychology?" The truth is I didn't think much about it and was brash enough to say so. But I was intrigued to know why he would call to ask me. The reason, as soon became clear, is that he had been approached by Mr. Mac about the possibility of creating a research program in parapsychology which he was willing to support very generously. The disturbing thing is that Mr. Mac was insistent that the program be located in the School of Medicine and further that it should be associated with the Department of Anatomy & Neurobiology. Even more disturbing was that he had indicated that he wanted me to head it up. I was about to protest that there was no way that I could possibly participate in something that I regarded as completely phony when Bill said: "You know, Max, the University never says 'No' to Mr. Mac, and while I respect and share to some degree your skepticism, I wonder if you would be willing to read a book that has apparently caught Mr. Mac's imagination. It's by two physicists from SRI (formerly the Stanford Research Institute) and is about a phenomenon they call 'remote viewing.'

If it was difficult for the University to say no to Mr. Mac, it was impossible for me not to agree to a request like this from Bill Danforth. In due course, a copy of the book arrived on my desk and over the following weekend I read it. As I expected, the book was wholly unconvincing, and the claims it made were dubious to say the least. In essence the authors claimed that everyone has the capacity to receive images of a scene perceived by another individual at some remote location. In support of this claim, they had taken people to various locations in and around Palo Alto, CA, and asked them to concentrate on the scene before them. Concurrently, a second group of individuals at some remote site were asked to concentrate on visual images that came to mind and to record what they had "seen." These reports were then judged by a third party (probably the authors) and given a score based on how closely the report matched the original scene. On this basis they concluded that the reports were astonishingly accurate and calculated that the probability of their reports being due to "mere chance" were on the order of one in more than a billion. I was unimpressed. The reports given were extremely vague; most read something like this: "I see some grass in the foreground; there are clouds in the sky, and I think there is some water and a building to one side." My sense was that they could apply to almost any outdoor scene, and the judgment of the scorers seemed entirely arbitrary and in every case gave the remote viewer the benefit of the doubt. But the fact that the authors claimed that anyone could "remote view" immediately suggested a fairly simple set of experiments to test the validity of their idea.

I soon got back to the Chancellor and told him how the claims for remote vision could be tested, but suggested that if Mr. Mac wanted us to pursue it, we should insist that the "experiment" be done secretly, that someone else be involved (we settled on Sam Guze, who was Chairman of the Department of Psychiatry and Vice Chancellor for Medical Affairs), and, most importantly, that we not ask Mr. Mac to fund it. Bill said he would discuss this with Mr. Mac and Sam Guze, and in due course I was given the go-ahead.

We began by taking as a given that no special subjects were needed; we decided to use a number of truly "naïve" individuals who would only learn about the nature of the experiment just before participating. We felt it important also to eliminate most of the weaknesses in the SRI study by selecting in advance about a dozen views and photographing each scene from the position that the viewers would scan it. In an attempt to quantify the results, we placed in the viewer's field of view three objects: large cards cut into square, triangular, or circular shapes and colored red, green, or yellow. For each viewer, the site to be used and the mix of card was determined just before the start of each experiment using a set of random numbers. Either Sam or I then drove the viewing subject to the chosen site, told the subject where to stand and what to look at (including the three selected cards) for about 5 min at exactly the same time as the remote viewer was instructed to concentrate on any image that came to mind. The remote viewer sat in a quiet room adjacent to Sam's office. At the end of the session (usually after about 10 min) the remote viewer was asked what he/she had seen and then specifically questioned about anything unusual (i.e., the cards) that they may have seen. Finally, they were presented with photographs of all 12 scenes and asked to indicate if any of them corresponded to the image they had seen.

It came as no surprise to Sam and me that not one of the remote viewers came up with anything approaching the correct scene. A number "guessed" that it was the famous Gateway Arch (which we had deliberately excluded from the selected scenes), and none mentioned the cards or anything remotely like them. We repeated the experiment about ten times and finally abandoned it when, quite by chance, one of the subjects, an attractive young woman, while standing on a corner viewing the St. Louis Cathedral was propositioned by two passing motorists (we had not known that this particular location was commonly used by some of the city's streetwalkers!).

Sam and I decided that I should let Mr. Mac know the result of the experiment, and so on the following Saturday afternoon I went to his home for "tea." Mr. Mac was a generous host and a careful listener. I recounted what we had done, why we had tried to make the experiment more rigorous than that done by the group at SRI, and our conclusion that we had found no evidence at all for "remote viewing." When I finished, he thanked me, said he was impressed at the way the experiment had been done, but then added that he wasn't really surprised at the outcome because he had never accepted the idea that everyone has the capacity for remote viewing. He believed it was a unique ability and was sure that there were individuals who had the ability. Would we, he asked, be willing to try the experiment again, only this time with a subject who was known to have the "ability?" He had heard that the CIA employed such individuals and that there was some concern that the United States, by failing to explore this area fully, was falling behind the Soviets. When I said that we would, although I remained skeptical, he picked up the phone at his desk and placed a call to Stansfield Turner, the Director of the CIA.

A few minutes later, Mr. Turner returned the call. After hearing what Mr. Mac was interested in, Mr. Turner said he would have two or three of the Agency's experts fly out to St. Louis to brief Mr. Mac about their experience in this area and to give him the name of one of their most useful subjects. I was impressed that Mr. Mac had such clout, but declined his invitation to be present at this briefing. Several days later, Mr. Mac called me to say that he had been given the name and telephone number of one of the CIA's most respected subjects and to ask if I would contact him.

With Bill Danforth and Sam Guze's approval, I called the man in question. After identifying myself and saying that we would like him to visit St. Louis (at our expense and with the promise of a fairly generous honorarium), he said he would be delighted to participate in such an experiment and was especially pleased that a respected university was prepared to take the subject of remote viewing seriously. I responded by saying that while in general the experiment we hoped to conduct followed the lines of the SRI study (with which he was familiar), we would be introducing a few additional elements that would enable us to determine whether the reported "viewing" was statistically significant and not merely random. Before I had a chance to elaborate on this or to describe exactly what changes were planned, he erupted quite violently. "There is no way I would participate in such a sham; it's obvious you have 'negative psi' and I can tell from your voice that your 'negative psi' would block any chance that the signals from the viewer would reach me." With that he slammed down the receiver—end of conversation, end of experiment.

The following Saturday afternoon I met again with Mr. Mac to tell him what had happened. He seemed disappointed that we had not been able to carry out the test and reiterated that he still believed that such extrasensory phenomena existed. Apparently, while he was an undergraduate at Princeton he had taken a trip across the country. One evening, he found himself in a small, Midwestern town, and, having nothing better to do, he explored the local library. A book on parapsychology caught his eye, and before the library closed, he had read enough to convince himself that this was the most exciting field he had encountered. On returning to Princeton, he told his faculty advisor that he wanted to drop Engineering and major in Psychology with a view to study extrasensory perception (ESP) and other paranormal phenomena. Fortunately perhaps for aeronautical engineering, his advisor rejected this idea out-of-hand (advisors could do that in those days). But ever since then he had remained interested in the field and, as I later learned, had from time to time contributed to various parapsychological studies at other institutions.

Concealing my skepticism, I said, "Would you agree, Mr. Mac, that such phenomena as ESP and 'remote viewing' must ultimately be mediated by the human brain?"

"I agree with that," he answered, and immediately I saw an opening. "Perhaps the problem lies in the fact that we don't know enough about how our brains work. We may be trying to understand the paranormal when we still know very little about the normal functioning of the brain. It's like trying to put a man into space or on the moon, before Kitty Hawk has left the ground."

"Now you're talking my language," he said, sitting up and slapping his thighs as he often did when he was excited. He continued, "You might be right. I need to think about this."

I don't know if my comments had really struck home. I do know that a few weeks later, Mr. Mac invited a group of neuroscientists to make a presentation about research opportunities in the brain sciences; and some months later, by which time I had left Washington University for the Salk Institute, Mr. Mac gave $10 million to endow a program on Higher Brain Function under the Directorship of my good friend, Sid Goldring, Chairman of the Department of Neurosurgery.

That concluded my "foray" into parapsychology, but a year or two after I had moved to San Diego, our son, Stephen, who had remained in St. Louis, sent me a cutting out of the local newspaper that provides an interesting afterword. Apparently, a faculty member in the Physics Department at Washington University had thought of a "fool-proof" psychokinesis experiment that had impressed Mr. Mac sufficiently for him to underwrite its testing (to the tune of $500,000). When an advertisement was placed seeking volunteers to participate in the experiment, "James Rande, the Magician," who has made a career of debunking such things, had two of his student magicians apply. Some time later, the faculty member announced that he had discovered two subjects who displayed extraordinary psychokinetic power in his experiment. Hearing of this, Rande contacted him and urged that he not publish his finding because this was just the sort of thing that lent itself to a magician's sleight of hand. Unfortunately for the faculty member, for the University, and for Mr. Mac, this rather pointed warning was ignored. You can imagine how embarrassed they all must have felt when Rande's two students came forward to explain how they had fooled the fool-proof test. For myself, I was glad that we had conducted our experiment without fanfare and that I had asked for no financial support. It was more than 10 years before I told a few close friends about this episode, and this is the first time it has seen the light of day.

The Salk Institute

In the early 1970s, Roy Vagelos and I were being recruited by other institutions—Roy to develop Biochemistry at Princeton and I to create a joint Department of Anatomy and Physiology at Stanford. Neither of us felt disaffected at WUMS, but we were concerned about the quality of the School's graduate programs and the perceived contrast in the quality of the basic science departments at the Medical School and the Biology Department on the main campus of the University. Bill Danforth responded to this concern forthrightly with imagination and remarkable generosity. As a result of his efforts the University created a Division of Biology and Biomedical Science that brought together, under one administrative structure, the Biology Department and the five basic science departments at the Medical School. Several new faculty positions were approved, and five new, interdepartmental graduate programs were created that more closely paralleled the structure of modern biology than the traditional departmental academic programs. Roy was appointed Director of the new Division, and with the considerable enthusiasm of most of the faculty there was an almost immediate improvement in the quality of the graduate students who began applying for admission. When, some three years later, Roy left Washington University to become Vice President for Research at Merck, I was asked to succeed him and continued in this role until 1980 when I moved to the Salk Institute.

Quite by chance, my later move to the Salk Institute also derived from the summer spent at CSH. The following spring, in 1973, at the urging of the Salk faculty members who had taken the neuroscience course, the President of the Salk, Fred de Hoffman, invited me to spend five or six weeks of the coming summer in La Jolla. Here, I gave an extended series of seminars on different aspects of neuroscience (including lectures/demonstrations on the human brain) that were well received and attracted a number of faculty and postdoctoral scientists from both the Salk and the University of California, San Diego (UCSD). The following year I was surprised to be invited to become a non-resident fellow of the Institute (a group corresponding roughly to an external scientific advisory board). Among the other non-resident fellows at the time was Steve Kuffler, and each year Steve and I spent an enjoyable 10 days meeting the group of neuroscience faculty, attending the Institute's annual meeting at which all new appointments and promotions were approved, and walking along the lovely beaches of La Jolla.

When I joined WUMS in 1968, I had indicated to the Dean and the Selection Committee that I felt one should not view a Chairmanship as a life sentence and that a term of about 10 years was long enough. At the end of the 10 years I reminded the Dean of this and said that I would like to consider stepping down from the Department Chair and the Directorship of the Division. It was certainly not because I was frustrated or disaffected. The Department was going well, I had terrific colleagues, and we enjoyed living in St. Louis and had made many lasting friendships. But I felt it was time to do something different and, in particular, to return to near full-time research. WUMS seemed willing to accommodate me in whatever way it could, but I soon realized that only by making a "clean break" could I truly escape being involved in the University's affairs.

As it happened, just about this time Mr. Sol Price (founder of the famous "Price Clubs," now Costco) approached the Salk Institute about the possibility of the Weingart Foundation, on which he served as Chairman and CEO, making a substantial gift for the creation of a new neurobiology laboratory at the Institute. Although neuroscience activities at the Salk had grown significantly within the previous few years, especially with Francis Crick's decision to move from Cambridge to La Jolla and the recruitment of Floyd Bloom's large group in pharmacology, basic endocrinology, and neurophysiology, the offer from the Weingart Foundation was too good to pass up. Within a matter of some weeks, Fred de Hoffman, Francis Crick, and Steve Kuffler persuaded me to move my group from St. Louis to the Salk as soon as the new laboratories could be constructed.

I was singularly fortunate at the time to have several very able young colleagues in the Department who had been with me for two or three years and, in Dennis O'Leary, a quite remarkable graduate student, all of whom were keen to move to California. Collectively, their work embraced most of the various strands we had been working on over the years, and, at the same time, the new space that was provided allowed us to consider adding a new dimension in cortical physiology. We were also greatly helped by being invited to become an active participant in the Clayton Foundation for Biomedical Research, a Texas-based medical research organization that was required to spend a significant proportion of assets in medical research in the state of California. The generous and stable support provided by the Clayton Foundation assured us that we could expand our activities in new directions, and it is a privilege here to acknowledge the generosity of the Trustees of the Foundation and the confidence they placed not only in my group, but in the Salk Institute as a whole, which they continue to support.

Among those who moved with me from St. Louis was Larry Swanson, who on completing his postdoctoral fellowship had stayed on as a Research Assistant Professor and had been joined recently by a postdoctoral fellow of his own, Paul Sawchenko. Larry and Paul continued their detailed analyses of the connections of several regions of the basal forebrain and hypothalamus. Because of their considerable neuroanatomical expertise at the Salk, they were soon in much demand from the peptide biologists for help and from some of the molecular biologists like Geoff Rosenfeld and Ron Evans who were working on the early development of the anterior pituitary. Larry subsequently moved to the University of Southern California, but Paul moved steadily up the academic ranks to a full Professorship with his own productive laboratory, where over the years he has had several significant contributions, many in collaboration with Wylie Vale and his colleagues. Among his other contributions of note was the development, with one of my postdoctoral fellows, Chip Gerfen, of the use of the kidney bean lectin, Phaseolus vulgaris-leucoagglutinin (PHA-L), which combines all the best features of the other axonal tracing with a level of detail of axonal and dendritic organization seen in the very best Golgi preparations. Since its publication, this approach has proved to be a most useful neuroanatomical method, as indicated by the frequency with which it is cited.

Another member of our group who moved with us from St. Louis to La Jolla was David Amaral. Before joining the lab in St. Louis, David had done a careful analysis using the Golgi technique of the structures of the neurons in the rat hilus. This region had never been carefully examined since the classic Golgi work on the hippocampus by Cajal and his student, Lorente de Nó. David's reexamination provided a number of new insights, and his work on the structure of the neurons in the rat hilus became a classic in its own right.

In our lab David extended our project on the connections of the primate hippocampus and parahippocampal region, bringing to this work a level of thoroughness and attention to detail that has characterized his studies ever since. At the Salk David continued his primate work and initiated an important collaboration with Larry Squire and Stuart Zola-Morgan, which included some interesting studies on the human brain. David left the Salk after several years for a position at Stony Brook and then settled at UC Davis, where he now directs a major program on autism.

Two others moving with us from St. Louis rounded out our group. These were Brent Stanfield, who as an undergraduate had worked with Gary Lynch and Carl Cotman at UC Irvine and had for personal reasons been with me successively as a graduate student and postdoctoral fellow, and Dennis O'Leary, my last graduate student, who had started his studies in St. Louis, but moved with us to complete his experiments at the Salk, returning to Washington University only to defend his dissertation. Until moving into science administration at the NIH in the late 1990s, Brent had carried out several studies on plasticity in the hippocampus following the selective removal of various efferent pathways. He was also the first person to show beyond doubt that some proportion of the cells generated in the adult dentate gyrus are indeed neurons and that their axons could be integrated into the existing mossy fiber system that links the dentate gyrus to the *regio inferior* of the hippocampus. Dennis did his thesis work on the development of the visual system in both chicks and rats. In addition, Dennis and Brent established a very productive collaboration involving studies of various aspects of neural plasticity and development, which continued for a number of years. When I left the Salk, Dennis came with me back to Washington University, where he established his own lab and independent reputation and where he stayed for a few years before the Salk attracted him back to La Jolla where he remains today.

Joining the group from St. Louis at the Salk was Richard Andersen from Vernon Mountcastle's group, where he had begun working on the functional properties of neurons in the parietal cortex of awake, behaving monkeys. Richard's initial work at the Salk was concerned with how the properties of visually responsive neurons in the parietal cortex were influenced by the angle of gaze. The success of this initial work soon led to his recruitment, first to MIT and later to Cal Tech, where he continues to direct a large and vigorous research group.

Shortly after our arrival in La Jolla, we heard from Han Kuypers at Rotterdam that he and his colleagues were using a number of fluorescent dyes, with different emission spectra, which were readily taken up by axon terminals and retrogradely transported to the cell bodies where they bound to different cellular components. They provided us with samples of two such dyes, nuclear yellow, which labeled nuclei brightly yellow, and true blue, which in the fluorescent microscope labeled the cytoplasm a brilliant blue. Together they made it possible for the first time to experimentally identify distant axon collateral pathways. Injections of each dye into putative collateral projection sites could, after a survival period of a few days, enable one to detect "doubly-labeled neurons" if axon collaterals were present. Larry Swanson, Paul Sawchenko, and I immediately set about testing the usefulness of this approach to resolve a long-standing problem in the hippocampus. Previous work from our lab and others had established the basic organization of the projections of each of the two major regions of the Ammon's horn (or hippocampus proper), originally termed the *regio superior* and *regio inferior* by Cajal. In the case of the *regio inferior*, David Gottlieb and I had also shown that there is a striking feature in the efferent projections: the region projects to identical sites on the two sides. Furthermore, the ipsilateral association and crossed (or commissural) projections follow identical courses and terminate in the same subregions. This, of course, raised the questions whether the *regio superior* consisted of a single population of neurons, each of which sent collaterals to all the field's known projection sites, or if neighboring cells projected independently to each site. In Larry and Paul's hands, the new double-labeling method resolved the issue straightforwardly and unequivocally. All the many projections of the *regio inferior* arise as collaterals of a single and uniform population of pyramidal neurons.

For our developmental studies we soon found that the new dyes offered yet another advantage: they were essentially non-biodegradable. This meant that one could follow the fates of cells (and their connections) over long periods of time. Brent Stanfield, Dennis O'Leary, and I first used this approach to resolve another long-standing issue in cortical development, namely, whether changes in connections that occur in the course of development are due to the deaths of some cells within a population of interest or if they could be due to the selective elimination of certain early formed collateral projections while the parent cells (and their other axon collaterals) persisted.

Naturally occurring cell death and selective synapse elimination had both been described in many regions of the nervous system, but in a number of others it was not clear which phenomenon accounted for the observed changes over the course of development. For example, as Innocenti and his colleagues had shown, early in postnatal life all regions of the cerebral cortex appear to extend callosal projections to the opposite cerebral hemisphere. Later, however, many regions clearly lack such callosal projections, and the question that arises is: Is the early "exuberant projection" (to use Innocenti's apt phrase) refined by the death of a proportion of the cells in specific regions or to the selective loss of their callosal branches with the persistence of the neurons themselves? By labeling the entire early cohort of neurons with early callosal projections with one dye shortly after birth, and by allowing the animals to survive beyond the refinement period (at about 3–4 weeks postnatally in rats) and then labeling extensively with a second dye, Brent and Dennis were able to show that, as far as can be judged, many if not all the original cells survive and maintain their other projections, although their early callosal projections can no longer be demonstrated. This somewhat unexpected but very satisfying finding provided a decisive observation that connectional refinements in the CNS can involve the selective elimination of specific, long-range axon collaterals and not just terminal branches as had been thought for sometime. Brent and Dennis quickly extended this initial set of findings to a number of other cortical projections, and this phenomenon of collateral elimination has proven to be a fundamental principle in the development of the cerebral cortex.

The Howard Hughes Medical Institute

The six years I spent at the Salk Institute were among the most enjoyable of my career. It was a privilege to be associated with so many outstanding colleagues, to get to know and spend many hours discussing neuroscience with Francis Crick, and to be able to assist some other colleagues such as Ron Evans, Steve Heinemann, and Jim Patrick as they established themselves among the early group of molecular neuroscientists. However, in the summer of 1986, I was lured back to Washington University as Provost and Executive Vice-Chancellor. This, I had thought, was to be my last academic position. But within two years I became convinced that academic administration on such a broad front made it virtually impossible to keep abreast with biomedical research. Fortunately, as I became convinced of this, I was approached by Purnell Choppin (who had just been appointed President of the Howard Hughes Medical Institute [HHMI]) about the possibility of my joining the HHMI in the position he himself had occupied as Vice-President and Chief Scientific Officer.

I had been associated with HHMI since the fall of 1983, when it considered starting a fourth research program in neuroscience to complement the longer established programs in Metabolic Regulation, Genetics, and Immunology. Before launching the new program, the Medical Advisory Board (MAB) invited a group of neuroscientists to meet with them at the Institute's New Headquarters in Coconut Grove, FL. This meeting confirmed the decision to go forward and set up neuroscience research groups at the MGH, Columbia University College of Physicians and Surgeons, UCSF, Hopkins, and Yale.

Shortly after the meeting in Coconut Grove, I had a telephone call from Dr. George Thorn, Chairman of the MAB, asking if I would join the MAB for a few months while the program was being established. I readily agreed, since it seemed that this new infusion of support for the field could have a major impact, given the magnitude of the Institute's endowment. (This had been established for the first time by the decision of the Trustees to sell the Institute's sole asset, the Hughes Aircraft Company, to General Motors for just over $5 billion.)

Several months later, Don Fredrickson, who had been appointed President of the HHMI, visited each of the MAB members about the possibility of establishing yet another research program; this resulted in the appointment of a number of outstanding X-ray crystallographers at several sites where HHMI had established relationships. It was during my meeting with Don Frederickson that the possibility of beginning a joint UCSD/Salk Institute HHMI unit was first raised, and in due course Ron Evans and Larry Swanson at Salk and Geoff Rosenfeld (and later Charles Zucker) at UCSD were appointed as investigators.

The evident success of HHMI's research programs from the time they were reorganized in the mid-1980s has been the subject of much discussion by others. Here, it will perhaps suffice to say that it obviously involved a number of related factors. Included among these are the size of its endowment and the resources this made possible; the careful selection of those appointed as investigators and the fact that they were all subject to rigorous scientific review by knowledgeable panels of experts; and the considerable assistance provided to the HHMI by the many universities, medical schools, and research institutions with which it was associated. An especially important factor was the decision to broaden the pool from which the HHMI could draw investigators from an initial relatively small number of medical schools to "competitions" open to essentially all research universities and research institutions. Equally important was the strong commitment of the Trustees to ensure that the primary focus of the HHMI be the support of biomedical research, both basic and clinical of the highest caliber.

One word about the HHMI's neuroscience program may be of particular relevance in the present context. This was the decision to concentrate the HHMI's efforts initially in the areas of cellular, molecular, and developmental neuroscience. Given that these areas showed the greatest prospect for rapid (and substantial) progress in the 1980s, in retrospect, this decision was clearly a wise one. However, it was also recognized that in time the program should be broadened to include systems neuroscience and beyond this cognitive neuroscience more generally. This expansion began in the early 1990s with the appointment of several investigators working on different aspects of sensory perception, learning, memory, and computational neuroscience. Since no constraints were placed on what investigators would pursue, the program provided a degree of flexibility that enabled individuals to move into new areas to avail themselves of new techniques and even to completely change direction. Their success in this speaks for itself, but it would be misleading if I were not to say that it has been especially gratifying to observe how the program has developed and to have had the opportunity to play some part in its evolution.

As biomedical research continues to provide us with greater understanding and with powerful new tools, the scientific community has, I think, a dual responsibility. One is to push forward the frontiers to make medical advances possible, to understand what cancer is, to develop new ways of treating cancer, to prevent heart disease, and to develop ways of preventing, ultimately, disorders such as Alzheimer's disease and depression. But science also has a second responsibility to society, which is to point out what we need to be concerned about as a society and to bring to bear humane, balanced, and thoughtful ways of dealing with the advances that come from biomedical research. Scientists need to speak to these issues.

Basic science is concerned with trying to understand the underlying basis of disorders, and it does that by trying to understand the underlying basis of normal biological processes. But out of that understanding come ways to prevent and ultimately, I think, to overcome the devastating disorders that affect humanity, recognizing of course that mortality is a reality of life and that we have to learn as a society to face death with equanimity, humanity, and dignity.

Selected Bibliography

Andersen RA, Asanuma C, Cowan WM. Callosal and prefrontal associational projecting cell populations in area 7a of the macaque monkey: A study using retrogradely transported fluorescent dyes. *J Comp Neurol* 1985;232:443–455.

Amaral DG, Avendano C, Cowan WM. The effects of neonatal 6-hydroxydopamine treatment on morphological plasticity in the dentate gyrus of the rat following entorhinal lesions. *J Comp Neurol* 1980;194:171–191.

Amaral DG, Cowan WM. Subcortical afferents to the hippocampal formation in the monkey. *J Comp Neurol* 1980;189:573–591.

Amaral DG, Insausti R, Cowan, WM. Evidence for a direct projection from the superior temporal gyrus to the entorhinal cortex in the monkey. *Brain Res* 1983;275:263–277.

Amaral DG, Insauti R, Cowan WM. The commissural connections of the monkey hippocampal formation. *J Comp Neurol* 1984;224:307–336.

Amaral DG, Insausti R, Cowan, W.M. The entorhinal cortex of the monkey: I. Cytoarchitectonic organization. *J Comp Neurol* 1987;264:326–355.

Amaral DG, Veazey RB, Cowan WM. Some observations on hypothalamo-amygdaloid connections in the monkey. *Brain Res* 1982;252:13–27.

Asanuma C, Andersen RA, Cowan WM. The thalamic relations of the caudal inferior parietal lobule and the lateral prefrontal cortex in monkeys: Divergent cortical projections from cell clusters in the medial pulvinar nucleus. *J Comp Neurol* 1985;241:357–381.

Asanuma C, Ohkawa R, Stanfield BB, Cowan WM. Observations on the development of certain ascending inputs to the thalamus in rats. I. Postnatal development. *Brain Res* 1988;41:159–170.

Avendano C, Cowan WM. A study of glial cell proliferation in the molecular layer of the dentate gyrus of the rat following interruption of the ventral hippocampal commissure. *Anat Embryol* 1979;157:347–366.

Banker GA, Cowan WM. Rat hippocampal neurons in dispersed cell culture. *Brain Res* 1977;126:397–425.

Banker GA, Cowan WM. Further observations on hippocampal neurons in dispersed cell culture. *J Comp Neurol* 1979;187:469–494.

Boss BD, Gozes I, Cowan WM. The survival of dentate gyrus neurons in dissociated culture. *Brain Res* 1987;433:199–218.

Boss BD, Peterson GM, Cowan WM. On the number of neurons in the dentate gyrus of the rat. *Brain Res* 1985;338:144–150.

Boss BD, Turlejski K, Stanfield BB, Cowan, WM. On the numbers of neurons in fields CA1 and CA3 of the hippocampus of Sprague-Dawley and Wistar rats. *Brain Res* 1987;406:280–287.

Carman JB, Cowan WM, Powell TPS. The organization of the cortico-striate connexions in the rabbit. *Brain* 1953;86:525–562.

Carman JB, Cowan WM, Powell TPS. The cortical projection upon the claustrum. *J Neurol Neurosurg Psychiatr* 1964;27:46–51.

Carman JB, Cowan WM, Powell TPS. Cortical connexions of the thalamic reticular nucleus. *J Anat (Lond)* 1964;98:587–598.

Carman JB, Cowan WM, Powell TPS, Webster KE. A bilateral cortico-striate projection. *J Neurol Psychiatr* 1965;28:71–77.

Cartwright CA, Simantov R, Cowan WM, Hunter T, Eckhart W. pp60C-src expression in the developing rat brain. *Proc Natl Acad Sci USA* 1988;85:3348–3352.

Cicero TJ, Cowan WM, Moore BW. Changes in the concentrations of the two brain specific proteins, S-100 and 14-3- during the development of the avian optic tectum. *Brain Res* 1970;24:1–10.

Cicero TJ, Cowan WM, Moore BW, Suntzeff V. The cellular localization of the two brain specific proteins S-100 and 14-3-2. *Brain Res* 1969;18:25–34.

Clairborne BJ, Amaral DG, Cowan WM. A light and electron microscopic analysis of the mossy fibers of the rat dentate gyrus. *J Comp Neurol* 1986;246:435–458.

Clairborne BJ, Amaral DG, Cowan WM. Quantitative, three-dimensional analysis of granule cell dendrites in the rat dentate gyrus. *J Comp Neurol* 1990;302:206–219.

Clarke PGH, Cowan WM. Ectopic neurons and aberrant connections during neuronal development. *Proc Natl Acad Sci USA* 1975;72:4455–4458.

Clarke PGH, Cowan WM. The development of the isthmo-optic tract in the chick, with special reference to the occurrence and correction of developmental errors in the location and connections of isthmo-optic neurons. *J Comp Neurol* 1976;167:143–163.

Clarke PGH, Rogers LA, Cowan WM. The time of origin and the pattern of survival of neurons in the isthmo-optic nucleus of the chick. *J Comp Neurol* 1976;167:125–141.

Cobb WA, Cowan WM, Powell TPS, Wright MK. The relation between photically evoked specific responses and strychnine spikes in the visual cortex of the cat. *J Physiol* 1955a;129:305–315.

Cobb WA, Cowan WM, Powell TPS, Wright MK. Some observations on the interaction between evoked strychnine spikes and specific responses in the visual cortex of the cat. *J Physiol* 1955b;128:54.

Cobb WA, Cowan WM, Powell TPS, Wright MK. Intra-cortical excitation following strychnine spikes. *J Physiol* 1955c;129:316–324.

Cowan WM. Centrifugal fibres to the avian retina. *Br Med Bull* 1970a;26:112–118.

Cowan WM. Anterograde and retrograde transneuronal degeneration in the central and peripheral nervous system. In Nauta WJH, Ebbesson SOE, eds. *Contemporary research methods in neuroanatomy.* Heidelberg: Springer-Verlag, 1970b.

Cowan WM. Neuronal death as a regulative mechanism in the control of cell number in the nervous system. In Rockstein M, Sussman ML, eds. *Development and aging in the nervous system.* New York: Academic Press, 1973;19–41.

Cowan WM. The development of the brain. *Sci Am* 1979;241:113–133.

Cowan WM. The development of the vertebrate central nervous system: An overview. In Garrod DR, Feldman J, eds. *Development in the nervous system.* Cambridge: University Press, 1981;3–33.

Cowan WM. The development of the nervous system. In Asbury AK, McKhann GM, McDonald WI, eds. *Diseases of the nervous system: clinical neurobiology.* Philadelphia: WB Saunders, 1992;5–24.

Cowan WM. Innovation and health reform: How much biomedical research is enough? In Raymond SU, ed. *Enterprise, excellence and efficiency: Priorities for health care policy,* New York Academy of Sciences, 1995;25–33.

Cowan WM. The emergence of modern neuroanatomy and developmental neurobiology. *Neuron* 1998;20:413–426.

Cowan WM, Adamson L, Powell TPS. An experimental study of the avian visual system. *J Anat* 1961;95:545–563.

Cowan WM, Clarke PGH. The development of the isthmo-optic nucleus. *Brain Behav Evol* 1976;13:345–375.

Cowan WM, Cuenod M. The use of axonal transport for the study of neuronal connections: A retrospective survey. In Cowan WM, Cuenod M, eds. *The use of axonal transport for studies of neuronal connectivity*. International Symposium, Gwatt-Thun, Switzerland, July, 1974, Amsterdam: Elsevier, 1975;1–24.

Cowan WM, Fawcett JW, O'Leary DDM, Stanfield BB. Regressive events in neurogenesis. *Science* 1984;225:1258–1265.

Cowan WM, Fawcett JW, O'Leary DDM, Stanfield BB. Regressive events in neurogenesis. In *Neuroscience*. Washington, DC: Amer. Assoc. Adv. Science, 1985; 13–29.

Cowan WM, Finger TE. Regeneration and regulation in the developing central nervous system with special reference to the reconstitution of the optic tectum of the chick following removal of the mesencephalic alar plate. In Spitzer NC, ed. *Current topics in neurobiology, vol. 5.* New York: Plenum Press, 1982;377–415.

Cowan WM, Gottlieb DI, Hendrickson AE, Price JL, Woolsey TA. The autoradiographic demonstration of axonal connections in the central nervous system. *Brain Res* 1972;37:21–51.

Cowan WM, Guillery RW, Powell TPS. The origin of the mammilary peduncle and other hypothalamic connexions from the midbrain. *J Anat (Lond)* 1964;98: 345–363.

Cowan WM, Harter DH, Kandel ER. The emergence of modern neuroscience: Some implications for neurology and psychiatry. *Annu Rev Neurosci* 2000;23:343–391.

Cowan WM, Kandel ER. A brief history of synapses and synaptic transmission. In Cowan WM, Südhoff TC, Stevens CF, eds. *Synapses*, Baltimore, MD: Johns Hopkins University Press, 2000;1–87.

Cowan WM, Kopnisky KL, Hyman SE. The human genome project and its impact on psychiatry. *Annu Rev Neurosci* 2002;25:1–50.

Cowan WM, Martin AH, Wenger E. Mitotic patterns in the optic tectum of the chick during normal development and after early removal of the optic vesicle. *J Exp Zool* 1968;169:71–92.

Cowan WM, O'Leary DDM. Cell death and process elimination: The role of regressive phenomena in the development of the vertebrate nervous system. In Isselbacher KJ, ed. *Medical science and society: Symposium celebrating the Harvard Medical School bicentennial*. New York: Wiley, 1984;643–668.

Cowan WM, Powell TPS. An experimental study of the relation between the medial mammillary nucleus and the cingulate cortex. *Proc R Soc Lond Ser B* 1954;143:114–125.

Cowan WM, Powell TPS. The projection of the midline and intralaminar nuclei of the thalamus of the rabbit. *J Neurol Neurosurg Psychiatr* 1955a;18:266–279.

Cowan WM, Powell TPS. Use of the "Glees Technique" in the hypothalamus. *Nature (Lond)* 1955b;176:1124.

Cowan WM, Powell TPS. The organization of the hippocampal projection system. VI Congress Federatif International d'Anatomie, Paris, 1956a;184–185.

Cowan WM, Powell TPS. A note on terminal degeneration in the hypothalamus. *J Anat* 1956b;90:188–192.

Cowan WM, Powell TPS. Centrifugal fibres to the retina in the pigeon. *Nature* 1962;194:487.

Cowan WM, Powell TPS. Centrifugal fibres in the avian visual system. *Proc R Soc Lond Ser B* 1963;198:232–252.

Cowan WM, Powell TPS. Strio-pallidal projection in the monkey. *J Neurol Neurosurg Psychiatr* 1966;29:426–439.

Cowan WM, Raisman G, Powell TPS. The connexions of the amygdala. *J Neurol Neurosurg Psychiatr* 1965;28:137–151.

Cowan WM, Stanfield BB, Amaral DG. Further observations on the development of the dentate gyrus. In Cowan WM, ed. *Studies in developmental biology.* New York: Oxford University Press, 1981;395–435.

Cowan WM, Stanfield BB, Kishi K. The development of the dentate gyrus. In Hunt RK, ed. *Current topics in developmental biology. vol. 15.* New York: Academic Press, 1980;103–157.

Cowan WM, Wann DF. A computer system for the measurement of cell and nuclear sizes. *J Micros* 1973;99:331–348.

Cowan WM, Wenger E. Cell loss in the trochlear nucleus of the chick during normal development and after radical extirpation of the optic vesicle. *J Exp Zool* 1967;164:267–280.

Cowan WM, Wenger E. The development of the nucleus of origin of centrifugal fibers to the retina in the chick. *J Comp Neurol* 1968a;133:207–240.

Cowan WM, Wenger E. Degeneration in the nucleus of origin of preganglionic fibers of the chick ciliary ganglion following early removal of the optic vesicle. *J Exp Zool* 1968b;168:105–124.

Cowan WM, Woolsey TA, Wann DF, Dierker ML. The computer analysis of Golgi-impregnated neurons. In Santini M, ed. *Golgi centennial symposium, perspectives in neurobiology.* Pavia & Milan, Italy, September, 1973, New York: Raven Press, 1975;81–85.

Crespo D, O'Leary DDM, Cowan WM. Changes in the numbers of optic nerve axons during late prenatal and postnatal development of the albino rat. *Dev Brain Res* 1985;19:129–134.

Crespo D, Stanfield BB, Cowan WM. Evidence that late-generated granule cells do not simply replace earlier formed neurons in the rat dentate gyrus. *Exp Brain Res* 1986;62:541–548.

Crossland WJ, Cowan WM, Kelly JP. Observations on the transport of labeled proteins in the visual system of the chick. *Brain Res* 1973;56:77–105.

Crossland WJ, Cowan WM, Rogers LA. Studies on the development of the chick optic tectum. IV. An autoradiography study of the development of retino-tectal connections. *Brain Res* 1975;91:1–23.

Crossland WJ, Cowan WM, Rogers LA, Kelly JP. The specification of the retino-tectal projection in the chick. *J Comp Neurol* 1974;155:127–164.

Crossland WJ, Currie JR, Rogers LA, Cowan WM. Evidence for a rapid phase of axoplasmic transport at early stages in the development of the visual system of the chick and frog. *Brain Res* 1974;78:483–489.

Cuenod M, Cowan WM. Some future developments in the use of axonal transport mechanisms for tracing pathways in the central nervous system. In Cowan WM, Cuenod M, eds. *The use of axonal transport for studies of neuronal connectivity.* International Symposium, Gwatt-Thun, Switzerland, July, 1974, Amsterdam: Elsevier, 1975;338–346.

Currie J, Cowan WM. Some observations on the early development of the optic tectum in the frog (Rana pipiens), with special reference to the effects of early eye removal on mitotic activity in the larval tectum. *J Comp Neurol* 1974a;156:123–142.

Currie J, Cowan WM. Evidence for the late development of the uncrossed retinotha-lamic projections in the frog, Rana pipiens. *Brain Res* 1974b;71:133–139.

Currie J, Cowan WM. The development of the retino-tectal projection in Rana pipiens. *Dev Biol* 1975;46:103–119.

Dent JA, Galvin NJ, Stanfield BB, Cowan WM. The mode of termination of the hypothalamic projection to the dentate gyrus: An EM autoradiographic study. *Brain Res* 1983;258:1–10.

Dowling JB, Cowan WM. An electron microscope study of normal and degenerating centrifugal fiber terminals in the pigeon retina. *Z Zellforsch* 1966;71:14–28.

Fawcett JW, Cowan WM. On the formation of eye dominance stripes and patches in the doubly innervated optic tectum of the chick. *Dev Brain Res* 1985;17:147–163.

Fawcett JW, O'Leary DDM, Cowan WM. Activity and the control of ganglion cell death in the rat retina. *Proc Natl Acad Sci USA* 1984;81:5589–5593.

Fentress JC, Stanfield BB, Cowan WM. Observations on the development of the striatum in mice and rats. *Anat Embryol* 1981;163:275–298.

Fox CA, Rafols JA, Cowan WM. Computer measurements of axis cylinder diameters of radial fibers and "comb" bundle fibers. *J Comp Neurol* 1974;159:201–223.

Fricke R, Cowan WM. An autoradiographic study of the development of the entorhi-nal and commissural afferents to the dentate gyrus of the rat. *J Comp Neurol* 1977;173:231–250.

Fricke R, Cowan WM. An autoradiographic study of the commissural and ipsilat-eral hippocampo-dentate projections in the adult rat. *J Comp Neurol* 1978;181:253–270.

Fry FJ, Cowan WM. A study of retrograde cell degeneration in the lateral mammillary nucleus of the cat, with special reference to the role of axonal branching in the preservation of the cell. *J Comp Neurol* 1972;144:1–24.

Gerfen CR, O'Leary DDM, Cowan WM. A note on the transneuronal transport of wheat germ agglutinen-conjugated horseradish peroxidase in the avian and rodent visual system. *Exp Brain Res* 1982;48:443–448.

Gottlieb DI, Cowan WM. On the distribution of axonal terminals containing speroidal and flattened synaptic vesicles in the hippocampus and dentate gyrus of the rat and cat. *Z Zellforsch* 1972a;129:413–429.

Gottlieb DI, Cowan WM. Evidence for a temporal factor in the occupation of available synaptic sites during the development of the dentate gyrus. *Brain Res* 1972b;41:452–456.

Gottlieb DI, Cowan WM. Autoradiographic studies of the commissural and ipsilateral association connections of the hippocampus and dentate gyrus of the rat. I. The commissural connections. *J Comp Neurol* 1973;149:393–422.

Haan EA, Boss BD, Cowan WM. Production and characterization of monoclonal antibodies against the "brain-specific" proteins 14-3-2 and S-100. *Proc Natl Acad Sci USA* 1982;79:7585–7589.

Hagbarth KE, Kerr DIB. Central influences on spinal afferent conduction. *J Neurophysiol* 1954;17:295–307.

Hendrickson AE, Cowan WM. Changes in the rate of axoplasmic transport during postnatal development of the rabbit's optic nerve and tract. *Exp Neurol* 1971;30:403–422.

Hendrickson AE, Wagoner N, Cowan WM. An autoradiographic and electron microscopic study of retino-hypothalamic connections. *Z Zellforsch* 1972;135:1–26.

Hunt RK, Cowan WM. The chemoaffinity hypothesis: An appreciation of Roger W. Sperry's contributions to developmental biology. In Trevarthen C, ed. *Brain circuits and functions of the mind*, Cambridge, UK: Cambridge University Press, 1990;19–74.

Insausti R, Amaral DG, Cowan WM. The entorhinal cortex of the monkey: II. Cortical afferents. *J Comp Neurol* 1987a;264:356–395.

Insausti R, Amaral DG, Cowan WM. The entorhinal cortex of the monkey: III. Subcortical afferents. *J Comp Neurol* 1987b;264:396–408.

Insausti R, Blakemore C, Cowan WM. Ganglion cell death during development of ipsilateral retino-collicular projection in golden hamster. *Nature* 1984;308: 362–365.

Insausti R, Blakemore C, Cowan WM. Postnatal development of the ipsilateral retinocollicular projection and the effects of unilateral enucleation in the golden hamster. *J Comp Neurol* 1985;234:393–409.

Kelly JP, Cowan WM. Studies on the development of the chick optic tectum. III. Effects of early eye removal. *Brain Res* 1972;42:263–288.

Kishi K, Stanfield BB, Cowan WM. A note on the distribution of glial cells in the molecular layer of the dentate gyrus. *Brain Res* 1979;4:35–41.

Kishi K, Stanfield BB, Cowan WM. A quantitative EM autoradiographic study of the commissural and associational connections of the dentate gyrus in the rat. *Anat Embryol* 1980;160:173–196.

Kopnisky KL, Cowan WM, Hyman SE. Levels of analysis in psychiatric research. *Dev Psychopathol* 2002;14:437–461.

Laatsch RH, Cowan WM. A structural specialization at nodes of Ranvier in the central nervous system. *Nature* 1966a;210:757–758.

Laatsch RH, Cowan WM. Electron microscopic studies of the dentate gyrus of the rat. I. Normal structure with special reference to synaptic organization. *J Comp Neurol* 1966b;128:359–396.

Laatsch RH, Cowan WM. Electron microscopic studies of the dentate gyrus of the rat. II. Degeneration of commissural afferents. *J Comp Neurol* 1967;130:241–262.

LaVail JH, Cowan WM. The development of the chick optic tectum. I. Normal morphology and cytoarchitectonic development. *Brain Res* 1971a;28:421–441.

LaVail JH, Cowan WM. The development of the chick optic tectum. II. Autoradiographic studies. *Brain Res* 1971b;28:391–419.

Matter-Sadzinski L, Matter J-M, Cowan WM. The selection of retinal ganglion cells that extend their axons for gene expression analysis. In Piatigorsky J, Shinohara T, Zelenka PS, eds. *Molecular biology of the eye—Genes, vision, and ocular disease.* New York: A. R. Liss, 1988;269–276.

Matthews MR, Cowan WM, Powell TPS. Transneural cell degeneration in the lateral geniculate nucleus in the macaque monkey. *J Anat* 1960;94:145–169.

McGill JI, Powell TPS, Cowan WM. The retinal representation upon the optic tectum and isthmo-optic nucleus in the pigeon. *J Anat (Lond)* 1966a;100:5–33.

McGill JI, Powell TPS, Cowan WM. The organization of the projection of the centrifugal fibres to the retina in the pigeon. *J Anat (Lond)* 1966b;100:35–49.

O'Leary DDM, Cowan WM. Further studies on the development of the isthmo-optic nucleus with special reference to the occurrence and fate of ectopic and ipsilaterally projecting neurons. *J Comp Neurol* 1982;212:399–416.

O'Leary DDM, Cowan WM. Topographic organization of certain tectal afferent and efferent connections can develop normally in the absence of retinal input. *Proc Natl Acad Sci USA* 1983;80:6131–6135.

O'Leary DDM, Cowan WM. Survival of isthmo-optic neurons after early removal of one eye. *Dev Brain Res* 1984;12:293–310.

O'Leary DDM, Crespo D, Fawcett JW, Cowan WM. The effect of intraocular tetrodoxin on the postnatal reduction in numbers of optic nerve axons in the rat. *Brain Res* 1986;30:96–103.

O'Leary DDM, Fawcett JW, Cowan WM. Topographic targeting errors in the retinocollicular projection and their elimination by selective ganglion cell death. *J Neurosci* 1986;6:3692–3705.

O'Leary DDM, Fricke RA, Stanfield BB, Cowan WM. Changes in the associational afferents to the dentate gyrus in the absence of its commissural input. *Anat Embryol* 1979;156:283–299.

O'Leary DDM, Gerfen CR, Cowan WM. The development and restriction of the ipsilateral retinofugal projection in the chick. *Dev Brain Res* 1983;10:93–109.

O'Leary DDM, Stanfield BB, Cowan WM. Evidence for the sprouting of the associational fibers to the dentate gyrus following removal of the commissural afferents in adult rats. *Embryology* 1980;159:151–161.

O'Leary DDM, Stanfield BB, Cowan WM. Evidence that the early postnatal restriction of the cells of origin of the callosal projection is due to the elimination of axonal collaterals rather than to the death of neurons. *Dev Brain Res* 1981;1:607–617.

Powell TPS, Cowan WM. The connexions of the midline and intralaminar nuclei of the thalamus of the rat. *J Anat (Lond)* 1954a;88:307–319.

Powell TPS, Cowan WM. The origin of the mamillo-thalamic tract in the rat. *J Anat* 1954b;88:489–497.

Powell TPS, Cowan WM. An experimental study of the efferent connexions of the hippocampus. *Brain* 1955;78:115–132.

Powell TPS, Cowan WM. The projection of the midline and intralaminar nuclei of the thalamus. VI Congress Federatif International d'Anatomie, Paris, 1956a.

Powell TPS, Cowan WM. A study of thalamo-striate relations in monkey. *Brain* 1956b;79:364–390.

Powell TPS, Cowan WM. The thalamo-striate projection in the avian brain. *J Anat* 1957;91:571.

Powell TPS, Cowan WM. The thalamic projection upon the telencephalon in the pigeon (*Columba livia*). *J Anat* 1961;95:78–109.

Powell TPS, Cowan WM. An experimental study of the projection of the cochlea. *J Anat* 1962;96:269–284.

Powell TPS, Cowan WM. Centrifugal fibres in the lateral olfactory tract. *Nature* 1963;199:1296–1297.

Powell TPS, Cowan WM, Raisman G. Olfactory relationships of the diecephalon. *Nature* 1963;199:710–712.

Powell TPS, Cowan WM, Raisman G. The central olfactory connexions. *J Anat (Lond)* 1965;99:791–813.

Powell TPS, Guillery RW, Cowan WM. A quantitative study of the fornix-mammillo-thalamic tract system. *J Anat* 1957;91:419–437.

Raisman G, Cowan WM, Powell TPS. The extrinsic afferent, association and commissural fibres of the hippocampus. *Brain* 1965;88:963–996.

Raisman G, Cowan WM, Powell TPS. An experimental analysis of the efferent projection of the hippocampus. *Brain* 1966;89:83–108.

Rickmann M, Amaral DG, Cowan WM. Organization of radial glial cells during the development of the rat dentate gyrus. *J Comp Neurol* 1987;264:449–479.

Rogers LA, Cowan WM. The development of the mesencephalic-nucleus of the trigeminal nerve in the chick. *J Comp Neurol* 1973;147:291–320.

Rothman S, Cowan WM. A scanning electron microscope study of the *in vitro* development of dissociated hippocampal cells. *J Comp Neurol* 1981;195:141–155.

Saper CB, Loewy AD, Swanson LW, Cowan WM. Direct hypothalamo-autonomic connections. *Brain Res* 1976;117:305–312.

Saper CB, Swanson LW, Cowan WM. The efferent connections of the ventromedial nucleus of the hypothalamus of the rat. *J Comp Neurol* 1976;169:409–442.

Saper CB, Swanson LW, Cowan WM. The efferent connections of the anterior hypothalamic area of the rat, cat and monkey. *J Comp Neurol* 1978;182:575–600.

Saper CB, Swanson LW, Cowan WM. An autoradiographic study of the efferent connections of the lateral hypothalamic area in the rat. *J Comp Neurol* 1979;183:689–706.

Saper CB, Swanson LW, Cowan WM. Some efferent connections of the rostral hypothalamus in the squirrel monkey (*Saimiri sciureus*) and cat. *J Comp Neurol* 1979;184:205–242.

Schlessinger AR, Cowan WM, Gottlieb DI. An autoradiographic study of the time of origin and the pattern of granule cell migration in the dentate gyrus of the rat. *J Comp Neurol* 1975;159:149–175.

Schlessinger AR, Cowan WM, Swanson LW. The time of origin of neurons in Ammon's horn and the associated retrohippocampal fields. *Anat Embryol* 1978;154:153–173.

Stanfield BB, Caviness VS Jr, Cowan WM. The organization of certain afferents to the hippocampus and dentate gyrus in normal and reeler mice. *J Comp Neurol* 1979;185:461–484.

Stanfield B, Cowan WM. Evidence for a change in the retinohypothalamic projection in the rat following early removal of one eye. *Brain Res* 1976;109:129–136.

Stanfield BB, Cowan WM. The morphology of the hippocampus and dentate gyrus in normal and reeler mice. *J Comp Neurol* 1979a;185:393–422.

Stanfield BB, Cowan WM. The development of the hippocampus and dentate gyrus in normal and reeler mice. *J Comp Neurol* 1979b;185:423–460.

Stanfield BB, Cowan WM. Evidence for the sprouting of entorhinal afferents into the "hippocampal zone" of the molecular layer of the dentate gyrus. *Anat Embryol* 1979c;156:37–52.

Stanfield BB, Cowan WM. The sprouting of septal afferents to the dentate gyrus after lesions of the entorhinal cortex in adult rats. *Brain Res* 1982;232:162–170.

Stanfield BB, Cowan WM. An EM autoradiography study of the hypothalamic-hippocampal projection. *Brain Res* 1984;309:229–307.

Stanfield BB, Cowan WM. The development of the hippocampal region. In Peters A, Jones EG, eds. *Cerebral cortex vol. 7: The development and maturation of the cerebral cortex.* New York: Plenum Press, 1988;91–131.

Stanfield BB, Wyss JM, Cowan WM. The projection of the supramammillary region upon the dentate gyrus in normal and reeler mice. *Brain Res* 1980;198:196–203.

Swanson LW, Cowan WM. The efferent connections of the suprachiasmatic nucleus of the hypothalamus. *J Comp Neurol* 1975a;160:1–12.

Swanson LW, Cowan WM. Hippocampo-hypothalamic connections: Origin in subicular cortex not Ammon's horn. *Science* 1975b;189:303–304.

Swanson LW, Cowan WM. A note on the connections and development of the nucleus accumbens. *Brain Res* 1975c;92:324–330.

Swanson LW, Cowan WM. An autoradiographic study of the organization of the efferent connections of the hippocampal formation in the rat. *J Comp Neurol* 1977;172:49–84.

Swanson LW, Cowan WM. The connections of the septal region in the rat. *J Comp Neurol* 1979;186:621–655.

Swanson LW, Cowan WM, Jones EG. An autoradiographic study of the efferent connections of the ventral lateral geniculate nucleus in the albino rat and the cat. *J Comp Neurol* 1974;156:143–164.

Swanson LW, Lindstrom J, Tzartos S, Schmued LC, O'Leary DDM, Cowan WM. Immunohistochemical localization of monoclonal antibodies to the nicotinic acetylcholine receptor in the midbrain of the chick. *Proc Natl Acad Sci USA* 1983;80:4532–4536.

Swanson LW, Sawchenko PE, Cowan WM. Evidence that the commissural, associational and septal projections of the *regio inferior* of the hippocampus arise from the same neurons. *Brain Res* 1980;197:207–212.

Swanson LW, Sawchenko PE, Cowan WM. Evidence for collateral projections by neurons in Ammon's horn, the dentate gyrus, and the subiculum: A multiple retrograde labeling study in the rat. *J Neurosci* 1981;1:548–559.

Swanson LW, Wyss JM, Cowan WM. An autoradiographic study of the organization of intrahippocampal association pathways in the rat. *J Comp Neurol* 1978;181: 681–716.

Wann DF, Cowan WM. An image processing system for the analysis of neuroanatomical data. Proceedings of the Computer Image Processing and Recognition Symposium, Columbia, Missouri 1972;411–419.

Wann DF, Price JL, Cowan WM, Agulnek MA. An automated system for counting silver grains in autoradiographs. *Brain Res* 1974;81:31–58.

Wann DF, Woolsey TA, Dierker ML, Cowan WM. An on-line digital computer system for the semi-automatic analysis of Golgi-impregnated neurons. *IEEE Trans Biomed Eng* 1973;BME-20:233–247.

Walicke P, Cowan WM, Ueno N, Baird A, Guillemin R. Fibroblast growth factor promotes the survival of dissociated hippocampal neurons and enhances neurite extension. *Proc Natl Acad Sci USA* 1986;83:3012–3016.

Willard MB, Cowan WM, Vagelos PR. The polypeptide composition of intra-axonally transported proteins: evidence for four transport velocities. *Proc Natl Acad Soc USA* 1974;71:2183–2187.

Wyss JM, Stanfield BB, Cowan WM. Structural abnormalities in the olfactory bulb of the reeler mouse. *Brain Res* 1980;188:566–571.

Wyss JM, Swanson LW, Cowan WM. A study of subcortical afferents to the hippocampal formation in the rat. *Neuroscience* 1979a;4:463–476.

Wyss JM, Swanson LW, Cowan WM. Evidence for an input to the molecular layer and the stratum granulosum of the dentate gyrus from the supramammillary region of the hypothalamus. *Anat Embryol* 1979b;156:165–176.

Wyss JM, Swanson LW, Cowan WM. The organization of the fimbria, dorsal fornix and ventral hippocampal commissure in the rat. *Anat Embryol* 1980;158: 303–316.

Veazey RB, Amaral DG, Cowan, WM. The morphology and connections of the posterior hypothalamus in the cynomologus monkey *(Macaca fascicularis)* I. Cytoarchitectonic organization. *J Comp Neurol* 1982a;207:114–134.

Veazey RB, Amaral DB, Cowan WM. The morphology and connections of the posterior hypothalamus in the cynomologus monkey *(Macaca fascicularis)* II. An autoradiographic study of the efferent connections. *J Comp Neurol* 1982b;107:135–156.

Veening JG, Swanson LW, Cowan WM, Nieuwenhuys R, Geeraedts LMG. The medial forebrain bundle of the rat. II. An autoradiographic study of the topography of the major descending and ascending components. *J Comp Neurol* 1982;206: 82–108.

John E. Dowling

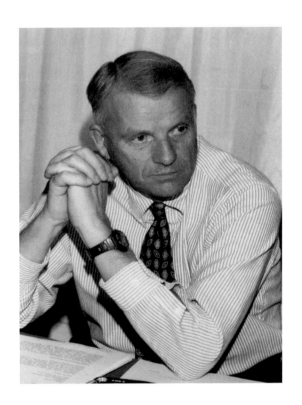

John E. Dowling

BORN:
Pawtucket, Rhode Island
August 31, 1935

EDUCATION:
Harvard College, A.B. (Biology, 1957)
Harvard Medical School (1957–1959)
Harvard University, Ph.D. (Biology, 1961)

APPOINTMENTS:
Harvard University (1961)
Johns Hopkins University (1964)
Harvard University (1971)
Chairman, Department of Biology,
    Harvard University (1975–1978)
Associate Dean of the Faculty of Arts and Sciences,
    Harvard University (1980–1984)
Master, Leverett House, Harvard University (1981–1998)
Maria Moors Cabot Professor of Natural Science (1987–2001)
Harvard College Professor, Harvard University (1999)
Llura and Gordon Gund Professor of Neurosciences,
    Harvard University (2001)

HONORS AND AWARDS (SELECTED):
Friedenwald Medal, Association for Research in Vision and
    Ophthalmology (1970)
American Academy of Arts and Sciences (1972)
National Academy of Sciences, USA (1976)
Retina Research Foundation Award of Merit (1981)
M.D. (Hon.) University of Lund, Sweden (1982)
Alcon Research Institute Recognition Award (1986)
Prentice Medal, American Academy of Optometry (1991)
American Philosophical Society (1992)
Von Sallman Prize in Vision and Ophthalmology (1992)
The Helen Keller Prize for Vision Research (2000)
Llura Liggett Gund Award for Lifetime Achievement (2001)

John Dowling has studied the retina his entire career. He is best known for his detailed analysis of synaptic circuitry of the retina and its functional organization. His laboratory has also focused attention on retinal pharmacology, particularly the role of dopamine in retinal function, and, recently, on retinal development and genetics.

John E. Dowling

I have always enjoyed reading about scientists and their discoveries. As a college student, Sinclair Lewis' *Arrowsmith* left an indelible impression, and then later Cajal's *Recollections of My Life* was inspiring—even exciting—to read. But there are many, many more books—biographies, autobiographies, and even some historical fiction—about scientists that I have devoured. As I sit down to write this brief essay on my own life as a scientist, I ask myself what made these books so much fun to read, and how do I make this piece interesting to others and perhaps as instructive as many of the books I found so fascinating?

Some melding of one's personal and scientific life is important to recount, but beyond that, one's philosophy of doing science, how particular lines of research were taken up, and how one becomes a scientist and manages a scientific life. Perhaps I should start with the latter to put into context what is to come. How did I end up spending a life studying the retina? Clearly, my mentor, George Wald, was instrumental and that story will come. But simple curiosity as to how things work has played an enormous role in directing my scientific life. I have never felt that I am particularly brilliant, but I do find myself mulling things over again and again, seeking an explanation or possible answer to a scientific puzzle and then trying to think of a way to establish my idea. Much of my success, without a doubt, has come from my students and co-workers who arrived in the laboratory with wonderful skills or ideas, and my contribution to their work has been to encourage them, to give them free rein, and to help focus their efforts on the most significant questions. Those working in the laboratory have also learned as much from each other as from me, and I always encourage multidisciplinary approaches and collaborations to crack open a problem. At any one time in the lab, we are carrying out anatomical, physiological, pharmacological, and now genetic approaches to the problems at hand. An interactive laboratory is a happy and productive one, and I count virtually everyone who has been in the laboratory as a good friend. For my 65th birthday, my former students held a symposium in my honor, and about 90 of the 100 or so people who have been in the laboratory over the years attended. That tribute was most gratifying. As a last point for those starting out in science, over the years I have made every effort not to compete with my former students. The projects they undertake in my laboratory are theirs; they take them with them. If my laboratory continues to work on the same or similar problem, it is as a collaboration or, at the very least, with a continuous exchange of information between the labs. A consequence of this is that my laboratory is always moving on to new areas of research. The downside is that sometimes I feel something is not being finished that was started in the lab. But, that is a penalty I think worth taking—to make sure the next generation has the opportunity to develop an area of research.

The Beginnings: George Wald, Vitamin A Deficiency, and Visual Adaptation

I was born in Rhode Island, the fourth of five children. My father was a physician, an ophthalmologist, and my mother was trained as a chemist. Education was always emphasized in the family, and from the sixth grade onward, I attended a private school. However, studying was not my forte, and I was a mediocre student at best, until my junior and senior years. Chemistry awakened me academically in my junior year—my first A ever— and that then carried over into college.

Curiosity about things and building things consumed much of my time growing up. I had a small room in our basement where I could construct elaborate structures with erector sets; make my electric train layout ever more complicated; and build model boats, cars, and planes with electric or gas engines. Sports, especially competitive ones, were an enduring interest, but a bout with polio when I was 16 left me permanently lame in one leg and altered my activities from baseball, football, hockey, and skiing to golf, squash, and sailing, which I enjoy to this day. Extracurricular activities at school occupied too much of my time, but also may have been the reason I was admitted to Harvard University as an undergraduate. In my senior year of high school I was president of the class, editor-in-chief of the school newspaper, and captain of the golf team. This trait of getting involved in too many things is still with me; I wish I could say "no" more often when asked to serve on a committee or to take on another responsibility.

I arrived at Harvard determined to focus on academics, and it was a new world for me. I had fair success and was pointed toward medicine as a career. But all that changed in my junior year when I took biochemistry from George Wald. He was mesmerizing, especially in the second semester which was devoted to topics in biochemistry. I can still feel the excitement he generated in me when he talked about Albert Szent-Györgyi's famous experiments with glycerinated muscle fibers. That they would contract when ATP was added seemed miraculous to me, getting at the essence of life.

Halfway through that second semester, I asked George (then Professor Wald to me and for many years thereafter) if I could undertake a senior project in his laboratory beginning that summer. I was accepted into the laboratory and that changed my life. George proposed that I work on vitamin A deficiency in rats to determine why after prolonged deficiency, recovery was often incomplete upon refeeding of vitamin A. Earlier studies by Katherine Tansley and others in England had suggested that photoreceptors degenerate in prolonged vitamin A deficiency, and Ruth Hubbard in the Wald lab had shown that opsin (without attached vitamin A aldehyde) was much less stable than is rhodopsin. George surmised that the lack of complete recovery was due to irreversible photoreceptor degeneration. So I began a series of biochemical measurements, mapping out what happens to a rat on a deficient diet. First, liver stores of vitamin A decrease, then blood stores decline and with that rhodopsin levels. Some time later (~2 weeks), opsin levels begin to decline, and so Wald's hypothesis seemed correct. Opsin is an important structural component of the outer segment of the photoreceptor, and degeneration of photoreceptors occurs as opsin levels decline.

But I was curious as to what effect the loss of rhodopsin had on the rat's vision. How could this be determined? Donald Kennedy, eventually to become Head of the Food and Drug Administration (FDA) and President of Stanford University, was just completing his Ph.D. in the Biology Department, recording the electroretinogram (ERG) of the frog. Don agreed to record the ERG of a rat in his setup, and it was clear that this was the way to go. I inherited much of Don's equipment when he left, moved it upstairs to a darkroom, and began my electrophysiological studies. I found that as the visual pigment levels decline, the light sensitivity of the eye decreases, as one would expect, but it did so logarithmically! This was new and suggested a relationship between visual pigment levels in a photoreceptor and visual sensitivity, a contentious issue at the time. The next question was whether a similar relationship exists during light and dark adaptation, but those measurements were not made for another year. My first paper reporting the studies carried out as an undergraduate were published in the *Proceedings of the National Academy of Sciences (PNAS)* in 1958.

My senior year at Harvard was spent mainly in the Wald laboratory, and I found research immensely satisfying and fun. But I also remained determined to go to medical school and enrolled at the Harvard Medical School in the fall of 1957. I soon found I was missing the Wald lab and so began spending free afternoons in Cambridge. The following summer is when I examined the role of visual pigment levels in light and dark adaptation and also mapped out the exchange of vitamin A between the retina and pigment epithelium during light and dark adaptation. This resulted in a *Nature* paper published in 1960. The second year of medical school was spent split between Cambridge and Boston, and a new observation I made led me to take a year's leave of absence from medical school to work on it.

This was the finding that vitamin A acid (now called retinoic acid) could prevent animals from dying from vitamin A deficiency, but did not prevent them from going blind. In other words, retinoic acid can fulfill all of the somatic functions of vitamin A—growth, tissue maintenance, and so forth—but cannot be reduced in the body to vitamin A aldehyde (now called retinal) which is essential for vision. Thus, with retinoic acid it was possible to isolate vitamin A deficiency to the eye and photoreceptors. This enabled me to complete elegantly my original project that I began with Wald. I could show that with prolonged vitamin A deficiency, photoreceptors were indeed lost and that in such retinas complete recovery did not occur after vitamin A refeeding.

Again, though, curiosity about an aspect of the project led me to another technique that eventually would play a major role in my research career, namely electron microscopy. What did vitamin A-deficient photoreceptors look like? Ian Gibbons had just joined the Harvard Biology Department and was in charge of a new electron microscope facility. Why not learn how to do electron microscopy and find out? I did just that and thus began my anatomical studies. A *PNAS* paper reporting our retinoic acid studies was published in 1960 and included biochemical, electrophysiological, and electron microscopic observations.

Retinoic acid (RA) has become a most important molecule for understanding development, and 10 years ago we revisited RA in terms of its role in retinal and photoreceptor development. But how did I come to use it in the first place? In 1957, R.A. Morton's classic book on vitamin A appeared, and Ruth Hubbard read in it that whereas vitamin A deficiency symptoms could be reversed in animals dosed with RA, never could one find traces of RA in the animal's tissues. This suggested that RA could not be converted back to retinal or vitamin A in biological tissues, the molecules essential for vision. She suggested I try vitamin A acid in my experiments, and, as they say, the rest is history.

An opportunity arose while in medical school that led me into yet another area of lifetime interest, namely inherited retinal degenerations. Richard Sidman was my Instructor in Neuropathology at Harvard Medical School and he had read my first paper on vitamin A deficiency. He had recently brought into this country rats with an inherited retinal dystrophy—the RCS (Royal College of Surgeons) rats—and he wondered if they might have a deficit in vitamin A metabolism. We began a collaboration that resulted in a *Journal of Cell Biology* paper in 1962. Although we found no evidence that the defect in the RCS rat was caused by a deficit in vitamin A metabolism, several inherited retinal degenerations in man have now been shown to be caused by such genetic defects. But I am now getting ahead of my story.

During my year leave of absence from medical school, as the story of RA unfolded, George Wald suggested that I consider obtaining a Ph.D. Since I had had two years of medical school training, had been an undergraduate in the Biology Department, and had done, in his opinion, enough research for a thesis, George believed I could quickly qualify for the degree. An amusing story resulted from my attempt a few days later to enroll in the Graduate School of Arts and Sciences (GSAS) at Harvard. When I approached the receptionist asking for the application forms for graduate study, I was told in a somewhat contemptuous voice that since the deadline for admission for the following year was the next day, there was no way I could complete the application process in time. I then said I was not seeking admission for the following year, but for the next semester (only two weeks off!) and that I believed Professor Wald had spoken to the GSAS Dean on my behalf. The receptionist disappeared into the Dean's office, but reappeared a short time later with the forms and a red face! I entered graduate school in February 1960, took qualifying exams in April, and wrote my thesis over the summer and into the fall. The degree was granted in January 1961.

I fully expected to return to medical school the following year, but, again, George intervened. He was undertaking a new introductory undergraduate course in biology at Harvard, designed for both scientists and non-scientists, that would emphasize the unity of life at the molecular level. This course was to replace the traditional botany and zoology courses that focused on the differences among organisms. He asked if I would join him and a small cadre of young biologists to help design and teach the course. The offer was too tempting to refuse, and I extended my leave of absence from medical school—now in its 43rd year!

The course, entitled "The Nature of Living Things," began that year, and I was appointed an Instructor in the Department beginning in February 1961. I was promoted to Assistant Professor in July and given laboratory space adjacent to the Wald laboratory. And so, my independent research career began. Initially, I followed up on and extended the research projects I had begun as an undergraduate and graduate student, as well as completed the study on the RCS rats with Richard Sidman. With Ruth Hubbard, I looked at the formation and utilization of 11-cis vitamin A in eye tissues, as well as the effects of brilliant light flashes on the ERG in light and dark adaptation. With Ian Gibbons, I studied the fine structure of the pigment epithelium, and then, when Richard Cone was visiting from the University of Chicago, I extended my observations on the mechanisms underlying light and dark adaptation, showing that there are both neural and photochemical components at play.

Up to that point (1963), virtually all of my research had been carried out on the rat, a rod-dominated animal. What about cones? Do cones light and dark adapt like rods? How different is their fine structure? Curiosity about these questions was to lead me far beyond photoreceptors, light and dark adaptation, and vitamin A deficiency and to one of the most fruitful collaborations of my career. Ground squirrel retinas contain mainly cones, and I thought they would be ideal animals to study. But, how would I obtain some? Charles Lyman at Harvard Medical School was studying hibernation in ground squirrels and was the obvious source. A call to Charles resulted in the promise of some animals, but he mentioned that a visitor to our department from England, teaching Jack Welch's Invertebrate Zoology course that year while Jack was on sabbatical leave, was also interested in ground squirrels and why didn't we share animals? That was my introduction to Brian Boycott.

Brian was then interested in synaptic plasticity and wished to follow up on an old observation that spines on cerebellar Purkinje cells change shape during hibernation. His laboratory was just down the hall, and so we began to take the bus over to the medical school to pick up animals and tissues. In my lab, I recorded the ground squirrel ERG during light and dark adaptation, and then I began to study the fine structure of the photoreceptors by electron microscopy. What caught my eye were the photoreceptor terminals and the fact that on occasion I could trace a process back from the photoreceptor terminal to its cell of origin. Photoreceptor-bipolar cell contacts were expected and seen, but I could also identify processes from horizontal cells synapsing with the photoreceptor cells. Horizontal cells were very much a mystery then—indeed, some thought they were glial cells—but the fact that they were receiving input from photoreceptor cells clearly indicated they were neuronal.

What was the neuronal circuitry of the outer retina? I began to discuss this with Brian on our medical school trips and started to learn more about synapses and synaptic circuitry. We mused that it was important to learn more about the horizontal and bipolar cells of the ground squirrel retina by light microscopy and Golgi staining, techniques with which Brian was expert. At the same time, Brian had found significant changes in the cerebellar (Purkinje cell) spines during hibernation at the light microscopic level, but he recognized that these changes needed to be studied by electron microscopy—something I could do. The next step was obvious: we join forces and share each others' expertise.

We made substantial progress on both fronts, but curiously we never formally published either study. (Several years later, Roger West in our laboratory revisited the ground squirrel retina and did publish several papers on its cellular and synaptic organization.) Brian returned to England at the end of the year, and the next year, I moved to The Wilmer Institute at Johns Hopkins University. I had been an Assistant Professor in the Harvard Biology Department for three years, and, as was then the custom, assistant professors were seldom promoted at Harvard. A tempting offer from Ed Maumenee, Chief of Ophthalmology at the Wilmer, to occupy magnificent new space in the Woods Research Building was too good to pass up, and so I moved to Baltimore in June 1964.

The Early Wilmer Years: Retinal Circuitry and Single Cell Recordings

During my last year as an Assistant Professor at Harvard, George Wald was on sabbatical leave in England, and so my teaching responsibilities were considerable. I did stay in contact with Brian, who was becoming more and more interested in the retina, but who also felt that to make progress with understanding retinal circuitry, the ground squirrel was not the place to start; too little was known about its cells. Since Polyak's 1941 book *The Retina* provided a wealth of material on the primate retina and its cells, we thought perhaps we should begin there. Brian visited the Wilmer in July 1964 for a few weeks, the first of many such visits over the next 10 years. During that first visit we studied what ground squirrel material he had prepared, but also fixed some monkey retinas for both light and electron microscopy, and it was this material that set us on our course.

I first looked at the foveal cones—about which virtually nothing was known at the electron microscopic level. A paper in *Science* early in 1965 described the photoreceptor outer and inner segment structure, but also, tantalizing, the structure of the foveal cone photoreceptor synapses which seemed simple compared to the ground squirrel photoreceptor synapses and, perhaps, easier to analyze. I began to focus on identifying retinal synapses in both plexiform layers. Ribbon synapses in photoreceptors were well known, but ribbon synapses were also present in the inner plexiform layer (IPL). In what cells were they? A particularly well-fixed piece of human retina, provided us by Ed Maumenee from an eye surgically removed for melanoma, gave us the answer and much more. Large bipolar cell terminals could be readily identified in the human IPL, and they made abundant ribbon synapses. Conventional synapses were also seen in the IPL. The obvious question was what cell makes these? Again, the piece of human retina provided the answer. I could follow processes from amacrine cells into the IPL where they made such conventional synapses. We reported these first results at the annual Cold Spring Harbor Laboratory Symposium in the spring of 1965 and with them a tentative diagram of the synaptic circuitry of the IPL (Fig. 1).

Fritoff Sjostrand was Chair of the session at the Cold Spring Harbor meeting at which I presented our findings, and following the presentation, he expressed contempt for our wiring diagram. He chastised us for not carrying out serial section studies (of which he was then master). He said sitting on one's rear end and doing the hard work was necessary before drawing any such diagram. I replied that sitting on one's behind and thinking hard about one's observations was equally valid, which brought down the house but lost me the friendship of Sjostrand. He never spoke to me again.

In London, Brian was making new observations at the light microscope level on the primate retina, whereas in Baltimore, I extended the electron microscopic (EM) observations (even carrying out some limited serial section analyses). Brian was then visiting twice a year, and when he was in Baltimore, it was intense but exciting. We published our electron microscopic studies on the primate retina (with much grander diagrams) in the *Proceedings of the Royal Society* in 1966 (Dowling and Boycott, 1966), but the light

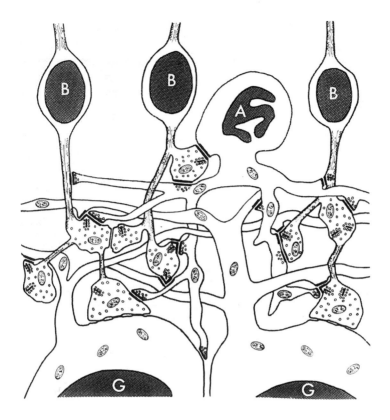

Fig. 1. Our summary diagram of the synaptic organization of the primate IPL layer presented at the 1965 Cold Spring Harbor Symposium. B, bipolar cells; A, amacrine cell; and G, ganglion cells. (From Dowling JE, Boycott BB. *Cold Spring Harbor Symp Quant Biol* 1965;30:393–402. With permission.)

microscopic paper did not appear until 1969. The latter was a massive tome, 75 pages in length, published in the *Physiological Transactions of the Royal Society*. It went through 12 drafts and had over 100 micrographs and figures.

My lab at Johns Hopkins was also growing. George Weinstein, an ophthalmologist, first joined us and carried out a marvelous study on light and dark adaptation of the isolated rat retina, making simultaneous physiological and biochemical measurements. Helga Kolb soon arrived from Geoff Arden's laboratory in London, and she wanted to do anatomical studies. Brian and I thought combining the light and electron microscopic observations by studying Golgi-stained cells in the electron microscope (a technique pioneered by Bill Stell at the National Institutes of Health) was the next logical step to take, and it yielded wonderful results. An early result was the discovery of a second type of midget bipolar cell in the primate retina—the

flat midget cell—which was the first hint that information from photoreceptors to bipolar cells was divided into two pathways, ON and OFF pathways.
But at that point we knew nothing of the physiology of bipolar cells so that
realization was some time off. Helga studied the connections of all of the
outer plexiform layer cells, providing for the first time quantitative data
with regard to the number of connections made between photoreceptor and
bipolar or horizontal cells. Her paper in the *Philosophical Transactions* in
1970 was submitted for a Ph.D. from the University of Bristol.

Following a lecture I gave at Johns Hopkins on the synaptic organization of the primate retina, a new graduate student, trained as an electrical
engineer at MIT, came to my office asking if I thought it possible to build
a theoretical model of the retina. My answer was that since we knew virtually nothing of the electrical responses of the retinal cells, it was too early
to model the retina, but why didn't he, for his graduate work, make such
recordings from the mudpuppy retina. I had been introduced to the mudpuppy retina by Paul Brown of the Wald lab when I was still at Harvard;
he was taking advantage of the mudpuppy's large photoreceptor cells for
microspectrophotometric measurements. But what impressed me then was
that all of the retinal cells were large, and this might be an ideal retina
from which to record the responses of single cells. Alexander Bortoff of the
State University of New York at Albany had been making some intracellular
recordings from the mudpuppy retina, and so the project seemed feasible.

The graduate student called back a few days later to say he would like
to try the project and that is how Frank Werblin joined the lab. Frank
was soon recording intracellularly from the mudpuppy cells, but the critical
step was to stain the recorded cells. This was accomplished with the use of
Niagara Sky Blue, and soon Frank identified and characterized the electrical
responses of all of the retinal neurons. His was a spectacular thesis reporting
for the first time that there are both ON- and OFF-center bipolar cells, that
bipolar cells have a center-surround organization, and that many amacrine
cells respond transiently at the on and off of illumination. His results
were subsequently published in the *Journal of Neurophysiology* in 1969
(Fig. 2).

In the meantime, I was continuing my anatomical studies, first on the
frog retina and then on mudpuppy. Clearly, retinas vary in their synaptic
circuitry, and I began to explore whether the variations in synaptic circuitry
could be correlated with complexity of ganglion cell responses. It had been
appreciated for some time that cold-blooded vertebrates such as frogs had
many ganglion cells with complex receptive field properties such as movement and direction sensitivity. This must be correlated with differences in
circuitry. But how was this done?

Electron microscopic studies soon showed that there were many more
amacrine cell (conventional) synapses in the IPL compared to bipolar (ribbon) synapses in frog as compared to primates and that there were abundant

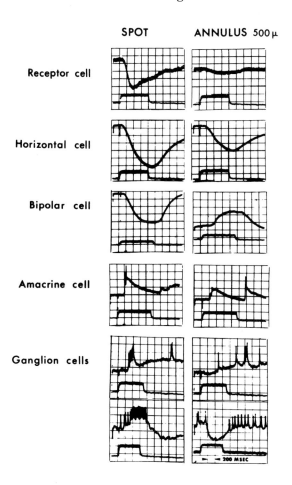

Fig. 2. Intracellular recordings from mudpuppy retinal cells to a spot of light (left) and annulus (right). (From Werblin FS, Dowling JE. *J Neurophysiol* 1969;255:339–355. With permission.)

serial and reciprocal synaptic arrangements made by the amacrine cell processes in the frog retina. This implicated the amacrine cells as playing a pivotal role in generating complex ganglion cell responses such as movement and direction selectivity, and Werblin's recordings from amacrine cells, showing that many of them respond transiently at the onset and offset of illumination—that is, they are highly movement sensitive—strongly supported this interpretation. Mark Dubin, another Johns Hopkins graduate student, eventually extended these studies to a number of species, providing quantitative measurement of synaptic frequencies and densities in the IPL.

The Marine Biological Laboratory: Horseshoe Crabs, Skates, and Teaching

The years at Johns Hopkins were exceptionally productive and fruitful. I did miss teaching, although I was an affiliate member of the Biophysics Department on the Homewood Campus of Johns Hopkins and taught a graduate seminar there. One day, Francis (Spike) Carlson, Chairman of the Biophysics Department, called to say that the Marine Biological Laboratory (MBL) wished to establish a Neurobiology Course and would I consider teaching such a course there? I knew little of the MBL, so Spike suggested I spend a summer in Woods Hole, MA, and become acquainted with the laboratory. I did that, beginning the summer of 1967, and I have been returning to Woods Hole and the MBL ever since.

That first summer I decided to learn how to record intracellularly from neurons. I recorded from photoreceptor (retinular) and second-order (eccentric) cells in horseshoe crab eyes and discovered a second type of discrete potential in the retinular cells. This is a regenerative potential that serves as an amplifying mechanism, ensuring that the absorption of a single photon in the retinular cell results in the generation of a nerve impulse in the eccentric cell. I spent a second summer recording from the *Limulus* eye, but then the following summer began another exceptionally fruitful collaboration with Harris Ripps, then of New York University and now of the University of Illinois School of Medicine in Chicago. Harris is an expert in visual pigment measurements and also has a long-standing interest in light and dark adaptation. We surmised that studying these processes in an animal that had only rods could be useful, and the early literature suggested that certain marine elasmobranches, including dogfish, had only rods. We first looked at dogfish, but discovered they have some cones. However, the other common elasmobranchs in Woods Hole, the winter and summer skates, did turn out to have pure rod retinas, and we spent nearly a decade of summers studying the retina of these animals and mapping out light and dark adaptation processes at all levels of the retina. The photoreceptors in the skate, although being classic rods in the dark-adapted retina, adopt cone-like behaviors when the eye is light adapted. Many of the features of photoreceptor light and dark adaptation were first revealed in the skate, and we showed that there are adaptation mechanisms at play proximal to the receptors. Another important finding we made in the skate was that horizontal cells hyperpolarize and lose light responsiveness when synaptic transmission from the photoreceptors is blocked with Mg^{2+}. This provided direct evidence that the photoreceptors release an excitatory neurotransmitter in the dark and that the hyperpolarizing response of horizontal cells in the light is due to a decrease in transmitter release from the photoreceptors. We eventually published 14 papers based on our summers' collaborative efforts.

Teaching soon became a prominent part of my Woods Hole experience. Michael Bennett of the Albert Einstein School of Medicine and I initiated the Neurobiology Course at the MBL in the summer of 1970, and we taught the course for five years before turning the reins over to others. The Neurobiology Course at the MBL is now one of the mainstays there. In the 1980s I helped David Papermaster establish a training course in vision at the MBL, and then in the mid-1990s Nancy Hopkins from MIT and I began a short course on the Neural Development and Behavior of Zebrafish, my most recent research interest.

I continued to maintain a summer laboratory at the MBL until the mid-1990s, when my laboratory began to raise zebrafish in The Biological Laboratories at Harvard. It then became difficult to justify setting up a summer lab at the MBL when we had more fish at Harvard (~30,000) than were available at any one time at the MBL. I continue to come to the MBL to teach and write, and for the past few years I have been involved administratively at the laboratory, serving at the present time as President of the Corporation.

The Later Wilmer Years: Functional Retinal Organization

A number of students and postdoctoral fellows eventually joined the lab at Johns Hopkins and contributed significantly. Bob Frank, an ophthalmology resident, looked at the effects of rhodopsin photoproducts on visual sensitivity. Dwight Burkhardt discovered a new extracellular potential in the frog retina—the proximal negative response (PNR)—and provided evidence that it derives from amacrine cells. Bob Miller recorded intracellularly from the glial (Müller) cells in the mudpuppy retina, found that they respond when the retina is illuminated, and provided some of the first evidence that Müller cell responses contribute to the ERG.

Les and Steve Fisher explored synaptic circuitry in the tadpole and cat eye, respectively, showing that there are significant changes in retinal synaptic organization during metamorphosis and that cat amacrine cells can make direct somato-somatic synapses on bipolar cells in the IPL. Gus Aguirre, a veterinarian, came to the lab to study dogs with inherited retinal degeneration, and Dick Chappell undertook a study of the dragonfly ocellus thought to be a "simple" retina. He recorded the electrical responses of the ocellar cells, whereas I examined the fine structure of the photoreceptors and synapses made in the ocellar synaptic plexus.

Those were wonderful and heady days at Johns Hopkins. On Thursdays at noon, the lab went *en masse* down to Lombard Street, lined with Jewish delicatessens, and the usual fare was a knish and corned beef sandwich washed down with a bottle of Cel-ray soda. Friday was seminar day, with lunch provided by Pat Sheppard, about whom I will say more shortly, followed by an informal talk. In the spring and fall, doubles tennis on the courts across the street from the Wilmer was often played, followed by beer and a sandwich at Frank's, a small pub-like bar a few blocks away. Sunday afternoons in the fall were spent watching the Baltimore Colts from the end zone—seats that Mark Dubin obtained by staying up all night at the stadium to ensure our obtaining them.

Pat Sheppard joined our lab shortly after I arrived in Baltimore and served as the lab's technician, accountant, artist, cook, procurer of material, and whatever. She cut marvelous sections for both light and electron microscopy and was responsible for all of the drawings we published. She fed us well before the Friday seminars and always seemed able to find what we needed for our experiments. The only time I saw her flustered was when Brian dashed in one day to ask if she could get him a box of rubbers. She did not know that rubbers in England are erasers. Pat ended up working for me for 27 years, retiring in 1991.

The Association for Research in Vision and Ophthalmology (ARVO) meeting (then the ARO meeting) became a mainstay for the lab beginning in the late 1960s. Until 1968, it was a small, mainly clinical meeting, but the ARO Trustees wanted it to expand. Several of us were asked how this might be done, and we proposed organizing sections that would represent various areas of eye and vision research. Paul Witkovsky from New York University, who had been spending time with us learning electron microscopy, and I organized a section on visual electrophysiology. The ARVO meeting eventually expanded beyond all expectations and now attracts over 8000 vision researchers each year to Ft. Lauderdale, FL, its present meeting site. In 1970, I was given the Friedenwald Award by ARVO, and I presented an overview of our lab's research to the attendees. It was well received and the published paper remains one of the most satisfying I have written.

In mid-1970, I was asked by the Biology Department at Harvard if I would like to return as full professor. It was a hard decision. Johns Hopkins had not only been generous to me, but the research had been going exceptionally well and many excellent students and postdoctoral fellows were coming to the lab. The deciding factor was the opportunity to teach undergraduates again and to be involved in college life. I returned to Harvard in June 1971, and that is where I have been since.

The Harvard Years—1970s: Dopamine, Pharmacology, and Interplexiform Cells

A number of people came with me to Harvard, including Pat Sheppard, Gordon Fain, Jochen Kleinschmidt, and Roger West. Ralph Nelson, a graduate student in Biophysics, decided to stay in Baltimore to finish his degree and his experiments on the electrical properties of mudpuppy retinal neurons. At Harvard, Gordon recorded intracellularly from the mudpuppy photoreceptors and showed definitively that rods have a higher sensitivity to light than do cones—by about 25 times. Jochen examined adaptation in gecko photoreceptors recorded intracellularly, and Roger undertook an analysis of the photoreceptors and synaptic input onto the ganglion cells in the ground squirrel retina.

In 1973, a visitor from Sweden joined the laboratory for a two-month stay, and once again a marvelous collaboration began that added another dimension to our research that continues to this day. Berndt Ehinger, an ophthalmologist, was interested in retinal pharmacology, particularly the role of monoamines in the retina. He was an expert with the Falk Hillarp method, which causes cells containing monoamines to fluoresce. He and others had observed what appeared to be a new type of cell in fish and New World Monkeys that sits among the amacrine cells, but extends processes into both plexiform layers of the retina. The color of the fluorescence suggested that these cells contain dopamine. But what are their synaptic connections? Berndt came to the lab to find out.

To identify the processes of the cells in the electron microscope, we took advantage of the fact that cells containing monoamines have robust reuptake systems that do not discriminate between the natural transmitter and certain analogs that can alter the fine structural appearance of the synaptic terminals. By feeding fish retinas one such analog, we were able to identify the synapses made by these cells and show that they are centrifugal in nature. They receive input in the IPL, whereas the bulk of their input is in the outer plexiform layer on horizontal cells. These cells were eventually called interplexiform cells, and they and dopamine have been studied in our lab ever since (Fig. 3).

Dopamine acts as a classic neuromodulator on horizontal cells, binding to D1 receptors and activating adenylate cyclase through a G-protein. The resulting increase in cyclic AMP activates protein kinase A (PKA), which modulates both glutamate and gap junctional channels in horizontal cells. Since those early days, the study of dopamine in the retina has become a virtual industry. Every retinal cell type responds to dopamine, and there are a variety of dopamine receptors in the retina whose activation can both increase or decrease cyclic AMP levels. The story gets more complicated yearly, and we still do not have a complete grasp of dopamine's overall role in the retina. Indeed, it appears as if dopamine must play multiple roles. Many people in the lab have studied the effects of dopamine on retinal cells over the years, including Bill Hedden, Rick Lasater, Keith Watling, Rob Van Buskirk, Andy Knapp, Doug McMahon, Stuart Mangel, Denis O'Brien, Pat O'Connor, Xiong-Li Yang, Tina Tornqvist, Osamu Umino and, most recently, Ethan Cohen, and all have added to the story.

Work in the laboratory during the 1970s was not focused entirely on dopamine and dopaminergic mechanisms. Curiosity about other neuroactive

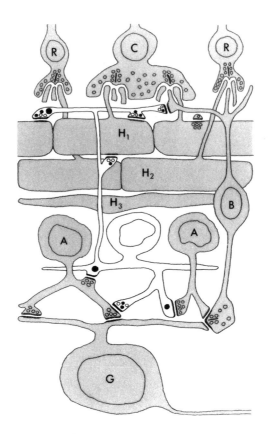

Fig. 3. Synaptic organization of the dopaminergic interplexiform cell in goldfish. The unshaded cell is the interplexiform cell. R, rods; C, cone; H_1, H_2, and H_3, horizontal cells; B, bipolar cell; A, amacrine cell; and G, ganglion cell. (From Dowling JE, Ehinger B. *Science* 1975;188:270–273. With permission.)

substances in the retina led us into studies of the amino acids as the principal excitatory and inhibitory neurotransmitters in the retina. Rick Lasater, Sam Wu, Mickey Ariel, Randy Glickman, Stuart Bloomfield, and Ido Perlman contributed here, as did Berndt Ehinger, who for many years paid us an annual visit. Dave Pepperberg and Stuart Lipton also continued work on photoreceptor adaptation, studying the effects of retinal, Ca^{2+}, and the cyclic nucleotides on these cells, while Geoff Gold, a physics graduate student at Harvard, carried out beautiful experiments, both anatomical and physiological, on the electrical coupling between photoreceptors.

Much of our work during the 1970s was physiological or anatomical and was carried out on fish retinas, both goldfish and skate. As the questions we were asking became more sophisticated, it became clear that we needed to know more about the molecules involved in synaptic transmission, particularly those involved in retinal neuromodulation. I was eligible for a sabbatical leave in 1978, my first at Harvard, and so I went to Cambridge, England for the year to work in Les Iversen's laboratory. I was awarded a Guggenheim Fellowship for the year and stayed at Churchill College where I was an Overseas Fellow. It was a marvelous year. I worked closely with Keith Watling, a young postdoctoral fellow in Iversen's laboratory, on the generation of cyclic AMP in the retina. Watling came to the other Cambridge to work in my laboratory in the early 1980s, so our collaboration continued for several years.

I had returned to Harvard in 1971 to become involved in undergraduate teaching. I was the only senior neurobiologist in our department at that time, and so in the spring of 1972 I initiated an introductory neurobiology course. Previously, faculty from the Neurobiology Department at Harvard Medical School had taught an upper level neurobiology course at the College, but I wanted to teach a more introductory course that would enable students in their sophomore year to be introduced to the field. The course was called Biology 25 and was equivalent in level to the Department's introductory cell, developmental, and molecular biology courses that students could take after introductory biology and chemistry courses. The course continues to this day, although it has changed somewhat as I will explain later. I was joined in teaching the course initially by Dave Hubel and Richard Sidman. Eventually, Dave retired from the course and then Dick, so for many years I taught it alone.

I also became more involved in administration at Harvard. I was Chair of the Department of Biology from 1975 to 1978 and elected to the Faculty Council in 1976. Henry Rosovsky, Dean of the Faculty of Arts and Sciences, asked if I would serve on the committee to revamp the General Education requirements at Harvard. From this committee came the Core Program which requires that all undergraduates take specially designed "Core" courses in fields outside of their area of specialty. I was concerned principally with the science part of the Core; all students not in a science concentration are required to this day to take two science courses before they graduate: one in the physical sciences and the other in the life sciences. I have team-taught two such courses for many years, first with Carroll Williams, a cell biologist and expert in insect hormones, and then with Howard Berg, a biophysicist interested in bacterial motility. In these courses, we have introduced non-science students to the exciting advances in molecular, cell, and neurobiology.

The 1980s: White Perch and Neuromodulation

It was becoming increasingly clear as our pharmacological experiments progressed that we needed a simpler system than the whole retina to understand how neuroactive substances were affecting neurons at the cell and molecular level. A few laboratories were beginning to isolate and culture retinal neurons, and this seemed to be a promising approach. We first isolated neurons, especially horizontal cells, from goldfish or carp retinas, but the results were often disappointing. Although the neurons would survive in culture for several days, they would usually round up, and it was difficult to distinguish subtypes of cells. Nevertheless, we were able to make a number of important observations with them. Rick Lasater, for example, showed that cultured horizontal cells respond selectively to L-glutamate and not to L-aspartate, providing some of the early evidence that the photoreceptor transmitter is L-glutamate. Rob Van Buskirk made partially purified carp horizontal cell preparations by velocity sedimentation procedures that enabled him and others in the laboratory to study the effects of dopamine, vasoactive intestinal peptide, and other substances on the generation of cyclic AMP in these cells. In Woods Hole, Lasater, Ripps, and I isolated skate retinal neurons and recorded from both horizontal and bipolar cells, but cultured skate horizontal cells, like carp horizontal cells, tended to round up in culture.

In the summer of 1981, I decided to spend my time at the MBL seeking a fish whose neurons would culture better. We had just bought a house on Oyster Pond, in Woods Hole, and this was our first summer on the pond. Our first weekend there, a friend of my wife was visiting with her 12-year-old son. He had a new fishing rod—a birthday gift—and wanted to try it. From the dock at the rear of the house, we soon found we could readily catch fish of 6–8 in. in length. I wasn't sure what they were, but catching them was great fun. On Monday, my first day in the lab, I decided to culture neurons from the retinas of these fish, now identified as white perch. I'll never forget my first look at the cultured neurons from the white perch— they were spectacular! I could, for example, identify four types of horizontal cells, and the cells maintained their shape for days to weeks (Fig. 4). I spent the rest of the summer trying other fish, but none worked as well as the white perch.

Needless to say, the white perch retina became the mainstay preparation in our laboratory for more than a decade. We would collect 200–300 each fall from Oyster Pond to use throughout the winter and spring. A number of important observations were made both in the 1980s and the early 1990s with isolated retinal neurons, as well as with the intact retina from the white perch. Rick Lasater and I showed that strong electrical coupling occurs between overlapping pairs of horizontal cells of the same morphological type, but not between overlapping pairs of cells of different morphological types, and that dopamine decreased the conductance of the electrical junctions of the coupled cells. Subsequently, Doug McMahon and Andy Knapp demonstrated that the reduced conductance induced by dopamine was the result mainly of a reduced open time of the gap junctional channels.

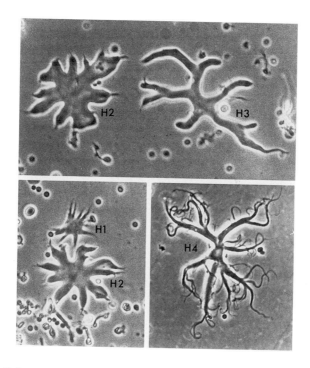

Fig. 4. Subtypes of horizontal cells observed in cultures of the white perch retina. The H_4 cell is connected exclusively to rods. The H_1, H_2, and H_3 cells are cone horizontal cells. (From Dowling JE, Pak MW, Lasater EM. *Brain Res* 1985;360:331–338. With permission.)

In the mid-1980s, it was generally believed that the principal effect of dopamine on horizontal cells was to modify the electrical coupling between adjacent cells. However, earlier Bill Hedden and then Stuart Mangel in our laboratory showed that dopamine reduced the responsiveness of horizontal cells to light in the intact fish retina when full-field illumination was used. This effect of dopamine cannot be explained by reduced coupling between cells, and so Andy Knapp looked to see if dopamine affected the horizontal cells' responsiveness to the photoreceptor transmitter, L-glutamate. He found that dopamine greatly enhances L-glutamate-gated conductances in cultured white perch horizontal cells, the first direct evidence for dopamine modulation of excitatory amino acid neurotransmission in the vertebrate central nervous system (CNS). Such modulation by dopamine has now been found in many parts of the CNS. Subsequently, Knapp and Karl Schmidt showed that dopamine exerts this effect on the glutamate channels by increasing the channel opening probability in response to a given concentration of agonist and also by increasing the duration of the channel open times somewhat. Emily Liman, at about the same time, showed that the enhancement of the excitatory amino acid currents in the horizontal cells was mediated via a cyclic AMP-dependent kinase (PKA).

The work of Mangel and, subsequently, of Xiong-Li Yang, Tina Tornqvist, and Bill Baldridge stimulated another line of research that continues to this day. Following prolonged dark adaptation, horizontal cell responses are suppressed, and light is needed to sensitize the cells. The extent of dark suppression of horizontal cells is influenced by the time of day. From these observations, Mangel in his own laboratory has demonstrated circadian clock regulation of horizontal cells and other retinal neurons. Dopamine is clearly involved in the circadian regulation of retinal neuronal responses, but the story is as yet incomplete. We do not yet understand very well the significance of dark suppression of horizontal cells, and the effects of dopamine on retinal cells are many and complex; indeed, effects of dopamine on every retinal cell type has been reported.

Two other studies from our laboratory utilizing the white perch retina deserve mention. Using cultured neurons, Haohua Qian discovered a novel GABA response from the rod (H_4) horizontal cells of the perch. This non-desensitizing, bicuculline-resistant GABA response was subsequently shown to be the result of activation of ligand-gated channels made up of rho (ρ) subunits. These ligand-gated channels have been called GABA$_c$ receptors and appear to play a particularly important role in the visual system. Isolation and cloning of the genes for the rho receptors in the white perch have now been accomplished by Qian, first working in our laboratory and later with Harris Ripps in Chicago. George Grant used slices of the white perch retina to study the generation of ON-bipolar responses in the white perch retina. For more than 30 years, it has been known that the ON-bipolar response generated by cones in fish is different from the ON-bipolar response generated by rods. The latter response has been shown to be linked to a metabotropic glutamate receptor and biochemical cascade that results in channel opening in the light, resulting in cell depolarization. But the cone ON-bipolar cells response is different; glutamate released in the dark directly hyperpolarizes the cell and the ON-light response results from relief of the hyperpolarization. Grant found that glutamate hyperpolarizes the bipolar cells by activating a glutamate transporter linked to a Cl^- channel. In the dark, Cl^- enters the bipolar cell, thus hyperpolarizing it. When the transporter is no longer activated by glutamate, i.e., in the light, and Cl^- no longer enters the cell, it depolarizes. This is a novel mechanism of generating a postsynaptic response, and it will be of interest to see if this mechanism occurs elsewhere in the brain. Kwoon Wong, a graduate student in the lab, is presently following up and extending Grant's work.

Teaching in both Bio 25 and the Core courses continued in the 1980s and, on an alternate year basis, I also led a graduate seminar. I was also drawn more into administration, both at Harvard and elsewhere. In 1980, Dean Rosovsky asked if I would serve as Associate Dean of the faculty to advise him on matters pertaining to the burgeoning biology activities at Harvard. I sat with a small group of Academic Deans, mainly over sandwich lunches in the Rosovsky office on Tuesdays, and we discussed faculty appointments, issues of the day, and new initiatives. It was an interesting experience of four years duration that convinced me that I did not want to go further in academic administration. I did accept in 1981 an administrative assignment as Master of Leverett House at Harvard that proved to be a delight. For the last three of their four years at Harvard, undergraduates live in 1 of the 12 residential units called Houses. They provide a small college atmosphere, having a dining hall, a library, music, theatre, and athletic facilities, and a staff of both academic and administrative personnel to provide advice, letters of recommendation for fellowships, graduate study, and so forth. Each House is led by a senior faculty member and his/her spouse, and they serve as Co-Masters. Judith and I served as Co-Masters of Leverett House for 17 years, until 1998.

Administrative activities outside of Harvard also began to take time. I was elected to the National Academy of Sciences in 1976 and shortly thereafter was asked to serve on the Assembly of Life Sciences, the oversight committee for life science, projects undertaken by the National Research Council at the request of the U.S. Government. I served two terms on the Assembly and then in the mid-1980s served as chair of the committee, then called the Commission of Life Sciences. I also served on the Council of the National Eye Institute, so for a few years I was going to Washington, D.C. once or twice a month. Again, I much enjoyed these experiences, but they also confirmed that I did not want to become a full-time administrator.

I was eligible for another sabbatical in the mid-1980s and decided to use the year to draw together in a book what had been learned about retinal mechanisms over the previous 25 years. I spent seven months in Okazaki, Japan, hosted by Ken Naka at the National Institute of Biology there. It was a memorable time. I wrote in the mornings and spent the afternoons working in the lab with Ken and his colleagues. The choice of Japan as a place to write the book was suggested by my wife Judith, who was becoming increasingly interested in the arts and culture of Japan. She was then in graduate school at Harvard, studying under Harvard's expert in Japanese art, John Rosenfield. She made many friends in Japan that year and brought back some wonderful objects to sell. That turned into a flourishing Asian Art Gallery, first in Cambridge and now in Boston.

I titled my book *The Retina: An Approachable Part of the Brain,* and it was well received. I found writing the book most enjoyable. So I then embarked on writing an introductory textbook on neuroscience, based on my course Biology 25. Called *Neurons and Networks,* it is now in a second edition. A trade book on neuroscience, *Creating Mind,* followed and was published in the late 1990s. It did not become a best seller, but did get some nice reviews.

1990s: Zebrafish, Genetics, and Development

Toward the end of the 1980s, the white perch in Oyster Pond began to disappear, and so we cast around for a substitute fish. The closest relative to the white perch readily obtainable was the hybrid striped bass. These fish, a cross between striped bass and white bass (essentially landlocked white perch), were being raised for commercial purposes, and a large fishery raising them operated in western Massachusetts. When we began to use them in our experiments, I was astonished at how consistent our results became. Why? The obvious answer was that these fish were all raised under identical conditions and were of the same age and of the same genetic stock. It seemed clear to me that carrying out experiments on animals whose genetics, age, and environment could be controlled was the way to go.

Zebrafish as an experimental model were introduced back in the 1970s by George Streisinger at the University of Oregon, but it was not until the early 1990s that a number of groups recognized their potential. We began to examine the eyes of zebrafish at that time, first looking at the effects of retinoic acid (RA) on retinal development. This work, carried out mainly by George Hyatt, Ellen Schmitt, and Nick Marsh-Armstrong, found that RA is critical for early retinal development, especially of the ventral retina. Too much RA at an early stage of eye development results in an apparent duplication of the retina, whereas block of RA synthesis early on results in an eye with no ventral retina (Fig. 5). These experiments were some of the first to show that the ventral and dorsal parts of the retina are quite distinct, especially with regard to development.

A collaboration with Wally Gilbert's groups at Harvard was undertaken to see if we could mutagenize zebrafish using insertional viral methods. In this we failed, but in the mid-1990s efficient methods for mutagenizing zebrafish chemically became available, and Sue Brockerhoff, Jim Hurley, and Jim Fadool began to look for functional and developmental mutations in zebrafish that were eye specific. To this end, Sue developed a behavioral test, based on the optokinetic reflex (OKR), that enabled her to examine visual function in 5-day-old larval fish. She eventually isolated a number of mutants that were completely or partially blind or even color blind. Jim Fadool isolated several developmental mutants, a number of which were worked on subsequently by newer members of the team, including Brian Link and Tristan Darland. A second behavioral test, based on the escape response, was developed by Lei Li, another postdoctoral fellow, that enables us to examine visual behavior in adult fish. Fish with slow inherited retinal degenerations were found with this test, which also permitted us to study dark adaptation and the effects of the circadian clock on visual responsiveness.

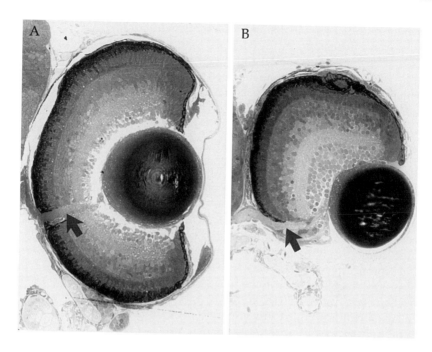

Fig. 5. The effect of blocking RA synthesis by citral on development of the zebrafish eye. In the citral-treated eye (B), no ventral retina is present. The control (A) is a 5-day-old eye. The arrow in each micrograph points to the optic nerve. (From Marsh-Armstrong N, et al. *Proc Natl Acad Sci USA* 1994;91:7286–7290. With permission.)

We continue to work on zebrafish and I remain confident that they have much to teach us. Not only can the ERG be recorded from the zebrafish eye, but slices of the zebrafish retina can be made, making it possible to examine the responses of single retinal neurons. The opportunity to carry out anatomical, physiological, and pharmacological studies on retinas from animals whose genetics can be manipulated presents a wonderful opportunity. But only time will tell us how far the zebrafish can take us.

As one becomes an elder statesman in a field, invitations to join boards pour in and, as I noted earlier, I say "yes" too often. Thus, in the 1990s I was on the board of over 20 organizations at one time or another, and some I still sit on. All were interesting, but they do take time. I also served as President of ARVO in the mid-1990s and on the Council of the National Academy of Sciences. I continued to teach my introductory neurobiology course and core courses and became involved in a new interdisciplinary program at Harvard called Mind, Brain, and Behavior (MBB). This interfaculty initiative was set up by the University President to inquire as to what impact modern neuroscience is having, or might have, on other academic disciplines. I was primarily involved in establishing an undergraduate program in MBB, and today we have five participating concentrations; Biology, Computer Science, History of Science, Philosophy, and Psychology. My introductory neurobiology course is taken by everyone in the program, and because of the diversity of students taking the course with varied backgrounds, it has broadened considerably and is now entitled "Behavioral Neuroscience."

Epilogue

At this point in my life, I remain active with a full laboratory and teaching schedule. I intend to stay full time for several more years, but then I think it is important to scale back and allow the resources I am using to go to younger scientists. I believe our research is still of high quality, but then I am reminded of something Henry Rosovsky said to me when I was Associate Dean at Harvard: "Whenever I talk to one of our scientists, he tells me he is doing the best work of his career. That can't be true!" There are several reasons why scientists believe the work they are presently doing is the best of their careers, but of course, Henry is correct.

What have I left out of this account? My indebtedness to many people, but especially to my wife of 28 years, Judith, who has been so supportive. Her only complaint has been that I do too many things, and she is almost certainly correct. It is the second marriage for both of us, and we have his, hers, and our own children—all of whom are now grown and doing their own thing (none in science, by the way). I have had an assistant at Harvard, Stephanie Levinson, for more than 25 years, and she has contributed to the laboratory and our research in innumerable ways. Many at Johns Hopkins and Harvard have served us well, and a number are mentioned in this piece. But there are others who have played important roles and they are not forgotten.

It has been a full and fortunate life, with many "ups" and very few "downs." Cajal said in *Recollections of My Life* that "The retina has always shown itself to be generous with me," and I feel exactly the same. Some 30 years ago, I rashly predicted that the retina would be pretty much understood in 25 years. I now recognize how wrong I was, but the field has come far, and I am delighted to have been part of this adventure. When I began, little was known of the mechanisms underlying light and dark adaptation and the relationship, if any, between visual pigment levels and visual sensitivity. Retinoic acid was unappreciated as a biologically important molecule. Retinal synapses and circuitry were virtually unknown, and the electrical responses of the retinal neurons were mysterious, save for those of the ganglion cells.

Today not only has much progress been made on these issues, but many others as well. The major excitatory and inhibitory neurotransmitters in the retina are identified, and we realize that the majority of neuroactive substances in the retina serve as neuromodulators—not initiating retinal activity but modifying it; in response to light conditions, time of day, and so forth. Clues as to how the retina develops from unspecified precursor cells have emerged and so on and so forth. Many investigators and laboratories have contributed to our present understanding of this tiny piece of the brain. Not that all of the mysteries are solved—far from it—but the progress made over the past 50 years is satisfying. I only wish I could be present in 2050 to hear then of the understanding of this "approachable part of the brain."

Selected Bibliography

Allwardt B, Lall AB, Brockerhoff SE, Dowling JE. Synapse formation is arrested in retinal photoreceptors of the zebrafish *nrc* mutant. *J Neurosci* 2001;21:2330–2342.

Armett-Kibel C, Meinertzhagen IA, Dowling JE. Cellular and synaptic organization in the lamina of the dragonfly *Sympetrum rubicundulum. Proc R Soc Lond Ser B* 1977;196:385–413.

Boycott BB, Dowling JE. Organization of the primate retina: Light microscopy. *Philos Trans R Soc Lond Ser B* 1969;255:109–184.

Boycott BB, Dowling JE, Fisher SK, Kolb H, Laties AM. Interplexiform cells of the mammalian retina and their comparison with catecholamine-containing retinal cells. *Proc R Soc Lond Ser B* 1975;191:353–368.

Brockerhoff SE, Hurley JB, Janssen-Bienhold U, Neuhauss SC, Driever W, Dowling JE. A behavioral screen for isolating zebrafish mutants with visual system defects. *Proc Natl Acad Sci USA* 1995;92:10545–10549.

Brockerhoff SE, Hurley JB, Niemi GA, Dowling JE. A new form of inherited red-blindness in zebrafish. *J Neurosci* 1997;17:4236–4242.

Chappell RL, Dowling JE. Neural organization of the ocellus of the dragonfly. I. Intracellular electrical activity. *J Gen Physiol* 1972;60:121–147.

Darland T, Dowling JE. Behavioral screening for cocaine sensitivity in mutagenized zebrafish. *Proc Natl Acad Sci USA* 2001;8:11691–11696.

Dowling JE. Chemistry of visual adaptation in the rat. *Nature* 1960;188:114–118.

Dowling JE. Neural and photochemical mechanisms of visual adaptation in the rat. *J Gen Physiol* 1963;46:1287–1301.

Dowling JE. Foveal receptors of the monkey retina: Fine structure. *Science* 1965; 147:57–59.

Dowling JE. Discrete potentials in the dark-adapted eye of *Limulus. Nature* 1968;217:28–31.

Dowling JE. Synaptic organization of the frog retina: An electron microscopic analysis comparing the retinas of frogs and primates. *Proc R Soc Lond Ser B* 1968b; 170:205–228.

Dowling JE. Organization of vertebrate retinas. Friedenwald Lecture. *Invest Ophthal Vis Sci* 1970;9:655–680.

Dowling JE, Boycott BB. Neural connections of the retina: Fine structure of the inner plexiform layer. *Cold Spring Harbor Symp Quant Biol* 1965;30:393–402.

Dowling JE, Boycott BB. Organization of the primate retina: Electron microscopy. *Proc R Soc Lond Ser B* 1966;166:80–111.

Dowling JE, Chappell RL. Neural organization of the dragonfly ocellus. II. Synaptic structure. *J Gen Physiol* 1972;60:148–165.

Dowling JE, Cowan WM. An electron microscope study of normal and degenerating centrifugal fiber terminals in the pigeon retina. *Zeitsch Zellforsch* 1966;71: 14–28.

Dowling JE, Ehinger B. Synaptic organization of the amine-containing interplexiform cells of the goldfish and *Cebus* monkey retinas. *Science* 1975;188:270–273.

Dowling JE, Ehinger B. The interplexiform cell system. I. Synapses of the dopaminergic neurons of the goldfish retina. *Proc R Soc Lond Ser B* 1978;201:7–26.

Dowling JE, Gibbons IR. The fine structure of the pigment epithelium in the albino rat. *J Cell Biol* 1962;14:459–474.

Dowling JE, Hubbard R. Effects of brilliant flashes on light and dark adaptation. *Nature* 1963;199:972–975.

Dowling JE, Pak MW, Lasater EM. White perch horizontal cells in culture: Methods, morphology and process growth. *Brain Res* 1985;360:331–338.

Dowling JE, Ripps H. Visual adaptation in the retina of the skate. *J Gen Physiol* 1970;56:491–520.

Dowling JE, Ripps H. S-potentials in the skate retina. Intracellular recordings during light and dark adaptation. *J Gen Physiol* 1971;58:163–189.

Dowling JE, Ripps H. Adaptation in skate photoreceptors. *J Gen Physiol* 1972;60: 698–719.

Dowling JE, Ripps H. Effect of magnesium on horizontal cell activity in the skate retina. *Nature* 1973;242:101–103.

Dowling JE, Sidman RL. Inherited retinal dystrophy in the rat. *J Cell Biol* 1962;14:73–109.

Dowling JE, Wald G. Vitamin A deficiency and night blindness. *Proc Natl Acad Sci USA* 1958;44:648–661.

Dowling JE, Wald G. The biological function of vitamin A acid. *Proc Natl Acad Sci USA* 1960;46:587–608.

Dowling JE, Watling KJ. Dopaminergic mechanisms in the teleost retina. II. Factors affecting the accumulation of cyclic AMP in pieces of intact carp retina. *J Neurochem* 1981;36(2):569–579.

Dowling JE, Werblin FS. Organization of retina of the mudpuppy, *Necturus maculosus*: I. Synaptic structure. *J Neurophysiol* 1969;255:315–338.

Ehinger B, Otterson OP, Storm-Mathisen J, Dowling JE. Bipolar cells in the turtle retina are strongly immunoreactive for glutamate, *Proc Natl Acad Sci USA* 1988;85:8321–8325.

Fadool JM, Brockerhoff SE, Hyatt GA, Dowling JE. Mutations affecting eye morphology in the developing zebrafish (*Danio rerio*). *Dev Genet* 1997;20:288–295.

Fain GL, Dowling JE. Intracellular recordings from single rods and cones in the mudpuppy retina. *Science* 1973;180:1178–1181.

Frank RN, Dowling, JE. Rhodopsin photoproducts: Effects on electroretinogram sensitivity in isolated perfused rat retina. *Science* 1968;161:487–489.

Gold GH, Dowling JE. Photoreceptor coupling in the retina of the toad *Bufo marinus*. I. Anatomy. *J Neurophysiol* 1079;42:292–310.

Grant G, Dowling JE. A glutamate-activated chloride current in cone driven ON-bipolar cells of the white perch retina. *J Neurosci* 1995;15:3852–3862.

Grant G, Dowling JE. On bipolar cell responses in the teleost retina are generated by two distinct mechanisms. *J Neurophysiol* 1996;76:3842–3849.

Green DG, Dowling JE, Siegel IM, Ripps H. Retinal mechanisms of visual adaptation in the skate. *J Gen Physiol* 1975;65:483–502.

Hedden WL, Dowling JE. The interplexiform cell system. II. Effects of dopamine on goldfish retinal neurons. *Proc R Soc Lond Ser B* 1978;201:27–55.

Hubbard R, Dowling JE. Formation and utilization of 11-cis vitamin A by the eye tissues during light and dark adaptation. *Nature* 1962;193:341–343.

Hyatt GA, Schmitt EA, Fadool JM, Dowling JE. Retinoic acid alters photoreceptor development *in vivo*. *Proc Natl Acad Sci USA* 1996;93:13298–13303.

Hyatt GA, Schmitt EA, Marsh-Armstrong NR, Dowling JE. Retinoic acid-induced duplication of the zebrafish retina. *Proc Natl Acad Sci USA* 1992;89:8293–8297.

Hyatt GA, Schmitt EA, Marsh-Armstrong N, McCaffery P, Dräger U, Dowling JE. Retinoic acid establishes ventral retinal characteristics. *Development* 1996;122:195–204.

Kleinschmidt J, Dowling JE. Intracellular recordings from Gecko photoreceptors during light and dark adaptation. *J Gen Physiol* 1975;66:617–648.

Knapp AG, Dowling JE. Dopamine enhances excitatory amino acid-gated conductances in cultured retinal horizontal cells. *Nature* 1987;325:437–439.

Knapp AG, Schmidt KF, Dowling JE. Dopamine modulates the kinetics of ion channels gated by excitatory amino acids in retinal horizontal cells. *Proc Natl Acad Sci USA* 1990;87:767–771.

Kolb H, Boycott BB, Dowling JE. A second type of midget bipolar cell in the primate retina. *Phil Trans R Soc Lond Ser B* 1969;255:176–184.

Lasater EM, Dowling JE. Carp horizontal cells in culture respond selectively to L-glutamate and its agonists. *Proc Natl Acad Sci USA* 1982;79:936–940.

Lasater EM, Dowling JE. Dopamine decreases the conductance of the electrical junctions between cultured retina horizontal cells. *Proc Natl Acad Sci USA* 1989;82:3025–3029.

Lasater EM, Dowling JE, Ripps H. Pharmacological properties of isolated horizontal and bipolar cells from the skate retina. *J Neurosci* 1984;4:1966–1975.

Lasater EM, Watling KJ, Dowling JE. Vasoactive intestinal peptide induces cAMP accumulation and membrane potential changes in isolated carp horizontal cells. *Science* 1983;221:1070–1072.

Li L, Dowling JE. A dominant form of inherited retinal degeneration caused by a non-photoreceptor cell-specific mutation. *Proc Natl Acad Sci USA* 1997;94:11645–11650.

Li L, Dowling JE. Disruption of the olfactoretinal centrifugal pathway may relate to the visual system defect in *night blindness b* mutant zebrafish. *J Neurosci* 2000;20:1883–1892.

Link BA, Fadool JM, Malicki J, Dowling JE. The zebrafish *young* mutation acts non-cell autonomously to uncouple differentiation from specifications for all retinal cells. *Development* 2000;127:2177–2188.

Lipton SA, Rasmussen H, Dowling JE. Electrical and adaptive properties of rod photoreceptors in *Bufo marinus*. II. Effects of cyclic nucleotides and prostaglandins. *J Gen Physiol* 1977;70:771–791.

Mangel SC, Dowling JE. Responsiveness and receptive field size of carp horizontal cells are reduced by prolonged darkness and dopamine. *Science* 1985;229:1107–1109.

Marsh-Armstrong N, McCaffery P, Gilbert W, Dowling JE, Dräger UC. Retinoic acid is necessary for development of the ventral retina in zebrafish. *Proc Natl Acad Sci USA* 1994;91:7286–7290.

McMahon DG, Knapp AG, Dowling JE. Horizontal cell gap junctions: Single-channel conductance and modulation by dopamine. *Proc Natl Acad Sci USA* 1989;86:7639–7643.

Miller RF, Dowling JE. Intracellular responses of the Müller (glial) cells of mudpuppy retina: Their relation to the b-wave of the electroretinogram. *J Neurophysiol* 1970;33:323–341.

Pepperberg D, Lurie M, Brown PK, Dowling JE. Visual adaptation: Effects of externally applied retinal on the light-adapted, isolated skate retina. *Science* 1976;91:394–396.

Peterson RT, Link BA, Dowling JE, Schreiber SL. Small molecule developmental screens reveal the logic and timing of vertebrate development. *Proc Natl Acad Sci USA* 2000;97:12965–12969.

Pu GA, Dowling JE. Anatomical and physiological characteristics of the pineal photoreceptor cell in the larval lamprey, *Petromycon marina*. *J Neurophysiol* 1981;46:1018–1038.

Qian H, Dowling JE. Novel GABA responses from rod-driven retinal horizontal cells. *Nature* 1993;361:162–164.

Rodrigues P, Dowling JE. Dopamine induce neurite retraction in retinal horizontal cells via diacylglycerol and protein kinase C. *Proc Natl Acad Sci USA* 1990;87:9693–9697.

Sakai H, Naka K-I, Dowling JE. Ganglion cell dendrites are presynaptic in the catfish retina. *Nature* 1986;319:495–497.

Schmitt EA, Dowling JE. Early retinal development in the zebrafish, *Danio rerio*. A light- and electron-microscopical analysis. *J Comp Neurol* 1999;404:515–536.

Umino O, Dowling JE. Dopamine release from interplexiform cells in the retina: Effects of GnRH, FMRFamide, bicuculline and enkephalin on horizontal cell activity. *J Neurosci* 1991;11:3034–3045.

Van Buskirk R, Dowling JE. Isolated horizontal cells from carp retina demonstrate dopamine-dependent accumulation of cyclic AMP. *Proc Natl Acad Sci USA* 1981;78:7825–7829.

Watling KJ, Dowling JE. Dopaminergic mechanisms in the teleost retina. I. Dopamine-sensitive adenylate cyclase in the homogenates of carp retina: Effects of agonists, antagonists and ergots. *J Neurochem* 1981;36(2):559–569.

Watling KJ, Dowling JE, Iversen LL. Dopamine receptors in the retina may all be linked to adenylate cyclase. *Nature* 1979;281:578–580.

Weinstein GW, Hobson RR, Dowling JE. Light and dark adaptation in the isolated rat retina. *Nature* 1967;215:134–138.

Werblin FS, Dowling JE. Organization of the retina of the mudpuppy, *Necturus maculosus*. II. Intracellular recording. *J Neurophysiol* 1969;255:339–355.

West RW, Dowling JE. Synapses onto different morphological types of retina ganglion cells. *Science* 1972;178:510–512.

Yang X-L, Tornqvist K, Dowling JE. Modulation of cone horizontal cell activity in the teleost fish retina. II. Role of interplexiform cells and dopamine in regulating light responsiveness. *J Neurosci* 1988;8:2268–2278.

Zucker CL, Dowling JE. Centrifugal fibers synapse on interplexiform cells in teleost retina. *Nature* 1987;330:166–168.

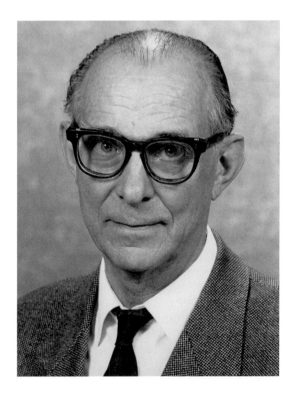

Oleh Hornykiewicz

BORN:

Sykhiw (formerly Poland, now Ukraine)
November 17, 1926

EDUCATION:

University of Vienna, M.D. (1951)

APPOINTMENTS:

Department of Pharmacology, University of Vienna (1951)
Professor of Pharmacology, University of Toronto (1968)
Professor of Biochemical Pharmacology, University of
Vienna (1976)
Professor Emeritus, University of Toronto (1992)
Professor Emeritus, University of Vienna (1995)

HONORS AND AWARDS (SELECTED):

Höchst Foundation Award, University of Vienna (1965)
Gold Medal, Canadian Parkinson's Disease Association
(1970)
Gardner Foundation Award, Canada (1972)
Ludwig Schunk Prize, Justus Liebig University, Germany
(1974)
Wolf Prize, Israel (1979)
Lifetime Achievement Award, Clark Institute of
Psychiatry, Canada (1992)
Ludwig Wittgenstein Prize, Austria (1993)
Kardinal-Innitzer Prize, Austria (1997)
Billroth-Medaille, Gesellschaft der Ärzte in Wein,
Austria (2001)

*Oleh Hornykiewicz is best known for his discovery of the dopamine deficit in
the brain of patients with Parkinson's disease and the initiation of the
L-dopa treatment of this disorder. His chemical work in the freshly frozen
autopsied human brain opened a new field of neuroscience research aimed
directly at finding the neurotransmitter-related biochemical causes as well
as rational treatments of neurological and psychiatric brain disorders.*

Oleh Hornykiewicz

Some Thoughts on Memories

We all are slaves to our memories. Writing an autobiography has been rightly seen as a way of freeing oneself of the grip of the remembered past. In reality, committing memories, the good and the bad, to paper rarely achieves that goal. Too often is the written record a tangle of "fact and fiction." True, many, perhaps all, events experienced in the past are deposited in our brain as accurate, lifelike pictures and episodes. However, only in some rare "moments of vision" are we able to draw on them: what we usually get when "calling to mind" the past are only various fragments of the real events. As a writer of your autobiography, you find yourself in the somewhat bizarre position of acting the part of interpreter of your own past. That is how our memories make the task of producing a useful, or meaningful (or true?), personal record so arduous a labor. We are indeed slaves to our memories. And yet, are not our memories said to be our second, possibly our only real, life?

Be that as it may, about six years ago, when Larry Squire—then as now Editor-in-Chief of the series *The History of Neuroscience in Autobiography*— asked me to contribute to Volume 2, I agreed, but, full of doubts, could not bring myself to write a single line. Asked a year or so ago to try my hand at it again, the sense of obligation, together with a touch of vanity, got the better of me, and here I find myself writing, foolishly, what I consider to be bits and pieces of my remembered past.

My Birthplace Sykhiv (Sichów)

All things considered, I have had a simple, uncomplicated life. Born on November 17, 1926, as the youngest of three boys into a fourth-generation family of Catholic priests (Eastern-[Byzantine]Rite Ukrainian Catholic; married priesthood), I spent my early childhood in a rural environment. Sichów, my birthplace (now Sykhiv), was a tiny community on the outskirts of Lwów (now Lviv), the capital of the then southeastern province of Poland, an area which until the end of World War I was a part of the Austrian Hapsburg Monarchy, known as eastern Galicia; in September 1939, Lwów became part of the Soviet Union and is now the westernmost provincial capital of the independent state of the Ukraine. In Sykhiv, my father served the spiritual and sacramental needs of little more than a few dozen Ukrainian Catholic families; his main professional activities as youth educator were in Lviv, where he taught Catholic doctrine (including church history and philosophy) in high schools (gymnasia) and teachers' colleges. My mother, the descendant of an old and by then impoverished landed gentry, managed the (very modest) parochial economy and looked after the social and educational needs and well-being of the women folk and their young.

The picture of what for me represents my birthplace stands out clearly and distinctly in my mind—the parochial house, built by my father, where I was born; close by, surrounded by high fir trees, the little, nearly 300-year-old wooden church of The Holy Trinity, where I was baptized; the shady orchard with patches of pale-blue forget-me-nots in the tall, freely growing grass around the plum, pear, and apple trees; the large, sunny rose and flower garden behind the parish house, set up and lovingly cared for by my mother; and, separated from the fenced-in flower garden by a narrow dirt road, the small, but never still railroad station. All these were my early playgrounds, the world of my childhood.

Lviv (Lwów)

Moving to Lviv (in 1933 or 1934, at about the time of my reaching school age) was no shock to me. The bustling activity of the "big city" (about 200,000 inhabitants at that time) immediately captivated me, converting me forever into a confirmed city dweller. I liked school, and I was lucky to have had excellent teachers (in the Markian Shashkevych School). Many years later, when studying medicine in Vienna, I was once more to recognize how important good teachers were for one's (good) choices in life.

With warm feelings, I recall the long summer vacations, always spent in the country: the beauty of the mountains; the broad, inviting forms of the foothills; the wheat fields in the endless plains; the large, festive family gatherings; merriment with the innumerable cousins—I once counted more than 40, first degree, of them. Despite these holiday pleasures, I liked coming back to the busy city. Lwów of that time remains in my memory a cheerful place, full of joy of life and gaiety. The world as I saw it appeared to me a good place in which to be. Of course, I could not help noticing the homeless, the large number of street beggars, and the emaciated street acrobats, often using for their acrobatic stunts children my age and younger. Today, I would easily recognize behind all this the poverty, the misery and the despair. At that time, for me—the not-yet-teenager—all this was part of the world as it was, a world to be explored and looked at in wonder.

World War II, Part One (Lviv)

On September 1, 1939, the happy, carefree period of my childhood came abruptly to an end with the outbreak of the war, triggered by the German

attack on Poland. When after less than three weeks Poland surrendered
to Germany, the non-aggression pact concluded a few weeks earlier (in
August 1939) between Hitler and Stalin came into effect, and the Soviet
army entered Lviv. Overnight, the gay, light-hearted city was transformed
into a gloomy and desolate place: denunciations; arrests; dark rumors; a
shortage of food; and endless political meetings (also for us school children),
invariably ending with "spontaneous" messages of gratitude to Comrade
Stalin. Quite desperate was the situation of the officers of the Polish army
caught between two merciless enemies. I remember how one of them, our
next-door neighbor (major of artillery), had been desparately beseeching my
father—himself in a state of despair—to advise him what to do with himself
and his family. Hardly 6 months later, more than 4000 Polish officers would
be murdered at Katyn by Stalin's secret police. Was our neighbour one of
them? We never heard of him, of his wife, or their daughter (Halka; about
my age) again.

My father immediately lost his job and faced the prospect of vanishing,
like many members of the intelligentsia and the clergy, in Stalin's dungeons
or forced labor camps. We only were saved from that fate by my mother
having Austrian ancestors. This entitled us to leave (hand luggage only!) the
by now hermetically sealed off country, with Vienna as our final destination
(where my father's brother, our dearest uncle Myron, lived permanently).

Friends, home, hard-earned savings and possessions, and personal property and belongings, all that was left behind, never to be recovered. Not a
bad lesson for a boy, just turned 13, about the vanity and futility of striving
after security and material possessions.

World War II, Part Two (Vienna)

We arrived in Vienna, which (like the rest of Austria) was already part of
Hitler's Germany, in February 1940. Six months later, I started school again
after overcoming the initial obstacle posed by my complete ignorance of
the German language (which despite the Austrian ancestry raised doubt
about my ethnic "suitability") and my lung tuberculosis which I and my
elder brother had contracted in one of the "resettlement camps" we had
been staying at for months before we were allowed to go to Vienna. (As
late as 1967, when I moved to Canada, I was required to go, for the first
three years, to medical checkups [chest X-ray; sputum] at Toronto's Gage
[Environmental Health] Institute.)

After quickly getting a grasp of the German language, I plunged head
over heels into the world of (printed) knowledge, literature, and poetry, now
all wide open to me. But knowledge of German also acquainted me with
Hitler's political system and ideology; the hate propaganda against political,
ethnic, and religious "enemies"; the absolute control of all media; no free
speech; widespread fear of police informers and overzealous neighbors; and

again and again, people disappearing in the concentration camps. To me, now in my most susceptible and sensitive years, to watch the agony and despair of the Jewish population was deeply disturbing: to see their personal debasement, their defencelessness against being taken away, crammed in open trucks, to their final fate, the concentration camps. My father and my mother were appalled at what they saw and showed it to us, their children, unmistakably.

To my great relief, I found that school was mainly concerned with imparting knowledge rather than propagating Nazi ideology. In this, my school (the former "Sperlgasse"-Realgymnasium Wien II) may have been an exception. Before Hitler occupied Austria, the majority of pupils in this school had been Jewish (with Sigmund Freud, at one time, being one of them). By 1940, the Jewish pupils were gone, but their non-Jewish classmates and several moderate teachers had remained, and with them, the multi-ethnic spirit had also stayed. Apart from lessons on (ridiculously distorted) European history (hostile to Austria and the Hapsburgs), which could not be taken seriously, the most openly ideological subject taught was the new "race biology," presented to us with all the dangerous, because so scientific "genetic evidence" (and selected heritable diseases as examples); the implication of all this being that the "health and purity of the (Germanic) race" could be best preserved by eliminating all those carrying the "bad" and the "inferior" genes. When I see the present-day contagious enthusiasm for all research having to do with "the genes," and when I stop and think of the possibility of the "genetic mentality" coming, in whatever guise, to life again, I wonder and I worry.

As the eastern front began to crumble, huge crowds of refugees from the east poured into Vienna, adding to the many problems in the city. In 1943 and 1944, the bombing of Vienna began (Americans coming at daytime, British by night). This brought the until then distant war and the mountains of dead it had already cost right to my doorstep. Soon, our school was hit and we had to move to another school (which proved virulently Nazi), only to be bombed out of there again. Destruction and ruins were everywhere; I watched, stupefied, the Vienna State Opera House burn for two days and two nights. Much time was spent in (mostly inadequate) air-raid shelters which, when hit, turned into mass graves. In the end, death was everywhere, affecting practically every family, appearing more normal than staying alive. Paradoxically, it was the awareness of the "collective misery" that provided some alleviation of the personal grief—the only way one could keep functioning during that time. (To me, though, the loss of my elder brother three months after being sent, not yet 19 years old, to the eastern front has remained an open wound to this day.)

On April 5, 1945, the Soviet forces reached the outskirts of Vienna. The ensuing 9 days of fierce street fighting left nearly 40,000 dead soldiers (Soviet plus German) scattered in the streets and surrounds of the city. But then, the nightmare of the Hitler regime was over, and we could breathe freely again and leave the darkness of the subterranean shelters; "it was from there that we emerged/to see—again—the stars" (Dante, 1980). During that period, on the eve of the final act, I concluded my high school education.

Horas Non Numero Nisi Serenas

My growing up in the shadow of World War II raises the question: What became of my youth, of what is said to be the "best years" of our life? Is it possible for me to recall anything of that time besides its horrors? Strange as it sounds, I find in my memory of that time many happy moments, which I do not think could be dismissed as a subconscious attempt at escaping from reality. I well remember the exhilaration of reading, in the original tongue, again and again the poetry of Schiller and Hölderlin and Goethe's *Faust*, his *Wilhelm Meister*, and his *Wahlverwandtschaften*. To my mind come the evenings in the Vienna State Opera that step by step made me understand and love music—ever since my steady companion (along with poetry). I recall my fascination with Vienna's historical past and the thrill of the first friendships. Also, there was the experience of nature, so plentiful around Vienna. With surprise I noticed how unmoved nature remained in the face of the war, continuing to give freely of her attractions. I can see with my mind's eye in all intensity scenes such as lying on sunny summer days in the tall grass on the banks of the river Danube, daydreaming while watching the tug boats pass by, struggling up-river, smoothly gliding down or sitting on the slopes of the Wienerwald, so feminine in their soft contours, lost in thought, taking in the picture of the beautiful city below, resting there as in the hollow of one's hand. What a wondrous thing our memory is! It registers, as Penfield (1975) tells us, every detail of our past experiences, yet when left to itself, it prefers—like the sundial—to count the sunny moments only.

Medical Studies

Initially, the political uncertainty at the end of the war, the desperate food situation (one of our best teachers, in German and Latin, starved during those months literally to death in his one-room flat near Vienna), and the continuous harassment by the Soviet authorities, so well described by Graham Green (1971) in his story *The Third Man*, produced a rather gloomy after-war atmosphere. But gradually, the positive influence of the newly gained freedom made itself felt and some aspects of normal life could be resumed.

It was in this atmosphere of the just beginning recovery from the total ruin and destruction that I enrolled, in October 1945, as a student of medicine at the University of Vienna. Before being admitted, however, we had to do something like two weeks of "rubble shovelling" (to help clean up

Vienna's ruins) and pass a medical checkup. When I stepped on the scales in the examining room, my weight was, to the doctor's alarm, not more than 48 kg (ca. 106 lb). Instantly, they gave me (for the whole term) a ticket for a free daily bowl of soup (provided for by the American Quakers).

My choice of "Medicine" was greatly influenced by my eldest brother who, seven years my senior, was already a medical doctor. Since I affectionately admired him, nothing appeared to me more desirable than being like him. Attending the lecture courses turned out to be no simple matter. Like the rest of Vienna, the medical buildings and lecture theatres were half in ruins, and the few intact ones were hopelessly overcrowded. There was a shortage of lab space and teaching staff. Everyone was trying to get his "Dr.med." (M.D.) as fast as possible, to be among the first to compete for the few paid internship positions in the city hospitals. The whole atmosphere—not necessarily conducive to good schooling—was that of a "struggle for the survival of the quickest."

Three Teachers

Three teachers in my medical years decisively influenced my research career. Friedrich Wessely, replacing the (for political reasons) dismissed professor of "Chemistry for Medical Students," was our teacher on that subject. A full-blooded, high-calibre organic chemist and Head of the University's Organic Chemistry laboratories, Wessely gained our affection by his uncompromising commitment to teaching. When at the end of the first winter term he noticed that we had understood next to nothing of his high-level chemistry, he gave us during the bitterly cold February 1946 term break an extra crash course, making us scribble on the blackboard all sorts of formulas, equations, and chemical reactions—with numb fingers, winter coats on, and all this for a full four weeks in the totally unheated lecture theatre.

Friedrich Ehmann was my teacher in neuroanatomy and brain development. Thin, kyphoscoliotic, short of breath, and cyanotic with heart disease, he was an example of competence, knowledge, and dedication. Exact and crystal clear, his lectures could have gone to print just as they were delivered. His standing phrase introducing important summary statements and conclusions, "la-dies-and-gentle-men-eve-ry-word-is-im-por-tant," became proverbial with us.

Finally, there was Franz von Brücke, our teacher in pharmacology and toxicology. Combining wide knowledge in both experimental medicine and biology with personal research experience and a special gift for speech, Brücke was able to communicate as no one else the excitement of pharmacological research and its relevance for the patient. With his classical education, ranging from ancient languages to literature to arts to philosophy, and his familiarity with the history of medicine, he succeeded in making us realize how much medicine was part of the great human cultural endeavor, not just a scientific guest. Who could not be fascinated by his reading to us from Homer's *Odyssey* the lines pertaining to the use of opium ("one of the drugs given to the daughter of Zeus [Helen] by an Egyptian woman") for the purpose of alleviating mental suffering (Homer, 1991).

Vienna's Pharmacology, Part One

After obtaining my degree in medicine in July 1951, I immediately joined the Pharmacological Institute of the University of Vienna. It was for me an easy decision because the Head of that Institute was no other than Professor Franz von Brücke, my much admired teacher in pharmacology. For the first 10 months, though, I alternated between working from 3:00 PM to late at night in pharmacology as a "voluntary research assistant without salary" and serving from 7:00 AM to 2:00 PM as a "temporary intern" in the Rudolfs-Hospital. The clinical work earned me something like $20 a month, which enabled me, at last, to go now and then to a café (coffee house) and twice a month on standing room or cheap seats to an opera or concert.

A Good Place to Visit

From Brücke's lectures, I already had an idea about the great tradition of the Institute, in its modern form established by Hans Horst Meyer, one of the internationally leading pharmacologists at the beginning of the last century. Thus, I was aware that Meyer's collaborators in this Institute included names to be found in every encyclopedia, such as George H. Whipple, Cornelius Heymans, Carl Cori, Otto Loewi, and Alfred Frölilich. In the course of the 16 years I spent in that Institute, practically all prominent pharmacologists and physiologists of the time stopped in Vienna to visit our laboratories. I well remember Ernst Pick, Hans Heller, (Sir) Henry Dale, Carl Cori, Hans Molitor, Guiseppe Moruzzi, Otto Loewi, Wilhelm Feldberg, Cornelius Heymans, Stephen Kuffler, Hermann Blaschko, (Sir) John Gaddum, Harold Burn, Klaus Unna, Julius Axelrod, David Nachmansohn, and Henry Barcroft—the list could be continued *ad libitum*.

A regular visitor was Professor Ulf von Euler, the physiologist at Stockholm's Karolinska Institute, who had relatives in Vienna (of the same name). (I also remember the visit of his famous father, Hans von Euler-Chelpin, already in his 90s, and his wife, Baroness Uggles, Ulf's step-mother). On his visits, Ulf von Euler used to take friendly interest in my dopamine/Parkinson findings, ending the conversations—as many others in later years—with the remark: "Your discoveries should be recognized." I have always wondered what he meant by that.

A Good Place to Work

The great number of prominent visitors from around the world was not surprising considering the research that was being carried out in our laboratories. Practically all important branches of pharmacology were represented: heart and kidney; motor end plate, development of new muscle relaxants; hormone research; autonomic, especially catecholamine, and CNS pharmacology; drug metabolism and drug development (especially noteworthy were the studies on new broncholytics, using the guinea pig bronchospasm method, which became famous in connection with the discovery, made in our institute [Heribert Konzett, Richard Rössler], of the broncholytic activity of isoprenaline, furnishing the basis for Raymond Ahlquist's classification of adrenoceptors in alpha and beta type); EEG recordings and single cell recordings in the brain of awake rabbits; heart–lung preparations; and, last but not least, the application of the technique of sympathetic denervation of various organs and tissues. When, in 1961, Georg Hertting (from our Institute, later Head of Pharmacology at the Freiburg University, Germany) applied the latter method in Axelrod's lab in Bethesda, it provided the first and definitive proof of the presynaptic "re-uptake" of synaptically released noradrenaline (Hertting and Axelrod, 1961). This discovery fundamentally changed our concepts of synaptic neurotransmitter dynamics.

The Voice of a Dissenter

For young people like me, the prominent visitors, the high activity of the many research groups, and the atmosphere filled with ideas were greatly stimulating, giving rise to high motivation and enthusiasm for research. In the course of time, I found, however, one strong dissenter from my positive view of Vienna's pharmacology of the time. This was at a reception given by "Pergamon's" Captain Maxwell during the 1975 International Pharmacology Congress in Helsinki, at which also von Euler's pharmacological colleague at the Karolinska, known for his influence with the Nobel committee in physiology and medicine, was present. When I introduced myself to him, he greeted me with the words: "Vienna pharmacology?—a bad institution, no good research out of there." I thought this a somewhat subjective way of "evaluating" my former (or any other) institution, wondering about the reason behind the unusual choice of words for that wholesale stricture. But then, this episode allowed me to catch a (first) glimpse of the human factor even high-profile institutions and committees are burdened with.

My First Laboratory Work

I was introduced to experimental work by Adolf Lindner, Brücke's most senior assistant. Lindner was a friendly, fatherly person, good-humoured and open to relaxed conversations. He was a skillful experimentalist, and he

had a particularly inventive mind, holding many patents for novel therapeutic agents and procedures. Lindner's method of testing the aptitude of
newcomers was to give them, without further help or comment, J.H. Burn's
textbook (in English!) on *Biological Standardization* and let them chew on
it (especially its statistics part). Many beginners would sooner than later
quietly leave the lab, never to be seen again. It was on Lindner's advice that,
years later, I applied for a British Council Scholarship that brought me to
Oxford.

My first experimental work (together with the unforgettable Gustav
Niebauer, later Head of Dermatology at Vienna's University) was on the
enzymatic activity of human plasma, which we found to oxidize many
polyphenols, including substances of physiological interest, such as dopa
and the catecholamines formed from it. We termed this activity polyphenol
oxidase and suggested that it contained copper as its prosthetic group. It soon
turned out that our enzymatic activity was identical to the laccase activity
of ceruloplasmin which Holmberg and Laurell had previously isolated from
pig plasma. Important for my later work with the human brain and its diseases was a study I did together with the neurologists Heimo Gastagger and
Helmut Tschabitscher on our copper-containing plasma enzyme in patients
with Wilson's disease, a well-known disorder of copper metabolism with
(hepato-lenticular) degeneration of the basal ganglia. In this disorder the
polyphenol oxidase activity in the patients' plasma was low (like the levels of ceruloplasmin, as had earlier been shown by Scheinberg and Gitlin).
Thus, it came about that, right in my first postdoctoral work, the influence
of all three of my favorite teachers had made itself felt: Franz von Brücke
(pharmacology, where I worked), Friedrich Wessely (my bent for chemical
problems), and Friedrich Ehmann (my feeling at home in the human brain).
Moreover, right in the beginning of my experimental research career, I came
directly in touch with a biochemical problem in a basal ganglia disease. Was
it only chance that, years later, this study proved a very useful introduction
to my work on dopamine in Parkinson's disease brain?

The Oxford Interlude

Oxford Pharmacology

The 16 years of my stay in Vienna's Pharmacological Institute were
interrupted by a stay, from September 1956 to February 1958, in the
Pharmacological Department of Oxford University (with a British Council Scholarship), where I worked in Hermann (Hugh) Blaschko's laboratory.
The department, under the direction of the very dynamic Professor Harold
J. Burn, was at that time probably the most productive British pharmacological institution, humming with research activities and new ideas. Even
before joining this Institute, I knew the names of its senior researchers: in

addition to Burn and Blaschko, Edith Bülbring (like Blaschko, an emigrée from Berlin), John Walker, Miles Vaughan Williams, and Raymond Ing (the chemist). The place was full of visiting scientists from all over the world. Since some of the senior members of Oxford's pharmacology were also members of well-known Oxford colleges, they often associated with distinguished scientists from abroad that were spending their sabbaticals in the respective colleges. I well remember the occasion when Professor Burn, a member of Balliol College, brought to lunch (regularly served in the department's library) a senior American visitor. Somehow, I found myself sitting next to him. Desperate to say something, I asked him what he was presently working on. Smiling, he replied that he was "trying to find out why the sky is blue." After that I kept my mouth shut, taking his answer as a rebuke for my silly question. Later, I learned that this was exactly what he was trying to figure out—his name was Harold Urey, the famous chemist from Chicago, the discoverer of deuterium.

Meeting Fellow Scientists—and a Healthy Rule about
"Abstracts"

Brücke, who obviously knew personally most of his British colleagues, gave me over a dozen letters of introduction; this enabled me to visit and meet personally senior researchers and heads of the main research laboratories in Great Britain. Other occasions to meet fellow scientists, both British and those from other countries working in British laboratories, were the famous meetings of the Physiological Society. I enjoyed the high level of the presentations and the lively discussions (with [Sir] Henry Dale and Edgar [Lord] Adrian still very much active). I also remember how impressed I was by the rule of the Society that gave its members the power to veto the publication of any of the "abstracts" (in the *Journal of Physiology*) of the papers just presented. I actually witnessed such a thing happen, when Sir Lindor Brown (physiologist, London) objected to an "abstract" on the grounds that it was "of no use." If the rule were made universal and applied today, I wonder what would happen to those fat volumes of "Abstracts" of the many oversized meetings, nowadays so popular.

Social Life

Of course, it would not have been the Oxford of the 1950s if, in addition to high academic activities, there would not have been an equally busy social life going on "day and night." There were countless receptions, dinners, and parties. The latter were civilized when given in respectable settings and, more often, less civilized (not to say, "wild") parties took place in the "digs" (private accomodations) of the younger (visiting) generation. I still have a vivid memory of the party at which one of our company made too fast, "spirited" a start, and after about 90 min had to be "revived," not too successfully, by being placed, as he was, in the bathtub filled with cold water.

Helping Blood Platelets to Take up Catecholamines

A few days after I arrived in Oxford (September 1956), Blaschko went on an extended lecture tour. During his absence, I kept myself busy by helping to measure adrenaline and noradrenaline uptake into isolated blood platelets in Gustav Born's research lab (in the old Radcliff Observatory). Gustav was a combination of sharp scientific intellect, high musical talent (excellent flute player), and great sense of humor, soon becoming the world leader in blood platelet research. He was of great help to me in those first weeks of my stay in Oxford, introducing me to some of the peculiarities of that famous place.

Oxford, Continued: Dopamine Has Its Own Physiological Role in the Body

Blaschko's Idea

When Blaschko returned from his lecture tour, he immediately started to draw my attention to dopamine, a substance so named just four years earlier by Sir Henry Dale, replacing the unwieldy 3,4-dihydroxyphenylethylamine or the misleading 3-hydroxytyramine. Until then, dopamine had been regarded as a mere metabolic intermediate in the synthesis of noradrenaline in the body. Blaschko, in contrast, conceived the idea that dopamine must have "some regulating functions of its own which are not yet known." He expressed this idea in a lecture entitled "Metabolism and Storage of Biogenic Amines," which he had given in the fall of 1956 (on the occasion of Arthur Stoll's, the famous Sandoz [Basel] chemist, 70th birthday) before the Swiss Society of Physiology, Biochemistry, and Pharmacology (Blaschko, 1957). Although Blaschko based his idea upon observations known to other prominent catecholamine researchers, such as Heinz Schümann and Ulf von Euler, none of them had come up with the right conclusion. This instance very aptly characterizes Blaschko: low key, kind, interested in people, and with an exquisite sense of humor. Blaschko had, in addition to a phenomenal memory, a very precise, penetrating mind, coming up with surprising solutions to seemingly insoluble problems.

Convinced of the correctness of his hypothesis, Blaschko asked me to test it experimentally. He referred me to experiments done 15 years earlier by Peter Holtz in Germany, the discoverer of dopa decarboxylase, who in 1942 had noticed that in the rabbit and the guinea pig, dopamine had an effect on the arterial blood pressure opposite to that of adrenaline: instead of raising the blood pressure, as adrenaline did, dopamine lowered it (Holtz and Credner, 1942). Could this be due to dopamine having a physiological role different from that of adrenaline and noradrenaline?

My First Dopamine Study

Despite the Oxford busy social life, I found enough time to carry out Blaschko's idea. With my thorough training in Vienna's Pharmacological Institute, I found the experiments easy to do. When repeating the experiments of Holtz, I also used iproniazid, the first *in vivo* effective monoamine oxidase inhibitor. According to Holtz, inhibition of dopamine's metabolism by that enzyme should have abolished the, as he thought, "unspecific" vasodepressor effect of dopamine. However, I found that the opposite was true: iproniazid potentiated the fall in blood pressure produced by dopamine. I also tested L-dopa, the amino acid from which dopamine is formed in the body. L-dopa behaved exactly like dopamine. These results convinced both Blaschko and me that dopamine had its own physiological role in the body, different from that of the other two naturally occurring catecholamines, adrenaline and noradrenaline.

About six months later, my Oxford scholarship came to an end. Before leaving Oxford, in February 1958, to rejoin Vienna's Pharmacological Institute, Blaschko gave me the advice to continue working with dopamine, which he considered to have a "bright future." Blaschko's prediction was, once more, to come true, this time in my laboratory in Vienna.

Vienna's Pharmacology, Part Two: Mostly Dopamine and Mostly Parkinson's Disease

Focus on Brain Dopamine

Taking Blaschko's advice to heart, and having convinced myself of dopamine's own biological activity in the periphery, I thought it would be worth looking into dopamine's role in the brain. It so happened that my dopamine study in Oxford, which I had finished in early summer 1957, coincided in time with other dopamine studies that immediately focused the attention on the brain. In the August 3, 1957, issue of *Nature*, Kathleen Montagu from the Runwell laboratory in Wickford, near London, had reported, for the first time, on the occurrence of dopamine in the brain of various species, including humans. In the November 16, 1957, issue of *Nature*, Hans Weil-Malherbe, Head of the Runwell laboratory, followed up Montagu's paper by a study on the intracellular distribution of dopamine in the rabbit brain stem. At the same time, the antireserpine effect (in rabbits) of the dopamine and noradrenaline precursor L-dopa was for the first time described by Peter Holtz in Germany (in the September/October 1957 issue of *Naunyn-Schmiedebergs Archiv fuer Experimentelle Pathologic und*

Pharmakologic) and by Arvid Carlsson in Sweden (in the November 30, 1957, issue of *Nature*).

My decision to go into the brain was reinforced, practically immediately after my arrival in Vienna (February 1958), by reports published by both Carlsson in the February 28, 1958, issue of *Science* and Weil-Malherbe in the May 24, 1958, issue of *Nature* that confirmed once more the occurrence of dopamine in the animal brain and showed that reserpine removed the dopamine from the brain and that L-dopa restored its brain levels.

Starting with Brain Dopamine (in the Rat)

After my return from Oxford, I obtained my first fully salaried position in Vienna's Pharmacological Institute as a "Universitäts-Assistent," which entitled me to my own research group. However, for my first dopamine analyses, I lacked a sensitive detection apparatus, such as the just then developed Aminco-Bowman spectrofluorimeter. Therefore, I settled on the colorimetric adrenochrome reaction for catecholamines of von Euler and Hamberg, which I adapted for measurement of dopamine in brain extracts, combining it with the separation procedure for catecholamines developed in Carlsson's laboratory (Dowex columns).

The first study, which I did with my first postdoctoral collaborator Georg Holzer, dealt with the effect of monoamine oxidase inhibitors (iproniazid, harmine), as well as cataleptogenic agents (bulbocapnine, chlorpromazine), and cocaine on dopamine levels in the whole rat brain. We found that only monoamine oxidase inhibitors changed (increased) brain dopamine; the time course of the effect suggested a rather high turnover rate of the dopamine in the rat brain. This we interpreted as favoring a physiological role of the amine in brain function.

The Emergence of the Dopamine/Parkinson's Disease Idea

What could be the role of dopamine in brain function? In the January 15, 1959, issue of *Experientia*, Bertler and Rosengren (from Carlsson's laboratory in Lund) published an exciting observation. Patterning themselves on Marthe Vogt's exemplary study on the regional distribution of noradrenaline in the dog brain, Bertler and Rosengren found, also in the dog, that dopamine, in contrast to noradrenaline, was highly concentrated in the corpus striatum (Bertler and Rosengren, 1959a). This observation immediately gave brain dopamine a functional significance. Connecting the striatal localization of dopamine with the brain dopamine-depleting and parkinsonism-inducing effects of reserpine, it now was possible to say, as Bertler and Rosengren did, that the "results favour[ed] the assumption that dopamine is connected with the function of the striatum and thus with the control of movement."

For me, the direction of my own research was now very clear. With all the evidence available from animal experiments, the one thing that needed to be done was to leave the animal brain and the reserpine model and go directly to the human brain. As it soon turned out, this was the decisive step. I was already familiar with basal ganglia, i.e., Wilson's disease from my first postdoctoral work in the early 1950s; and my very recent dopamine/L-dopa studies in Oxford and now in Vienna was just the right introduction to this as yet unchartered field of research. Thus, the idea of connecting the observations from laboratory animals with human basal ganglia diseases, especially Parkinson's disease, came—after reading the Bertler and Rosengren 1959 *Experientia* report—very naturally to me. In the same year, Carlsson's report on the Bertler and Rosengren data appeared in the *Pharmacological Reviews* (vol. 11, part II). However, much to my regret, I could not benefit from any of Carlsson's ideas; by the time his article came out in print (end of June 1959), we in Vienna were already well into our Parkinson/dopamine work, with results in the first two patients (low striatal dopamine) already in our hands.

Fresh Postmortem Brain Material: Its Rise from the Scorned to the Most Treasured

At the time when I started working with fresh autopsied human brain, studies in such material of chemically unstable neurotransmitter substances, including catecholamines and their related enzymes, had been rare. They had been traditionally viewed with great suspicion as to their usefulness and scientific significance. Many senior colleagues, including knowledgeable biochemists, tried to dissuade me from "wasting my time on such half-decomposed, dirty material." However, this was the only material that could possibly be used for the study I had in mind. Today, fresh human brain material is highly valued as a source of information on human brain diseases that cannot be obtained from animal models. Several human brain tissue banks in many countries now exist, supplying research labs with sometimes very rare and precious material. This radical reversal of opinion has been primarily the result of the unexpected success of our dopamine studies in the Parkinson brain and the subsequent introduction of dopamine replacement with L-dopa.

The Dopamine/Parkinson's Disease Work Begins

The Source (of the Material)

In order to carry out my project, a suitable source of fresh autopsied human brains had to be found. It was not difficult to obtain autopsied non-neurological control brains from the University's Pathological Institute.

The best source for Parkinson material was the pathology unit of Vienna's largest City Hospital "Wien-Lainz" with its attached large Home for the Aged, where many Parkinson patients were chronically housed. However, the clinician in charge of the neurology unit of that nursing facility, Walther Birkmayer, was not on the best of terms with me at that time. Fortunately, my next postdoctoral collaborator in training, replacing Georg Holzer, was Herbert Ehringer, a very capable, hardworking, and ambitious young man. What made Ehringer so essential was that he had, from his student days, a good relationship with the chief prosector of the "Lainz" pathology, Stephan Wuketich, who readily agreed to supply us with the necessary brain material.

The Discovery

In April 1959, about eight weeks after reading the Bertler and Rosengren report in *Experientia*, we received the first brain of a patient who had died with Parkinson's disease. After carrying the samples of the caudate nucleus and putamen of this patient, together with control samples, through the extraction procedure, the thrilling moment of performing the von Euler and Hamberg color (iodine) reaction arrived. Instead of the pink color in the control samples, indicating presence of dopamine, the reaction vials containing the Parkinson material showed hardly a tinge of pink discoloration. For the first time ever, and before even placing the reaction vials into the colorimeter, I could see the brain dopamine deficiency in Parkinson's disease literally with my own naked eye!

The Study

By late spring of 1960, within little more than 12 months, we had collected and analyzed the brains of 17 non-neurological controls; 2 patients with Huntington's disease; 6 patients with extrapyramidal disorders of unknown etiology; and 6 Parkinson brains (4 postencephalitic, and 2 idiopathic disease). Two neonate brains and one infant brain were also examined. Of all the 14 cases with extrapyramidal disease, only the 6 Parkinson's disease cases had a severe loss of dopamine in the caudate nucleus and putamen. The results of this study were published in the December 15, 1960, issue of the *Klinische Wochenschrift*. Ever since that time, this discovery has provided a rational basis, and a point of departure, for all the following modern research into mechanisms, causes, and treatment of Parkinson's disease.

It is worth noting that our observations were made by means of a simple, only moderately sensitive, colorimetric method; they did not require any complicated, ultra-modern machinery or out-of-the-way chemistry. This shows that sophisticated methodology, although sometimes of great help, is not an essential component of discovery. The simple method we had used matched perfectly the clear idea on which the study was based, resulting in that irreducible simplicity that is an unfailing mark of the true and durable.

On Conceiving an Idea: The Beginnings of the L-Dopa Era

The discovery of the dopamine deficiency in the Parkinson brain was, quite logically, the basis for the next stage of what came to be known as "the dopamine miracle," that is, the step from the human brain homogenate to the patient. This step marked the beginnings of the dopamine replacement era of Parkinson's disease treatment with L-dopa.

It has often been noted that even what later appears as an obvious idea requires the right moment to be conceived. In mid-October 1960, two months before our report on the dopamine discovery came out in print, the idea struck me that it should be possible to improve the motor deficits of Parkinson's disease by replacing the missing brain dopamine. At that time, I was revisiting Blaschko's laboratory in Oxford, among other things correcting the proofs of our dopamine paper, which had been forwarded to me from Vienna. Was it the influence of the ideas—still lingering in the lab's atmosphere?—of my previous dopamine/L-dopa work done there that put the instant thought into my mind of using L-dopa as the dopamine-replacing drug of choice in the patients? What a splendid neurophilosophical topic would the true life of ideas, and the world they inhabit, make!

Looking for a Neurologist: On the Usefulness of Vienna's Cafés

In order to carry out my idea, I needed the help of a neurologist. My immediate choice fell on Walther Birkmayer. Birkmayer was a clinical neurologist with a sharp diagnostic eye and considerable drug-testing experience, especially with anticholinergics in Parkinson patients. Since he was in charge of the neurological ward of Vienna's largest Home for the Aged Wien-Lainz, he had access to many chronically housed patients with parkinsonism. Birkmayer had an engaging personality and was easy to motivate, and, in addition, he was very eager to find a way into research. These qualities suggested him to me as an ideal partner for carrying out my L-dopa idea. On the other hand, Birkmayer had many enemies in Vienna's medical faculty (especially because of his political past); therefore, it required an act of balance to work with him and yet remain on good terms with the others.

Following the first successful L-dopa trials, Birkmayer and I had five years (1961–1966) of a productive and amicable working relationship. We regularly met, sometimes twice weekly, in order to plan the next set of the rapidly progressing clinical trials. I taught Birkmayer monoamine biochemistry, myself turning into something like a clinical pharmacologist. Initially, we met in my office in the Pharmacological Institute, but after a while Brücke disliked Birkmayer's presence in "his" Institute. We then moved our sessions to the "Café Schwarzspanier," not an uncommon Viennese answer to

all kinds of space problems. In the past, several Viennese artists/bohemiens
had been known to have actually lived in cafés; one of them, a noted writer,
even ended his life in his café. The Café Schwarzspanier was a very convenient meeting place for me, as it was located in a housing complex just
around the corner from the Pharmacological Institute. On the site of the
housing complex stood, until 1903, the house in which Beethoven had
spent the last 18 months of his life and in which he died in 1827. The
Café Schwarzspanier also is no more; it closed its doors sometime in the
1970s.

It Is Impossible to Suppress an Idea

Tyrants, dictators, and oppressive regimes are all well aware of, and bemoan,
the fact that ideas, once brought into the world, cannot be indefinitely suppressed, let alone killed. This is also attested, on an infinitely smaller scale,
by the initial fate of my L-dopa idea.

At the beginning of November 1960, immediately after returning from
my visit with Blaschko, I contacted Birkmayer about the possibility of
an L-dopa trial on his ward. Despite the clear rationale for my proposal,
Birkmayer would not listen to me. There were two reasons for that. First,
at that early time, dopamine as a chemical compound of physiological interest, as well as its possible involvement in basal ganglia function, was quite
alien to Birkmayer's thinking. Second, his unwillingness to collaborate
with me went back to a grudge he bore me when in the spring of 1958 I
rejected, with a flimsy excuse, his suggestion to analyze the brains of patients
with Parkinson's disease, coming to autopsy from his ward, for changes in
hypothalamic serotonin, an idea that to me lacked scientific stringency.

After several reminders and pressure "from above," especially from
Brücke, in July 1961, nearly nine months later, Birkmayer finally gave
L-dopa intravenously to his first few patients. The intravenous (iv) route
suggested itself for two reasons. First, it was the most economical route,
considering the small amounts (about 2 g) of L-dopa with which I was able
to supply Birkmayer. Second, iv L-dopa had been tried in humans as early
as the 1940s and found basically safe. In the immediate past, Degkwitz, a
neuropsychiatrist at the University of Frankfurt in Germany, had used iv
L-dopa in an attempt to counteract, *inter alia*, the reserpine "sedation" in
psychiatric patients.

The Dopamine/L-Dopa Miracle

The effect of iv L-dopa in our first patients was spectacular. Akinesia,
the most disabling of the motor deficits, responded most dramatically.
Birkmayer instantly forgot his grudge against me and became a zealous
convert. We started our first L-dopa trials in July 1961. In August, we made

a documentary film with five patients. Eight weeks later we sent in our first report entitled "The L-Dopa Effect on Akinesia in Parkinsonism" to the *Wiener Klinische Wochenschrift* for publication. This report appeared in print in the November 10, 1961, issue of the journal. In the evening of the same day, I presented in the scientific session of the "Gesellschaft der Ärzte in Wien" for the first time my dopamine/Parkinism brain study in a lecture with the title "Biochemical-Pharmacological Foundations of the Clinical use of L-Dihydroxyphenylalanine in Parkinsonsm." My lecture was followed by Birkmayer showing the film and commenting on the clinical observations.

Today, it is generally agreed that the initiation of the treatment of Parkinson's disease with L-dopa represented one of the triumphs of pharmacology of our time. L-dopa's unprecedented success proved, for the first time, that therapeutic neurotransmitter replacement in a chronic, progressive, degenerative brain disease (until then regarded as basically untreatable) was indeed possible. This provided, apart from the benefit to the patients, a stimulus for analogous studies of many other brain disorders, both neurological and psychiatric. As John Hardy (National Institutes of Health, Bethesda) put it in a recent letter to me, "L-dopa's discovery was the defining finding for transmitter-based therapeutics."

The Simple and Logical Is Not Always the Most Obvious

I have stressed the logical, rational nature of the steps leading to the discoveries about dopamine and L-dopa in Parkinson's disease. Easy as they were to take and carry out, at that time, these steps were not as obvious to everyone as they appear today. Two of the most striking examples may serve to illustrate this point. First, in Carlsson's laboratory in Lund, Bertler and Rosengren followed up their crucial January 1959 study in the dog by measuring, without delay, dopamine in the normal human postmortem brain (Bertler and Rosengren, 1959b). However, they apparently did not attempt to obtain and analyze Parkinson brains, despite the fact that pathological material is easier to obtain than brain material from control cases. Second, in 1960, Degkwitz, as mentioned, had used iv L-dopa in psychiatric patients (Degkwitz et al., 1961). He was the first to show that L-dopa abolished the reserpine "sedation" in humans—a state that must have included the well-known reserpine akinesia. Stangely enough, the idea of trying to counteract the Parkinson akinesia with L-dopa had not occurred to him. Both these examples clearly illustrate how restricted, one-way thinking can influence the direction of one's work. At that time, not only leading dopamine laboratories, but also knowledgeable clinical experimenters were so deeply preoccupied with reserpine and its central actions, be it in animals or in patients, that all of them overlooked and missed the most obvious.

All Too Human?

The amicable and highly successful working relationship between Birkmayer and me, which could have turned into something like friendship, did not last. In the course of time, Birkmayer, who could have rested on his own major clinical achievements, developed his own version—contrary to historical fact—of the events leading to the use of L-dopa. Taught as I had been to respect the academic code and to acknowledge other people's work and ideas, I found Birkmayer's behavior discouraging, and I put our relationship on ice. It is amazing to see how often this disregard of intellectual property repeats itself, right to this day, in academic circles. To see this happen has always been deeply saddening to me. Is it the lack of proper judgement or an unhealthy ambition that drives people to such behavior? Or is this due to a slow subconscious process of reinterpretation of reality in one's own favor, to the point of the individuals, in fact, believing in what they are saying? How difficult is it to read and understand the hidden thoughts and motives of others—and how much could be said about it!

Dark Days and Years for Dopamine

The quick success of the steps "from brain homogenate to treatment" would have been expected to immediately establish brain dopamine's role in brain function, particularly in Parkinson's disease. This, however, was not the case. Despite all the evidence from animal experiments, especially those with reserpine, and the human brain, especially Parkinson's disease—both of which I found to be compelling—it took many years before dopamine was recognized as a brain neurotransmitter in its own right and its role in Parkinson's disease was accepted. Why was this so?

The main reason for the neglect of brain dopamine in the first half of the 1960s was the controversy, starting around 1956, between Bernard Brodie (NIH, Bethesda) and Arvid Carlsson (Lund/Göteborg) about how to explain reserpine's central "sedative" or "tranquilizing" effects. Brodie had advanced the brain serotonin hypothesis, whereas Carlsson saw more reason for the role of brain "catecholamines." Today, it is difficult to understand why the discoveries about brain dopamine, made between 1957 and 1960, had not immediately put an end to the debate, or at least changed it into a "serotonin–dopamine" dispute. Quite to the contrary, the debate continued well into the mid-1960s, with dopamine, if not completely ignored, being lumped together with noradrenaline as "the catecholamine(s)." Also, the existence of dopamine receptors in the brain, distinct from noradrenaline receptors, was sometimes forgotten. Also, dopamine's crucial and so plainly evident role in reserpine parkinsonism and Parkinson's disease was for several years discredited by the claim that the direct (synthetic) noradrenaline precursor 3,4-dihydroxyphenylserine (dops) actually had central actions similar to those of L-dopa. Curiously, it was Marthe Vogt, probably the astutest brain researcher of the time, but not particularly a friend of dopamine, who in 1960, during one of the fiercest battles, had the insight to remind the combatants that one "could explain the effect of dopamine on an entirely different basis from the effects of the other catecholamines..." and therefore she was "not quite certain that we are right in lumping together experiments in which the [brain] dopamine level is up and others in which the noradrenaline level is up" (Vogt, 1960).

Coming to the Rescue of Brain Dopamine

I felt very unhappy about so many influential people being so deeply preoccupied with this debate. My attitude was that of a "dopamine purist." I did not see any need for any other monoamine, be it serotonin or noradrenaline, in order to explain Parkinson's disease and reserpine parkinsonism (in the debate usually misnamed "reserpine sedation" or "tranquilization"). I felt that any "admixure" was detrimental to the significance and uniqueness of all the dopamine/L-dopa observations. However, my opinion was not sufficient to change the minds of the "dogmatists." Fortunately, I found two strong allies: Theodore (Ted) Sourkes and Guy Everett.

Ted Sourkes, at McGill's Allan Memorial Institute of Psychiatry in Montreal, was a seasoned catecholamine researcher with a long, distinguished record. He came early to the brain dopamine field when, in 1961, he found, together with the clinical neurologist André Barbeau (of the Université de Montréal), low urinary excretion of dopamine in patients with Parkinson's disease and, as a consequence of that, suggested to Barbeau (independently from us in Vienna) the oral use of L-dopa. After that, Sourkes and the neurophysiologist Louis Poirier (of Laval University in Quebec City) were the first to reproduce, in the primate, the main symptoms of parkinsonism by lesioning the substantia nigra, correlating them with the dopamine loss in the striatum, and thus producing evidence for a nigrostriatal dopamine pathway in the primate.

The other strong dopamine advocate, Guy Everett, was the neuropharmacologist at the Abbot Laboratories in Chicago. In a series of pharmacological experiments (in rodents), Everett demonstrated that locomotor behavior was under the control of brain dopamine, with no involvement of noradrenaline. By this, he also disproved the notion that dops, i.e., the noradrenaline formed from it, had L-dopa-like central effects. He also coined for the mistreated dopamine the term "the Cinderella of the biogenic amines" (Everett, 1970). Since both Sourkes and Everett were competent and highly respected researchers, their observations could not be lightly dismissed. But in the end, the fruitless "serotonin–catecholamine" debate was terminated and decided in favor of brain dopamine by the unprecedented success of the L-dopa therapy.

"You Have Got the Necessary Brains": Human Brain Studies, Continued

When, in the summer of 1961 Ted Sourkes visited me in Vienna, we also discussed the difficult dopamine situation. In the course of the discussion, I asked Ted, in passing, whether he thought it worthwhile for me to continue with the human brain studies. "Yes, carry on with this work," he said, humorously adding, "you have got the necessary brains for it." Thus encouraged, we continued this line of research and found the results quite rewarding.

At the end of 1960, Ehringer moved to the University of Innsbruck and was replaced by Hanno (Hans) Bernheimer, who was very good with chemical methodology and a skillful brain dissectionist. With his help, I concentrated on what I thought was important. I provided evidence for the existence of a nigrostriatal dopamine pathway in the human brain, at that time shown only in animal brain. We showed, by measuring dopamine's metabolite homovanillic acid, that in Parkinson's disease the remaining dopamine neurones in the striatum were highly overactive; this observation gave rise to the very familiar concept today of the compensatory (adaptive) capacity of the remaining neurones, so as to maintain striatal function despite major neuronal losses. We compared, in a large collaborative study, the degree of substantia nigra cell loss with the loss of striatal dopamine and established a cause-effect relationship between the severity of Parkinson symptoms and the degree of striatal dopamine loss; we also demonstrated this by studying the dopamine levels separately in the right and the left striatum in a case with unilateral parkinsonism. With Hans-Jörg Lisch (who replaced Bernheimer in 1966), I traced the course of the nigrostriatal dopamine neurons in the human brain by studying the distribution of homovanillic acid within the internal capsule. Last, but not least, we showed, together with Walther Birkmayer, that the L-dopa effect in the Parkinson patient was specific and not mimicked by any of the other catecholamine- or L-dopa-like substances, including the ill-famed dops.

No Language Barrier for Brain Dopamine

Scientific work published in the Western World in languages other than English is said to be at risk of being totally ignored. This cannot be said of our observations published in German; they immediately attracted the attention of many English-speaking colleagues. In February 1961, only eight weeks after our brain dopamine/Parkinson paper came out in print, Ted Sourkes contacted me by letter, and a couple of weeks later, so did André Barbeau. Many others wrote to me asking for information; among them were Bill (W.G.) Clark, Charles Markham, David Marsden (at that time still a medical student), Pat McGeer, Isamu Sano, Erminio Costa, Michael Pare,

Everardus Ariens, Morris Aprison, Guy Everett, Mel Yahr, Wilhelm Raab, Harold Himwich, Donald Calne, George Selby, Sidney Udenfriend, and Melvin vanWoert. The first visitor was Ted Sourkes, who in August 1961 already came to Vienna to see me in my laboratory. In September 1965, I had a visit from Melvin Yahr and Roger Duvoisin (from Columbia University's neurology department). Other visitors, as far as I remember, included André Barbeau, Merton Sandler, Leo Hollister, and Melvin vanWoert.

Bill Clark, the biochemist turned (psycho)pharmacologist in Los Angeles, proved himself a diligent reader of (German) footnotes. In his letter of January 28, 1964, he asked me for the L-dopa film, which we had offered on a loan basis to interested people in a footnote in our 1962 paper written in German. He showed the film to his neurological friend Charles Markham, who, in April 1964, wrote to me, saying that "there is no question that the second and third patient showed greater mobility after L-dopa." Markham, a highly successful and very circumspect L-dopa expert, was among the first in the United States to use oral L-dopa.

In 1966, Donald Calne became seriously interested in repeating our iv L-dopa trials in London. He wrote and asked me about the best source of L-dopa for iv use. A little later, Calne was the first in Great Britain to publish on the therapeutic efficacy of oral L-dopa and the first to demonstrate, in 1973, the anti-Parkinson action of bromocriptine, the first clinically useful dopamine agonist. Donald and I became close friends in the course of our wanderings that brought us both to Canada: Donald to Vancouver and me to Toronto.

When vanWoert came to see me in October 1966, he gave me a copy of an as yet unpublished manuscript, written together with George Cotzias and L.M. Schiffer, reporting their spectacular results with high oral doses of D,L-dopa given to Parkinson patients in daily increasing amounts. Reading this report, which subsequently came out in the February 16, 1967, issue of *New England Journal of Medicine*, I realized that at last L-dopa had reached the New World.

First Contacts With the New World

The New World opened its doors to me for the first time in November 1965. Sidney Udenfriend (NIH, Bethesda) had sent me an invitation on behalf of Melvin Yahr and Erminio Costa, who were organizing a symposium on the "Biochemistry and Pharmacology of the Basal Ganglia." This was on the occasion of the opening of the William Black Lecture Hall at Columbia University's Parkinson's Disease Information and Research Center in New York City. It was at that symposium that I gave my first formal North American lecture (followed by an interview with the press, together with Arvid Carlsson) on my work on dopamine, L-dopa, and Parkinson' disease. However, already two weeks earlier I had spoken about our results in a seminar in Canada, little knowing that soon this country would become my second (or third?) home; this was upon Ted Sourkes' invitation, who had asked me to speak in his lab at Montreal's Allan Memorial Institute of Psychiatry at McGill.

At the Columbia symposium in New York I was greatly impressed with meeting so many prominent North American scientists. "A sky full of stars." There were such senior people as Herbert Jasper of the McGill Neurological Institute, Columbia's Houston Merritt and David Nachmansohn, Wally Nauta (from MIT, Boston), Seymour Kety (from NIH, Bethesda), George Koelle (University of Philadelphia), and George Palade (Rockefeller University, New York), among others. Brodie, Udenfriend, Costa, and Carlsson were already known to me from the serotonin–catecholamine debates. I knew Sourkes and Yahr from their visits to my Vienna laboratory. I met Everett there for the first time. Mel Yahr, the main organizer of the symposium, was the first neurologist worldwide to test (in 1968/1969) the anti-Parkinson efficacy of L-dopa in a double-blind study. He became the leading neurologist, and the driving force, of clinical Parkinson's disease research, first at Columbia and then at New York's Mount Sinai School of Medicine. Mel and I developed a close, friendly relationship over the many years of our continuous contacts and exchange of ideas.

Trying to Put Dopamine on the Agenda of "Big Labs": Support from an Unexpected Direction

The Columbia meeting was also the starting point for a collaboration between Sidney Udenfriend at Bethesda and me in Vienna. At that time, Udenfriend was studying and characterizing, for the first time, the enzyme tyrosine hydroxylase. He agreed to measure this rate-limiting enzyme in our human normal and Parkinson brains. For several months I was supplying him with postmortem brain material. However, there were, at that time, too many technical problems with measuring the enzyme in human postmortem material which could not be solved on such an across-the-Atlantic basis. However, we continued our friendly relationship and years later shared, to our pleasant surprise, the Research Award of the City of Hope National Medical Center, Duarte (Los Angeles), where Eugene Roberts, of GABA fame, was Head of Neurosciences, and the wonderful Rachmiel Levine was Research Director.

Another important collaboration I had started in the mid-1960s was that with Rolf Hassler, the eminent Parkinson researcher and director of the Max-Planck Institute for Brain Research in Frankfurt, Germany. Hassler kept supplying me with brain samples taken from cats in which he had made various midbrain, including substantia nigra, lesions. However, when, in 1965, I voiced the view that there existed, in humans, a nigrostriatal dopamine pathway, Hassler terminated all contacts with me: he was strictly opposed to the idea of such a fiber connection. Years later we established tacitly a truce, but to my regret never regained our former easy relationship. What a pity to lose over such matters a potential friend!

While my attempts to put dopamine and Parkinson's disease on the agenda of internationally highly respected laboratories had, at most, doubtful results, the cause of brain dopamine received support from an unexpected direction. In July 1964, George H. Acheson (University of Cincinnati, OH), the Editorial Chairman of the renowned *Pharmacological Reviews*, asked me to write an article on "the interesting aspects of dopamine in the brain." He stressed that the article should point to the future rather than review the past. My essay, which I boldly entitled "Dopamine (3-Hydroxytyramine) and Brain Function," appeared in June 1966. It was indeed written for the future, putting brain dopamine definitively on the map of brain research at a time when the word "neuroscience" was not yet what it is today. I consider this article as the successful conclusion of my "human brain dopamine era" in Vienna's Pharmacological Institute. To this day I admire Acheson's foresight in requesting such a review in the "darkest days" of dopamine. It shows how a good editor can decisively help in advancing the progress of research and influence its direction.

Enough Time for Some "Real" Pharmacology

During all those dopamine/parkinsonism years, there was enough time to do some "real" pharmacology. Together with Ehringer and Klaus Lechner, we studied the effect of neuroleptics on the catecholamine and serotonin metabolism in the rat brain. With Alfred Springer and A. Aigner, I examined the effect of inhibition of dopamine-β-hydroxylase on the locomotor effects of L-dopa. Adrenergic tolerance was investigated with Hubert Obenaus (who later became Head of Toxicology at Vienna's Sandoz Research Institute— and godfather of one of my children). And with Walter Kobinger (Later Director of Pharmacology at the Ernst Boehringer Research Institut in Vienna), we studied the role of medullary cholinergic mechanisms in the regulation of the carotid sinus reflex and blood pressure. We developed an intricate method for injection of drugs into the internal carotid artery in the rat (later used in the Netherlands by my Vienna collaborator Pieter van Zwieten). Ever since, Walter and I have continued and deepened our close and friendly relationship.

My 10 Years in Toronto (1967–1977)

In the fall of 1967, I received an offer from the University of Toronto. Although at that time Brücke was in reasonably good health and about 10 years from retirement, people in the Institute were already getting into the starting holes for the race for his position. It was as if they had sensed that

Brücke's post would soon be vacant. (Brücke died, unexpectedly, two-and-a-half years later, in the spring of 1970.) The relaxed atmosphere in the Institute, so typical and enjoyable until then, changed. Since I have never been good at races for positions, I welcomed the opportunity to move to Toronto to become, to my own surpise, a (neuro)psychopharmacologist.

The way I came to psychopharmacology was very simple. In September 1966, Toronto's pharmacologist Werner Kalow had heard me speak on my dopamine/parkinsonism work at the Biberach (Germany) laboratories of Boehringer Ingelheim (where, for a year or two, he, Kalow, was Director of Medical Research). He contacted Harvey Stancer, the biochemical psychiatrist at the just then opened Clarke Institute of Psychiatry at the University of Toronto. Soon afterward, I was offered the position of Head of the Clarke's (as yet completely empty) Psychopharmacology Division. I accepted, and thus, thanks to dopamine, I could rightly call myself, for at least 10 years, something like a psychopharmacologist. (Here I may add that I was not completely unprepared for that position. A few years earlier, I had written, together with Brücke, a book on the *Pharmacology of Psychotherapeutic Drugs*, published in 1966 in German and in 1969 in English.)

I moved to the North American continent at the best possible time. In February 1967, George Cotzias published his landmark report on the strong, sustained anti-Parkinson effect of high oral doses of D,L-dopa (Cotzias, van Woert, and Schiffer, 1967). This produced quite a stir in the North American neurological research community. Thus, when 10 months later, in October 1967, I made a fresh start in Toronto, the atmosphere was just right for my interest in dopamine and Parkinson's disease.

New World, New Colleagues

Settling down in Toronto was made easy for me by the very helpful attitude of the colleagues at the Clarke Institute (with the always available Harvey Stancer next door in the neurochemistry section), as well as in the departments of pharmacology and neurology. I was soon appointed full professor with tenure in pharmacology and later in psychiatry. I immediately liked the atmosphere in the Clarke Institute and its just then appointed new Director Robin Hunter (also Head of the Department of Psychiatry), whose honest and straightforward character suited me. Werner Kalow, now the newly appointed Head of the Pharmacology Department and pioneer of the new research field of "pharmacogenetics," greatly contributed to my own and my family's feeling of being at home in Toronto; for newcomers like us, his advice and help with the smaller and bigger problems were invaluable. I liked and respected Clifford (Rick) Richardson, Head of the University's Neurology Department. He was a real gentleman, kind, modest, and self-disciplined, and his name was already known to me from the "Steele-Richardson-Olszewski Syndrome" (progressive supranuclear palsy). With the active help of the people in Toronto, as well as throughout the United States and Canada (e.g., Ted Sourkes in Montreal), I soon found my way around North America. I liked and admired the enthusiasm and the open-mindedness of my fellow scientists and their readiness to recognize and acknowledge other people's achievements. I could not have wished for better colleagues.

More New Colleagues

I was surprised at how quickly my presence in Toronto was detected. Soon, I had to satisfy innumerable requests for invited lectures and research seminars, organizing committee meetings, congresses, and symposia all over the North American continent; sitting on grant committees, going on site visits, and evaluating grant applications for the MRC (Canada) and the NIH; and more than half a dozen memberships of medical advisory boards of various foundations. In the latter capacity, I was able to meet with practically everyone prominent in neuroscience in North America. There was Milton Wexler's "Hereditary Disease (H.D.) Foundation" in Los Angeles; Sam Belzberg's "Dystonia Research Foundation" (with John Menkes [Los Angeles] as Research Director); the "Committee to Combat Huntington's Disease" in New York with Marjorie Guthrie, the admirable and lovable wife of Woody Guthrie; and several Parkinson's Disease Foundations, both in Canada and in the United States. In addition, there were the lay patient societies and organizations. To all this should be added the visitors that came to see me at the Clarke Institute to discuss questions of mutual interest. I remember the day when Hirotaro Narabayashi, the renowned neurologist (from Tokyo), came to see me (when visiting his neurosurgical colleague, the admirable Ron Tasker, at the Toronto General Hospital). Narabayashi's visit was the beginning of our very close relationship that lasted until his death in 2001. Seymour Kety, one of the great "fathers of neuroscience," I had met already at Mel Yahr's symposium in 1965. Subsequently, I came to admire Kety's clear and unerring judgement, his wide horizon, and his ability to see things in a larger context. His "knowledge of things" and awareness of its philosophical underpinnings made many of our conversations a special pleasure and gain for me.

Research at the Clarke Institute's Division of Psychopharmacology

It was easy for me to do research at the Clarke Institute. I found that the colleagues in the other research sections, most of them psychiatrists, were very pleasant people with whom I soon developed friendly relationships and from whom I learned a great deal about that dimension of the human brain that we could not claim to see or measure (yet) in our test tubes.

The Right Drug for the Wrong Reason?

I soon resumed my dopamine/Parkinson research work. This became, in my view, a necessity when I noticed that seasoned brain researchers, who had spent all their lives tackling frustratingly difficult problems, found the whole brain dopamine/Parkinson business irritatingly simple and the dopamine-substitution explanation for L-dopa's "miraculous" effect outright unbelievable. Catchy, but distinctly jaundiced phrases were coined by distinguished brain scientists, such as that L-dopa was "the right therapy for the wrong reason" (Ward, 1970; Jasper, 1970). Doubts about L-dopa as a physiological replacement of dopamine were expressed by stating that "since L-dopa floods the brain with dopamine, to relate its [antiparkinson] effects to the natural function of dopamine neurons may be quite erroneous" (Vogt, 1973). Failure of some investigators to detect in the human brain significant activity of dopa decarboxylase, the enzyme responsible for dopamine formation, appeared to justify the skepticism. Challenged by these doubts, the first problem I attacked was the presence of dopa decarboxylase in the human brain. With my extremely motivated and able Ph.D. student, Kenneth G. Lloyd, who came to me from Ted Sourkes' laboratory, we demonstrated that dopa decarboxylase was definitively present in the human brain in amounts comparable to the amounts found in other mammals' brains and with an analogous regional distribution. Thus, finding out, and adhering to, the proper assay conditions, skillfully established by Ken Lloyd, was all that was needed to save the normal human brain from the deplorable fate of having some abnormal, rather mysterious, catecholamine synthetic pathway.

We followed up, logically, this dopa decarboxylase enzyme work by measuring the activity of tyrosine hydroxylase in the human brain (something I had tried to do while still in Vienna in 1965/1966 with Sidney Udenfriend) and demonstrated that both these dopamine synthetic enzymes were greatly reduced in the Parkinson brain.

Encouraged by this success, we proceeded to demonstrate the dopamine-replacing nature of L-dopa treatment. This we achieved by directly showing that patients treated with L-dopa had more dopamine in the striatum than untreated patients, with the highest dopamine levels shortly after the last premortem dose of L-dopa. The publication of this study, in 1975, silenced all doubts about L-dopa therapy and dopamine replacement.

A Plethora of Ideas to Test

In the course of time, we extended the work in the human brain in many directions. We studied (Ken Lloyd) the GABA receptors and the adenylyl cyclase-coupled dopamine receptors (Masato Shibuya) in the Parkinson brain; the striatal D-2 dopamine receptors in Parkinson's disease (Phil Seeman, Irene Farley, Ali Rajput) and schizophrenia (Phil Seeman, Irene Farley, Walle Tourtellotte); regional monoamine, especially brain serotonin distribution in depression (Ken Lloyd, Irene Farley), using brains of suicide victims; and regional noradrenaline levels (Irene Farley, Kathleen Price) in brains of patients with paranoid schizophrenia. We also measured (Vladimir Hachinsky) homovanillic acid in the CSF of patients with cerebral infarction. There was also all the work in animal models, such as regional monoamine studies in rhesus monkeys on long-term neuroleptic drug therapy (George Paulson [Columbus, OH], Kathleen Price); the influence of brain dopamine mechanisms on rat EMG (Detlef Bieger); the effect of morphine (Klaus Kuschinsky) and met-enkephalin and β-endorphin (Stuart Bernie, Ken Koffer) on striatal dopamine and catalepsy; the role of corpus striatum in morphine catalepsy (Ken Koffer); the relationship between the striatum, the substantia nigra, and epileptic seizure activity (Ruggero Fariello, Masato Shibuya, Ken Lloyd); the effect of chronic neuroleptic or L-dopa administration in rats on the GABA levels in the substantia nigra (Ken Lloyd); and the selective anti-dopaminergic action (in the rat) of γ-hydroxybutyric acid (Krishna Menon, Detlef Bieger). We would sooner be short of time than of ideas to be tested experimentally.

An especially important achievement of our work in Toronto was a study of neurotransmitters, especially dopamine, in the brain of patients with Lesch-Nyhan syndrome. The results of this study provided a neurochemical reference standard for the transgenic animal model used today in studying this X-linked inherited metabolic brain disorder. This study also for the first time showed that loss of striatal dopamine was not necessarily connected with loss of nigral dopamine cell bodies—a situation later most dramatically and consequentially demonstrated by our study of a unique case of dopa-responsive (Segawa) dystonia.

Having the Best of Both Worlds: Commuting Between Vienna and Toronto (1977–Present)

In 1976/1977, I moved back to Vienna to head the Institute of Biochemical Pharmacology, newly established at the Faculty of Medicine of the University of Vienna. As is so often the case, we returned to Vienna for family reasons. We, that is my family and I, still count the 10 years we spent in Toronto as among the happiest years of our life together. The people who were so generous and hospitable, the excellent colleagues, the friendly neighbors, and the easy way to raise children all contributed to our feeling happy and very much at home in Canada. And then there was, again, the allure of nature: intense, boundless, and bountiful.

Vienna: Institute of Biochemical Pharmacology

Right from the beginning of my work in Vienna, we devoted most of our time to work with neurotoxins and with the search for mechanisms of neurodegeneration. We studied three neurotoxins: kainic acid, ethylcholine aziridinium (AF64A), and 1-methyl-4-phenyl-1,2,3,6-tetrahydropyridine (MPTP).

Kainic Acid

We started working with kainic acid when Günther Sperk (now Professor of Pharmacology at the University of Innsbruck) returned, in 1977, from his postdoctoral stay with Ross Baldessarini at the Mailman Research Center, McLean Hospital (Belmont, MA) and joined my laboratory. Soon, Michael Berger started as my Ph.D. student, joined us, and a little later Halina Baran, another of my very active Ph.D. students. Many of the studies were done in collaboration with the renowned neuropathologist Franz Seitelberger and his collaborator Hans Lassmann. Kainic acid served as a reliable excitotoxin to produce, in the rat, biochemical and morphological changes in the striatum, typical of Huntington's disease. As an epileptogenic agent, kainic acid allowed us to study the brain changes during generalized seizures and provided an especially valuable model of temporal lobe (limbic) epilepsy.

AF64A

This neurotoxin was brought to my laboratory by Heide Hörtnagl from Israel Hanin's place at the University of Pittsburgh (PA), where she had spent two years with a research fellowship. We used this agent to selectively lesion the brain cholinergic neurones, especially in the hippocampal formation. By thus imitating (in the rat) the cholinergic deficits typical of Alzheimer's disease, the analogous changes in several brain transmitter systems as well as neuropeptides could be analyzed under controlled experimental conditions. In this model, we also could clarify the role of glucocorticoids in the cholinergic degeneration in the rat hippocampus.

MPTP

MPTP was the third neurotoxin Christian Pifl and I used in connection with my continuing interest in Parkinson's disease. We did these studies in cooperation with Günther Schingnitz at Boehringer-Ingelheim's CNS pharmacology laboratory (Germany). They supplied us with brains of rhesus monkeys treated acutely or chronically with MPTP. In these studies, we established the effect of this parkinsonism-inducing dopamine neurotoxin on the regional patterns of several brain neurotransmitters (in addition to dopamine) throughout the primate brain. When Christian Pifl returned from a two-year fellowship in Marc Caron's laboratory at Duke University (Durham, NC), we continued with our interest in MPTP by studying in cell cultures the role of the specific cell membrane dopamine transporter in the phenomenon of neurodegeneration.

New Drugs for Parkinson's Disease: Back to Human Disease

An especially pleasant cooperation developed, in the 1980s, between my laboratory (Christian Pifl, Heide Hörtnagl) and Walter Kobinger and Ludwig Pichler from the pharmacology laboratory at Vienna's Ernst Boehringer Research Institute. The result of this collaboration was the introduction in the treatment of Parkinson's disease of a new class of (non-ergoline) direct dopamine agonists (i.e., B-HT 920, talipexol, in Japan; in the Western Hemisphere, the chemically closely related pramipexol).

Although my laboratory in Vienna was meant to do work exclusively in animals, this rule was broken when the neurologist Elfriede Sluga offered us valuable amyotrophic lateral sclerosis material. Susanne Malessa, Oswald Bertel, and Michael Berger used this material to study the spinal cord changes in glutamatergic, monoaminergic, and cholinergic parameters in this neurodegenerative condition.

Full-time animal work notwithstanding, my laboratory (especially Heide Hörtnagl) found time for collaborative research in patients. These studies served as a reminder for those of my collaborators doing exclusively animal work that in medical research it is, in the end, the patient that counts.

Toronto: the Human Brain Laboratory

The Birth of a New Research Facility

When I moved to Vienna, a considerable number of valuable, freshly frozen human brains that we had collected during the 10 years of my stay at the Clarke Institute remained in the Institute. Initially, work with this material was continued by Ken Lloyd. When in 1978 Ken moved to Synthelabo in Paris, I offered to Fred Lowy, the Head of the Clarke Institute at that time, to continue this work. Lowy liked the idea and I became the Head of the Clarke Institute's newly created "Human Brain Laboratory," commuting for more than 10 years between Vienna and Toronto. I divided the research work between animal experiments in Vienna and human brain work in Toronto. This enabled me to direct the easy-to-plan-ahead postmortem brain research work in Toronto, without requiring my continuous presence there. In 1980, Stephen Kish joined me from Tom Perry's laboratory in Vancouver, and soon he was able to take responsibility for the day-to-day operations of my new laboratory in the Clarke Institute.

Specific Striatal Dopamine Patterns and the Etiology of Parkinson's Disease

In the human brain laboratory we first concentrated on studying brain dopamine and other transmitters (including serotonin, noradrenaline,

GABA, glutamate, and cholinacetyl transferase) in brain disorders other than idiopathic Parkinson's disease, but accompanied by parkinsonian symptomatology. The results of these studies proved crucial when we tried to test the various hypotheses, just then put forward, postulating multiple causes of nigral cell death, thus implying a "multifactorial" etiology of Parkinson's disease. This, for us, amounted to the question: Had the striatal dopamine loss in Parkinson's disease a constant and typical pattern, or was it unpredictably variable as would be expected if multiple causative factors were involved? We carried out an elaborate inter- and subregional analysis of the dopamine patterns in the Parkinson striatum, showing that indeed Parkinson's disease had a very characteristic and constant striatal dopamine pattern. Since none of the other brain disorders with parkinsonian symptomatology mimicked the Parkinson pattern, we concluded that Parkinson's disease must have a specific etiology. By studying the striatal dopamine patterns during normal ageing, we also could disprove another idea on the possible etiology of Parkinson's disease, i.e., the "pathologically accelerated ageing of nigral dopamine neurones" hypothesis.

Beyond Parkinson's Disease

In the course of our human brain studies, we were the first, or among the first, to characterize biochemically many brain disorders other than idiopathic Parkinson's disease, among them heredity parkinsonism-dementia, neuronal intranuclear inclusion body disorders, Lesch-Nyhan syndrome, Down's syndrome, olivo-ponto-cerebellar-atrophy, fatal hyper-thermia syndrome, (human) narcolepsy, progressive supranuclear palsy, dialysis encephalopathy, cortico-basal ganglionic degeneration, spinocere-bellar ataxia, Huntington's disease, dementia-parkinsonism-motoneuron disease, and dystonia musculorum deformans.

To this list (that reads like a textbook of neurology) should be added a unique case (supplied by Ali Rajput) of dopa-responsive (Segawa) dystonia. Our corresponding study was the starting point for an in-depth search, including in the Clarke Institute (Yoshiaki Furukawa and Steve Kish), of the cause of this inborn (GTP cyclohydrolase I gene mutation) disorder affecting the nigrostriatal dopamine system.

Three Special Reasons for the Success of My Human Brain Laboratory

Apart from Steve Kish, who, being the right person in the right place, was gradually taking over—very successfully—my duties, a major reason for the success of my human brain laboratory had to do with another specific individual, Vivian Rakoff, Head of the Clarke Institute from 1980 to 1990. During each of my working stays at the human brain laboratory, Rakoff regularly offered me his support, asking me if there was anything extra he could do for my laboratory. He was crucial in helping me to maintain the technial staff (Kathleen Price-Shannak and others), add laboratory space and new equipment, and make Steve Kish stay at the Clarke Institute, so as to manage our daily human brain work. Moreover, the pleasure of the countless conversations with Vivian, enjoying his brilliant gift of speech and the poetic resonance of his spoken word, made these 10 years unforgettable for me.

And then, there was the indispensable Ali Rajput, Head of Neurology at the University of Saskatchewan at Saskatoon. For more than two decades, Rajput had been systematically collecting frozen brains of patients he himself had seen and treated for prolonged periods of time; these included, in addition to Parkinson patients, many other, quite rare conditions. Rajput offered me his collaboration, including his vast experience and neurological knowledge. Without his unique brain material we would not have been able to do even one-tenth of our human brain research. Over the many years of our collaboration, Ali and I developed an ever closer relationship, both professional and—for me especially precious—personal. We continue our collaboration in Ali's neurology research laboratory in Saskatoon.

Finally, there was my own expertise which I had acquired in the many years of collecting fresh, autopsied human brains and the knowledge of how to handle and dissect them in the frozen state. Especially important was the experience I gained in identifying and isolating the various regions of the brain from 2- to 3-mm thick (frozen) slices, always cut by hand. In the beginning, Riley's unsurpassed *Atlas of the Basal Ganglia, Brain Stem and Spinal Cord* and Olszewski and Baxter's *Cytoarchitecture of the Human Brain Stem* were of great help; later, I could do without them. It was as if, with time, the human brain had started speaking to me in a language I could ever better understand. My know-how was important for our studies which crucially depended on the correct identification and reproducibility of the brain regions dissected, some of them ill-defined or without definite borders. When in the late 1970s the idea of human brain tissue banks emerged, Earl Usdin (NIMH) and Tom Chase (NINDS) asked me to host an NI Health-sponsored "International Human Brain Dissection Workshop." The workshop took place September 14–15, 1979, in Vienna and was attended by experts from all over the world. To be asked to organize this workshop was an exquisite gesture of recognition of our contributions to this field.

On Having Reached "the Top"

When, as a fledgling M.D., I started in research, nothing appeared to me more desirable than advancing to a higher position and one day reaching the top. In my youthful inexperience, I thought that this would give me the highest degree of freedom of doing research as I pleased, without any obstacles, exclusively for myself. Later, when by good fortune I reached whatever was possible in my profession, I made a, possibly not too surprising, discovery: I realized that the opposite of what I imagined was true. When I review the beginnings of my career in research, I now see that it had been then that I had the greatest freedom, in the sense that, basically, I was responsible only for my own research, concerned with my own progress only. The higher I rose, the more of my time I had to give to the young people in the laboratory: helping them with formulating scientific concepts; teaching them (self) critical judgement; introducing them to the idea of the scientific method; trying to awaken in them the sense of wonder and reverence for nature, the object of all our inquiries; and, finally, taking responsibility for their actual research work, knowing how important it was for their future. Sometimes, all this was easy enough; sometimes, much sensibility was called for; and sometimes, a firmer guiding hand was required. All in all, the less they felt my hand, the more successful I considered my guidance. In short, in the course of my life in research, my efforts shifted from working for myself to serving others. Although to some this may appear a great pity, I think it is right: to pass on what one has received.

Arriving at the "Finishing Post"

When, in November 1991, I turned 65 and became Professor Emeritus at the University of Toronto, I could turn over to Steve Kish a well-organized, productive, widely known, and, in its way, unique research facility. Steve has since continued, at the highest level, the research tradition in my Clarke "creation," now renamed the "Human Neurochemical Pathology Laboratory."

In Vienna, I became Professor Emeritus in 1995, but I continued as acting Head of the Institute until February 1999. In that year, my Institute, together with the other three brain research laboratories, became part of the Institute for Brain Research, a newly founded research facility at our medical faculty—an idea I had been fighting for during the preceding 15 years. During those years, I could not avoid venturing into faculty politics. For the first time in my academic career I let myself be dragged into something like quarrels with colleagues; this happened when I tried to give the new Institute a structure that would guarantee its research as high a scientific standard as possible. Since my ideas would have meant both a change in the existing regulations on faculty structure and a shakeup within our brain research community, I suffered, not suprisingly, defeat on both fronts: "Nec Hercules contra plures!" The Institute opened its doors in early summer 2000. With peace and harmony long since restored, I am confident that the research done there will soon reach the goal I have envisaged for it.

People I Would Have Liked to Meet

As mentioned, I was lucky enough to meet, on my wanderings, and interact with practically everyone in my field of research and with most researchers of my generation in the other fields of neuroscience. Yet there are three individuals whom I would have liked to meet for very specific reasons.

Wilhelm Raab, a former Viennese and later Professor of Experimental Medicine at the University of Vermont at Burlington, was the first to discover, in the late 1940s, a catecholamine-like compound in the animal and human brain, with highest concentrations in the basal ganglia (caudate nucleus). Raab also was the first to inject (i.p.) D,L-dopa in order to increase the level of his new compound in the rat brain. He analyzed the caudate nucleus of 10 psychotic patients, but, unpardonably, did not think of looking at even a single Parkinson brain. I would have liked to talk to Raab, the inventive all-round experimentalist gifted with genius, to find out what kind of person he was, to hear his views on the conceiving of extraordinary ideas (of which he had so many) and on the process of discovery, and possibly also to talk with him about the bitter reality of the missed opportunities as the darker side of life as a researcher. A few months before I could visit him, Raab died in 1970 at the age of 75 "of a self-inflicted bullet wound" (*JAMA* 1970; 214: 2348).

I could have easily met the Vienna-educated Erwin Chargaff, later at the Biochemistry Department at Columbia University, at Mel Yahr's 1965 symposium at Columbia; he was a discussant of Holger Hydén's presentation. However, I missed him at the meeting. I heard him speak many years earlier in Vienna at the International Biochemistry Congress in the summer of 1958. I remember my satisfaction when Chargaff mentioned, in his opening lecture, Blaise Pascal, my favourite "thinking reed." I also remember him pondering over the fact that "with the increase in the radius of our ever expanding sphere of knowledge, also the circumference of the unknown that surrounds us, increases." I would have liked to hear Chargaff's ideas about what he thought knowledge was, how he would distinguish it from understanding, and whether amassing knowledge really led to greater understanding; I would also have questioned him about his worries and concerns about the direction in which the present-day science is moving.

I would have had little opportunity to meet Oxford's distinguished physiologist (Sir) Charles Sherrington. He died in 1952, more than four years before my time in Oxford. When reading his treatise *Man on His Nature*, I was struck most of all by the absolute honesty with which Sherrington, the scientist, posed his fundamental questions about the human condition (Sherrington, 1940). I do not think that these questions have been fully answered yet, not even by his famous pupil (Sir) John Eccles, in my opinion. I would have liked to listen to Sherrington-the-poet's musings about the intriguing, but not too rare, association between the poetic and the scientific mind, and about his problems with the scientific mind of Goethe, the poet; hear what he thought today, against the background of his *Man on His Nature* of 1940, about the enigma of that "mindful" brain of ours, priding itself on perceiving everything there is in nature but itself being a piece of the nature perceived; and what he would have to say about the prospects and promises of the now apparently established discipline of *neurophilosophy*, as the newest and most challenging branch of our present-day neuroscience.

Looking Back

Looking back at the years I spent in research, first in Vienna and then in Toronto, and finally on both sides of the Atlantic, I am surprised to see that I have achieved everything I could have wished for. I feel happy that I so much enjoyed what I have been doing during the more than 50 years and I knew how to do. The support and recognition I received for my work, I have accepted with gratitude, as a charming reminder to do more and better. Yet the time I spent in research would, without a doubt, have meant much less to me without the friends I made during all those years; I have just recently been reminded of how many of them I do have (see, Rajput, 2001).

Coda

Apart from mentioning, here and there, my family, I have not yet said anything about my private life during the time I spent in research. The happiest part of it was, quite simply, life with my wife Christina. I married Christina in 1962. She bore me four children, a girl and three boys, each of whom I am affectionately proud of, and she has accompanied and supported me on all my wanderings and in all my endeavours for more than 40 years now. Before, however, falling into the trap of stereotypes or trivialities, I will let Robert Louis Stevenson speak for me. In his account on *An Inland Voyage*, Stevenson (1992) writes: "We asked him [Bazin, the innkeeper] how he managed in La Fère. 'I am married', he said, 'and I have my pretty children ...' We sat in front of the door ... Madame Bazin came out after a while; she was tired with her day's work, I suppose; and she nestled up to her husband and laid her head upon his breast. He had his arm about her and kept gently patting her shoulder. I think Bazin was right, and he was really married. Of how few people can the same be said!"

Having come to an end with my simple and uncomplicated life's story, what remains for me to do is give thanks—as the day is drawing to a close and the shadows lengthen—to all those mentioned in my account and the many others, although unmentioned, yet so close to the heart of my memory.

I cannot think of a better way of taking leave of you all than, as many years ago, with the lines of W. H. Auden (1991):

Fondly I ponder You all:
without You I couldn't have managed
even my weakest of lines.

Selected Bibliography

Baran H, Lassmann H, Sperk G, Seitelberger F, Hornykiewicz O. Effect of mannitol treatment on brain neurotransmitter markers in kainic acid-induced epilepsy. *Neuroscience* 1987;21:679–684.

Barolin GS, Bernheimer H, Hornykiewicz O. Side differences in brain dopamine (3-hydroxytyramine) levels in a case with hemiparkinsonism. (In German) *Schweiz Arch Neurol Neurochir Psychiatr* 1964;94:241–248.

Berger ML, Lassmann H, Hornykiewicz O. Limbic seizures without brain damage after injection of low doses of kainic acid into the amygdala of freely moving rats. *Brain Res* 1989;489:261–272.

Berger M, Sperk G, Hornykiewicz O. Serotonergic devenervation partially protects rat striatum from kainic acid toxicity. *Nature* 1982;299:254–256.

Bernheimer H, Birkmayer W, Hornykiewicz O, Jellinger K, Seitelberger F. Brain dopamine and the syndromes of Parkinson and Huntington: Clinical, morphological and neurochemical correlations. *J Neurol Sci* 1973;20:415–455.

Birkmayer W, Hornykiewicz O. The effect of L-3,4-dihydroxyphenylalanine (= DOPA) on the Parkinsonian akinesia. (In German) *Wien Klin Wochenschr* 1961;73:787–788. (Republished in English translation in *Parkinsonism Related Disorders* 1998;4:59–60.)

Birkmayer W, Hornykiewicz O. The effect of L-dihydroxyphenylalanine (= L-DOPA) in the Parkinsonian syndrome in man: On the pathogenesis and treatment of Parkinsonian akinesia. (In German) *Arch Psychiatr Gesamte Neurol* 1962;203: 560–564.

Bernheimer H, Hornykiewicz O. Decreased concentration of homovanillic acid in the brain of Parkinsonian patients: Result of a disturbance of central metabolism of dopamine. (In German) *Klin Wochenschr* 1965;43:711–715.

Born GVR, Hornykiewicz O, Stafford A. The uptake of adrenaline and noradrenaline by blood platelets of the pig. *Br J Pharmacol* 1958;13:411–414.

Ehringer H, Hornykiewicz O. Distribution of noradrenaline and dopamine (3-hydroxytyramine) in human brain: Their behaviour in extrapyramidal system diseases. (In German) *Klin Wochenschr* 1960;38:1236–1239. (Republished in English translation in *Parkinsonism Related Disorders* 1998;4:53–57).

Farley I, Price KS, McCullough E, Deck JHN, Hordynski W, Hornykiewicz O. Norepinephrine in chronic paranoid schizophrenia: Above-normal levels in limbic forebrain. *Science* 1978;200:456–458.

Furukawa Y, Shimadzu M, Rajput AH, Shimizu Y, Tagawa T, Mori H, Yokogochi M, Narabayashi N, Hornykiewicz O, Mizuno Y, Kish SJ. GTP-cyclohydrolase I gene mutations in hereditary progressive and dopa-responsive dystonia. *Ann Neurol* 1996;39:609–617.

Gastager H, Hornykiewicz O, Tschabitscher H. Copper and *p*-polyphenol oxidase in the blood serum of cases with clinically manifest and sub-clinical forms of hepatolenticular disease. (In German) *Wien Zeitschr Nervenheilkd* 1954;9: 312–319.

Hinzen D, Hornykiewicz O, Kobinger W, Pichler L, Pifl C, Schingnitz G. The dopamine autoreceptor agonist B-HT 920 stimulates denervated postsynaptic brain dopamine receptors in rodent and primate models of Parkinson's disease: A novel approach to treatment. *Eur J Pharmacol* 1986;131:75–86.

Holzer G, Hornykiewicz O. Dopamine (hydroxytyramine) metabolism in the rat brain. (In German) *Naunyn-Schmiedeberg's Arch Exp Pathol Pharmakol* 1959;237:27–33.

Hornykiewicz O. The action of dopamine on the arterial blood pressure of the guinea-pig. *Br J Pharmacol* 1958;13:91–94.

Hornykiewicz O. Topography and behaviour of noradrenaline and dopamine (3-hydroxytyramine) in the substantia nigra of normal and Parkinsonian patients. (In German) *Wien Klin Wochenschr* 1963;75:309–312.

Hornykiewicz O. Dopamine (3-hydroxytyramine) and brain function. *Pharmacol Rev* 1966a;18:925–964.

Hornykiewicz O. Metabolism of brain dopamine in human Parkinsonism: Neurochemical and clinical aspects. In Costa E, Cote LJ, Yahr MD, eds. *Biochemistry and pharmacology of the basal ganglia.* Proc. of the 2nd Symposium of the Parkinson's Disease Information and Research Center, Columbia University, New York, 1965. Hewlett, NY:Raven Press, 1966b;171–181.

Hornykiewicz O. Parkinson's disease: From brain homogenate to treatment. *Fed Proc* 1973;32:183–190.

Hornykiewicz O. Psychopharmacological implications of dopamine and dopamine antagonists: A critical evaluation of current evidence. *Annu Rev Pharmacol Toxicol* 1977;17:545–559.

Hornykiewicz O. From dopamine to Parkinson's disease: A personal research record. In Samson F, Adelman G, eds. *The neurosciences: paths of discovery, II.* New York: Birkhäuser, 1992;125–147.

Hornykiewicz O. Levodopa in the 1960s: Starting point Vienna. In Poewe W, Lees AJ, eds. *20 years of Madopar—new avenues.* Basle: Editiones Roche, 1994;11–27.

Hornykiewicz O. Dopamine miracle: From brain homogenate to dopamine replacement. *Movement Disorders* 2002a;17:501–508.

Hornykiewicz O. Brain dopamine: A historical perspective. In DiChiara G, ed. *Handbook of experimental pharmacology, vol. 154/I: Dopamine in the CNS I.* Berlin: Springer-Verlag, 2002b;1–22.

Hornykiewicz O, Kish SJ. Biochemical pathophysiology of Parkinson's disease. *Adv Neurol* 1986;45:19–34.

Hornykiewicz O, Kish SJ, Becker LE, Farley I, Shannak K. Brain neurotransmitters in dystonia musculorum deformans. *New Engl J Med* 1986;315:347–353.

Hornykiewicz O, Lisch HJ, Springer A. Homovanillic acid in different regions of the human brain: Attempt at localizing central dopamine fibres. *Brain Res* 1968;11:662–671.

Hornykiewicz O, Niebauer G. The polyphenol oxidase in the human blood serum. (In German) *Arch Exp Pathol Pharmakol* 1953;218:448–456.

Hörtnagl H, Berger ML, Havelec L, Hornykiewicz O. Role of glucocorticoids in the cholinergic degeneration in rat hippocampus induced by ethylcholine arizidinium (AF64A). *J Neurosci* 1993;13:2939–2945.

Hörtnagl H, Berger ML, Reither H, Hornykiewicz O. Cholinergic deficit induced by ethylcholine aziridinium (AF64A) in rat hippocampus: Effect on glutamatergic systems. *Naunyn-Schmiedeberg's Arch Pharmacol* 1991;344:213–219.

Kish SJ, Chang LJ, Mirchandani L, Shannak K, Hornykiewicz O. Progressive supranuclear palsy: Relationship between extrapyramidal disturbances, dementia, and brain neurotransmitter markers. *Ann Neurol* 1985;18:530–536.

Kish SJ, Karlinsky H, Becker L, Gilbert J, Rebbetoy M, Chang LJ, DiStefano L, Hornykiewicz O. Down's syndrome individuals begin life with normal levels of brain cholinergic markers. *J Neurochem* 1989;52:1183–1187.

Kish SJ, Perry TL, Hornykiewicz O. Benzodiazepine receptor binding in cerebellar cortex: Observations in olivopontocerebellar atrophy. *J Neurochem* 1984;42: 466–469.

Kish SJ, Rajput A, Gilbert J, Rozdilsky B, Chang LJ, Shannak K, Hornykiewicz O. Elevated γ-aminobutyric acid level in striatal but not extrastriatal brain regions in Parkinson's disease: Correlation with striatal dopamine loss. *Ann Neurol* 1986;20:26–31.

Kish SJ, Shannak K, Hornykiewicz O. Uneven pattern of dopamine loss in the striatum of patients with idiopathic Parkinson's disease. Pathophysiologic and clinical implications. *New Engl J Med* 1988;318:876–880.

Kish SJ, Shannak KS, Perry TL, Hornykiewicz O. Neuronal [3H]benzodiazepine binding and levels of GABA, glutamate, and taurine are normal in Huntington's disease cerebellum. *J Neurochem* 1983;41:1495–1497.

Kish SJ, Shannak K, Rajput A, Deck JHN, Hornykiewicz O. Aging produces a specific pattern of striatal dopamine loss: Implications for the etiology of idiopathic Parkinson's disease. *J Neurochem* 1992;58:642–648.

Lee T, Seeman P, Rajput A, Farley IJ, Hornykiewicz O. Receptor basis for dopaminergic supersensitivity in Parkinson's disease. *Nature* 1978;273:59–61.

Lee T, Seeman P, Tourtellotte WW, Farley IJ, Hornykiewicz O. Binding of 3H-neuroleptics and 3H-apomorphine in schizophrenic brains. *Nature* 1978;274:897–900.

Lloyd KG, Davidson L, Hornykiewicz O. The neurochemistry of Parkinson's disease: Effect of L-dopa therapy. *J Pharmacol Exp Ther* 1975;195:453–464.

Lloyd K, Hornykiewicz O. Occurrence and distribution of L-DOPA decarboxylase in the human brain. *Brain Res* 1970a;22:426–428.

Lloyd K, Hornykiewicz O. Parkinson's disease: Activity of L-Dopa decarboxylase in discrete brain regions. *Science* 1970b;170:1212–1213.

Lloyd KG, Hornykiewicz O. Occurrence and distribution of aromatic L-amino acid (L-DOPA) decarboxylase in the human brain. *J Neurochem* 1972;19:1549–1559.

Lloyd KG, Hornykiewicz O, Davidson L, Shannak K, Farley I, Goldstein M, Shibuya M, Kelley WN, Fox IH. Biochemical evidence of dysfunction of brain neurotransmitters in the Lesch-Nyhan syndrome. *New Engl J Med* 1981;305:1106–1111.

Pifl Ch, Hornykiewicz O, Giros B, Caron MG. Catecholamine transporters and 1-methyl-4-phenyl-1,2,3,6-tetrahydropyridine neurotoxicity: Studies comparing the cloned human noradrenaline and human dopamine transporter. *J Pharmacol Exp Ther* 1996;277:1437–1443.

Pifl Ch, Nanoff Ch, Schingnitz G, Schütz W, Hornykiewicz O. Sensitization of dopamine-stimulated adenylyl cyclase in the striatum of 1-methyl-4-phenyl-1,2,3,6-tetrahydropyridine-treated rhesus monkeys and patients with idiopathic Parkinson's disease. *J Neurochem* 1992;58:1997–2004.

Pifl Ch, Schingnitz G, Hornykiewicz O. The neurotoxin MPTP does not reproduce in the rhesus monkey the interregional pattern of striatal dopamine loss typical of human idiopathic Parkinson's disease. *Neurosci Lett* 1988;92:228–233.

Pifl Ch, Schingnitz G, Hornykiewicz O. Effect of 1-methyl-4-phenyl-1,2,3,6-tetrahydropyridine on the regional distribution of brain monoamines in the rhesus monkey. *Neuroscience* 1991;44:591–605.

Pifl C, Zezula J, Spittler A, Kattinger A, Reither H, Caron MG, Hornykiewicz O. Antiproliferative action of dopamine and norepinephrine in neuroblastoma cells expressing the human dopamine transporter. *FASEB J* 2001;15:1607–1609.

Rajput AH, Gibb WRG, Zhong XH, Shannak KS, Kish S, Chang LG, Hornykiewicz O. Dopa-responsive dystonia: Pathological and biochemical observations in a case. *Ann Neurol* 1994;35:396–402.

Sperk G, Berger M, Hörtnagl H, Hornykiewicz O. Kainic acid-induced changes of serotonin and dopamine metabolism in the striatum and substantia nigra of the rat. *Eur J Pharmacol* 1981;74:279–286.

Sperk G, Lassmann H, Baran H, Kish SJ, Seitelberger F, Hornykiewicz O. Kainic acid-induced seizures: Neurochemical and histopathological changes. *Neuroscience* 1983;10:1301–1315.

Sperk G, Lassmann H, Baran H, Seitelberger F, Hornykiewicz O. Kainic acid-induced seizures: Dose-relationship of behavioural, neurochemical and histopathological changes. *Brain Res* 1985;338:289–295.

Literature Cited in the Text

Auden WH. A thanksgiving. In Mendelson E, ed. *Collected poems*. New York:Vintage Books-Random House Inc., 1991.

Bertler Å, Rosengren E. Occurrence and distribution of dopamine in brain and other tissues. *Experientia* 1959a;15:10–11.

Bertler Å, Rosengren E. On the distribution in brain of monoamines and of eznymes responsible for their formation. *Experientia* 1959b;15:382–383.

Blaschko H. Metabolism and storage of biogenic amines. *Experientia* 1957;13:9–12.

Cotzias GC, van Woert MH, Schiffer LM. Aromatic amino acids and modification of parkinsonism. *New Engl J Med* 1967;276:374–379.

Dante Alighieri. *The divine comedy*, Inferno, Canto XXXIV, verses 138–139. Verse translation by Mandelbaum A. New York: Bantam Books, 1980.

Degkwitz R, Frowein R, Kulenkampff C, Mohs U. Über die Wirkungen des L-DOPA beim Menschen und deren Beeinflussung durch Reserpin, Chlorpromazin, Iproniazid und Vitamin B6. *Klin Wochenschr* 1961;73:787–788.

Everett GM. Evidence for dopamine as a central neuromodulator: Neurological and behavioral implications. In Barbeau A, McDowell FH, eds. *L-dopa and parkinsonism*. Philadelphia: FA Davis, 1970;364–368.

Green G. The third man. In *The third man and the fallen idol*. London-New York: Penguin Books, 1971.

Hertting G, Axelrod J. Fate of tritiated noradrenaline at the sympathetic nerve endings. *Nature* 1961;192:172–173.

Holtz P, Credner K. Die enzymatische Entstehung von Oxytyramin im Organismus und die physiologische Bedeutung der Dopadecarboxylase. *Arch Exp Pathol Pharmakol* 1942;200:356–388.

Homer. *Odyssey*, Book 4, verses 219–230. Translated by Rien EV. London-New York: Penguin Books, 1991.

Jasper HH. Neurophysiological mechanisms in parkinsonism. In Barbeau A, McDowell FH, eds. *L-dopa and parkinsonism*. Philadelphia: FA Davis, 1970; 408–411.

Penfield W. *The mystery of the mind*. Princeton, NJ: Princeton University Press, 1975.

Rajput AH. Open letter to the committee on the Nobel Prize in medicine. *Parkinsonism and Related Disorders* 2001;7:149–155 (see also, *Science* 2000;291:567–569).

Sherrington CS. *Man on his nature*. London: Cambridge University Press, 1940.

Stevenson RL. An inland voyage. In *Travels with a donkey in the Cevennes and selected travel writings*. The World's Classics, Oxford-New York: Oxford University Press, 1992.

Vogt M. Discussion. In Vane JR, Wolstenholme GEW, O'Connor M, eds. *Adrenergic mechanisms*. Ciba Foundation Symposium, London: Churchill, 1960;578.

Vogt M. Functional aspects of the role of catecholamines in the central nervous system. *Br Med Bull* 1973;29:168–172.

Ward AA. Physiological implications in the dyskinesias. In Barbeau A, McDowell FH, eds. *L-dopa and parkinsonism*. Philadelphia: FA Davis, 1970;151–159.

Andrew Huxley

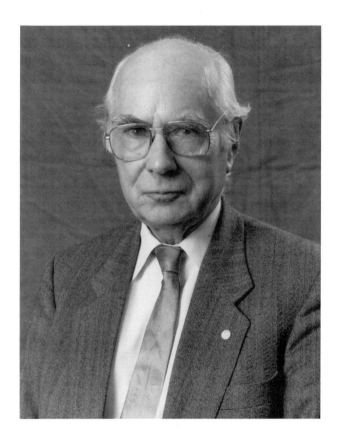

Andrew F. Huxley

BORN:

Hampstead, London, UK
November 22, 1917

EDUCATION:

University College School, London (1925)
Westminster School, London (1930)
Cambridge University, Trinity College, B.A. (1939)

APPOINTMENTS:

Operational Research, Anti-Aircraft Command (1940)
Fellow Trinity College, Cambridge (1941–1960, 1990–)
Operational Research, Admiralty, London (1942)
Physiology Department, Cambridge, Demonstrator (1945)
Assistant Director of Research (1951)
Reader in Experimental Biophysics (1959)
Jodrell Professor and Head of Department of Physiology,
University College London (1960)
Royal Society Research Professor (1969–1983)
President of the Royal Society (1980–1985)
Master of Trinity College, Cambridge (1984–1990)

HONORS AND AWARDS:

Fellow of the Royal Society (1955)
Nobel Prize in Physiology or Medicine (1963)
Copley Medal, Royal Society (1973)
Knight Bachelor (1974)
Honorary Sc.D., Cambridge (1978)
Foreign Associate, National Academy of Sciences USA
(1979)
Order of Merit, UK (1983)
Grand Cordon of the Sacred Treasure, Japan (1995)

*Andrew Huxley studied nerve conduction in the squid giant fiber jointly
with Alan Hodgkin and in myelinated fibers with Robert Stampfli. Later,
he turned to muscle contraction, proposing the sliding-filament theory
simultaneously with H.E. Huxley and contributing to both theoretical and
experimental studies.*

Andrew F. Huxley

T he Huxley family into which I was born is well known for three of its members: my grandfather Thomas Henry Huxley (1825–1895), the 19th-century biologist, and two of my half-brothers, Julian Huxley (1887–1975), biologist, and Aldous Huxley (1894–1963), novelist. Huxley is not a common surname, but it is also not very rare; it is the name of a village in Cheshire in northwestern England. I am not detectably related to Dr. Hugh Huxley, and it is pure coincidence that, in the same year, he and I independently got onto the idea that muscle contraction takes place by relative sliding motion of two sets of filaments. Leonard G.H. Huxley, a physicist who became Vice-Chancellor of the Australian National University in Canberra, was my third cousin.

T.H. Huxley wrote a short autobiography which includes the following passage:

As I grew older, my great desire was to be a mechanical engineer, but the Fates were against this; and, while very young, I commenced the study of Medicine under a medical brother-in-law. But, though the Institute of Mechanical Engineers would certainly not own me, I am not sure that I have not, all along, been a sort of mechanical engineer in *partibus infidelium*.... The only part of my professional course which really and deeply interested me was Physiology, which is the mechanical engineering of living machines.

Much of the same could be said of me: my boyhood interests were mainly mechanical, and I entered Cambridge University with the intention of specializing in physics and becoming an engineer. My subsequent interest in physiology is exactly described by the phrase "the mechanical engineering of living machines," and a substantial part of my work has been the design and construction of instruments needed for my research.

T.H. Huxley is best remembered as "Darwin's bulldog," on account of his vigorous defence of the theory of evolution by natural selection after the publication of Charles Darwin's *Origin of Species*. His interest in physiology continued throughout his life. Although he never did any original research in physiology, he was influential through lectures and a small textbook and especially through stimulating the development of physiology as an independent subject in England. It was on the strength of his advice that Trinity College in 1870 started Cambridge physiology by appointing Michael Foster as a teaching Fellow in the subject, thus establishing a strong tradition in physiology which I found when I entered the college as an undergraduate in 1935. It was also on his advice that T.J.P. Jodrell gave money to University College London to establish a full-time professorship of physiology (the first in England); I held that post from 1960 to 1969. T.H. Huxley's own research was in comparative anatomy and palaeontology; he was also very influential as a promoter of science and education and through his many lectures and essays on a wide variety of topics.

T.H. Huxley coined the word "agnostic" to describe his own position in relation to the existence of a deity. He was explicitly not an atheist, taking the view that there was no way of getting reliable knowledge of the existence or the nature of any deity. My father followed him in this respect and so have I.

My father Leonard (1860–1933) was the second of his three sons; the eldest died at the age of four and the youngest became a doctor who made a successful career as a first-rate physician and general practitioner, but was not responsible for any particular advance in medicine. His son Michael was in the Foreign Office, but left in order to found the Geographical Magazine. Of the daughters of T.H. Huxley, the eldest married an architect, Frederick Waller. Sir Crispin Tickell (formerly Ambassador to Mexico and British Permanent Representative to the United Nations, and Warden of Green College, Oxford 1990–1997) is their great-grandson. The second was herself a talented painter and married the well-known painter John Collier, but died after having one daughter; Collier later married T.H. Huxley's youngest daughter and their son Laurence was in the Foreign Office and became Ambassador to Norway. Another daughter married Alfred Eckersley, an engineer and builder of railways in Mexico and South America. Their three sons were all important figures in the early days of radio: Thomas was elected as a Fellow of the Royal Society for his theoretical work on transmission and reflection of radio waves, Peter was chief engineer to the British Broadcasting Corporation, and Roger was on its programme side.

My father was a classical scholar and for some years taught Latin and Greek, first at St Andrews University and then at Charterhouse School, a well-known boy's school in Surrey, south of London. He then turned to a literary career, writing several biographies, notably, the standard *Life and Letters* of T.H. Huxley (published in 1900), followed by a similar life of Joseph Hooker, one of the leading botanists of the 19th century and a very close friend both of Charles Darwin and of T.H. Huxley. He then worked for the publishers Smith Elder until that firm came to an end in 1916 with the suicide of its head, Reginald Smith (son-in-law, not son, of the George Smith who had built the reputation of the firm in the 19th century). The business was taken over by another long-standing publishing firm, John Murray, and my father worked for them until the end of his life as a reader and later as editor of the *Cornhill*, a literary magazine. Although in no way a professional scientist, he was very knowledgeable about science, not only the biology that he had learned from his father and from writing his father's life, but he was familiar with physics and chemistry at an elementary level. He was a lover of the countryside and knew most of the birds and wild flowers that we came across when out for a walk. He was a keen gardener.

Much about the Huxley family is to be found in *The Huxleys* by Ronald Clark.

My father and his first wife, Julia Frances Arnold, were married in 1885. She was a granddaughter of Thomas Arnold who, as Headmaster of Rugby School, had set a new standard for schooling in England early in the 19th century. Her eldest sister was Mary Ward (Mrs. Humphry Ward), novelist and social reformer, whose daughter Janet became the wife of the historian George Trevelyan. This connection was very important to me, since I came to know them and other members of the Trevelyan family closely as a result of it.

The eldest son of my father's first marriage was Julian Huxley, another biologist whose interests were mainly in animal behavior, in animal development, and in evolution, but who also became well known for his essays on a wide range of public questions. His interests in biology were very different from mine, and I do not think that I was much influenced by him in that respect. Their third son was Aldous Huxley, the novelist. Julian and Aldous were a generation older than myself, so they were like uncles to me and to my one full brother David (1915–1992, later a lawyer who spent his working life in Bermuda and in the United States). I saw them often until Aldous's move to the United States in 1939 and Julian's death in 1975. Both were very good company, though in different styles: Julian was full of stories and very entertaining; Aldous was quieter, but his conversation was always full of interest.

Julia Huxley died in 1908, and four years later my father married Rosalind Bruce as his second wife. She was 30 years his junior and survived him by more than 60 years, dying in 1994 at the age of 104. Her father William Wallace Bruce, who died in 1907, had been a successful London merchant, importing from the West Indies and the Mediterranean and with interests in shipping. He retired at the age of 45 and devoted himself to social matters. He was elected as a member of the London County Council, serving on its Finance Committee and its Housing Committee. He was deeply involved in slum clearance, notably, in the Seven Dials district of London. He was also a Major in the Artists' Corps of Volunteers. His father was born in Northern Ireland and had come to London after spending several years as a merchant in Demerara, where he became a member of the government and Councillor of the Supreme Court of Civil and Criminal Justice. His forebears had included several Presbyterian and Unitarian ministers distinguished enough to be included in the Dictionary of National Biography. My mother's maternal grandfather was Thomas Fielding Johnson, who owned and ran a spinning mill in Leicester. He gave the land and the initial building (previously a lunatic asylum) for the University College of Leicester (later Leicester University) and was also a notable benefactor to the Leicester Infirmary.

My mother had strong native intelligence, but was not of an intellectual turn of mind and had not been at a university. She was very skillful with her hands, particularly in wood-carving and needlework, and she encouraged my brother and myself in woodwork and metalwork, which stood me in good stead during my research career. She was brought up as a Unitarian, but did not continue as a churchgoer after her marriage.

Boyhood

I was born (1917) and brought up in Hampstead (north London). My interests were mainly mechanical. My brother and I played a lot with a set of wooden bricks; we made things with Meccano, a toy consisting of metal strips and plates with holes through which they could be joined with nuts and bolts, together with rods, wheels, and cogs so that an unlimited range of working models could be constructed; and we played with clockwork trains ($1\frac{1}{4}$ in. gauge). I made things for the railway from wood and metal. My parents bought for us a metal-turning, screw-cutting treadle lathe (Drummond 4 in. round-bed) which I still possess; I have used it throughout my career for making my own apparatus. In my teens, I added several features to it: divisions on the movements, two four-start worm gears to obtain finer automatic feeds, and a clutch on the main shaft so that a screw-cutting tool would automatically return to the correct position to deepen the thread it was cutting after disconnecting and re-engaging the clutch.

Microscopes were another boyhood interest. When I was about 12, my parents gave my brother and me a small microscope (top magnification of about 200X), and later, I had the use of two 19th-century microscopes that had belonged to members of my mother's family. I learnt about microscopes and microscopy from *The Microscope: A Practical Handbook* by L.H. Drew & L. Wright which was given to me by my half-brother Julian. Toward the end of my schooldays, I chose as a prize *Applications of Interferometry* by W. Ewart Williams, by which I was introduced to the concept of an interference microscope (this bore fruit later when I developed an interference microscope for the research on muscle which I started when Hodgkin and I had finished our work on nerves). I do not think I began taking photographs down a microscope until my student days at Cambridge.

For many years, I collected butterflies and moths (often rearing them from caterpillars), both on weekend expeditions, in our Hampstead garden, and when we were on holiday. This was, I think, a pure collector's instinct. In the same way, one summer I collected ferns, and another summer, I collected grasses, sedges, and rushes. I did not have much interest in living things as such; for most of my childhood we had no pets, though later on we had a cat. I was once given a nest of ants between two sheets of glass, so that one could watch their activities; I kept this for some years, feeding the ants with sugar solution. I watched them with interest, but not systematically. I remember reading *Ants, Bees and Wasps* by Sir John Lubbock (Lord Avebury).

We spent our summer holidays at Connel Ferry, near Oban, on the west coast of Scotland, where my mother's mother owned a holiday house; sometimes we stayed in that house, but sometimes it was occupied by other branches of the family and we then rented another house in the same village. We had a rowing boat with an outboard motor on Loch Etive, but did not sail. Our main occupations were picnicking with boat(s) or car(s), often jointly with uncles, aunts, and cousins; climbing the hills (no rock climbing); and coarse fishing in the loch. At Easter, we often went to other houses that my grandmother rented for use by her daughters and their families, first at Thorpeness near Aldeburgh on the east coast of England and later at Felpham near Bognor on the south coast. At Easter 1931, my grandmother took my parents, my brother, and myself on a Hellenic cruise during which we visited cities on the Dalmatian coast and most of the famous sites in Greece and Sicily, preceded by a few days in Venice and finishing with a few days in the south of France. Until my father's death in 1933, my parents regularly spent a couple of weeks in Switzerland each winter for skating (English-style figure skating) and another two weeks in May touring in the northwest of Scotland.

We often drove out of London for the day at weekends, usually either to the parts of Surrey that my father had known when he was a Master at Charterhouse and when his first wife was Headmistress of the girls' school Prior's Field that she had founded (and where we often dropped in for tea) or to Ivinghoe and Ashridge on the Chiltern Hills, northwest of London, near Albury where Mrs. Humphry Ward, sister of my father's first wife, had lived.

Schooling

I was never at a boarding school. Before going to school, I was taught for about a year (1924–1925) by a governess, who came because my brother was kept at home after an attack of measles followed by pneumonia. I then went to University College School in Hampstead, junior branch 1925–1929 and senior branch 1929–1930. My parents then moved me (as they had moved my brother) to Westminster School, where I had the main part of my secondary schooling (1930–1935). It had originated as a school attached to the monastery of which Westminster Abbey was the church, and after the monastery was dissolved by Henry VIII, the school was refounded by Queen Elizabeth I and became one of the leading schools in Britain. I was elected to a non-residential scholarship at the end of my first year.

For my first two years (including one year after taking School Certificate) I did classics and reached the point of enjoying much of the Latin and Greek literature that we read, but my real interests were clearly in the sciences and my parents persuaded the headmaster (with some difficulty) to allow me to switch to the science side. I was extremely well taught in physics by J.S. Rudwick (father of M.J.S. Rudwick, well known as a historian of geology); I was also well taught in mathematics. I did not find chemistry interesting and had only a small amount of biology. I was not particularly good at games; we played soccer in the winter and I played tennis in the summer. I also played a good deal of Eton fives (a ball game in which the players hit the [hard] ball with their hands in a court modeled on the space between two buttresses of a building at Eton School). I was often the youngest in my form. I won several book prizes for being top of my form and also several prizes for pieces of good work, in the shape of Maundy money (silver penny, twopenny, threepenny, and fourpenny pieces, not in general circulation but minted primarily for distribution by the King or Queen to the poor at an ancient ceremony on Maundy Thursday, the day before Good Friday).

University Education, 1935–1939

In those days, there were closed scholarships from Westminster School to Christ Church, Oxford, and closed exhibitions to Trinity College, Cambridge (all such awards have since been abolished). My brother went to Christ Church in 1934 with one of the scholarships to read PPE (politics, philosophy, and economics), but I went to Trinity, Cambridge in the next year with one of the exhibitions and a major open scholarship, won in examinations in physics, chemistry, and mathematics. My father and all my half-brothers had also been at Oxford (Balliol College), but the choice of Cambridge for me was partly because of its higher reputation at that time for science, partly because my mother (this was after my father's death) thought it would be better for me to be at a different place from my elder brother and partly because of our friendship with George Trevelyan, he being then Regius Professor of Modern History at Cambridge and a Fellow of Trinity College. The choice turned out to be of great importance for my career as I went up with the intention of specializing in physics; if I had gone to Oxford I would not have had the opportunity of switching to physiology, as I did with no difficulty at Cambridge.

At Cambridge University, the courses for degrees ("triposes") are divided into two parts, with much flexibility allowing for change after Part I. For Part I (the first two years of the course in natural sciences) it was natural for me to take physics and chemistry as whole subjects (two-year courses) and mathematics as a half-subject. The regulations required me to take a third experimental science, and I chose physiology on the advice of Ben Delisle Burns (1915–2001, later a distinguished neurophysiologist) who had been a boyhood friend in Hampstead and was then an undergraduate at King's College, Cambridge: he told me that physiology was a lively subject in which even in the first year newly discovered things, and things still controversial, were taught, unlike the situation in physics or chemistry. At Cambridge (as also at Oxford) an important part of the teaching consists of spending an hour a week, either alone or with one or two other undergraduates, with a member of the teaching staff of the College. Most of these "supervisions" that I was given were in physiology, and these were given by William Rushton and F.J.W. (Jack) Roughton, both Fellows of the Royal Society and well known for their research, respectively, in nerve conduction and color vision and in the carriage of gases by the blood. I found the subject much more stimulating than physics or chemistry, partly because of their teaching and partly because the course in physics did not take me far beyond what I had learned at Westminster. Another Fellow of Trinity College and Lecturer in the Department of Physiology who influenced me toward switching to physiology was Glenn A. Millikan, son of R.A. Millikan who determined the charge on the electron by the oil-drop experiment. He was an exceptionally friendly and lively person who was extremely good to many undergraduates of my generation. He allowed me to assist him in a small way with his experiments, measuring changes in the oxygenation of myoglobin in active muscles by a photoelectric method and later in the development of a spectrophotometer for biochemical use (never completed on account of the war). Millikan married the elder of the two daughters of George Mallory who was killed on Mt. Everest. At the outbreak of war they moved to the United States, where he held a post at Vanderbilt University. He developed a photoelectric device for measuring the oxygenation of the blood of aircraft pilots. Sadly, he was killed in a climbing accident shortly after the war.

My interest in physiology was also stimulated by other members of Trinity College a few years older than myself whom I met socially through living in the same college, notably, Alan Hodgkin (1914–1998; a Junior Research Fellow from October 1936 and Master of the College, 1978–1984) and David K. Hill, an undergraduate one year senior to me who followed his father A.V. Hill as a distinguished muscle physiologist. Others were R.L.M. Synge (inventor of partition chromatography with A.J.P. Martin, Nobel Prize, 1952); John Kendrew (collaborator of Max Perutz in the determination of protein structure, Nobel Prize, 1962); J.H. Humphrey, M.R. Pollock, and P.G.H. Gell (all of these later became Fellows of the Royal Society); A.H. Gordon and B.M. Wright (later of the National Institute for Medical Research); and E.D. Barlow (later psychiatrist, Head of the London Zoo, and Chairman of Cambridge Scientific Instrument Co., founded by his grandfather Horace Darwin).

As a result of these influences, I decided toward the end of my second year to do Part II of the Tripos in physiology, not physics. I was advised by

E.D. Adrian (later Lord Adrian, President of the Royal Society and Master of Trinity College) to become medically qualified, largely for career reasons since at that time nearly all University posts in physiology were held by medically qualified persons. My Part I work covered the requirement for preclinical study in physiology, but I had not studied anatomy, so I spent the academic year 1937–1938 dissecting the human body. I had one year of clinical study (1939–1940), but this was stopped by the bombing of London and that was when I started my war work. As I shall tell later, this was in anti-aircraft and naval gunnery; this came about through the influence of A.V. Hill, whom I had gotten to know through his son David. A.V. Hill was a leading figure in muscle research throughout the first half of the 20th century (Nobel Prize, 1923); he influenced my career in several ways.

I spent part of the summer of 1938 in the laboratory of Jack Roughton, helping with experiments on his rapid reaction apparatus. Britton Chance was also in the same laboratory at the time. He spent part of his time adding a photoelectric detector to Roughton's apparatus and the rest of it in developing a servo pick-off from a magnetic compass as part of an automatic pilot for a sailing boat; both of these activities led on to fields in which he later became world famous.

I took the Part II course in physiology in 1938–1939. There were only 12 of us taking that course; 3 of us later became Fellows of the Royal Society (J.A.B. Gray, later Head of the Medical Research Council, J.C. Waterlow, later Professor of Nutrition at the London School of Hygiene and Tropical Medicine, and myself). Our main lecturers were E.D. Adrian (who had become Head of the Department in 1937), William Rushton, Jack Roughton, Bryan Matthews, Basil Verney, Nevill Willmer, and Wilhelm Feldberg, who were members of the departmental staff. Members of other departments from whom we had occasional lectures included G.S. Adair, J. Hammond, F.H.A. Marshall, and D. Keilin. All of these either already were or later became Fellows of the Royal Society.

At the end of my Part II year (summer of 1939), I had invitations to join in research work both from Nevill Willmer, distinguished both in cytology and in vision studies, and from Alan Hodgkin, who had already carried out several important pieces of research on nerve conduction. Although considerably attracted to Willmer's work on account of my interest in microscopy, I accepted Hodgkin's invitation, partly because I had gotten to know him personally and he was nearer to me in age and partly because nerve conduction was a field in which my knowledge of physics would be useful.

First Research, Summer 1939

Hodgkin moved his equipment to the Marine Laboratory at Plymouth early in the summer vacation of 1939 with the intention of doing experiments on the giant nerve fibers of squids, and I joined him in early August. He first suggested that I should measure the viscosity of the axoplasm by suspending the fiber from a cannula and dropping mercury down; this was abortive because the mercury drops stopped as soon as they entered the fiber, the axoplasm being a gel and not a liquid as we had supposed. Having gotten the fiber suspended in this way, Hodgkin suggested pushing an electrode down inside so as to record the membrane potential directly between axoplasm and external fluid. We used a saline-filled glass tube containing a chlorided silver wire to make a non-polarizable electrode and Hodgkin's direct-coupled amplifier with cathode-follower input, so that the steady resting potential could be recorded as well as the action potential. We immediately found that the amplitude of the action potential was much greater than the resting potential, so that the internal potential went considerably positive at the peak of the action potential. This was contrary to the then current belief, although Hodgkin already had hints of an "overshoot" from external recordings on single fibers from crabs and lobsters, but this was not published until later.

The outbreak of war seemed imminent, so we left Plymouth on August 30, two days before Hitler invaded Poland. We wrote a short note that was published as a letter to *Nature* reporting the result, but with almost no discussion of its significance. I wrote a slightly longer account which I submitted to Trinity College as a dissertation for a junior Research Fellowship; wartime regulations allowed the Electors to award these Fellowships without the usual full-length dissertation. I was awarded one in 1941. A full-length paper written almost entirely by Hodgkin, but under both names appeared in the *Journal of Physiology* in 1945; in it we suggested four possible explanations for the overshoot, all of them wrong. We were both familiar with the experiment carried out in the United States in 1937 by K.S. (Kacy) Cole and Howard Curtis which showed a great increase in the conductance of the membrane during the action potential, implying an increase in permeability to ions, and we ought to have realized that this increase in permeability was highly specific for sodium ions, allowing them to enter by diffusion down their concentration gradient, carrying their positive charge inwards. If either of us had known the paper of Overton (1902: On the indispensability of sodium (or lithium) ions . . .), I am sure that we would have reached this conclusion immediately in 1939.

Curtis and Cole also recorded the action potential internally from giant fibers of squid in the summer of 1939 at Woods Hole, MA, but they used a bare platinum electrode with indeterminate junction potential and a capacity-coupled amplifier, so they could not record the resting potential and therefore did not recognize the overshoot.

Medical Studies

When I finished undergraduate work in 1939, I was intending to do a couple of years' research before going to a hospital for my clinical studies. With the outbreak of war, however, it seemed right to go ahead at once toward a medical qualification, but I had not gotten a place at a clinical medical school. Several others in Cambridge were in the same situation, so John Ryle, then Regius Professor of Physic at Cambridge, ran an introductory clinical course for us at Addenbrooke's Hospital, Cambridge, for the first six months of the war. My other main teacher was the nutritionist R.A. McCance; for the first three months of the war, he and his colleague Elsie Widdowson ran an experiment on rationing and I was one of their subjects. Our diet was similar to the ration diet that was available throughout the war: not restricted for total calories (bread and potatoes were not rationed in Britain until after the end of the war), but the amounts of meat, fats, milk, and sugar were much more severely restricted in our experiment than in wartime rations. Healthy young males like myself stayed perfectly fit on this diet; at New Year in 1940 some of us, including McCance, Widdowson, and myself, spent a week in the Lake District taking very vigorous exercise, which we were perfectly able to do. The only disadvantage of the diet was that we had to chew bread much of the time while we were walking and climbing.

I then spent six months as a clinical student at University College Hospital in London, under the surgeon Gwynne Williams and the physician and clinical scientist Sir Thomas Lewis, famous for his studies of cardiac arrhythmias and of pain. Teaching there stopped at the end of September 1940 on account of the bombing of London, and I was moved into operational research for the Anti-Aircraft Command. I found clinical study very interesting, and I do not know whether I would have returned to physiology if I had completed a medical course or whether I would have made a career in clinical work. As things turned out, most of my life has been spent in posts where I was teaching medical students, and I am very glad to have had even that single year of clinical study since it enabled me to see how different the attitude of a clinician has to be from that of a scientist: the clinician has to make immediate decisions, often on slender evidence, while the scientist has (almost) unlimited time.

War Work

A.V. Hill had led the team that developed anti-aircraft gunnery in World War I. With this background, he was in touch with General Pile, C-in-C AA Command in the summer of 1940, and felt that Pile needed scientific advice. Hill introduced Patrick Blackett (discoverer of the positron; Nobel Prize, 1948) to Pile, who appointed him as Scientific Adviser. Blackett needed assistants. All physicists and mathematicians were already busy on war work so Hill provided him with a team of physiologists: Leonard Bayliss, a lecturer in physiology at University College London and son of the famous Sir William Bayliss; Hill's son David; and through him, myself. We had all taken physics in Part I of the Natural Sciences Tripos at Cambridge, which was very adequate for dealing with the sort of problems that we were faced with, and our acquaintance with biology was probably a better background than physics for trying to deal with the huge uncertainties of war. Radar sets working on a wavelength of 3 m were already deployed at most of the gunsites around London, and most of our work was devising ways of using the very imprecise data from these radars for controlling the guns, with all the predictors being designed on the assumption that enemy aircraft would be picked up in searchlight beams and could be tracked with high precision with optical telescopes.

Blackett moved from AA Command to Coastal Command of the Royal Air Force, where he was busy with anti-submarine warfare, and Basil Schonland, a South African famous for his studies of lightning, took over our unit. Blackett moved again, to the Admiralty, where he was Chief Adviser on Operational Research and was again engaged mostly on anti-submarine warfare. In 1942, he got me transferred to the Admiralty to work in the Gunnery Division of the Naval Staff. I was nominally under Sir Ralph Fowler, famous as a pioneer of statistical mechanics, but he had already had a stroke and only came in occasionally; nevertheless, he was still a formidable character. Much of my work was scientific advice to the gunnery officers of whom the Division was composed, but there was a certain amount of what could properly be called operational research: I was on board several warships while they were carrying out gunnery trials, and I crossed the English Channel four days after the invasion of France to examine the damage done to defences by the naval bombardments. I stayed on at the Admiralty for a few months after the end of the war, writing up my wartime activities for my successors, and returned to Cambridge at the beginning of 1946. I found my war work interesting, and I benefitted afterwards from experience that I had gained in statistics and numerical solution of equations and in the theory of servo mechanisms which I had come across in connection with the automatic control of gun turrets.

For some years after the war, I was an Associate Member of the Ordnance Board, the body responsible for the design and testing of guns.

Marriage

At a dance in January 1946 I met my future wife, Jocelyn Richenda Gammell Pease (she uses the name Richenda), who was then a second-year undergraduate at Newnham College, Cambridge. She had spent three years during the war in the United States, with the family of Charles Dunbar (later Secretary of the Brookhaven Research Laboratory) in Cambridge, MA. There she attended the Buckingham School as a day girl. We became engaged in the summer of 1946, but did not marry until July 1947 when she had finished as an undergraduate.

Her father was Michael Stewart Pease (1890–1966), a geneticist who worked on poultry and was well known for developing autosexing breeds (breeds in which the plumage was noticeably different in the two sexes immediately after hatching). His father was Edward Reynolds Pease, a founding member of the Fabian Society and for many years its Secretary, who came from a Quaker family but became an atheist and left the Quakers (Richenda is a Quaker name). Joseph Pease, a direct ancestor, was a notable figure in the development of railways in the mid-19th century.

My wife's mother's maiden name was Helen Bowen Wedgwood (1895–1981), the eldest child of Josiah, 1st Baron Wedgwood and previously for many years M.P. for Stoke-on-Trent, and Ethel Bowen, daughter of Judge Bowen. She had been an undergraduate at Newnham and was, for many years, a Justice of the Peace and a County Councillor. Through the Wedgwoods, my wife was connected with the Darwins, a circumstance that led to our meeting: the dance at which we met was at the home of Sir Alan and Lady Barlow, she being a granddaughter of Charles Darwin. Richenda's mother had known her as a distant cousin, while I knew two of the Barlow sons as undergraduates at Trinity College.

My wife's elder brother is the nuclear physicist R. Sebastian Pease, F.R.S.

Although my wife read Natural Sciences at Cambridge, she did not make a career in science. She has been active in many voluntary capacities, for many years as a Justice of the Peace, a chairman of school governors, and Chairman of the Bedfordshire, Cambridgeshire and Peterborough Wildlife Trust, etc. We have six children: our one son Stewart (born 1949) is an engineer, one of our daughters is a botanist, and another is a molecular geneticist. My wife is an excellent hostess, and I have depended greatly on her in the periods when I had to do a lot of entertaining as President of the Royal Society and as Master of Trinity College, Cambridge.

Research on Nerve at Cambridge and Plymouth, 1946–1952

I returned to Cambridge to take up my Fellowship at the beginning of 1946 and joined Hodgkin again; he had returned immediately after the end of hostilities. The idea that the overshoot of the action potential might be due to entry of sodium ions had come to me as a result of hearing the Croonian Lecture by August Krogh (famous mainly for his studies of the capillary circulation) at the Royal Society in October 1945; he reported work in Scandinavia during the war using radioactive tracers which had shown that cell membranes were not totally impermeable to sodium ions as had been generally supposed (Krogh, 1946). From then on, the sodium hypothesis was under active discussion between Hodgkin and myself. There were several difficulties in the idea. First, Curtis and Cole in the United States had repeated their intracellular recordings, but used a non-polarizable electrode and a direct-coupled amplifier. They recorded an overshoot much too large to be explained by sodium entry (later admitted to be due to overcompensation for lag due to resistance and capacitance of the electrode and input circuit). Second, they had stated that resting and action potential were unchanged in a solution which did not contain sodium. Third, it was then believed that the selective permeability to potassium ions, responsible for the resting potential, was due to the hydrated potassium ion being smaller than the hydrated sodium ion, and this made it difficult to imagine that a membrane could be more permeable to sodium than to the smaller potassium ions.

We did not attempt direct tests of the sodium theory at once because it was clear that these would be best done on the giant nerve fiber of the squid, which was available in Britain only at Plymouth; the laboratory there had been badly damaged by bombing in the war so experiments were not possible in the summer of 1946. The relevant experiments were done by Hodgkin with Bernard Katz in the summer of 1947; I did not join them because I was married that summer and was occupied with our honeymoon and with visits to members of the family. Meanwhile, in 1946, 1947, and the early part of 1948, I computed (with a hand-cranked Brunsviga calculator) several action potentials on a variety of assumptions about the way in which the ions penetrated the membrane, either as free ions or in combination with a "carrier" anion confined to the membrane. In some cases the carrier was buffered by combination with another ion (Ca^{2+} or H^+) present at a higher concentration on one side of the membrane than the other, causing either inactivation of the sodium permeability or a delay in the rise of the potassium permeability. We did not consider the possibility to which we were later led by our voltage-clamp work and that has since been confirmed by more specific experiments, namely, that the ions pass through "gates" that are opened or closed by change of membrane potential.

This work was not published at the time, but it was a useful guide when we did our experiments with the voltage clamp in 1948 and 1949. I have recently (2002) published an account of the speculations and calculations that we made in 1946–1948. They included several propagated action potentials as well as the simpler "membrane action potentials" in which the potential change is constrained to have the same time course at all points in the area of membrane considered. Strictly, the equations governing a propagated action potential are partial differential equations since distance along the fiber and time are both independent variables. It would not have been practicable to compute the solution to such equations with a hand calculator, so we converted them into a set of simultaneous ordinary differential equations by assuming a constant velocity. The solution for the internal potential would then go toward plus infinity or toward minus infinity according to whether the guessed velocity was greater or less than the true value, which was approached by successive approximation.

After our first season's work with the voltage clamp, I calculated one more action potential assuming that the ions crossed the membrane combined with a carrier, but with parameters adjusted to match the voltage-clamp results. This was published in our contribution to a meeting in Paris in 1949 (Hodgkin, Huxley, and Katz, 1949).

Later, in 1947, I was joined by Robert Stämpfli from Bern, who had been introduced to Hodgkin and me by Professor Alex von Muralt. He had taught himself to dissect single myelinated nerve fibers from the nerves of frogs, as had been done in the 1920s by Kato in Japan. Together, we gave strong additional evidence for saltatory transmission in those fibers. We also measured their resting and action potentials, finding an overshoot similar to that in the squid fiber and showing the dependence of the overshoot on the external sodium concentration.

Hodgkin and I (1947) used an indirect method to estimate the amount of potassium leaving a nerve fiber per impulse conducted, showing that it was sufficient for the charge carried to restore the resting potential after the action potential. Our publication contained the first mention of the idea that the rise of the action potential is due to the entry of sodium ions.

The Voltage Clamp

Both Hodgkin and Cole suspected that the all-or-none character of the nerve action potential was due to a current-voltage relation in the membrane that was continuous but included a region of negative slope which caused positive feedback and therefore instability. Such a feature would make it difficult to measure the current-voltage relation. I remember a discussion with Hodgkin, probably in 1945, in which he pointed out that it would be necessary to use electronic feedback to an internal electrode so as to control the internal potential ("voltage clamp") and to make it undergo stepwise changes. I replied that it would be just as good to feed current from a low-impedance source, but Hodgkin had realized that this would be an imperfect arrangement since the electrode would become polarized by the high current density that would be needed.

Early in the war, Cole suggested to J.H. Bartlett that he should perform an experiment of this type on the "iron wire model": it was well known that iron wire made passive by immersion in strong nitric or sulfuric acid would propagate an electric change when electrically stimulated in a way that had close analogies with nerve conduction. Bartlett (1945) used a low-resistance potentiometer to apply step changes of potential to a piece of iron made passive in this way and recorded the current with a D.C. amplifier and cathode-ray oscillograph; the experiments were only moderately successful.

Cole, together with M. Marmont, was the first to make experiments of this type on the squid giant fiber in the summer of 1947 (Cole, 1949). However, their experiments were limited: Marmont had originally devised the apparatus with the intention of controlling the membrane current and Cole had made an addition which made it possible to use it to control the internal potential. Using it in this voltage-control mode, they did show that the current-voltage relation is continuous with a region of negative slope (Cole, 1949), but they did not analyze the current into components carried by different ions; further, their apparatus was not a true voltage clamp since they controlled the current by feedback from the same internal electrode by which current was injected. This effectively provided a low-impedance source from which potential changes were applied to the internal electrode and the results were therefore distorted by electrode polarization, as Hodgkin had foreseen: the long-lasting outward current during what should have been a constant raised internal potential declined because the potential of the axoplasm did not follow perfectly the potential applied to the wire.

Hodgkin and I, together with Katz in the initial experiments, had our equipment running in 1948 (Hodgkin, Huxley, and Katz, 1952), but made our final series of measurements in 1949. By varying the external sodium concentration, we separated the membrane current into an inward component due to sodium entry and an outward component that we attributed to the exit of potassium ions. We further analyzed the mechanism of the permeability changes by applying a second step of potential. We fitted equations to the time courses of the permeability changes as functions of time and membrane potential and solved the resulting differential equations representing the behavior of the membrane when not controlled by feedback. EDSAC I, the first electronic computer in Cambridge (and one of the first in the world), was not available at the time because it was being upgraded, so I did the computations by hand as I had done in 1946–1948. The final result was satisfactorily similar to the action potentials recorded from the actual fibers. The results were published in 1952 (Hodgkin and Huxley, 1952a,b,c,d) and were the basis on which Hodgkin and I received shares in the Nobel Prize for Physiology or Medicine in 1963. Sir John Eccles also received a share in the prize for establishing that synaptic transmission depends on changes in ionic permeability; neither Hodgkin nor I ever worked with Eccles.

We confirmed that the outward component of membrane current is carried by potassium ions by comparing a steady outward current with the outward movement of radioactive potassium using fibers from the cuttlefish Sepia.

After analyzing and publishing the work with the voltage clamp, we could not see how to carry the analysis of excitation and conduction to a deeper level. We looked for "gating currents," i.e., the small currents now known to be carried across the membrane by movement of charged structures that open gates in response to membrane potential change, permitting the small ions to pass through. We could not detect them, partly because our measurements were not precise enough and partly because the very small gating currents were overlaid by the much larger currents carried by the ions and blockers such as tetrodotoxin were not yet available. The huge advances that have been made since have depended on advances in electronic techniques and in other branches of biology, notably, molecular genetics. Hodgkin and I therefore turned to other lines of work. Hodgkin turned to other aspects of nerve function such as the active transport of ions across the membrane by which the ion movements during activity are reversed and, later, the excitation of the rods and cones of the retina by light. I moved into investigations of muscle contraction. I did, however, continue with a small amount of theoretical work about nerve conduction (Huxley, 1959).

The set of equations that Hodgkin and I had produced was first put onto an electronic computer by Cole, Antosiewicz, and Rabinowife (1955). The result showed a discontinuity between stimuli that led only to a small active response by the fiber and stimuli that led to a full-sized action potential. It was clear to Hodgkin and me that the equations required that the response should be continuous, and I remember a conversation with Cole in which I failed to convince him of this. Later, however, he admitted that the apparent discontinuity was due to a computer error: the program asked it to divide zero by zero at a certain point in one of the equations describing the ionic permeabilities (Cole, 1958).

Research on Muscle at Cambridge, 1952–1960

I had become interested in muscle through being asked to take over the lectures on muscle to the final-year course in Physiology from David Hill, who moved from Cambridge to Plymouth in 1948. From the lecture notes that I inherited from him, I learned about the phenomenon known as the "reversal of striations," well described by 19th-century microscopists such as Engelmann (1881), but almost completely neglected since 1900. During contraction of fibers from limb muscles from insects, the region with highest refractive index changed from the A band to the vicinity of the Z line. This seemed to me to be something that might give a clue to the intimate mechanism of contraction, and it was attractive to me because of my interest in microscopy. The 19th century work did not show whether the phenomenon was related to activation or to development of tension or to shortening, because the insect fibers that had been studied (satisfactory for microscopy because of their small diameter and very broad striations) were not fully excitable. From the work of Ramsey and Street (1940), it was known that single fibers could be dissected from muscles of frogs in a fully excitable state, but these fibers were thick and had narrow striations and, therefore, it was virtually impossible to obtain a satisfactory image of their striations by ordinary light microscopy. Polarized light, with high-aperture illumination, does give a satisfactory optical section, but the 19th-century work had shown that the phenomenon does not show up with polarized light. Phase contrast shows refractive index differences well on thin specimens, but not on thick specimens such as these muscle fibers. What was needed was an interference microscope in which the light that had passed through the specimen was combined with coherent light that had bypassed the fiber; the path differences due to the refractive index differences in the fiber would then be converted to intensity differences by interference and could be observed by eye or by photography.

As mentioned in connection with my boyhood interests, I already had an idea for making such an instrument, based on a polarizing microscope, but incorporating a Wollaston prism below the condenser to separate the incident polarized light into two components with electric vectors at right angles and a second Wollaston prism above the objective to recombine the two beams, with the specimen being placed so that one of the beams passed through it while the other passed through an empty space in the field nearby. I took the idea to the microscope makers Messrs R. & J. Beck, who told me that the idea had already been patented by F.H. Smith (1947); commercial development was therefore impossible, but they were ready to make a single set of the necessary components for me. A low-power instrument of this type, with the objective and condenser each consisting of a simple doublet, was easily made by adding the Wollaston prisms to a standard polarizing microscope, but it did not have sufficient resolving power to be useful for studying the striations of frog muscle. With a high-power condenser and objective, however, the ideal positions for the prisms are inside the condenser and objective, so they have to be placed outside them with the result that the two beams are displaced laterally when they emerge from the upper prism, causing the image to be crossed by finely spaced interference fringes. It was therefore necessary to add further birefringent components to bring the two beams into superposition. The resulting instrument, with an objective of numerical aperture 0.9, functioned very well, even with white light (Huxley, 1954, 1957a). I made the parts for holding and adjusting the prisms myself, using the lathe that my parents had given to my brother and myself when I was about 12 years old. The movements had to have high precision: appreciable intensity changes were caused by a change of path difference between the two beams of 10 nm, corresponding to a displacement of the lower Wollaston prism by 1 μm.

In the work on frog muscle fibers with this microscope, I was joined by Rolf Niedergerke from Göttingen. Before we got around to stimulating a fiber to look for the reversal of striations, we noticed that when we stretched a fiber passively, all or nearly all the change of length took place in the I bands, the reverse of what was in the textbooks of that date. There was no visible change in the striations during isometric twitches or short tetani. These observations immediately suggested that the material that gave the high refractive index and birefringence to the A bands was in the form of rodlets which did not change their length when the fiber was stretched; the reversal of striations would then be attributable to crumpling or overlapping of the ends of these rodlets when the fiber shortened and they collided with the rodlets of the adjacent sarcomere. We recorded cinematographically the changes in the striations when strong local shortening was induced by application of steady current, and on one occasion the distinction between A and I bands became very indistinct and a narrow dense line appeared where the center of the A band had been; the reversal of striations did occur with further shortening when a second set of dense lines appeared at the positions of the Z lines. A natural interpretation of the first set of dense lines was that they were due to collision or crumpling of the ends of a second set of filaments in each I band and the outer parts of each adjacent A band, which slid into the A bands during shortening; this was the observation that suggested to us the idea of sliding filaments. However, in most of the contractions that we observed, this sequence of changes did not occur, but both A and I bands appeared to become progressively narrower. We therefore delayed publishing the result; it turned out later that the reason for the difference was that, in most cases, only the myofibrils near the surface were activated and the inside of the fiber shortened passively and the fibrils were thrown into waves so that the striations were foreshortened in the image (Huxley and Gordon, 1962). This was in the early part of 1953; I was not able to give much time to research as I was then Press Editor of the *Journal of Physiology* and also Secretary of the College Council, as well as having teaching duties (not very heavy).

I spent the summer of 1953 at the Marine Biological Laboratory at Woods Hole, supported by a Lalor Fellowship. There I met H.H. Weber of Tübingen (later of Heidelberg), who told me of the experiments by Wilhelm Hasselbach (1953) in his laboratory. He had dissolved away the myosin from fragmented muscle and examined the residue with the electron microscope, finding that the actin was in the form of filaments held together at their centers by the Z line. This immediately suggested that the second set of filaments that we postulated were composed of actin. A little later during that visit, I met Hugh Huxley (from the Cavendish Laboratory, Cambridge) and Jean Hanson (from the Department of Biophysics at King's College London), who had come to Woods Hole from MIT, where they were working in the laboratory of F.O. Schmitt. I told them of our observations with the interference microscope and our idea that length changes in muscle took place by relative sliding movements of two interdigitating sets of filaments. They showed me the electron micrographs of transverse sections of frog muscle that established the existence of two sets of filaments and that were published by Hugh Huxley later the same year, with a brief mention of the sliding-filament theory. They also showed me their phase micrographs of separated myofibrils treated with various solutions that showed, in agreement with Hasselbach's observation, that the additional material in the A bands was myosin. The main accounts of the evidence for sliding filaments by H.E. Huxley and Hanson (1954) and by myself with R. Niedergerke (1954)

appeared alongside in *Nature* the following year. Details of my work with
Niedergerke were published in 1958.

In our 1954 article, we proposed that relative force between filaments
of the two sets was generated by independent force generators distributed
throughout the region of overlap between the filaments. The basis for this
suggestion, which has been amply confirmed, was the observation by Ramsey
and Street (1940) that, over much of the range of initial length at which isometric contractions could be recorded, the tension developed was roughly
proportional to the amount of overlap of the two sets of filaments. However,
the lengths of the filaments were not accurately known, so it remained uncertain how close the proportionality between overlap and force was. I returned
to this problem several years later (see below).

In the summer of 1954 I spent a lot of time brooding on the nature of the
mechanism by which the independent force generators that we postulated in
each overlap zone produce force or sliding movement. A clue was provided by
Dorothy Needham (wife of biochemist and sinologist Joseph Needham), who
pointed out that the relation between rate of energy liberation and speed of
shortening found by A.V. Hill (1938) implied that repeated interactions took
place at each active site during a single contraction (Needham, 1950). Such
cyclic action is difficult to fit into the idea, universally accepted at that time,
that contraction takes place by shortening of continuous filaments, which
may be the reason why this suggestion did not immediately attract much
attention. In a sliding-filament process, however, it is natural to think in
terms of cyclic mechanisms since one cannot imagine a single interaction
between active sites on the filaments operating over a distance approaching
1 μm such as can occur in a single contraction. So I thought out a mechanism
in which a "side-piece," attached to the backbone of the thick filament by an
elastic connection, was able to attach to a site on the thin filament with a rate
constant that was moderate when the relative positions of the filaments were
such that the connection gave a positive contribution to overall tension, and
the rate constant for detachment was large after sliding motion had brought
it to a position where its contribution was negative. With a suitable choice
of parameters, this theory gave a good approximation to the relationships
established by A.V. Hill (1938). However, it was so speculative that I did not
consider publishing it until Bernard Katz, one of the editors of *Progress in
Biophysics and Biophysical Chemistry*, suggested that I write a contribution
to one of its issues. I accepted this invitation, and in early 1955, I submitted
a typescript containing the theory. I was very disappointed that the article
did not appear until nearly two years later (Huxley, 1957c).

The theory has remained useful, as its main kinetic assumptions are
probably roughly correct. It is now clear, however, that much or all of the
generation of force is due to more specific changes in the cross-bridge than
merely attaching in a position where the elastic element is stretched, but
this need not alter the kinetics greatly.

The theory was undermined when A.V. Hill (1964) showed that the rate of energy liberation did not increase with shortening speed over the whole range, as described in his 1938 paper, but passed through a maximum. However, I showed later that this feature can be explained if the initial attachment involves two steps.

Before leaving Germany, my colleague Rolf Niedergerke had become aware of some of the 19th century microscopy of muscle. I followed this up using the wonderful collection of reprints made by Michael Foster, which was then in the library of the Physiological Laboratory at Cambridge (it is now in the library of the Whipple Museum of the History of Science in Cambridge). I found that most of our observations had been well known in the latter part of the 19th century, though no one seems to have proposed a sliding-filament process. The old observations had been lost after 1900, chiefly because of a switch of interest to biochemical events and the argument that contraction must be a molecular process: molecules are not visible with the light microscope and, therefore, nothing important will be learned from what can be seen. This is set out in the small book that I published in 1980.

The Inward Spread of Activity in a Muscle Fiber

In late 1953, I was joined by Bob Taylor from the University of Illinois. We set out to look for changes in the light scattered and diffracted by frog muscle fibers activated by electric current under conditions where no action potentials are set up. We made a trough with a shape designed so that current was drawn uniformly from the fiber over a substantial length and set up a drum camera for recording the diffraction spectrum continuously. Nothing of great interest was emerging, so we switched to the question of how a change of potential difference across the surface membrane activates the contractile material at distances up to several tens of micrometres. This had become an acute problem in 1949 when A.V. Hill showed that the whole cross-section of each fiber began to contract within a few milliseconds after an action potential, a time too short to allow a hypothetical activator substance liberated at the membrane to reach the center of the fiber by simple diffusion.

With my interest in muscle structure, I was aware of papers showing that the Z lines in adjacent myofibrils were united to form a membrane ("Krause's membrane") that connected with the inside of the surface membrane (Enderlein, 1899). This suggested that this structure might conduct an influence (of unspecified nature) inward from the membrane. We tested this idea by reducing the membrane potential of a very small area of membrane by applying a saline-filled micropipette (tip diameter about 1 μm) to the surface of an isolated fiber from frog muscle and then applying a negative electric potential to the fluid in the pipette. We watched the fiber under a polarizing microscope so the anisotropic A bands were clearly visible; the Z lines were not visible, but their position was recognizable because it is at the middle of the non-birefringent I band. The result was just as we hoped: when the pipette was placed over an I band, we often saw a contraction, completely localized to that I band; but when the pipette was over an A band, we never saw a contraction. We recorded these local contractions with a cine camera, and we published a letter in *Nature* entitled "Function of Krause's Membrane."

We showed the film at a meeting of the Physiological Society. The electron microscopist J.D. Robertson was in the audience. He produced from his pocket a slide showing an electron micrograph of a longitudinal section of muscle which clearly showed a pair of tubules penetrating the fiber on either side of each Z membrane, so he suggested that inward conduction took place along these tubules and that our pipettes were not small enough to distinguish between the two members of each pair. However, his micrograph (Robertson, 1956) was from a muscle of a lizard, while our experiments were on fibers from frog muscle, so it was possible that both of us were right—as happens in many controversies in biology.

To resolve this problem, it was necessary to repeat our experiment using an optical system that shows the Z membranes. The interference microscope that I had developed for study of the changes in the striations did this, so Taylor and I repeated the experiment under this microscope on frog fibers and also on fibers from crab muscle with much broader striations. In a frog fiber, the Z line always remained central in the I band, even when the pipette was applied just to one side of it; however, in a crab fiber, the Z line was pulled across toward the side on which the pipette was placed. Later, in collaboration with Ralph Straub from Geneva, I repeated the experiment on fibers from lizard muscle and saw the same result as in crab muscle—not what one might have expected from the evolutionary relationships of those animals. If we had known of the paper of Golgi's pupil Veratti, published in 1902, we would have been aware of these differences in the system of transverse tubules, but it had been completely forgotten until rediscovered and reprinted in English translation (Veratti, 1961).

Indications of membrane structures inside muscle fibers were seen with the electron microscope at about the same time as our observations of local contractions, but the structures in frog muscle at the level of the Z line seen by Porter and Palade (1957) consisted of a row of vesicles, not a continuous structure. The Wellcome Trust provided an electron microscope for our department in 1957, and I studied the membrane systems of frog muscles with it, finding that, in some preparations, Porter's vesicles were replaced by a tubule (Huxley, 1959). At about the same time, Andersson-Cedergren demonstrated continuous tubules in mouse muscle, but they were in pairs flanking each Z line, like the tubules seen by Robertson in lizard muscle.

Thus, it became clear that inward conduction was taking place along these tubules, and the title of our letter to *Nature*, "Function of Krause's Membrane," was inappropriate. This is an example of the danger of relying on an apparent confirmation of a preconceived hypothesis, as emphasized in Karl Popper's book *Conjectures and Refutations*.

With the electron microscope, I looked for openings of these tubules to the extracellular space, but could not see any. Even now, such openings have rarely been seen in the skeletal muscles of frogs or mammals. In 1964, however, Makoto Endo in my laboratory showed that a fluorescent dye enters the tubules from the extracellular space, and Sally Page and Hugh Huxley independently showed with the electron microscope that large molecules can enter the tubules. It was only later that I found evidence from the late 19th century that Indian ink particles can enter the tubules of heart muscle (Nyström, 1897). These observations made it clear that changes of membrane potential can spread up the membranes of the tubules, causing liberation of the activator (calcium ions) close to the contractile material. These and other confusing observations are set out (Huxley, 1971) in my Croonian Lecture to the Royal Society.

For the local-activation experiments, I designed a micromanipulator; for electron microscopy, I designed an ultramicrotome. In both, I used crossed-strip hinges for the levers that gave the fine movements. These allow rotation about a single axis with no friction and no backlash, unlike ordinary pivots. I was pleased with myself for thinking up this type of pivot, but later found that there had been controversy about 1900 between the Cambridge Scientific Instrument Company and the National Physical Laboratory as to which of them had invented it first. Initially, both instruments were made for me by the workshop of the Engineering Department of Cambridge University; in both cases they also made a number of copies for other laboratories. The ultramicrotome was later manufactured by the Cambridge Scientific Instrument Co., which provided an important additional income when we were paying fees for the education of our six children.

The Maximum Length for Contraction

In 1958 I was joined by Lee Peachey, who had just completed his Ph.D. at the Rockefeller University under the pioneer electron microscopist Keith Porter. We returned to the problem of the relation between the tension generated by an isolated muscle fiber and the amount of overlap between the thick and thin filaments. As soon as we stretched an isolated fiber under a light microscope, we noticed that there were regions at both ends where the sarcomeres (the units of the striation pattern) were much less extended than in the middle of the fiber. This made measurements of tension ambiguous, but we were able to show that the middle part of the fiber was unable to shorten if it was stretched so far that there was no overlap as seen in our electron micrographs. There was, however, still overlap in the end regions, and if the tendon ends were held stationary, tension rose because the regions with overlap shortened, stretching the middle still further.

This showed that the relation between length and isometric tension could be found reliably only if precautions were taken to keep constant the length of a selected region in the middle of the fiber. This was the first problem to which I addressed myself after moving from Cambridge to University College London in 1960.

Move to University College London, 1960

Early in 1960, I was invited to accept the Chair of Physiology at University College London. I was then very comfortably established at Cambridge, with a teaching Fellowship at Trinity College and a Readership in the Physiology Department at University College London (both tenure positions), and we were living in an extremely attractive house in the picturesque village of Grantchester, a couple of miles outside Cambridge. Therefore, there was a strong temptation to stay where I was.

However, I also received a letter from A.V. Hill, whom I had gotten to know through his son David, as I said earlier. He was then working at University College London in his retirement. In this letter, A.V. said that he had been in a similar position in 1919, comfortably established in Cambridge following his return after World War I, when he was offered the Chair of Physiology at Manchester University. Lord Rutherford, the physicist, had just returned from Manchester to Cambridge, so A.V. asked his advice. He quoted this advice to me, saying that he had followed it and had never regretted doing so. The advice was: "Cambridge is a splendid place when you are young and Cambridge is a splendid place when you are old, but for the middle of your life for God's sake get out." So I entered into negotiations with University College and London University.

The only serious obstacle was that we wished to stay living in our Grantchester home, but this was over 50 miles from London and London University had a rule that its staff must live within 30 miles (in those days, professors and readers were appointed by the University, not by the College). Further, I was told that the University readily relaxed this rule in any direction except toward Oxford or Cambridge. The rule had been introduced because Oxford and Cambridge dons used to accept a chair in London University, but stay living in Oxford or Cambridge and turn up in London only occasionally for a lecture or a committee meeting. I assured them that I had no intention of behaving like that, and it was agreed that I could stay in our Grantchester home provided that I also had a London address and spent some nights there each week. I did not get a flat in London, but slept Monday, Tuesday, and Thursday nights in bed-and-breakfast places within walking distance of the College. I always traveled by train to London early on Monday, home Wednesday evening till Thursday morning, and home again on Friday evening. On this basis I saw at least as much of my family as I did when working in Cambridge, since in term time I gave tutorials from 6:00

till 8:00 PM three days each week and often dined in the College on those evenings, and at weekends I sometimes had teaching duties and often went to work in my laboratory. When I was staying in London in the routine that I adopted, I would get some supper and return to my office or my laboratory until nearly midnight, walk back to my bed-and-breakfast, and walk back to the department early next morning. In this way, I spent more hours in the department each week than anyone else. I am sure it is the best way of doing a London job.

Like A.V. Hill, I did not regret the move: University College London was a very friendly place, and I had opportunities there which I would not have had if I had stayed in Cambridge, as a relatively junior member of the department. As a former Fellow of Trinity College, I still had the right to take meals in the College and to bring guests to the college's "feasts," as guest nights are called in Cambridge.

I retired from headship of the department in 1969, when I was awarded one of the research professorships of the Royal Society. This provided not only my salary, but also generous allowances for research expenses, a secretary, and a technician. I still gave a few lectures, but I had no administrative duties. I stayed on at University College London until I was appointed Master of Trinity College, Cambridge, in 1984, as I shall tell later.

Research on Muscle at University College London, 1960–1984

As I have already mentioned, I returned once again to the problem of the length-tension relation in isolated muscle fibers from frogs. As Lee Peachey and I had found in our experiments at Cambridge, it was necessary to arrange that the middle region of a fiber was held at constant length during a contraction so as to avoid the extra tension that is given by sarcomeres with greater overlap near the ends of the fiber if the ends are held stationary. This required continuous measurement of the length of the selected region and feedback from this measurement to a motor which moved one tendon of the fiber so as to keep the length signal constant. I was joined for two years by Al Gordon who had just completed a Ph.D. in physics at Cornell, and we developed a device ("photo-electronic spot-follower") which detected the positions of two small pieces of gold leaf stuck to the isolated muscle fiber at the ends of a selected region within which the striation spacing was uniform. This gave a length signal from which we used feedback to a galvanometer movement to which one tendon of the fiber was attached. This development was completed in collaboration with Fred Julian from the Naval Medical Research Institute at Bethesda (1962–1965). We were then able to show a close proportionality between filament overlap and the tension developed on stimulation with the fiber held a series of lengths above that which gave the maximum tension (at shorter lengths, the tension fell away because the filaments of adjacent sarcomeres collided). We also showed that, over the same range, the speed of unloaded shortening was almost independent of overlap, as would be expected if the movement was being generated by independent active sites in the overlap zone.

The situation was confused for many years by the measurements by G.H. Pollack and his collaborators, who omitted to use feedback control of sarcomere length and found that substantial tension developed even when the fiber was stretched considerably beyond the length at which there ceased to be any overlap in most of the length of the fiber. When at last they did control the sarcomere length, they obtained results in close agreement with what we had published a quarter of a century before (Granzier and Pollack, 1990).

In 1967 I was joined by Bob Simmons. Originally trained in physics, he had been with David Phillips at the Royal Institution doing X-ray crystallography on enzymes, but came to University College to take a course designed to give some biological background to physicists and chemists who wished to make a career in biological research. For his project in this course, he worked with me, and our collaboration continued until he moved to King's College London 12 years later.

We settled down to investigating the mechanism of force generation in muscle by applying step changes of either tension or length to a fiber during a contraction. The first studies of transient responses of muscle had been made by Dick Podolsky using steps of tension. He had found that the response was a heavily damped oscillation of length, superposed on the steady shortening that followed the drop in tension. At first, we too tried to use tension steps so as to avoid complications due to changes in length of series elastic elements that would occur after the step itself if tension were not kept constant. We used negative feedback from a tension signal to the motor attached to one of the tendons to control the tension. We found an oscillatory response superposed on steady length change, as Podolsky had done, but under some conditions the oscillation was only very lightly damped (Armstrong, Huxley, and Julian, 1966). However, we found it too difficult to obtain satisfactory performance during the first few milliseconds after the step because of the non-linearity of the muscle properties. That was the immediate reason why we switched to steps of length, though in retrospect the results from length steps were easier to interpret. The response to a step decrease in length consisted of a series of decaying exponential terms, which indicated that the response of the contractile system is more directly related to length changes than to tension changes since the latter generate an oscillatory response.

We found that the response to a shortening step was composed of four phases: Phase 1, an almost linear decrease in tension simultaneous with the length; Phase 2, recovery in a few millseconds much of the way toward the original tension; Phase 3, a delay or actual reversal of the tension recovery; and Phase 4, slow recovery to the original tension.

Phase 2 appeared to represent the actual working stroke of the cross-bridges, and we found that its time course became more rapid the larger the shortening step was applied, and therefore the smaller the tension during Phase 2. We produced a theory of this acceleration on the basis that the working stroke in a cross-bridge consisted of one or a few stepwise events which stretched the elastic element in the cross-bridge and that the work done against this elasticity formed part of the activation energy for the step(s) (Huxley and Simmons, 1971). This theory is still useful, although it has had to be modified in its quantitative aspects as a result of improved measurements and evidence that there is appreciable compliance in the filaments themselves (Huxley and Tideswell, 1996).

We were joined in 1971 by Lincoln Ford, with a two-year fellowship from the NIH. After improving our equipment so as to obtain much better time resolution, we obtained our final series of measurements. We published four papers on the responses to length steps under various conditions: first, during the tension plateau of fibers at their normal length; second, on fibers stretched to various lengths; third, during steady shortening at various speeds; and fourth, during the rise of tension at the start of stimulation (Ford, Huxley, and Simmons, 1977, 1981, 1985, 1986). Lincoln returned for a month or so each year to help in preparing these papers, but our close collaboration ended with Ford's return to the United States in 1973, Simmons's move to King's College in 1979, and my becoming President of the Royal Society in 1980. As a result, we did not achieve what I had hoped for, namely, making a synthesis of our results into a comprehensive theory, as Hodgkin and I had done for nerve conduction in our papers of 1952.

Another very productive collaboration has been with Vincenzo Lombardi of the University of Florence and later with his colleague Gabriella Piazzesi. It began in October 1979 when Lombardi came to University College London for a nine-month visit. Lee Peachey was also with me at the time. Much of our work was developing a new device for obtaining a signal representing change in length of the selected segment of an isolated muscle fiber. We used the light diffracted by the striations, but not in the way that is commonly used, which is to estimate the spacing from the angle of the first diffraction line, since that method is subject to numerous artifacts. We devised a circuit which signaled the longitudinal displacement of an image of the striations, and the difference between the outputs of two of these circuits, one at each end of the selected segment of the fiber, gave the change of length. This apparatus turned out to be much more satisfactory than other methods and became the standard method in my laboratory and in Lombardi's. It gives a precision of about 1 in 10^5 of segment length, with a time lag of about 1 μs.

During that first visit, we also did one experiment on living fibers. This was designed to detect compliance in the thin filaments, and it appeared to confirm the conclusion reached by Ford, Simmons, and myself that such compliance was negligible. Perhaps fortunately, we did not publish it: more recent experiments by much more direct methods have shown clearly that the compliance is quite appreciable.

Since then, Lombardi came to collaborate for periods of a few weeks, usually twice each year. This continued throughout the period when I was President of the Royal Society or Master of Trinity and into my retirement until 1998, when I gave up my laboratory and sent my equipment to Florence for his use. We made further improvements to the equipment, including a miniaturized loudspeaker-type motor for changing the fiber length, which I made on the lathe that I have owned since boyhood. This gave steps complete in about 30 μs, as compared to 150 μs with previous motors. With these sharp steps, the effects of reflection of the traveling wave set up by the step were noticeable, and we devised circuits for shaping the command signal in order to reduce these effects.

Throughout, we have also had a continuous correspondence about his experimental work at Florence and drafts of his papers based on it.

Other Workers in My Laboratory

While I was Head of the Department at University College London, I usually had two or three others in my laboratory, working more or less independently on problems connected with muscle. A few of these were working for a Ph.D. and the others were postdocs. In contrast with present-day custom, I did not put my name on the papers reporting their work unless I had taken a very substantial part in the experiments. They included Saul Winegrad, Hugo Gonzalez-Serratos, Lucy Brown, Makoto Endo, Clara Franzini-Armstrong, Reinhard Rüdel, Stuart Taylor, Peter Heinl, Jan Lännergren, Russell Close, and Lydia Hill.

Resonance in the Cochlea

My father had received as an undergraduate prize a copy of Helmholtz's book on hearing (*Die Lehre von den Tonempfindungen...*), and I read parts of it when I was an undergraduate. I was impressed by his evidence for a resonance mechanism for pitch discrimination, and this impression was strengthened by Thomas Gold's dissertation which won for him a junior Research Fellowship at Trinity College (Gold and Pumphrey, 1948; this was the same Gold who later became well known in cosmology and geochemistry). Gold also argued that the sharpness of resonance would only be possible if there is a positive feedback process to counteract the damping due to the fluids in the cochlea. In the late 1950s, I contemplated switching my main line of research from muscle to the mechanism of the cochlea and I asked the advice of Bryan Matthews, then Head of the Physiology Department at Cambridge, who had done some experiments on the ear. He replied that the problems had been definitively solved: von Békésy had shown that the movements of fluids in the cochlea were not sharply tuned so that pitch discrimination must be done in the brain, and his conclusions had been confirmed by the electrical recordings of Hallowell Davis and Tasaki. I therefore stuck to my muscle work and was duly surprised when Nelson Kiang (1965) showed extremely sharply tuned responses in fibers of the auditory nerve when the blood circulation in the preparation was well maintained.

I never did any experimental work on the ear, but I did publish one theoretical paper (1969) in which I showed that true resonance might occur in a structure resembling the cochlea provided that the cochlear partition (basilar membrane plus organ of Corti) had appropriate mechanical properties. I do not believe that the suggestions in that article have been followed up. There is much emphasis now on the movements generated by the outer hair cells of the cochlea. These no doubt counteract damping as suggested by Gold more than half a century ago, but I am not aware that they have other effects on possible resonance.

My other contribution to the theory of hearing was to draw attention (1990a) to the beautiful experiments of Ernst Bárány (1938). Bryan Matthews had drawn my attention to his paper, which had shown beyond doubt that the important function of the ossicles is to reduce bone-conducted sound relative to air-conducted sound. This had been completely neglected, and all the textbooks stated that the function of the ossicles was to improve the matching between air and the fluids of the cochlea. This matching is achieved almost entirely by the large ratio of the area of the eardrum to the area of the footplate of the stapes, and it is beyond belief that evolution would have produced the elaborate system of ossicles when the same result could have been achieved by a small reduction in the area of the footplate of the stapes.

President of the Royal Society

The Royal Society is the equivalent in Britain of the National Academy of Sciences (NAS) in the United States, though of course much smaller. It supports and promotes science in many ways. It receives a substantial grant each year from the government, but this is spent on professorships, research fellowships, etc. awarded by the Royal Society. The Royal Society has sufficient funds of its own to remain independent of government with regards to its policy and the reports that it produces—nothing like as many as the NAS. Outside Britain, it has an important function in promoting international contacts through exchange schemes.

I did not have time for consecutive research while I was President of the Royal Society or Master of Trinity College, Cambridge, especially during the year when I held both of those offices (1984–1985). Work at the Royal Society took up about three days a week, and I made several trips abroad visiting the national academies of other countries. Although I gave up a few memberships of other bodies, I also had responsibilities in the International Union of Physiological Sciences, the Muscular Dystrophy Group of Great Britain, the Natural History Museum, the Science Museum, the Nature Conservancy Council, and the committee that advises the Home Office on experiments on living animals. Such time as I could find for research was mostly spent in finishing the analysis of the results that Bob Simmons, Lincoln Ford, and I had obtained and in writing the last two papers on that work, but, as I have already mentioned, I did occasionally get into the laboratory with Vincenzo Lombardi.

The one important innovation that was made during my time was the establishment of the junior research fellowships known as University Research Fellowships. At that time, very few vacancies were coming up for positions in the universities in Britain, partly because of cuts in government funding, but also because of the age structure in the universities that had been established in the 1960s. These fellowships are awarded to scientists, mathematicians, or engineers with a few years' postdoctoral experience and are tenable for up to 10 years, with the expectation that many of the holders will obtain university posts within that time. There are now over 300 holders of these appointments.

Another matter that took up a good deal of my time was resisting pressure from politically minded groups to break off scientific contacts with countries with totalitarian governments. For example, scientists from South Africa and from China had been prevented from attending certain international congresses, and the two most senior Soviet scientists wishing to attend the International Congress of Biochemistry in Australia in 1982 were denied visas (not for scientific reasons). This was the main topic of my annual address to the Royal Society in November 1982. My other addresses were concerned with unjustified criticisms of Darwinian evolution (1981); ethical questions such as experimentation on living animals (1983); government support of science and the universities (1984); and the fragmentation of biology (1985).

Master of Trinity College, Cambridge, 1984–1990

At most of the colleges in the universities of Oxford and Cambridge, the Head is elected by the Fellows of the college. In Trinity, however, our founder, King Henry VIII, laid down that its Head should be appointed by the King or Queen of England. The Fellows are consulted on the appointment, but they have no veto, and as a result they give the Master very much less power than in most other colleges, in case an unwelcome appointment might be made. Much of the work that heads of other colleges have to do is performed in Trinity by the Vice-Master, who is elected by the Fellows from among their number. The Master of Trinity is therefore to some extent a figurehead, though he is Chairman of the College Council and of any meeting of the

Fellows at which important decisions may be taken. He would be expected to take a leading part in dealing with any crisis that might arise in the College; fortunately, nothing of that sort happened during my tenure.

The Master when I was an undergraduate before the war was the physicist J.J. Thomson, who had discovered the electron in 1897. He was the last Master who was not subject to a retiring age, and he remained Master until his death in 1940 at the age of 83. His successors included George Trevelyan and Lord Adrian, whom I have mentioned in other connections, and my immediate predecessor was Alan Hodgkin, my mentor. As is customary, we moved into the Master's Lodge, which is a part of the college buildings. It is a splendid residence (and also very comfortable). The main entertaining rooms date from the beginning of the 17th century and provided a wonderful setting for the considerable amount of entertaining that we were expected to do, both of undergraduates and of senior members of the University, as well as one visit by the Duke of Edinburgh (Chancellor of the University); one by Princess Margaret, sister of the Queen; and two by the Princess Royal in her capacity as President of the British Olympic Committee when it held fund-raising dinners in the College.

Diffraction of Light by the Striations of Muscle

A very convenient way of estimating changes in the length of a segment of an isolated muscle fiber is to measure changes in the direction of one of the first-order beams in the diffraction pattern of laser light created by the striations. This technique is widely used on account of its simplicity, but, unless additional precautions are taken, it is subject to artifacts due to differences in the spacing and orientation of the striations in different "domains" within the fiber. During a visit to Lee Peachey in Philadelphia, I developed an optical device to recognize these domains. They diffract in slightly different directions and therefore cause fine structure within each diffracted beam. By using a mask with a hole to select a particular spot in this pattern, individual domains could be made visible and recorded photographically. This work led me to look into the theory of light diffraction by a thick striated structure. Several conclusions emerged, such as the existence of particular thicknesses at which the intensity of a diffracted beam drops to zero. However, these results are of only limited use in interpreting the diffraction pattern from a muscle fiber since the theory assumes a perfectly regular structure.

Retirement, 1990–

When I retired from the Mastership, we moved back to our house in Grantchester, where I am now writing this. I continued a little experimental work in collaboration with Vincenzo Lombardi and his colleague Gabriella Piazzesi from Florence, but I did not have a full-time collaborator. For some years, I had as a research assistant, Simon Tideswell, who was skilled in computers, and we published two papers based on simulations of transient responses. The first paper (1996) gave a fairly good simulation of the tension time course after step changes of length. The second paper (1997) dealt with a phenomenon discovered by Lombardi and known as the rapid recovery of the power stroke and provided a fresh explanation based on the attachment of the second head of myosin molecules of which only one head had previously been attached to the actin filament.

When Lincoln Ford, Bob Simmons, and I were analyzing our records of the tension changes in response to stepwise shortening, we needed four exponential terms to fit the early phase of tension recovery (Phase 2), but the simulations in the 1996 paper by Tideswell and me gave a time course much closer to a single exponential term. Julien Davis, however, fits Phase 2 with only two exponential terms, and he has recently suggested to me that the reason for the difference is that we took Phase 2 as being represented by deviations from a straight line fitted to the beginning of Phase 3, while he takes deviations from the curve obtained by fitting exponential terms to Phases 3 and 4. His procedure is probably better justified than ours, and I am planning to re-analyze some of our records by his method.

I remain very busy, refereeing papers submitted to journals, grant applications, and proposals for promotion or for prizes. I am writing obituaries and a few articles, largely historical such as this one. I try to keep up with the progress on muscle contraction by reading, by visiting to former colleagues, and by attending conferences and symposia in the field, though I am restricting the amount of long-distance travel that I undertake.

Many things are still uncertain about the way in which a myosin molecule pulls on an actin filament to make a muscle contract, and I still spend time thinking about this problem. It remains to be seen whether I shall have any ideas that are worth publishing.

Selected Bibliography

Bárány E. A contribution to the physiology of bone conduction. *Acta Oto-Laryngol* 1938;Suppl. 26:1–223.

Bartlett JH. Transient anode phenomena. *Trans Electrochem Soc* 1945;87:521–545.

Cole KS. Dynamic electrical characteristics of the squid axon membrane. *Arch Sci Physiol* 1949;3:255–258.

Cole KS, Antosiewicz HA, Rabinowitz P. Automatic computation of nerve excitation. *J Soc Ind Appl Math* 1955;3:153.

Cole KS. Membrane excitation of the Hodgkin-Huxley axon. Preliminary corrections. *J Appl Physiol* 1958;12:129–130.

Enderlein G. Beitrag zur Kenntniss des Baues der quergestreiften Muskeln bei den Insekten. *Arch Mikrosk Anat* 1899;55:144–150.

Engelmann TW. Ueber den faserigen Bau der contractilen Substanzen, mit besonderer Berücksichtigung der glatten und doppelt schräggestreiften Muskelfasern. *Pflügers Arch Gesamte Physiol* 1881;25:538–565.

Gold T, Pumphrey RJ. Hearing. I. The cochlea as a frequency analyser. Hearing. II. The physical basis of the action of the cochlea. *Proc R Soc Lond Ser B* 1948;135:462–491 and 492–498.

Granzier HLM, Pollack GH. The descending limb of the force-sarcomere length relation of the frog revisited. *J Physiol* 1990;421:595–615.

Hasselbach W. Elektronenmikroskopische Untersuchungen an Muskelfibrillen bei totaler und partieller Extraktion des L-Myosins. *Z Naturforsch* 1953;8b:449–454.

Hill AV. The heat of shortening and the dynamic constants of muscle. *Proc R Soc Lond Ser B* 1938;126:136–195.

Hill AV. The abrupt transition from rest to activity in muscle. *Proc R Soc Lond Ser B* 1949;136:399–420.

Hill AV. The effect of load on the heat of shortening of muscle. *Proc R Soc Lond Ser B* 1964;159:297–318.

Huxley HE, Hanson J. Changes in the cross-striations of muscle during contraction and stretch and their structural interpretation. *Nature* 1954;173:973–976.

Kiang NY-S. *Discharge patterns of single fibers in the cat's auditory nerve.* MIT research monograph no. 35. Cambridge, MA: MIT Press, 1965; Chap. 7.

Krogh A. The active and passive exchanges of inorganic ions through the surfaces of living cells and through living membranes generally. *Proc R Soc Lond Ser B* 1946;133:140–200.

Needham DM. Myosin and adenosinetriphosphate in relation to muscle contraction. *Biochim Biophys Acta* 1950;4:42–49.

Nyström G. Ueber die Lymphbahnen des Herzens. *Arch Anat Physiol (Anat Abt)* 1897:361–378.

Overton E. Beiträge zur allgemeinen Muskel- und Nervenphysiologie. I Mittheilung. Ueber die Unentbehrlichkeit von Natrium-(oder Lithium-)Ionen für den Contractionsact des Muskels. *Pflügers Arch Gesamte Physiol* 1902;92:346–386.

Porter KR, Palade GE. Studies on the endoplasmic reticulum. III. Its form and distribution in striated muscle cells. *J Biophys Biochem Cytol* 1957;3:269–300.

Ramsey RW, Street SF. The isometric length-tension diagram of isolated skeletal muscle fibers of the frog. *J Cell Comp Physiol* 1940;15:11–34.

Robertson JD. Some features of the ultrastructure of reptilian skeletal muscle. *J Biophys Biochem Cytol* 1956;2:369–380.

Smith FH. 1947 British provisional patent specification no. 21996.

Veratti E. Investigations on the fine structure of striated muscle fiber. *J Biophys Biochem Cytol* 1961;10(Suppl.):1–59.

Selected Publications by A.F. Huxley

Book

Huxley AF. Reflections on muscle (based on the Sherrington Lectures, 1977). Liverpool: Liverpool University Press, 1980. Reprinted by Princeton, NJ: Princeton University Press.

Chapter in Book

Huxley AF. Looking back on muscle. In Hodgkin AL, Huxley AF, Feldberg W, Rushton WAH, Gregory RA, McCance RA eds. *The pursuit of nature. Informal essays on the history of physiology*. Cambridge, UK: Cambridge University Press, 1977;23–64.

Papers in Journals

Armstrong CM, Huxley AF, Julian FJ. Oscillatory responses in frog skeletal muscle fibres. *J Physiol* 1966;186:26–27P.

Brown LM, Gonzalez-Serratos H, Huxley AF. Structural studies of the waves in striated muscle fibres shortened passively below their slack length. *J Muscle Res Cell Motil* 1984;5:273–292.

Elliott GF, Huxley AF, Weis-Fogh T. On the structure of resilin. *J Mol Biol* 1965;13:791–795.

Ford LE, Huxley AF, Simmons RM. Tension responses to sudden length change in stimulated frog muscle fibres near slack length. *J Physiol* 1977;269:441–515.

Ford LE, Huxley AF, Simmons RM. The relation between stiffness and filament overlap in stimulated frog muscle fibres. *J Physiol* 1981;311:219–249.

Ford LE, Huxley AF, Simmons RM. Tension transients during steady shortening of frog muscle fibres. *J Physiol* 1985;361:131–150.

Ford LE, Huxley AF, Simmons RM. Tension transients during the rise of tetanic tension in frog muscle fibres. *J Physiol* 1986;372:595–609.

Gordon AM, Huxley AF, Julian FJ. Tension development in highly stretched vertebrate muscle fibres. *J Physiol* 1966a;184:143–169.

Gordon AM, Huxley AF, Julian FJ. The variation of tension with sarcomere length in vertebrate muscle fibres. *J Physiol* 1966b;184:170–192.

Hodgkin AL, Huxley AF. Action potentials recorded from inside a nerve fibre. *Nature* 1939;144:710.

Hodgkin AL, Huxley AF. Resting and action potentials in single nerve fibres. *J Physiol* 1945;104:176–195.

Hodgkin AL, Huxley AF. Potassium leakage from an active nerve fibre. *J Physiol* 1947;106:341–367.

Hodgkin AL, Huxley AF. Currents carried by sodium and potassium ions through the membrane of the giant axon of Loligo. *J Physiol* 1952a;116:449–472.

Hodgkin AL, Huxley AF. The components of membrane conductance in the giant axon of *Loligo. J Physiol* 1952b;116:473–496.

Hodgkin AL, Huxley AF. The dual effect of membrane potential on sodium conductance in the giant axon of *Loligo. J Physiol* 1952c;116:497–506.

Hodgkin AL, Huxley AF. A quantitative description of membrane current and its application to conduction and excitation in nerve. *J Physiol* 1952d;117:500–544.

Hodgkin AL, Huxley AF. Movement of radioactive potassium and membrane current in a giant axon. *J Physiol* 1953;121:403–414.

Hodgkin AL, Huxley AF, Katz B. Ionic currents underlying activity in the giant axon of the squid. *Arch Sci Physiol* 1949;3:129–150.

Hodgkin AL, Huxley AF, Katz B. Measurement of current-voltage relations in the membrane of the giant axon of *Loligo. J Physiol* 1952;116:424–448.

Huxley AF. Applications of an interference microscope. *J Physiol* 1952;117:52–53P.

Huxley AF. A high-power interference microscope. *J Physiol* 1954;125:11–13P.

Huxley AF. An ultramicrotome. *J Physiol* 1957a;137:73–74P.

Huxley AF. Das Interferenz-Mikroskop und seine Anwendung in der biologischen Forschung. *Verh Ges Dtsch Naturforscher Aertze* 1957b:102–109. Berlin: Springer-Verlag.

Huxley AF. Muscle structure and theories of contraction. *Prog Biophys Chem* 1957c;7:255–318.

Huxley AF. Ion movements during nerve activity. *Ann NY Acad Sci* 1959;81:221–246.

Huxley AF. A micromanipulator. *J Physiol* 1961;157:5–7P.

Huxley AF. A theoretical treatment of the reflexion of light by multilayer structures. *J Exp Biol* 1968;48:227–245.

Huxley AF. Is resonance possible in the cochlea after all? *Nature* 1969;221:935–940.

Huxley AF. The activation of striated muscle and its mechanical response (The Croonian Lecture for 1967). *Proc R Soc Lond Ser B* 1971;178:1–27.

Huxley AF. A note suggesting that the cross-bridge attachment during muscle contraction may take place in two stages. *Proc R Soc Lond Ser B* 1973;183:83–86.

Huxley AF. Muscular contraction (review lecture at meeting of the Physiological Society, Leeds University, 14–15 Dec. 1973). *J Physiol* 1974;243:1–43.

Huxley AF. Address of the President at the Anniversary Meeting, 30 November 1981. *Proc R Soc A* 1981;379:v–xx; *Proc R Soc Lond Ser B* 1981;214:137–152.

Huxley AF. Address of the President at the Anniversary Meeting, 30 November 1982. *Proc R Soc A* 1983;385:v–xvi; *Proc R Soc Lond Ser B* 1983;217:117–128.

Huxley AF. Address of the President at the Anniversary Meeting, 30 November 1983. *Proc R Soc A* 1984;391:215–230; *Proc R Soc Lond Ser B* 1984;220:383–398.

Huxley AF. Address of the President at the Anniversary Meeting, 30 November 1984. *Proc R Soc Lond Ser A* 1985;397:183–196.

Huxley AF. Address of the President at the Anniversary Meeting, 30 November 1985. *Science Public Affairs* 1986;1:1–2.

Huxley AF. Muscular contraction (prefatory chapter). *Annu Rev Physiol* 1988;50: 1–16.

Huxley AF. A theoretical treatment of diffraction of light by a striated muscle fibre. *Proc R Soc Lond Ser B* 1990a;241:65–71.

Huxley AF. Bone-conducted sound. *Nature* 1990b;343:28.

Huxley AF, From overshoot to voltage clamp. *Trends Neurosci* 2002;25:553–558.

Huxley AF, Gordon AM. Striation patterns in active and passive shortening of muscle. *Nature* 1962;193:280–281.

Huxley AF, Niedergerke R. Interference microscopy of living muscle fibres. *Nature* 1954;173:971–973.

Huxley AF, Niedergerke R. Measurement of the striations of isolated muscle fibres with the interference microscope. *J Physiol* 1958;144:403–425.

Huxley AF, Peachey LD. The maximum length for contraction in vertebrate striated muscle. *J Physiol* 1956;156:150–165.

Huxley AF, Simmons RM. Proposed mechanism of force generation in striated muscle. *Nature* 1971;233:533–538.

Huxley AF, Stämpfli R. Evidence for saltatory conduction in peripheral myelinated nerve fibres. *J Physiol* 1949;108:315–339.

Huxley AF, Stämpfli R. Effect of potassium and sodium on resting and action potentials of single myelinated nerve fibres. *J Physiol* 1951;112:496–508.

Huxley AF, Taylor RE. Local activation of striated muscle. *J Physiol* 1958;144:426–441.

Huxley AF, Tideswell S. Filament compliance and tension transients in muscle. *J Muscle Res Cell Motil* 1996;17:507–511.

Huxley AF, Tideswell S. Rapid regeneration of power stroke in contracting muscle by attachment of second myosin head. *J Muscle Res Cell Motil* 1997;18:111–114.

Huxley AF, Lombardi V, Peachey LD. A system for recording longitudinal displacements in a striated muscle fibre during contraction. *Boll Soc Ital Biol Sper* 1981;57:57–59.

Slawnych MP, Seow CY, Huxley AF, Ford LE. A program for developing a comprehensive mathematical description of the crossbridge cycle of muscle. *Biophys J* 1994;67:1669–1677.

Sundell CL, Peachey LD, Goldman YE, Gonzalez-Serratos H, Huxley AF. Visualization of domains in spatially filtered images of skeletal muscle. *Biophys J* 1986;49:262a.

JacSue Kehoe

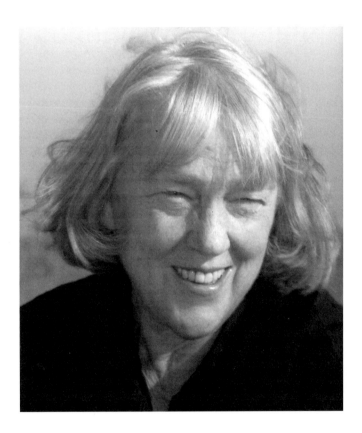

JacSue Kehoe

BORN:

Cleveland, Ohio
October 23, 1935

EDUCATION:

Northwestern University, B.A. (1957)
Brown University, Ph.D. (Psychology, 1961)

APPOINTMENTS:

Instructor, Brown University (1961)
NIMH Postdoctoral Fellow: Walter Reed Institute of
Research (1962–1964)
NATO Postdoctoral Fellow: L'Institut Marey, Paris
(1964–1965)
NSF Postdoctoral Fellow: L'Institut Marey, Paris
(1965–1967)
Centre National de la Recherche Scientifique (C.N.R.S.)
(1967–2001)
Emeritus Director of Research, C.N.R.S. (2001)

HONORS AND AWARDS:
Forbes Lectureship (1977)

JacSue Kehoe was among the first scientists to take advantage of the mollusc Aplysia for electrophysiological analysis of synaptic transmission. She demonstrated that a single transmitter could produce multiple, independent conductance changes in a single postsynaptic cell and characterized the synaptic actions of many neurotransmitters.

JacSue Kehoe

When looking at the first volume of the series of *The History of Neuroscience in Autobiography*, the idea of a résumé of my life following those of Sir Alan Hodgkin and Sir Bernard Katz seemed ridiculous. As the years and the volumes go by, however, and my gods have been succeeded by mere mortals, the idea seems less intimidating, although still, given my trajectory, less than evident. Obviously, affirmative action is still alive and well and must play a role in this choice. In view of the tortuous path I took to the field of neurobiology, and the somewhat atypical approach I have taken in my scientific endeavors, my contribution will at least add variety to those previously published in the series.

From Childhood to College

My life was much too normal, enjoyable, and uneventful to make good reading. In short, I was born to very understanding, generous, intelligent parents who provided unfailing support for their three children and a loving home environment, of which many of my school friends were jealous. I was the third and last child—a status I thoroughly enjoyed, since I was not subject to the tighter parental reins and higher expectations that are typically reserved for the eldest.

Our father, with a mother and younger sister for whom he had to provide, was obliged to become full-time breadwinner of the family at age 16 when he graduated from high school. He had already been working as station master of the local train station by the age of 12. His lack of formal education was, nevertheless, undetectable thanks to his lively intelligence and avid curiosity. Our mother, on the other hand, was anticipating a much later generation. Although she was born at the end of the 19th century, the daughter of a shoe salesman, after graduating from university she began doctoral studies. Health problems did not permit her to complete the program, but even the idea of going for a Ph.D. was very atypical for women at that time. More typical, however, was her tendency to put her role as mother and homemaker in first place. Although she was a high-school English teacher until she retired at age 70, she insisted that we list her profession as "homemaker" whenever we were required to fill out forms. This curious request might also have reflected a deference to my father who, on the academic front, could not compete with her credentials. Although she clearly had crossed the professional frontier, she held very strongly to the woman's role as spectator rather than participant in anything bordering on what was at the time strictly a man's world (e.g., politics, finances, etc.).

My parents started their family shortly after the Wall Street stock market crash, but their jobs were not affected by the consequent Great Depression. Nor did either of the two world wars directly affect our family's well-being. My father was too young to be called up for World War I and was too old for World War II. The only other male family member of their generation, my mother's brother, was likewise out of sync with the draft. However, World War II did affect my father's job, since Chrysler Corporation, for which he worked at the time, joined the war effort and he was moved for the "duration" from a Detroit suburb to Evansville, IN. There my father could realize his dream of living in the country (a dream my mother clearly did not share) where we were put in the typical country school in which two grade levels functioned simultaneously in one classroom and where the school term ended in May so the children could participate in the farming activities. We were exempt from such activities, since, although we had a 14-acre "farm," the stables and cow barn were inhabited exclusively by rabbits, stray cats, dogs, rats, and a goat named Sammy. My father drove into the city each day for work, while the rest of us were bussed off to school (whether for teaching or being taught).

Between the ages of 6 and 10, my awareness of the war was limited to the hunt for milkweed pods used for making life jackets for the sailors (at least that is what we were told); collecting tinfoil from chewing-gum wrappers (I never knew for what purpose); and learning what we could about the ongoing, faraway battles from radio broadcasts and from newsreels when we went to the cinema. I remember celebrating VJ day by harnessing Sammy to a wagon and having her pull me in the rain down the local country roads. The most personal impact that the faraway war had on me occurred upon the return from hostilities of our school bus driver whose joyful expansiveness had been transformed into a tightly guarded sadness following his years in the midst of the conflict. Distinctly different and more dramatic pictures of these years have been drawn by many scientists of my generation, who were much closer to and much more affected by the war.

When the "war effort" was over, we moved to Ohio and to the city. School, which had been for me until that time more of a social activity than an academic pursuit, became a bit more of the latter with the return to an urban environment. My academic interests were still much more affected by the personality of the teacher than they were by the subject matter. That changed, however, in junior high school, where I encountered dramatic arts. From my early experiences helping direct school plays (as assistant to the dramatic arts' teacher), I started for the first time thinking along the lines of "when I grow up…" A major influence in affirming this orientation was the nearby presence of an excellent summer Shakespeare theater at Antioch

College in Yellow Springs, OH—close enough to Dayton, where we lived, so that I could regularly make the trip on my bicycle. I was indeed bitten, and it was because of the certainty in my choice that science subjects rapidly disappeared from my course load.

Consequently, in high school, I was clearly already headed away from, rather than toward, a scientific career. Meanwhile, my sister (the eldest of the lot) was following in the academic and educational footsteps of our mother, heading for a teaching career via Ohio State University (at $90 per quarter tuition, as I recall). My brother, the meat of the children's sandwich, was headed for the sciences with enthusiasm and excellence and was off to Deep Springs College ($0.0 per year), participating in a generally successful experiment in education begun by L.L. Nunn in 1917 which still nourishes the academic elite, in spite of one of its peculiarities—the obligation of manual labor as part of the curriculum.

On the other hand, when I was ready to fulfill my dreams of becoming a theater director, Northwestern University, the private institution which housed the most renowned spot for university theater training, was not so financially welcoming as the institutions chosen by my siblings. Consequently, I felt an obligation to work to earn my room and board. This I did, with a number of other theater students, by living and working in an "old ladies' home" as it was called at that time, but which has surely since found a substitute label. The so-called "home" offered room and board to Northwestern students in exchange for work as kitchen aides and waitresses. That meant rising at 6:00 AM to serve prunes and other less crucial breakfast items and, of course, to perform various chores at prescheduled hours during the day.

From Theater to Experimental Psychology

My first two years in speech school were unfortunately not very captivating (including courses in "lighting effects," "make up," etc.). These two years also revealed to me the ferocious competition in the field, making me realize that I was unlikely to become the director of the best Shakespearean theater on the continent. Given that realization, and the fact that I knew I did not want to direct community theater in Podunk, I slowly began readjusting my career orientation, while never losing my love of theater. Slowly, I say, since I had no clear alternative in mind. I tried a geology course, because I had always been drawn to the notion of reading history with rocks as my book, but I quickly realized that such "reading in the field" was not open to women at that time, and sitting in an office was not what I was looking for when leaning toward geology. I also dabbled a bit in life sciences by taking an introductory biology course and a course in what was obviously still Mendelian genetics at the time.

The strongest common thread in all of my life's choices, though never expressed as such, was a constant underlying interest in animal and human behavior: observing it, understanding the variables that control it, and realizing how it could be modulated. This was clearly something that fascinated me in my short "career" directing plays: bringing out of people what they themselves did not know was in them. At least at that time, I was clearly more interested in the behavior of humans than in the behavior of the molecules of which they were constituted. This probably led me in my junior year of college to my first course in experimental psychology, and it was there that I was bitten a second time around.

My scientific debut revolved around a question that has become a very "hot" topic in neurobiology in the last few decades: memory and forgetting. My mentor, Benton J. Underwood, was one of the leading experimental psychologists interested in that field at that time. The experiments I performed for my honor's thesis involved using humans as subjects and nonsense syllables "à la Ebbinghaus" as the material to be learned and forgotten. My conversion to experimental psychology also added 20 more hours a week workload—20 hr waiting tables plus 20 hr analyzing data for professors in the Psychology Department. I do not recommend such a regime to others: though being motivated more by my courses in experimental psychology than by those in theatrical make up, I went through my last two years of college in a more or less comatose state, going to bed at 2:00 AM and rising to serve breakfast at 6:00 AM. But it was worth it. I was finally fully engaged in what I was doing and enjoying it.

From Experimental Psychology to Neurophysiology

The first real external manifestation of my latent interest in biology came when I had to choose a department of experimental psychology for graduate work. I homed in on either McGill University, where Hebb was the major attraction, or Brown University, where the program in so-called physiological psychology was very strong. I recognized that for understanding memory and other aspects of behavior it was clearly necessary to know the fundamentals concerning the functioning of the nervous system. Because the policy of both departments was to have a limited number of students, and since no graduate student was scheduled to leave the department at McGill that year, no one could enter. Consequently, I didn't have to make a decision myself, and I went off to graduate school at Brown, where Harold Schlosberg was then Chairman and an influential one at that. However, the physiological approach at Brown in the late 1950s was directed exclusively towards the study of sensory systems (either visual processes under Lorrin Riggs or the sensation of taste under Carl Pfaffmann), and I remained strongly attached to the study of memory, which at that time was being addressed exclusively by various methodologies used for the study of discrimination learning. At Brown, this methodology was primarily limited to the paradigm of positive reinforcement (in particular, Skinnerian) rather than that of so-called classical, aversive conditioning developed by Pavlov. For my Ph.D. thesis, I applied this methodology to the study, in pigeons, of paradigms used in the human studies of retention: proactive and retroactive inhibition.

Although for my final career destination I certainly would have profited enormously by a graduate school training concentrated on math, chemistry, and biology, I nevertheless continue to be thankful for the four years I spent at Brown in experimental psychology. It was a field that posed many questions of great interest to me, and I had the good fortune of spending my graduate school years with enthusiastic colleagues, both students and faculty, from whom I learned a great deal. Furthermore, I found the training I received to be very useful and "transferable" to other scientific disciplines, as well as to life itself. I remain particularly indebted to J.W. Kling (Jake) for the guidance he gave me in the acquisition of observational skills and in developing the notions of experimental control and methodological rigor. Whether such insistence is related specifically to experimental psychology or specifically to that department at that time, I don't know, but when I switched to biology, I found such considerations to be much less well developed. Other useful skills I brought with me were related to the necessity at that time to build all aspects of our experimental setups, using second-hand solenoid driven relays given to us by "Ma Bell" and stepping motors and the like purchased by weight on Canal Street in New York City. The shop work was obviously transferable, but by the time I fully entered neurobiology, transistors were replacing cathode tubes, and electronic circuits were replacing classical relay circuits.

A Few Rats and Squirrels Prior to Being Seduced by *Aplysia*

The year following my doctorate, I filled a temporary vacancy in Brown's Psychology Department, and then it was time to head for a job or a postdoctoral fellowship. I opted for the latter and will only mention briefly the kind of experience one could have, as a female candidate, at that time. Even though such might still exist now, it would be much more cleverly disguised, and I admit it was the first and last occasion upon which I felt directly confronted by a gender discrimination issue. In the interview I had for that postdoctoral position, I was bombarded with questions concerning an eventual marriage on my part, how I would anticipate handling a career once children came along, etc. Scientific questions seemed clearly secondary. Although I was obviously aware that such discrimination existed, up until that time my gender had never interfered with my career opportunities, so I was completely taken by surprise and left basically speechless. I was certainly not at all interested in pursuing a postdoctoral position with such a man, and

I believe the feeling was mutual. Instead I went off to a much more welcoming environment where the door to electrophysiology eventually opened fully for me.

I headed off to Washington, DC on a postdoctoral fellowship in Joseph Brady's lab at the Walter Reed Army Institute of Research headed by David Rioch. This lab was one of the first to put together a multidisciplinary group to study the biological bases of behavior. Again, however, I was still strictly a behaviorist and was continuing my studies of discrimination learning under the wing of William Hodos, who was studying the visual system of pigeons.

Although I was still fascinated by the questions that experimental psychology was posing at the time and spent part of the two years in Washington studying discrimination learning in rats and the parameters affecting hibernation in squirrels, I felt more and more pessimistic about being able to obtain answers that could go beyond the operational definitions which often fenced in our conclusions. This feeling, and the fortuitous presence of Felix Strumwasser in the lab next door to mine, resulted in a definitive change in my scientific orientation during the two years I spent in Washington, Felix was doing electrophysiological studies of circadian rhythms, using as one of his models a particular neuron in the central nervous system of *Aplysia californica* now known as R15, but labeled "parabolic burster" by Felix. Thanks to Felix's exclusive devotion to that very complicated neuron found in the abdominal ganglion, I was able to intercept the remaining ganglia of each *Aplysia* on their way to the trash can and use them for honing my skills as an electrophysiologist. With those ganglia, Felix's discarded cathode tube amplifier, and his very generous help, I began my studies of synaptic physiology.

From the United States to France: October 1964

The decision leading to my next move was influenced more by nonscientific motivations than by scientific ones. I was footloose and fancy-free and, until then, had had little money or time to be able to travel. I thought I should take the opportunity to do so before I was tied down by either personal or job constraints. The scientific justifications were hence the second to be taken into consideration. The opportunities suggested to me were going either to Santiago, Chile, where I would be experimenting on cats (a very unpleasant prospect for a cat lover to overcome); to Warsaw where Jerzy Konorski used electrophysiological techniques to answer questions posed mainly at that time by psychologists; or to Paris where I could continue to work on *Aplysia* in the Institut Marey directed by Alfred Fessard.

Although Paris, which I had already visited, seemed a less exotic destination than either Santiago or Warsaw, I had already developed an appreciation for molluscan neurons, and so I decided to go to France, where the *Aplysia* model for electrophysiological studies had been born. Arvanitaki started using that preparation in the early 1940s. However, the benefits of the *Aplysia* preparation as a model for the study of synaptic transmission became apparent only after the successive collaborations of Hersch Gerschenfeld and Eric Kandel with Ladislav Tauc at the Laboratoire de Physiologie Cellulaire in Paris. Twenty years prior to the development of the patch clamp, large cells were the only ones that offered the possibility of recording from a cell whose membrane potential could also be controlled by penetrating the neuron with more than one relatively low-resistance microelectrode. These same traits also made possible the early voltage clamping in these neurons, which permitted a much more analytical study of membrane responses to neurotransmitters. The second opportunity that gastropods, in general, and *Aplysia* neurons, in particular, offer is the ability to work on the "same," homologous neuron from one *Aplysia* to the next. Because of the relative ease of cell identification, it quickly became possible to identify both the pre- and postsynaptic elements of a synapse, thus offering a very valuable tool for the study of synaptic transmission.

So, on October 3, 1964, with a NATO Fellowship in my pocket, I was off to Paris on "le France" (the recently constructed ocean liner that had made its first transatlantic voyage in 1962) to continue discovering the glories of *Aplysia* neurons. The trip over was a nice break from the frenetic pace of my departure preparations. The weather was gorgeous; the food was excellent; and many good books later I arrived at Cherbourg, and my life in the "old world" began.

Friends from the Northwestern Psychology Department had put me in contact with a French couple, Michel and Danièle Gervais, who had managed the very difficult task of finding housing for me in Paris, right in the middle of St. Germain des Près. Although, at that time, housing was very scarce, and telephones essentially nonexistent for anyone renting an apartment, they managed to find both for me. American tourists were still bringing toilet paper with them when going to France—something which was indeed not necessary—but I certainly did experience a feeling of going back in time when arriving from the United States. The window sill was my refrigerator, and in the extremely cold winter of that year, it became my freezer. Only considerably later did I realize how close, in fact, we were at that time to the end of World War II and all that that implied for slowing down the modernization of France.

When I first came to the Institut Marey, on the edge of the Bois de Boulogne, and joined the Laboratoire de Neurophysiologie Cellulaire headed by Ladislav Tauc, I was surrounded exclusively by those for whom French was not their native language. This did not have a positive effect on my acquisition of French, since English was the common language of the lab. Although I successfully passed a French language exam as a graduate student, it was not because of any knowledge of French, but rather because of the alacrity with which I could manipulate a dictionary—the use of which was tolerated in such exams at Brown. Consequently, I came to Paris knowing, but mispronouncing, "bonjour" and "au revoir." To my chagrin, upon meeting the Head of the Institute, Alfred Fessard, I accidentally pulled out the inappropriate one and said au revoir. He very graciously asked if I would prefer speaking in English or in French. I repeat graciously because M. Fessard had also been assuming that the "JacSue Kehoe" who was coming to his institute was male and more akin to a "Jaku Su Kiho" of Japanese origin, hence much better equipped than an American woman, as the "a priori's" dictated at the time, to be an excellent neurophysiologist.

The location of the laboratory led to an interesting introduction to one aspect of Parisian life. When walking through the Bois de Boulogne to reach the lab, I often noticed cars slowing down and frequently lowering their windows in order to, I assumed, ask directions. My French was not up to understanding their requests, much less to answering them. I later learned that this was a pick-up zone for prostitutes, and in spite of my atypical attire for such a job (usually jeans and a sweatshirt), some drivers seemed to consider me a candidate.

L'Institut Marey: Changes in a Behavioral Reflex Correlated with Changes in Associated Synaptic Potentials

My first studies in the Institut Marey were performed under the direction of Jan Bruner, a Polish scientist who came to neurophysiology with a psychological bent, as did I, and was interested in "plastic changes" defined by his mentor, Jerzy Konorski. Janek and Ladislav Tauc had already begun a series of observations in *Aplysia* correlating the diminution in amplitude of a behavioral reflex (the retraction of tentacles in response to water drops falling on the head) with the diminution in associated central, excitatory postsynaptic potentials. Eric Kandel at the same time was beginning a series of studies paralleling the changes in the gill withdrawal reflex and postsynaptic potentials (PSP) in identified neurons in the abdominal ganglion using a similar paradigm. As history has shown, Eric made the right choice in persevering in those studies. His unswerving path, coupled with the aid of a vast array of collaborators and an impressive battery of scientific tools, led him to Stockholm.

L'Institut Marey: Cholinergic Synaptic Transmission

I, being less persevering and much less well equipped for the job, became diverted by some observations I made while studying so-called habituation and dishabituation of PSPs in the pleural ganglia of *Aplysia*. In an attempt to identify the neurotransmitter eliciting the PSPs that were "habituating" upon repetitive stimulation of the *Aplysia's* head, I applied curare to the solution bathing the ganglion. This did not answer the question that I was asking, since the PSPs were unaffected by this well-known cholinergic antagonist. However, the spontaneous synaptic activity—rare in the cells I was using for this study—changed, and a very dramatic hyperpolarizing wave repeatedly appeared. It was this that caught my attention, and the synapses generating that response became the centerpiece of my investigations for the next three years.

A year had passed by this time, and it was once again the period of the fall migration of the *Aplysia* group to Arcachon—a migration not dissimilar in some respects to that of American neurobiologists who, in the late spring, migrate to the Marine Biological Laboratory at Woods Hole, MA. As is the case for the move to Woods Hole in the United States, at both ends of the Arcachon "season" it was necessary to tear down, transport, and rebuild the experimental setups. However, the trip to Arcachon consisted of only about 10 "Aplysialogues" who went off to the Atlantic coast where *Aplysia* came to the shore at that time of year for their last hurrah.

Hersch Gerschenfeld came to join the lab for the fall "retreat," and at this time Philippe Ascher began his tenure as a full member of the laboratory. Leaving his cat preparation behind at the Faculté des Sciences, where he obtained his doctoral degree studying the startle reflex, Philippe began his studies on dopamine receptors in *Aplysia* neurons. His arrival had many repercussions on my life in France. He was the first native French speaker in the lab, and my insistence that, in spite of his fluent English, all our conversations be in French greatly facilitated at least my vocabulary if not my accent, which was beyond repair given the 30 years I had already acquired before I said my first au revoir. Second, Philippe, with his thorough scientific background, provided me a much needed counselor in anything chemical. His help was particularly indispensable when I was struggling to make solutions using impermeant replacements for Cl ions, and I still tremble at the thought of losing or gaining a few zeros when determining drug concentrations. There was a joke circulating at one time whose "hero" received a lot of empathy from me. It concerns the captain of a ship who, just before addressing his crew, would run down to his cabin; open a locked box; and take out, read, and then return a small piece of paper before going back up to the deck to talk with his men. He was beloved, and so no one dared confront him with the question as to the significance of this seeming superstition. But when he died, they forced open the box, only to find written on the paper: starboard, right; portside, left! My locked-up paper is for reminding me how many zeros for pico, nano, micro, and milli. Once my calculations are made, it is still up to Philippe to reassure me that they are right. However, in a much broader way, Philippe's vast scientific knowledge and his characteristic generosity in sharing it have provided an indispensable reservoir into which I have been able to dip throughout my career as a neuroscientist.

Let us return after this aside to my fascination with the hyperpolarizing synaptic response I described earlier. To further understand its origin and its mechanism, I put together my own experimental setup to begin trying to locate the presynaptic cell responsible for this intriguing synaptic activity. The response was particularly intriguing since, upon further observation, it was found to consist of two components: one rapid and the other more slowly developing and longer lasting. The slower component hyperpolarized the cell well beyond the equilibrium potential for Cl ions, suggesting that it was the result of a synaptically induced increase in potassium conductance—something not yet dogma in neuronal synaptology, although already known as a potent mechanism underlying cholinergic inhibition in heart cells.

Once the presynaptic neuron was finally localized, it became relatively easy to demonstrate that the transmitter being liberated was acetylcholine, thanks to there being a battery of pharmacological tools active on vertebrate cholinergic receptors and already known to be similarly effective on invertebrate receptors. Serendipity, however, once more played a significant role in permitting me to find the most elusive antagonist—that for blocking the receptor mediating the potassium-dependent response. That receptor refused categorization in the classification system used for defining cholinergic receptors at the time. Neither curare nor atropine blocked it, and neither nicotine nor muscarine activated it. In desperation I started pulling bottles off the shelf, and lo and behold the contents of one hand-labeled bottle, bearing the letters "BTM," selectively blocked the K-dependent response. But finding out what that mysterious substance might be required contacting Hersch Gerschenfeld who had left a variety of compounds on the shelf after his collaboration in Paris with Ladislav Tauc. This compound turned out to be a Smith Kline and French product, better known as SK&F 6890, βTM-10, or methyl-xylocholine. By whatever name, it was certainly not developed for interacting with cholinergic receptors, but rather as an adrenergic neuron blocker. Had I known that, I would never have tried it on that synapse! It was, however, a critical tool for showing that the K-dependent response elicited synaptically and that the response elicited by exogeneous ACh were mediated by the same receptor.

One of my first presentations of these results took place at a meeting of the French Physiological Society in Toulouse. There I described the pharmacological characteristics of the two receptors mediating the synaptic inhibitory response, as well as the ionic mechanisms underlying the changes in membrane potential induced by activation of these receptors. In the audience was Angelique Arvanitaki, who was not in such an angelical mood that day. She opened fire by dismissing the notion of ion channels as an Anglo-Saxon obsession and followed that with a chauvinistic attack (always more vigorous from converted immigrants) concerning my choice of using *A. californica*, which she considered to be less intelligent than the local species of the beast. Since the subject of my studies was not intelligence,

I had no particular opinion on that matter, but what became evident later in my studies of those receptors is that the receptor mediating the K-dependent response, i.e., the receptor that most interested me, was not expressed in the "local" species I later tested as an experimental preparation. I dare say that although I continue to be appreciative of the role Arvanitaki played in developing the *Aplysia* preparation as a model for electrophysiological studies, this "French" scientific experience did not encourage me to participate actively in the French Physiological Society thereafter.

In spite of Arvanitaki's lack of enthusiasm, I continued studying those elegant synaptic events which revealed (1) that more than one receptor for a neurotransmitter can co-exist on a given neuron; (2) that each of the receptors induced a different, independent conductance change (in this case, increases in Cl and K conductances, respectively); and (3) that the response to a given presynaptic neuron could be different for different postsynaptic cells. These findings, along with those concurrently coming out of Eric Kandel's lab, forced the recognition that a given transmitter could induce multiple, independent, membrane conductance changes in a single cell. The masking of the response mediated by one receptor by that of another receptor had led to many false interpretations about the mechanisms of neurotransmitter actions in many preparations.

Time for Important Decisions

The time had come when I was required to make active decisions about my future. I could no longer simply go with the flow. I had already overabused the generosity of the NSF and NIH, and I had a job in the United States waiting for a decision on my part. But I had a lingering sensation that I had not yet had my fill of France. This latter feeling led me to apply for a position in the Centre National de la Recherche Scientifique (C.N.R.S.), which, if successful, would permit me to work full time as a research scientist without mandatory teaching responsibilities. Given the limitations of my scientific background and the non-native character of my French, if I were to settle in France this definitely seemed like the best option for me (and for any student body). A successful entrance into this organization was soon followed by another important decision. I mentioned above the scientific savoir that Philippe kindly shared with all of us in the lab, but it was not only for that trait that I married Philippe in the fall of 1967. However, unlike Jim Watson who, in his recent autobiographical book, mixed in girls with genes and Gamow, I won't go into detail concerning the other criteria that helped me make an obviously complicated decision that entailed not only choosing a spouse, but simultaneously choosing a country.

In a delayed "honeymoon," we set off for the United States over the 1967 Christmas holidays so that Philippe could meet members of my family who were unable to attend our Paris wedding. En route to my parents' home, we visited the newly formed Neurobiology Laboratory at Harvard directed by Steve Kuffler. By that time part of my results were already published in *Nature*, and Steve had asked me to give a seminar. When I was in his office prior to giving my talk, he rather startled me with the comment, "So, you've realized your dream!" I certainly was not the "dreaming" kind; I functioned and still function much more on serendipity than on previously conceived dreams. But I later understood Steve's comment when seeing his somewhat similar attempts to analyze slow synaptic potentials in a much more recalcitrant mammalian ganglionic preparation that required considerably more effort.

Although my fare for our honeymoon was obviously not paid by the C.N.R.S., it was around this time when I was invited to a meeting in the United States and requested travel funds from the C.N.R.S. I was still in the lowest echelon on the C.N.R.S. ladder, so of course there would be no question of "first class travel." However, when I received what was supposed to be adequate financial assistance for making the trip, the restrictions they put upon my mode of travel support would have made it difficult for me to arrive on the other side of the Atlantic. Flying was not allowed; I was required to go by train!

May 1968

By this time, a few of us from the Institut Marey had moved to Gif sur Yvette, where much later the entire Institute was relocated in a new building. We, however, were in older buildings on the campus, and although rather isolated from the much denser activity in Paris, we could enjoy living for a year in the woods. This distance, however, did not keep us from a three-month's involvement with the others in our "home" lab during May 1968. In early 1967, the Laboratoire de Physiologie Cellulaire had already had a practice session for the student revolt of May 1968, so we were well prepared for the tumultuous events of the following year. Since the history of this general upheaval has been so widely documented, I will only give a brief description of the motivation leading young scientists to join this movement and mention how it dominated our lives for many months.

While the students in the United States were demanding that one "make love, not war!", in France, the students were pushing for an overhaul of the power structure of the French institutions. Within the framework of scientific laboratories, younger scientists such as we were making two major demands. The first demand was that the science should belong to those who, intellectually speaking, gave birth to the project and to those who actually did the science. In the hierarchical system in many European countries at that time, this was not always the case. Scientific results could basically be confiscated by those sitting at the top of the pyramid, without their having participated directly in the scientific project itself. Furthermore, since the system did not permit younger scientists to develop their own laboratories, they usually became older scientists stagnating in the same place in the pyramidal structure, bound to the scientific objectives of the chief. This was the background for the second demand: that younger scientists be given the right and the means of developing their own laboratories at a much earlier age, which would give them much more intellectual freedom in determining what science they actually could do and more recognition for having done it.

In practice, this period was occupied by unending "assemblées générales" at the Institut Marey where we were accused by the "higher ups" of being under the control of Moscow; with frequent street demonstrations first with students and later with workers as the "revolution" progressed; and with occasional visits to the Sorbonne where assemblies were taking place 24 hr a day. We also participated in study groups at the C.N.R.S. headquarters, where everyone participating, on both ends of the hierarchical pyramid we were trying to alter, was addressed in the informal "tu" form and the appellation "camarade" filled the discussion. We were, however, almost disappointed to find that the charter of the C.N.R.S. that we were intending to revise showed strong resemblance to what we had hoped to put in its place. It was clearly not the paper documents that needed to be revised, but rather the behavior adopted in applying the charter.

This period died down, as history books will tell you, and lives returned more or less to normal with a few scars in interpersonal relationships to remind us that the events had indeed occurred. Although much of the administration of French institutions rapidly returned to a "normal" pre-1968 functioning, repercussions of the 1968 student demands can be detected in the administrative structure of the post-1968 universities and, to some extent, in the nature of the interactions between colleagues of post-1968 generations.

Clearly, however, not all our hopes had been realized. As an example, it was in 1969 that, because of pressures instituted during the presidency of Charles de Gaulle, it was highly encouraged to have at least some publications in French. So I contributed a paper to the *Compte Rendu de l'Académie Française*. The paper was accepted, but only under the condition that I be listed in the index under the name of my husband: not only Ascher instead of Kehoe, but Mme. Philippe Ascher, instead of JacSue Ascher. I do hope that the few women who now are members of that hallowed institution have succeeded in changing that rule.

A Sabbatical Year at Downing Site, Cambridge, England: 1969

The fall of 1968 was occupied by the birth of our first son, David, and, two months afterwards, by our departure on our first "sabbatical." We were off to an old English farmhouse in a village of Cambridgeshire, where we lived with mice and dampness while doing research on Downing Site where Cambridge University's science departments were located. Taking our two-month old child and our *Aplysia* order forms with us, Philippe headed for the Pharmacology Department chaired by Arnold Burgen, and I was given hospitality by Gabriel Horn in the Anatomy Department. Both of us continued the work that we had, respectively, begun in Paris, surrounded by the lovely English countryside and aided by a wonderful woman, Sheila Coxall, who lived in our village and cared for David, our young son, while I was in the lab.

One repercussion of working in the lab of Gabriel Horn was that he arranged to include me as a visiting member of High Table at King's College in Cambridge. Today, that would seem evident and banal. However, in 1968 my admission to High Table, in fact, had some historical significance: it was the first time that a visiting female academic was given access, in her own right, to a Cambridge, all-male college. The advantages of this inclusion were mainly, for me, to be able to have use of the Combination Room, where I had the occasion to meet E.M. Forster and where a vast array of international newspapers were available daily. Most importantly, however, being a Visiting Fellow gave me access to the famous wine cellars of the College. My first attempts at ordering wine flustered the butler, who was not yet aware that a woman could possibly have such a right. What I was not given the right to have, however, was the snuff, a pleasure that the butler serving the cognac and port felt remained a man's prerogative. I didn't feel that it was a cause worth fighting for, so that frontier was left uncrossed.

One of my most marked memories of that year stems from the meeting of the Physiological Society at Cambridge, for which I had naively volunteered to do a demonstration. It was to take place on the top floor of the Physiology Department, but we didn't have the authorization to install our equipment there until the morning of the demonstrations. Philippe was back in France at that time, and I was still nursing my infant son. Luckily, I had an old graduate school friend, Joan Stevenson Hinde, who had also moved to the old world and lived close enough to us so that she could come to spend the night and be with David at 5:00 AM when I would be heading for Downing Site. Setting up the demonstration required moving all the equipment from the second floor of the Anatomy Department to the top floor of the Physiology Department—no small feat. No small feat also was the task I had set for myself, unexperienced in the ways of demonstrations. I stupidly decided to perform an experiment that had a probability of success under normal lab conditions of about one in five tries. The experiment involved simultaneous current clamp recordings from the cholinergic presynaptic neuron and from two postsynaptic neurons, while also injecting a potassium channel blocking agent in the presynaptic neuron and one of the follower cells. The K channel blocking agent was injected into the presynaptic neuron in order to induce a progressive increase in duration of the presynaptic action potential and, hence, a gradual increase in transmitter release. The increased release would then be reflected by an associated increase in the amplitude of both the Cl- and K-dependent elements of the postsynaptic response. The purpose of injecting the K channel blocking agent in the postsynaptic cell was to demonstrate the selective block of the K-dependent element of the response.

Setting up the demonstration was interrupted by periodic returns to the farmhouse to nurse David. However, the biggest frustration was trying to find the cells in a room where the sun's rays were attacking my setup with a vengeance. I was getting desperate because the time was rapidly approaching when the demonstration was to begin, and I still had not been able even to find the relevant neurons because of the sun's glare. Finally, as the morning wore on, the earth's movements improved my chances. The aggressive rays of the sun finally gave way to a simply well-lighted room, and I managed to do what was necessary by the time the crowds collected. In that crowd was Alan Hodgkin, who came to me at the end of my demonstration to offer his congratulations not only on my science, but also on my English. I do believe that to be a unique event: an Englishman complimenting an American on his/her English. Obviously, he had been drawn into this ignominious position by seeing my Paris address.

Our year's end in Cambridge was a difficult one. Philippe was operated on in England for what turned out to be a benign tumor on his thyroid; Philippe's father had his first of many heart attacks; and Philippe, David, and I all experienced the Asian flu that struck so hard in the winter of 1969, which also provided us with the experience of David's first and only fever convulsions. We all recovered from these physical aggressions, and that aspect of the winter in Cambridge left no serious repercussions. However, we also learned at that time that my father's prostate cancer, which he had hidden from all of us, had metastasized to bone, announcing his premature death that occurred the following spring.

Opening the Door to a Lab of Our Own

When I began describing our year in England, I said that we were on a "sabbatical year." In fact, it did start out like that, since we both had research positions at C.N.R.S. and no teaching obligations, which permitted us, without constraints, to change our workplace to a foreign lab. However, we were eager to have our own laboratory, and the only possibility to obtain independent space was for Philippe, who had the appropriate diplomas, to submit his candidacy for a position at the Faculty of Sciences, the predecessor of what was to become the Universities Paris VI and Paris VII. Consequently, when a position opened shortly after our arrival in England, Philippe made an about face and returned to make the traditional visits to those who would be voting on his application. It was a happy event when Philippe was offered the position, but that meant that he had to return to Paris from Cambridge once a week (during university sessions) to give his lectures. Furthermore, this good fortune seemed less good when the building program that was to make space available for us was halted as a consequence of the student revolt of May 1968. So Philippe had gained the teaching responsibilities without the lab space promised to accompany them. For me, an additional problem was that upon this offer to Philippe it seemed almost depressingly clear that in many respects our future was becoming completely predictable. Having lived in eight different states of the United States in my first 30 years, the idea of "sitting still" seemed a strange and perhaps monotonous one to me. But on the other hand, once you're in the 5th arrondissement of Paris, why would you want to move elsewhere?

Ecole Normale Supérieure—The Lab of Our Dreams

Soon after our return from England, we were fortunately offered space at Ecole Normale Supérieure—the French "Grande Ecole" where Philippe had done his predoctoral studies—so the problem of job responsibilities without space no longer existed. We started out, the two of us alone, with little in the way of equipment, but with 500 m^2 and a superb view of Paris. Unlike my scientific discoveries, this laboratory was indeed "dreamed of" and was definitely not serendipitous. We had carefully considered what kind of laboratory we wanted to establish—that is, the type that May 1968 had not yet brought into being. We had considered the criteria we wanted to use when selecting colleagues to join us, and the relationships we would encourage among the scientists themselves and between the scientists and the supporting staff. Soon we convinced many other groups to join us, and in a short time the lab was bristling with activity. But the story of that development is Philippe's to tell, since it is he who had the "political" and administrative responsibilities that permitted us to realize our dream, as well as the scientific breadth to make it a continuing success. I would just like to profit from this occasion to thank all the members of that lab (secretarial, technical, and scientific) for helping us develop and maintain the kind of environment we were determined to create. Without a similar desire on their part, it would have been much more difficult to reach our goal.

Summering at Cold Spring Harbor

While still at Cambridge, we had received a letter from James Watson, who, though still physically at Harvard University, had been named Director of the Cold Spring Harbor Laboratory of Molecular Biology where he had spent many happy and productive moments in earlier years. The story goes that Jim was hoping to obtain money for cancer research from the Sloan-Kettering Foundation, but had learned that their interests were being redirected toward neurobiology. So he, in turn, reoriented his grant proposal and requested, and received, funding for a summer program in neurobiology at Cold Spring Harbor. We were invited to teach the laboratory course in electrophysiology that was to accompany the theoretical course organized by the Neurobiology Department at Harvard. This program demanded six weeks presence at Cold Spring Harbor in the summer, three weeks of which, for us, involved the intensive direction of ten very bright and very motivated students. The course was designed for scientists in other disciplines who wished to collaborate with or become neurobiologists themselves. The idea was interesting, and the students were certain to be excellent. However, the only way that it would be possible for me to accept such an offer was to be accompanied by my child and his extraordinarily devoted baby-sitter, Nicasia Ayesta. Jim seemed amenable to this demand, and the result was that with Nicasia, my $2\frac{1}{2}$-year-old son David, and a 6-month-old foetus weighing me down, I left for our first of 15 summers at Cold Spring Harbor. All were exhausting, but worth the exhaustion. Nicasia also found these summer sessions enjoyable, after she eventually realized that the booming sounds that broke the silence of our first night on campus (where we were living in unlocked houses) were not guns being fired (she had read a lot about New York, and confused the city with the state), but rather fireworks in celebration of the Fourth of July.

Philippe pulled out of the course after the third season, since he had a heavy teaching load during the academic year, and thoroughly enjoyed replacing the summer teaching by reading in the Carnegie Library on the campus. By the fourth year the experimental course was altered. As a complement to the *Aplysia* ganglion preparation that I taught, we added the neuromuscular junction taught by Enrico Stefani and Dante Chiarandini.

These summers resulted in our children experiencing the thrill of walking on grass (an activity forbidden at the time in all Paris parks) and living their lives out of doors as opposed to within the walls of a Paris apartment. For us it provided friendships and scientific encounters with the current and future American neurobiology community. Finally, although our scientific interests did not yet overlap, we developed close and enduring friendships with many of the Cold Spring Harbor community, including Jim and Liz Watson, whose children were of similar ages to ours; Bill Udry, who as Managing Director had the task of finding housing for us each summer; and Helen Parker, whose work as Administrative Secretary was growing exponentially with the expansion taking place at Cold Spring Harbor under Jim's direction. Last, but far from least, I have been grateful for the opportunity to know Barbara McClintock, whose complete dedication to science was unique. She was in her cornfields throughout her career. Thanks to the appreciation that the Carnegie Institution of Washington had for her unstinting efforts over the period during which she was unable to convince many members of the scientific community of the importance of her findings, she was able to persevere unhindered, and without distraction, in the research that, many years later, was recognized by the Nobel Prize.

Erice, Sicily: 1973

During the years that followed the full publication of my studies on cholinergic synapses, I had on the docket a number of rather special international conferences where I was to describe those studies. Sir Bernard Katz had asked me to lecture at the International School of Biophysics, a two-week event in Erice, Sicily, scheduled for the spring of 1973. Although I had the greatest confidence in my data, which revealed a very clear picture of transmitter activation of two pharmacologically distinct membrane receptors, each of which controlled a distinct ion permeability in the membrane, I found it a bit frightening to be addressing students of biophysics who must surely have had a more acceptable view of how ions move across membranes or across anything as far as that goes. With no chemistry, physics, or biophysics in my background, I was certain that my imagination led to a rather personal view of the process, but I picked up the challenge in spite of it, deciding that as good as the students might be at understanding ion movements, they were likely unable to penetrate my imagination.

However, once again, I was certainly not ready to leave my sons (aged 1 and 4) for two to three weeks, so I was forced to add conditions to my acceptance, as had been done for Cold Spring Harbor, i.e., in this case, that Philippe be accepted as a student in the course and that we could also include Nicasia in our housing arrangements. The laboratory of Professor Borsellino in Camoglie, Italy, handled the administration of the International School of Biophysics, and they very generously made our participation as a family possible. It was an exciting course, a wonderful place in the clouds, and a precious opportunity to become acquainted with Professor Katz, one of the neuroscientists Philippe and I most admire.

Two Full-Time Jobs: Motherhood and Science

Participation in congresses where I presented the data on the cholinergic synapses continued, with trips to Israel and Leningrad leaving marked memories, not only because of the place and people involved, but also because in *both* instances I was obliged to leave my younger son in the process of coming down with scarlet fever and not at all happy to see his mother leave the country. In addition, during the trip to Israel, David, our older son, silently choked on a piece of meat and was only saved because Philippe's father, a doctor, noticed his blue face which had silently fallen onto his plate. Although I have always been thankful not to have been present, I have never been able to get rid of slight guilt feelings over not having been there to assume my maternal duties. David once did his best to encourage these guilt feelings. One morning when I was to leave for the lab, David developed a high fever which was quickly attributed to the onslaught of measles (against which vaccinations were not yet given in France). Once the diagnosis was made, I left him with the baby-sitter and went off to the lab. That evening upon my return David, in tears, said, "Maman, never *ever* leave me again when I'm ill!"

In the spring of 1975, when about to go off to a symposium in Leningrad, I tried to console my younger, 3-year-old son, Ivan, by telling him that when I returned I would be bringing him a Russian doll. It was only over a year later that I realized how much my departure had affected him when I heard him telling a story, as was his wont, to other children about a very sad child whose mother was leaving, but had promised that she would return with the gift of a Russian doll. Although a sad event for Ivan, the trip for me left fond memories since I was able to develop very close friendships with Ella Zeimal and Michel Michealson—the latter Head of the Pharmacological Laboratory of the Institute of Evolutionary Physiology and Biochemistry in Leningrad. The friendships were characterized by the intensity of relationships developed with Soviet scientists at that time who were hungry for contact with the outside world and who had to make the most of such occasions. The friendship with Michealson was abruptly shortened, however, since, even at the time of the symposium, he was already seriously ill with tuberculosis and was able to resist its aggression for only another few years.

Following a number of other symposia, I began to feel increasingly bothered by my frequent absences from the children. With the birth of the children, I found myself with two full-time jobs, since I was as fascinated by child rearing as I was by neurobiology. Although I, of course, could not be with them continually, I profited from the liberties offered by a pure research position in C.N.R.S., which permitted me to organize my own schedule to maximize the amount of time spent with my children. Until they reached school age, I put them to bed around midnight, so I was able to spend the evening with them, and I would go off to the lab when the baby-sitter arrived at 8:30 AM as they continued to sleep until noon. This permitted me to spend almost all of their waking hours with them, while permitting me to maintain a full research schedule. Since my C.N.R.S. position did not involve teaching responsibilities, and since I worked almost always alone, I was able to organize my time independently of others.

My involvement in child rearing was the major factor that made me limit my participation in conferences that required long distance travel. In addition, however, I had become bothered by the repeated presentations of data concerning a subject that had already become second place in my interests. Furthermore, given that I had no one replacing me at the experimental post when I was away, I could no longer spare the time that was needed to advance my studies on other synapses. Those synapses were more difficult to analyze since the transmitters mediating the synaptic activity remained an enigma. I was soon to realize the luck I had had by starting my synaptic studies with a synapse whose transmitter was possible to identify pharmacologically, and a transmitter for which the molluscan receptors resembled sufficiently those of their vertebrate friends so that pharmacological tools were available for dissecting the multiple elements of the synaptic events.

A Glimpse from Afar of the Political Situation in the United States: Mid-1970s

An interesting influx of mail arrived for me in the mid-1970s. I was clearly being courted to offer my candidacy to about 10 different biology and pharmacology departments, from New York University to Berkeley and throughout the United States. I am not certain exactly what new legislation had been enacted at that time, but it clearly had put in jeopardy the federal funding of many laboratories if they could be accused of discrimination on the basis of gender. I have also not followed the statistics that resulted from that affirmative action movement, but I do believe opportunities for women in American university science programs have improved since then. Although I greatly appreciated having been considered for such professional opportunities, I had no desire to leave my C.N.R.S. position in France or to force my family to change continents.

Noncholinergic Synapses and Other Transmitter Receptors

To the outside observer, little seems to unite the work I performed over the next 15 to 20 years in *Aplysia* neurons. However, all the questions I attempted to answer were stimulated by experiments designed to determine the transmitters being liberated at a number of synapses for which I had identified the pre- and postsynaptic neurons. This search led me to evaluate receptors for various amino acids, amines, and occasionally peptides, but unfortunately never did lead to the identification of the transmitters used at those synapses. For most of my synaptic studies following those on the cholinergic synapse I was therefore obliged to accept my failure to identify the transmitter involved and to live with the consequent limitations on the information I could obtain about certain aspects of the underlying mechanisms at those synapses.

A Glutamate Receptor Forces Me to Learn a New Trade

A very likely transmitter candidate for one set of the synapses I have been studying over the last 10 years is glutamate. However, since the pharmacological characteristics of the glutamate receptors on *Aplysia* neurons differ so markedly from those of mammalian glutamate receptors, it has been very difficult to find effective antagonists for the molluscan receptors. Nevertheless, the study of these receptors has not been without rewards.

Although in mammals, glutamate has been known as "an excitatory amino acid," it has long been known that glutamate can elicit, in invertebrate neurons, an inhibitory response by increasing Cl conductance via a receptor that appears to be related to the mammalian inhibitory glycine receptor. Furthermore, glutamate can also induce in some cells an increase in K conductance, as do essentially all other "classical" neurotransmitters tested on molluscan neurons. However, I found that the glutamate-induced K conductance, unlike the increase in K conductance activated by other transmitters in both mammals and molluscs (whether amines, amino acids, or peptides), does not require the intervention of a G-protein.

My conviction concerning the ionotropic nature of the glutamate-induced K conductance was reinforced by the discovery in 1999 of a glutamate-gated K channel in cyanobacteria (Chen et al.). This has encouraged me to reinforce the interpretation of my electrophysiological data by trying to pull out the proposed glutamate-gated K channel from *Aplysia* cDNA. Even if that receptor does indeed exist, my task will not be an easy one, since it is expressed in only a few *Aplysia* neurons. Nevertheless, the opportunity of learning some of the tricks of molecular biology has been fun and, hence, worth the effort. While honing my cloning skills by pulling out a more frequently expressed and better understood ionotropic receptor, I have managed to have some encouraging success. This success is surely due to the good training I received from Cristina Alberini during her month's visit to our lab in January 2001 and to the follow-up support generously offered by Jonathan Bradley, who was working in our laboratory until the summer of the same year. Both were very patient instructors indeed!

From the 5th Arrondissement to the 6th Arrondissement—2002

When Philippe's mandate as Director of the laboratory we had formed 31 years earlier expired, we wanted to make space for the incoming director and let the younger generations in the lab spread their wings. Fortunately for us, Alain Marty and Isabel Llano, previously members of our lab at Ecole Normale Supérieure, had just returned from Göttingen where they had spent six years in Erwin Neher's laboratory. They were in the process of setting up a new laboratory at the Université Paris V on the Rue des Saints Pères and were eager to have us join them. Although we have lost our view of the Val de Grâce, and the daily contact with our colleagues of "l'Ecole," we have gained the view of a gorgeous 18th century "hotel" that houses the Ecole des Ponts et Chaussées (renovated just in time for our arrival one year ago) and the company of a number of delightful young scientists working with Isabel and Alain.

For Better or For Worse: My Approach to Science and a Big Thanks to C.N.R.S. for Making It Possible

My real love in science has always been the experimental phase. As one sees and evaluates the data coming out of an experiment, there is not only the pleasure of finding answers to the questions being asked, but there are also new problems being exposed—exciting new avenues presenting themselves for further research. This love of the hands-on element in the scientific endeavor was the major reason for which I chose to work alone. Also, given my limited background in the general field of biology, I was hesitant to take on students who deserved wider scientific support than I could hope to offer them. Finally, having no constraints offered by the schedules of collaborators has permitted me the much desired flexibility to be able to organize my time as a function of my children's needs. Given my approach to science, my limited scientific background, and the demands made by active motherhood, I was very fortunate to have a pure research position such as only an organization like the C.N.R.S. can offer.

Except for a few brief visits from foreign colleagues, I only bent my "work alone, no-student" rule upon one occasion. When Eve Marder asked to come as a postdoctoral fellow, I felt from her application that all she would need was a month of training on the techniques I could teach her that would transfer well to her current experimental preparation, and since we had sufficient equipment and space at the time (1973), I could help her develop her own setup and let her fly on her own. This was done, and having Eve in the lab was a delight for everyone.

My personal career goal has been accomplished, since I was only look-ing for the kind of enjoyment and personal satisfaction I have consistently obtained over the years through solving each of the experimental problems as it was posed. However, my way of "doing" science is clearly often not the most effective means of having a serious impact on science or on other sci-entists. Being unable to follow up certain electrophysiological observations with supplementary biochemical analyses meant that some of these findings were more or less left in limbo. For anyone starting out in the field today, a multidisciplinary approach is clearly a must. However, if one judges by the way many laboratories function today, the change brought about by the multidisciplinary approach has not only affected the science, but has also altered the structural and social characteristics of laboratories themselves. To a certain extent, it is time for another May 1968.

Times have clearly changed since the period of my gods, who spent their career at the bench and whose enthusiasm and prestige were nourished strictly by the science they produced and not by empire building. It is clear that much of the transformation in neuroscience over the last 20 years was necessary as the discipline became much more expensive, with electrophysiology having become one of many approaches to the study of the brain. Modern genetics, molecular biology, neurochemistry, and modern imaging techniques have, in conjunction with electrophysiology, led to many extraordinary discoveries that would not have been possible without the marriage of the various disciplines. However, this marriage has also led to an exponential growth in budgets and often to an almost industrial approach to neursocience. For many scientists, the search for funds has often dominated the search for answers to scientific questions. The two or three colleagues at the bench have often become assembly lines of postdoctoral candidates reporting to higher ups, with the higher up resembling much more a chief executive officer than a scientific investigator or a thesis advisor. Furthermore, many recent scientific publications pass through Madison Avenue before arriving at Main Street. What used to be "Effects of This on That," which were then judged to be exciting or not by colleagues reading the findings in peer reviewed journals, are now often subject to the interests and "hype" of private publishers looking for more immediate satisfaction.

Finally, power has become a significant factor in our science, and as in many other situations, power can, and often does, corrupt. I find myself becoming an environmentalist who would like to breathe less polluted air, returning to the time when being among "well known" scientists was an exhilarating, positive experience. I do not think this is simply naive nostalgia. I truly believe that the times have changed: that the motivations and the mores of many in the community have changed and usually not for the better. Do we not have an obligation to try to reign in the negative "social" aspects occurring with the transformation of our field, while benefiting from the positive scientific progress it has permitted? Young scientists joining the field should be given the possibility of enjoying the excitement and enthusiasm of true scientific endeavor untainted by Madison Avenue and Wall Street.

Selected Bibliography

Kehoe JS. Pharmacological characteristics and ionic bases of a two component postsynaptic inhibition. *Nature* 1967;215:1503–1505.

Kehoe JS. Single presynaptic neurone mediates a two component postsynaptic inhibition. *Nature* 1969;221:866–868.

Kehoe JS. Ionic mechanisms of a two-component cholinergic inhibition in *Aplysia* neurones. *J Physiol* 1972;225:85–114.

Kehoe JS. Three acetylcholine receptors in *Aplysia* neurones. *J Physiol* 1972;225: 115–146.

Kehoe JS. The physiological role of three acetylcholine receptors in synaptic transmission in *Aplysia*. *J Physiol* 1972;225:147–142.

Kehoe JS. Electrogenic effects of neutral amino acids on neurons of *Aplysia californica*. *Cold Spring Harbor Symp Quant Biol* 1976;XL:145–155.

Kehoe JS. Transformation by concanavalin A of the response of molluscan neurones to L-glutamate. *Nature* 1978;274:866–869.

Kehoe J. Synaptic block of a calcium-activated potassium conductance in *Aplysia* neurones. *J Physiol (Lond)* 1985;369:439–474.

Kehoe J. Synaptic block of a transmitter-induced potassium conductance in *Aplysia* neurones. *J Physiol (Lond)* 1985;369:399–437.

Kehoe JS. Cyclic AMP-induced slow inward current in depolarized neurons of *Aplysia californica*. *J Neurosci* 1990;10:3194–3207.

Kehoe JS. Cyclic AMP-induced slow inward current: Its synaptic manifestion in *Aplysia* neurons. *J Neurosci* 1990;10:3208–3218.

Kehoe JS. Glutamate activates a K^+ conductance increase in *Aplysia* neurons that appears to be independent of G proteins. *Neuron* 1994;13:691–702.

Kehoe JS, Ascher P. Re-evaluation of the synaptic activation of an electrogenic sodium pump. *Nature* 1970;225:820–823.

Kehoe JS, McIntosh JM. Two distinct nicotinic receptors, one pharmacologically similar to the vertebrate a7-containing receptor, mediate Cl currents in *Aplysia* neurons. *J Neurosci* 1998;18:8198–8213.

Kehoe JS, Vulfius C. Independence of and interactions between GABA-. glutamate-. and acetylcholine-activated Cl conductances in *Aplysia* neurons. *J Neurosci* 2000;20:8585–8596.

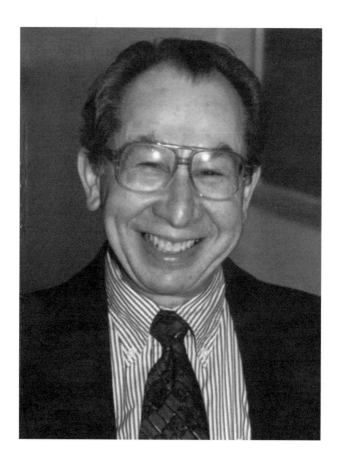

Edward A. Kravitz

BORN:
New York, New York
December 19, 1932

EDUCATION:
City College of New York, B.S. (1954)
University of Michigan, Ph.D. (Biological Chemistry, 1959)

APPOINTMENTS:
Postdoctoral Fellow, National Heart Institute (1958)
Harvard Medical School (1961)
George Packer Berry Professor of Neurobiology,
Harvard Medical School (1986)

HONORS AND AWARDS (SELECTED):
American Academy of Arts and Sciences (1976)
Einstein Visiting Fellow, Hebrew University (1981)
National Academy of Sciences, USA (1984)
Institute of Medicine (1986)
Governing Council, Institute of Medicine (1990–1994)
Humboldt Research Award (1992)
John S. Guggenheim Fellowship (1992)
A. Clifford Barger Lifetime Achievement in Mentoring
Award, Harvard Medical School (1998)
Education Award, Association of Neuroscience
Departments and Programs (2001)

In his early studies, Ed Kravitz and his collaborators demonstrated a transmitter role for GABA and established Procion Yellow as the first widely used dye for the determination of neuronal geometry. His studies with the amines serotonin and octopamine demonstrated their roles as synaptic modulators and led to studies exploring the function of amine neurons in complex patterns of behavior such as aggression. He has used invertebrate models, first lobsters and recently fruit flies, in order to bring genetic methods to the study of aggression. He has long been committed to education at the clinical/basic science interface and to the education of minorities in the sciences and medicine.

Edward A. Kravitz

My Life up to Now
"(3rd verse) I get up each morning and dust off my wits
Open the paper and read the obits
If I'm not there I know I'm not dead
So I eat a good breakfast and go back to bed

(chorus) How do I know my youth is all spent
My get up and go has got up and went
But in spite of it all I'm able to grin
And think of the places my get up has been."

"Get Up and Go," Song by Pete Seeger (1960)

I f I ever really get old, I will have this song as my anthem. "Get Up and Go" is a wonderful upbeat song about getting older that I first heard in a movie version ("Wasn't that a Time," American Roots Music, producer, 1982) of what turned out to be the Weaver's last performance at Carnegie Hall in 1981. I wish I had been at the concert. I must admit that I was apprehensive when asked to write an autobiography for *The History of Neuroscience in Autobiography, Volume 4*, because unless one is a serial killer or has sex with important people in prominent places, most scientists that I know tend to write their autobiographies near or at the ends of their active scientific lives. I don't feel any place near the end of my active scientific life, despite the attempts of deans and others to hasten the happening of that sorry event. I also worry about how I make anything I write into an accurate record of my career and not an interpretation of events designed to make me look good. Well, I suppose that is a problem with all autobiographies. In any event, here, without further apology, is my attempt to present an "accurate" portrayal of my career to the present day.

Roots and Childhood

Ada Machlus and Isadore Kravitz were married in Philadelphia, PA, in 1929, the city where they were born 20 years earlier. My mom had just graduated from high school and was working in a department store at the time: dad never finished high school. Shortly after the marriage, they moved to

New York where my brother Bill was born. I was born close to three years after that in December of 1932. We're actually not sure what the family name was. When dad was born, a doctor asked my grandfather for the family name: he said Koretsky, we think. The doctor told my grandfather that you could not raise an American boy with that name. Instead, they took my grandmother's family name, which was Kravitz.

Dad hit the New York job market at the start of the Great Depression. He co-owned a gas station for a while that supposedly was stolen from him by his partner, worked as a Western Union telegram delivery boy, and later sold Wearever aluminum pots and pans after cooking meals for groups of housewives in their homes. At some point during the 1930s, dad began working for his father in the garment industry. Samuel Kravitz ran a shop in downtown New York making expensive women's coats and suits as a subcontractor for other manufacturers. My father became a "cutter," which was the most important position in the shop. Large, heavy, multiply layered rolls of expensive, mostly woolen material were delivered to contractors along with patterns or forms used for cutting the pieces to be sewn into coats and suits by the "machine operators." The patterns developed by the manufacturer's cutters were used to calculate the numbers of coats and suits to be produced from the rolls of cloth supplied to the subcontractor. Standing in front of a huge, centrally located cutting table with the unrolled layers in front of him and with a large ceiling-mounted circular saw, dad always figured out how to get many more garments from each pattern than the numbers calculated by the manufacturers cutter. These were made into coats and suits that my grandfather sold privately at reduced market prices, but at huge profit for himself. Dad saw little of the "extra" money made by his father in this way.

As the expensive hand-crafted women's garment industry slowly died after World War II, dad played more and more of a role in keeping the earnings of his father and stepbrother coming in. First, my grandfather purchased a cluster of bungalows in Far Rockaway, NY, for summer rental by city dwellers escaping the New York heat. Dad became the caretaker for these bungalows, teaching himself plumbing, electrical wiring, carpentry, and painting along the way. In fact, there was nothing that dad could not do once he set his mind to it. He invented and patented a cigarette machine that delivered one cigarette at a time for a penny and that caught slugs (fake pennies). He invented an industrial-sized distilling apparatus to recapture purified perchlorethylene from waste dry cleaning fluid when the family purchased a series of dry cleaning stores in Harlem upon the demise of the garment industry shop. Dad subscribed to *Popular Science* and other science magazines of the day. One time I remember him being fascinated with and spending endless hours exploring magnetism after reading an article on the topic. He built an early crystal radio while still in Philadelphia, and we were among the first people in our Bronx neighborhood to own a television set. One year dad had to throw out unwelcome guests who had crowded into our living room to watch the New York Yankees in one of the first World Series to be televised and who refused to leave as the game went into extra innings. I suspect that with an education, dad would have been a great scientist or engineer, with his inquiring and agile mind, his uncanny ability to learn new things, and his knack of getting things to work.

Dad and mom together started the Bronx Chapter 85 of "The Mended Hearts" after dad's mitral valve replacement surgery in 1972. That too had an interesting history. The day dad was brought to his hospital room from intensive care, he overheard the nurses talking about a patient who was to undergo the same surgery and who was terrified at the prospect. Dad asked to be wheeled down to the patient's room, was helped to a sitting position at the foot of the bed, and said to the patient, "Hey, I had the same surgery 3 days ago, and look at me now." Apparently, that did the trick. The patient calmed down and underwent a very successful surgery. When dad's surgeon (Dr. Frater, who had been trained by Barnard) heard what he had done, he asked whether dad would be willing to start a chapter of The Mended Hearts at the hospital. Together, dad and mom gathered the necessary paperwork, and in June of 1973, Chapter 85 was chartered with dad as the president and mom as the secretary. The Mended Hearts is a national organization of former heart patients who individually visit cardiac surgery patients before and after surgery in hospital rooms and who hold regular group meetings in the hospitals as well. As dad's guest, I went to one of the meetings. Nurses, standing beside wheelchairs containing patients who were to undergo cardiac surgery in the days ahead, surrounded the room. Seated in the audience were former cardiac patients and their families. As each former patient stood up and listed the date and nature of their surgery, the faces of the waiting patients got brighter and brighter. It was positively inspirational. Dad was honored in 1979 by the Borough President of the Bronx for starting the first chapter in the borough and one of the first in New York City.

Mom was the one who raised me and my brother. She was the social chair of dad and mom's life together. Mom made the arrangements to see friends and family. Mom did the planning of summer vacations to the Catskill Mountains in New York, or later of summer vacations to Far Rockaway, or even later of vacations for the two of them to Florida. Mom was really a great organizer. I vividly remember her standing in her Brigadier General's outfit as a member of the Women's Volunteer Corps during World War II where she organized War Bond drives and collections of scrap metal and paper. She did the family finances and made sure that in the worst of times we were properly nourished and clothed. She picked the furniture and decorated the house. She wrote poetry and songs, none of which was ever published, and she played piano, although her lessons ended after her parents lost all their savings in the bank crashes of the 1920s. She also worked with and helped dad in the cleaning stores and was the mainstay of the Mended Hearts.

I remember her from my childhood as slender and glamorous, with long dark gently waving hair surrounding an angular, narrow, attractive face. She was the life of every party, dancing the evenings away and moving from table to table greeting friends and family. I remember her in later life, with white short cropped hair, not quite as slender or energetic, as the years and a reasonably hard life had taken their toll.

I was a smart kid growing up in a neighborhood and going to schools in which being smart was not appreciated. Schools did not know what to do with smart kids, so they had me skip grades, which invariably placed me in with older and bigger kids. The result was that I was in college at age 16, which was much too young to be in college. Before college I was with kids who did not associate with me because I was so young. My defenses against this were to develop a sharp tongue and quick wit and to become serious about sports. In grade school and high school, I played baseball as a catcher and basketball as a guard on neighborhood pick-up teams. In college, I played basketball for the 92nd Street "Y" team. After college, while at Sloan–Kettering for a year, I played third base in the city fast-pitch softball league. Sports was an important part of my youth, an enthusiasm that continues to the present day, when mostly I play tennis.

What I remember most about growing up in the Bronx was endless evenings sitting with friends on Mr. Hopengarten's newsstand outside the corner candy store. When chased from that perch, which happened nightly, we gathered around the corner to engage in noisy street games (Johnny on the Pony, Ring-o-levy-o, stoopball). Eventually, we were chased from those games as well. In fact, my friends and I seem to have spent an inordinate amount of our youth being moved from location to location over the neighborhood by complaints of storeowners, landlords, neighborhood residents, and the police, all of whom seemed to think we were creating disturbances. A favorite daytime game was stickball, which could be played in any of several ways. If enough kids were available, it was played with batters hitting on their own and other players spread out at positions roughly filling a narrow baseball diamond chalked out on Burke Avenue in the Bronx—a busy uphill main thoroughfare. It could also be played with a pitcher and one fielder and either an intact or split-in-half ball in the neighborhood back lot. In either case, the bats were broom handles pilfered from unsuspecting parents (since these were regularly confiscated by the police, we believed that there soon would be no intact brooms left in our neighborhood), and the balls were pink "Spaldeens," as they were called, until I eventually found out that they came from a box labeled "Spalding" in Mr. Hopengarten's store. When the Spaldeens split in half with use, they became the half balls used in backyard stickball. The police in New York seemed particularly intent on breaking up stickball games. The cry "chickie-da-cops" alerted us to throw the bat under the nearest car and gather in small groups chatting innocently. Somehow or other, the bats always were found by the relentless officers. Maybe it was the unusual placement of groups of three or four kids around home plate, first base, and the outfield that gave us away. I have no memory whatsoever of ever doing homework. I must have done some though, since I did graduate from various schools. Try as I might, I conjure up no images of me sitting in our small first floor one-bedroom apartment, burning midnight oil preparing for exams, or even doing any reading or school work.

College Days and Sloan-Kettering (1949–1954)

I did manage to get into college, barely passing the competitive examinations required for admission to the City College of New York (CCNY), after just making the honor roll at our neighborhood high school, Evander Childs High School in the Bronx. No one ever told me about the Bronx High School of Science or Stuyvesant High School where the brightest kids in the city went after completing eighth or ninth grades. College for me was a continuation of high school life, with evenings spent on Mr. Hopengarten's newsstand, me doing little home study, and my primary interests focused on girls and basketball (note to young folks: don't try to emulate this lifestyle—it just won't work these days).

One thing I vividly remember about college life was two summers working as a counselor in camps for handicapped children (Camp Oakhurst in Oakhurst, NJ, and Cradle Beach Camp in Angola, NY, on the shore of Lake Erie near Buffalo). I have never forgotten those young boys and girls dealing so bravely with devastating disorders such as muscular dystrophy, congenital birth defects, cerebral palsy, blindness, and epilepsy. Nor can I ever forget the way that most of the public reacted to outings with those children, looking the other way as we passed, offering us money, or hurrying by pretending not to see us or the children. Of course, some people opened their hearts to us and wanted to do something for the children. Like the time an operator of a "Dodgem Cars" attraction at an amusement park closed the ride to outsiders and gave us and the children the sole use of the ride in an environment where we would be safe. I have never seen a happier group of kids smashing into each other's cars on an amusement park ride. I am certain that the roots of my dedication to inspiring new generations of students to find solutions to neurological and psychiatric disorders are the two inspirational summers I spent working with these amazing youngsters.

I did get two A grades at CCNY. One was in basketball. The other was in Physical Chemistry, which was the toughest science course at the school and the only one I found challenging. As the end of college life approached, a difficult question loomed: What was I going to do with the rest of my life? Without much conviction, I applied to two medical schools and to be an officer in the U.S. Army Medical Corps: all three applications were rejected. Then I had a lucky break. I applied for and got a job as a Research Assistant to Dr. George Tarnowski, who had a small laboratory in the Chemotherapy Division at

Sloan–Kettering Hospital. My duties included injecting small pieces of solid tumors or Ehrlich ascites tumor cells into mice and then injecting drugs in what invariably turned out to be vain attempts to reduce the growth of the tumors. Dr. Tarnowski's laboratory adjoined another small laboratory where Dr. Lou Kaplan, a young biochemist, was studying the metabolic properties of mouse ascites tumor cells. Lou also played shortstop on the Sloan–Kettering softball team that played in the New York City Hospital League. With Lou's encouragment, I tried out for the team and ended up playing third base. Lou also encouraged me to do a research project. With Dr. Tarnowski's support, Lou's help, and the permission of the director of the chemotherapy unit (Dr. Christine Riley), I began a research project looking at amino acid metabolism in ascites tumor cells (mostly I remember breaking a lot of equipment). Once I started doing research, I was hooked. Finally, I had found something that excited me. That led to a night school course in biochemistry at CCNY, where I received an A grade, and applications to graduate programs in biological chemistry at Rutgers and the University of Michigan. Both accepted me, with the Michigan acceptance requiring that I maintain a B average in graduate school. I chose Michigan on the advice of the folks at Sloan-Kettering and quickly convinced the skeptics at Michigan that the risk was worth taking by maintaining an almost straight A average throughout my graduate career.

Start of My Life as a Scientist (1954–1959)

When I first arrived at the University of Michigan, Biological Chemistry was a department in transition. There was an older faculty (Adam Christman was the Chair) who were close to retirement age, who taught "classical" biochemistry, and who for the most part did not run active research programs. Saul Roseman (a distinguished investigator working on complex carbohydrate biosynthesis) was an exception, but he was not based in the West Medical Building that housed most of the department. Saul did play an important role in keeping me in graduate school, though, when a dispute broke out between me and my thesis advisor about storing solutions in volumetric flasks. Jim Hogg (carbohydrate biochemistry) and Merle Mason (tryptophan metabolism) also were active in research. There was a younger, newer faculty, who had recently been hired and whose numbers continued to grow during my graduate student years. These included Armand Guarino, a purine biochemist, who became my thesis advisor; Paul Srere, a carbohydrate pathway biochemist, who became a close friend and scientific mentor (Paul was the person who originally told me "the suit joke"—see below); Halvor Christensen, who was hired as the new Chairman of the Department soon after I arrived at Michigan; Robert (Bob) Greenberg, a nucleic acid chemist; Minor J. (Judd) Coon, who worked on intermediary metabolism; Bill Lands, a lipid chemist; and several others whose names escape me now. During my first year I received training in "classical" biochemistry: I crystallized proteolytic enzymes using the original methods and measured gas exchange with a Warburg apparatus. In seminar we debated issues like whether proteins or nucleic acids carried the genetic information. The student group was strong and cohesive, leading to many close and lasting friendships with my peers. Marshall Nirenberg, who won the Nobel Prize for cracking the genetic code a few years later while at NIH, was a few years ahead of me. Marshall and I shared an apartment on Huron Avenue for a while before he moved to NIH. Later, I heard that our house had been replaced by a church. I attach no significance to these two events. Joe Merrick, Chava Spivak, Halina Den, Milt and Sandra Schlesinger, and Usama Al-Khalidi formed my circle of friends. The qualifying exam for admission to Ph.D. candidacy was done in a novel way: one day during your second year of studies, a faculty member came up to you and said, "Your exam is now." I was advised that a good strategy for these exams was to get the faculty examiners arguing among themselves. By succeeding in doing that, I passed easily.

Armand gave me a free hand to work on whatever I desired. He hoped, of course, that it would be related to purine metabolism. I chose a project that probably was slightly larger than what he envisioned. I became interested in the question of how DNA was synthesized, which was not known at the time. What were the precursor molecules? How could I get at them? I made a few attempts to develop a cell-free system to study DNA biosynthesis by incubating 5′-deoxynucleotides, ATP, magnesium salts, and crude enzyme extracts from ascites tumor cells and other sources, but none of these worked. In order to do these experiments, I had to isolate the 5′-deoxynucleotides that I included in the incubations from DNA by hydrolysis, separating the nucleotides on ion-exchange columns. Sigma had started commercially supplying 5′-deoxynucleotides at that time, but supposedly Arthur Kornberg was buying out their entire supply. With the failure of my first experiments, I decided to try a different approach. Perhaps I could find and identify precursors if I used radioactive tracers in living cells under experimental conditions in which the cells were actively making DNA. I chose logarithmically growing *Escherichia coli*, which I knew had to be making large quantities of DNA, and added a short tracer pulse of radioactive guanine to the cultures. Periodically, I withdrew samples and separated them into acid soluble, RNA, and DNA pools to follow the radioactivity in the search for precursors. What I observed was that a large early peak of radioactivity appeared in the acid soluble pool, which was followed by a slower rise in radioactivity in the RNA fraction and a still slower and smaller rise in radioactivity in DNA. Thus, nothing particularly informative appeared regarding DNA biosynthesis; however, one very surprising result was obtained. I noticed that the counts in RNA were not stable, even though the literature of the day said that once synthesized RNA was stable and did not turn over. My counts went down by about 10% after the peak incorporation of radioactivity, and thereafter, the radioactivity in the RNA pool remained stable. I showed these results to many people, but everyone said that it was an artifact—that I was doing something wrong—that I shouldn't do anything with the results. Two years later, Astrachan and Volkin did a similar experiment using an only slightly different experimental system (bacteriophage-infected *E. coli*) and discovered messenger RNA. I've kept that notebook, with the original results, to remind me that when I talk to students about careers in science I should tell them not to necessarily listen to older and wiser advisors—at least not all the time.

My thesis research actually involved the role of inorganic phosphate in regulating the choice of pathways through which glucose would be metabolized in ascites tumor cells. The topic was selected after I accidentally discovered an inhibition by inorganic phosphate of the enzyme glucose-6-phosphate dehydrogenase, the first enzyme in the pentose-phosphate "shunt" pathway of metabolism. Extended discussions with Paul Srere helped sharpen the definition of the problem. The thesis described effects of inorganic phosphate on the choice of pathways of carbohydrate metabolism using (1) crude tumor cell extracts; (2) a reconstructed enzyme system in which I isolated and purified the rate-limiting enzymes in each of the pathways, combined them in amounts present in tissue extracts, and partially duplicated the effects I observed in the tissue extracts; and (3) intact tumor cells. This work led to one publication in *Science* and left me, once again, not knowing where I would go next. It is interesting that as I look back now at my thesis, I discuss "intracellular control factors" as important "compounds capable of governing the metabolic rates of various intracellular enzymic pathways." I also pointed out that multiple factors must be involved in regulating pathways of metabolism. Thus, from my earliest published work, I was interested in regulatory factors and their roles in pathway choice. As a budding biochemist, I focused on the roles such factors serve in choosing between metabolic pathways in a complex intracellular milieu. As a neuroscientist and now a neuroethologist, I have focused on extracellular regulatory factors (neurotransmitters and neurohormones), asking how they work at a cellular level (harking back to my biochemist days) and how they are involved in pathway choice and assembling patterns of behavior at an organismic level. My interest in the nervous system began in graduate school also, via endless arguments with philosophy graduate students about whether we ever could understand how nervous systems worked through biochemical or physiological studies.

What was I to do next though? Once again, Luck (now capitalized, since it seems to have played such a major role in my career) interceded. As I was starting to write up my thesis studies, Earl Stadtman, a distinguished biochemist from NIH, delivered a seminar in our department. I was so impressed with the beauty of his talk that I went up afterwards and asked if he had any postdoctoral openings. Earl said that one had just opened up and why didn't I apply. I did and was accepted.

A Year at NIH and an Offer from Steve (1959–1960)

During my last year of graduate study, I met and married Kathryn Anne Frakes, a lovely, lively, highly intelligent redhead who has been the love of my life, my lifelong companion, the mother of my two wonderful children, and my best friend. Immediately after we married, Kathryn and I, driving a 1950 Chevy sedan pulling a U-Haul van, headed to Bethesda, MD, and the start of postdoctoral studies in the Stadtman laboratory. The evening we arrived, the Stadtman's were having a party, to which we were invited. Immediately upon entering the Stadtman house, Kathryn was asked to dance and was whisked away by a distinguished European biochemist, leaving me to hang up our coats. On returning to the party, I noticed this distinguished gentleman (d.g.) sliding his hand up and down my new wife's back. Not knowing what to do on this my first evening in a new environment with my new wife, I cut in, much to Kathryn's relief. At that point the d.g. said, "I don't blame you." Thus began an interesting year at NIH.

Almost immediately after my arrival at NIH, Earl Stadman left on sabbatical to work with his friend and sometime competitor, Fyodor Lynen. That left P. Roy Vagelos in charge of the laboratory, and Roy and his wife Diana soon became wonderful friends of ours. In the Stadtman/Vagelos group I began work on the metabolism of the opium alkaloids. I had a vague notion that I was ultimately going to end up working in the nervous system and had developed a plan to move in that direction. The plan involved (1) learning how morphine and related alkaloids were synthesized and metabolized in plants as first steps toward learning how they functioned in the brain and (2) doing two additional postdoctoral stints after I finished my studies in the Stadtman laboratory with investigators working directly with nervous tissues. One of these postdocs was to be with David Nachmanson at Columbia University to learn how synapses worked. The second was to be with Oliver Lowry at Washington University in St. Louis, MO, to learn the elegant micromethods I felt would be required to study the biochemistry of single nerve cells. To the biochemists, Nachmanson was a martyr who was continually under attack from neurophysiologists because he had shown convincingly that their theories about how neurotransmission and the conduction of nerve impulses worked were wrong. Nachmanson believed that acetylcholine was involved both in transmission *and* in conduction, but he believed that the process did not involve the release of acetylcholine from presynaptic terminals or from any other sites. Instead, he believed that acetylcholine was synthesized and degraded within nerve cell membranes in a cyclical fashion and that this cycle generated *all* of the electrical signals recorded by neurophysiologists. Once again, Luck played her hand: none of these plans for postdoctoral training materialized.

For my studies on the biosynthesis of morphine alkaloids at the NIH, I had a field of opium poppies grown for me by the U.S. Department of Agriculture in Beltsville, MD. I also accumulated a collection of giant bottles of freeze-dried samples of the mold *Claviceps purpurea* for studies on the ergot alkaloids. I used leaves and roots of the poppy plants to study the biosynthesis of the opium alkaloids, but never began my planned studies with the mold samples. I was amused to hear, though, that about a year after I left the NIH, decontamination people in full body suits and masks were called upon to remove the harmless purple mold samples that I had left in the cold-room.

The move from the NIH to Harvard Medical School (HMS) came about as a result of a phone conversation between Steve Kuffler and Roy Vagelos. Steve had just moved from The Wilmer Institute at Johns Hopkins University to the Department of Pharmacology at HMS with Dave Hubel, Torsten Wiesel, Ed Furshpan, Dave Potter, and the ever-loyal electronics expert, Bob Bosler. Together they formed the Neurophysiology Laboratory in the Department of Pharmacology, with Steve as full Professor and everyone else in junior roles. Steve and Dave Potter already had begun a project aimed at identifying the inhibitory transmitter compound at crustacean neuromuscular junctions, with a biochemist colleague, Akira Kaji. Kaji left the project when the group moved to Harvard, and Steve began searching for a biochemist to continue this work. Steve also had begun to develop the philosophy that understanding the nervous system would take the combined efforts of investigators from many disciplines, including neurophysiologists, anatomists, and biochemists. In that vein, Steve was searching for a biochemist. Steve had obtained Roy's name from colleagues at NIH, and the phone call was to ask whether Roy was interested in joining the new group at Harvard. Roy said that he wasn't interested, but there was a guy in the group who kept giving journal club seminars on neurochemical topics and that he might be interested in the position. That led to a phone call to me from Steve, a chat at NIH when Steve was visiting, and an invitation to come to Boston to look at the job.

Discovery, Creation, and Political Activism (1960–1970)

A Visit to Boston and a Decision

A major snow storm was predicted for the day of my visit to Boston. I had prepared for the trip by reading, or trying to read, some of Steve's papers, which were full of incomprehensible squiggles, unfamiliar abbreviations, and cartoons. My biochemist colleagues gave me a list of things I should request in negotiating for the position. These included a salary of around $20,000; at least 1000 square feet of my own research space; $20,000 in startup money; and, above all, a position in Biochemistry and not in Pharmacology, where Steve's unit was located. None of the people I talked to before the visit had heard of Steve or any members of the group, and therefore, they urged great caution on my part in this non-biochemical environment. The snow storm hadn't yet started when I arrived in Boston and was greeted at the medical school by Dave Potter and Ed Furshpan, as Steve was otherwise engaged. Dave vigorously pumped my hand up and down and took long, striding steps around the office as he enthusiastically described the project of trying to identify the inhibitory transmitter compound at crustacean junctions. Ed, by contrast, gave the impression of someone trying to climb the walls and escape even while he told me about his Mauthner cell work. After this conversation, Dave took me down the hall to meet Dave Hubel and Torsten Wiesel. They too tried to explain their work to me, but to no avail. They asked what I was interested in though, and I told them that, among other things, I wanted to explore the biochemical basis of learning and memory. I noticed their sideway glances at each other as I talked about my plans. Then came the visit with Steve: I was completely unprepared for what followed next.

Steve patiently listened to my list of requirements. Then quietly, one by one, he dismissed them. Surprisingly, I wasn't the least bit offended by this. In later years I came to realize that Steve was the only person I'd ever known who could fire someone and have them walk out of his office with a smile on their face. Steve said that I didn't want a position in Biochemistry, because then I'd have to teach over there. Since I was only one year past my Ph.D., he offered me an Instructor's position in Pharmacology at a salary only slightly higher than the amount I was earning as an NIH postdoc (not very much, so I negotiated that up a little bit). "Space" he said, "you'll share with us." The most compelling argument for taking the position though was what Steve said next. "What you really want is the opportunity to see whether you're any good as a scientist. I can offer you five years of research support on an NIH Program Project Grant, and am happy to purchase any equipment you need. All I require is that you work on the nervous system." Of course, Steve also knew that if I had any sense, I'd join them on the project trying to identify the inhibitory transmitter compound at crustacean neuromuscular junctions.

After the meeting with Steve, I dropped in on my friend Howard Goldfine, then in the Microbiology Department. On our way back to his house in Cambridge, we got involved in a wild snowball fight with dozens of students who came pouring out of the freshman dormitories in Harvard Yard. Since I came to Boston without snow gear, I ended up thoroughly soaked by this diversion. I caught the last train leaving Boston before the storm closed down South Station, and on a long slow trip to Washington,

D.C., I had time to think about the offer from Steve. To this day, I'm not certain what clinched my decision to come to HMS. It just seemed to make sense. Here were a group of people who seemed to know a lot about the nervous system, and here was a golden opportunity to find out whether I was any good in the laboratory. Probably most important, though, was that I really liked the people I had just met and felt that this was a place I might fit in, learn a lot, and even serve an important role.

Discovery: GABA and Procion Yellow

GABA as a Transmitter Compound

Immediately after our move to Boston, Steve, Dave Potter, Ed Furspan, Bob Bosler, and Joseph Dudel (who was visiting with Steve at the time) packed up the laboratory and their families and headed to the Marine Biological Laboratory (MBL) in Woods Hole, MA, for the summer. Steve was the Director of a Training Program in Neurophysiology at the MBL that was the forerunner of the famous biophysics and neurobiology courses of later years at that Institution. Steve invited me to join the group, and somewhat reluctantly, Kathryn and I repacked our recently unpacked suitcases and headed to Cape Cod for a month. It was not an easy place to do biochemistry, with Steve's children cramming foul smelling bait in the same freezers and refrigerators in which I was trying to store tissue samples and reagents. Steve's laboratory also contained essentially no biochemical equipment. Still, the ambiance and environment were great, and the firm bonding between Steve and his "boys" (the academic world of the 1960s was very much a male-dominated world—it still is today, but fortunately things are getting better) that began during those early summers at the MBL ultimately previewed the creation of the first Neurobiology Department in the world.

The first project I worked on that summer involved a peptide as a possible neurotransmitter. Frank Belamarich (Boston University), Ian Cooke (Harvard), and Dave Potter working independently had shown that aqueous extracts of the pericardial organs of crustaceans (a crustacean nerve ring surrounding the heart, originally described by Alexandrowicz and later extensively studied by Don Maynard) contained a potent cardioexcitatory activity that was destroyed by proteolytic enzymes. With my biochemical background and supposed ability to purify proteins, this seemed a good starting project for me in the Kuffler group. Unfortunately, the peptide proved difficult to purify, and all purification steps I tried resulted in a complete loss of physiological activity. It was 25 years later (a little late to be pioneers in the field of peptides as transmitters) that we finally succeeded in purifying the peptide. Barry Trimmer, then a postdoctoral Fellow in my laboratory, used HPLC columns to isolate and sequence two FMRFamide-related peptides that accounted for most of the biological activity (TNRNFLRFamide and SDRNFLRFamide).

GABA is Not a Transmitter Compound?

In 1960 and 1961, Jack Eccles, David Curtis, Ernst Florey, Hugh McClellen, and other investigators proclaimed at two international congresses that GABA was not a transmitter compound in either vertebrate or invertebrate nervous systems. Florey's argument rested on his inability to find GABA in crustacean nervous tissues, while Eccles reported that there were significant differences between normal inhibitory mechanisms in the vertebrate spinal cord and the actions of externally applied GABA. This despite the fact that Florey was the first to suggest, *in print*, that GABA was a transmitter compound. He made the suggestion based on (1) pharmacological studies showing that GABA inhibited the firing of crustacean stretch receptor neurons (but many other substances also inhibited the firing of these cells) and (2) experiments carried out with Bazemore and Elliott showing that GABA contributed the bulk of the activity that blocked the firing of crustacean stretch receptor neurons in an extract from the vertebrate central nervous system (CNS) called Factor I. During the same period of time in which Florey first proclaimed that GABA was a transmitter compound and then that it was not, an outstanding series of neurophysiological studies appeared defining the ionic mechanism underlying inhibition in crustacean tissues and comparing that mechanism to the actions of bath-applied GABA. These studies by Fatt and Katz, Boistel and Fatt, Furshpan and Potter, Kuffler and Edwards, and Dudel and Kuffler demonstrated that the actions of GABA were identical to those of the natural inhibitory transmitter compound in crustacean tissues. Instead of claiming that GABA was a transmitter compound, however, this group of distinguished scientists cautioned that a number of essential experiments were missing and had to be done before GABA could be considered a transmitter compound. Of course, all these investigators *suspected* that GABA was a transmitter compound, but they were careful not to say so *in print*.

At the end of the summer, I began work on the GABA project. Despite claims to the contrary by Florey at both international congresses, Dave and Steve already had strong evidence that GABA was present in crustacean tissues. To demonstrate this, they dissected central and peripheral nervous tissues from 500 lobsters. They used acid extracts from these tissues in order to (1) separate physiologically active compounds by hanging curtain electrophoresis, (2) subdivide bioactive fractions using preparative paper chromatography, and (3) crystallize several of the active substances from the chromatograms. One of the compounds obtained in this way was GABA, and it represented about 30% of the inhibitory activity found in the original crude extracts. These procedures demonstrated convincingly that

GABA was present in central and peripheral nervous tissues of lobsters. To further confirm these observations, I felt it important to demonstrate that GABA actually was synthesized from glutamic acid in crustacean peripheral and central nervous tissues. This too flew in the face of published results, as Florey and Chapman reported that glutamic decarboxylase, the enzyme forming GABA from glutamate, was not present in crustacean tissues. Using radioactive glutamate labeled with C^{14} at different positions in the molecule, I showed that a particulate enzyme fraction from crustacean nervous tissues would convert glutamate to GABA and, as in vertebrates, that the mechanism involved removal of the carboxyl group as CO_2.

When I originally arrived in Boston, I carried a test tube of the organism *Pseudomonas fluorescens* (ATCC 13430), which had been grown on GABA as a sole carbon source, in my pocket. To grow on this unusual amino acid, high levels of a pair of enzymes that metabolized GABA were produced by this particular strain of the organism.

1. *GABA/glutamic transaminase*: GABA + α-ketoglutaric acid → glutamic acid + succinic semialdehyde
2. *Succinic semialdehyde dehydrogenase*: succinic semialdehyde + TPN → succinic acid + TPNH

In 1959, Jakoby and Scott had demonstrated that these enzymes offered the possibility of a rapid, sensitive, highly specific assay for GABA by measuring the amount of reduced pyridine nucleotide (TPNH) produced when GABA was metabolized through both steps (Jakoby and Scott, *J Biol Chem* 1959;234:937–940). Just before leaving the NIH, I visited the Jakoby laboratory to collect the culture. I knew that the cumbersome assay being used by Dave Potter to separate and identify GABA and other physiologically active compounds would have to be replaced by a faster, more sensitive, quantitative procedure for measuring GABA, and the enzyme assay offered that possibility. Our next step, therefore, which involved me, Dave, and Nico van Gelder (a second biochemist who arrived at HMS when I did), was to use the Jakoby and Scott enzyme assay to measure levels of GABA in peripheral axons. For our first studies using this procedure, we analyzed mixed nerve bundles containing excitatory, inhibitory, and sensory axons; then smaller bundles containing only excitatory and inhibitory axons; and finally, single inhibitory and excitatory axons. The relative concentrations of GABA in these tissues increased dramatically as we came closer to pure inhibitory axons, finally reaching the surprisingly high concentration of $0.1\,M$ in single inhibitory axon extracts.

We had fun during those early days preparing the enzymes used for the GABA assay (no kits were available), usually at the expense of new lab members. First, we grew up huge quantities of bacteria. Then, to extract proteins from the bacteria, we used the infamous "French Press." This device allowed one to subject concentrated suspensions of bacteria to thousands of pounds of pressure, then to drop the pressure to one atmosphere, thereby exploding the bacteria and yielding concentrated, highly active crude enzyme solutions. As each new person joined the Kuffler lab, we invited him or her to assist us in preparing our enzyme extracts. Their role would be to pump the handle of the enormous jack used to compress a plunger in the specially constructed steel cell containing the bacterial suspension. Of course, it got harder and harder to pump as the pressure within the cell grew higher, and when we released the contents of the cell to atmospheric pressure via a small valve at the bottom of the cell, the person manning the handle had to pump furiously to maintain the required high pressure within the cell. Our "volunteers" invariably ended up red-faced and exhausted. No one ever volunteered a second time.

During those early years in Boston, I learned many neurophysiological techniques: how to identify and dissect single axons (my first single excitatory and inhibitory axon dissections took 6 hr; by the end of several months they took about 20 min); how to use a physiological rig and record from single muscle fibers with intracellular electrodes; how to set up neuromuscular preparations for bioassays and for release experiments; and a little later in the mid-1960s, how to find and identify CNS neurons, a technique pioneered by Masanori Otsuka at the start of his sabbatical visit with us from Tokyo Medical and Dental University. Masanori joined the laboratory shortly after the completion of the experiments demonstrating the selective localization of GABA in crustacean inhibitory axons. In a set of elegant studies, he combined the physiological identification of neuronal cell bodies to map neuron position in central ganglia, with single cell biochemistry. In so doing, he generated the first detailed maps of the positions of physiologically identified neurons in an invertebrate central ganglion. When Masanori presented these results to a packed meeting room at a Federation of American Societies for Experimental Biology (FASEB) meeting (before the days of the Society for Neuroscience), 5 min of applause followed his talk, something I never had heard before at a national meeting.

Only two substances, acetylcholine and norepinephrine, were recognized as transmitter compounds in the mid-1960s. We knew that by adding a third compound to that list we would be doing something of great importance. We also knew that the most essential experiment, the release experiment, remained to be done. We had to show that GABA was released by inhibitory and not by excitatory nerve stimulation. We also understood that to really be a transmitter compound, enough GABA had to be released to exactly duplicate the effects of inhibitory nerve stimulation. That particular requirement, however, had not at the time and still has not been satisfied for any transmitter compound at any junction. Moreover, in studies with Les Iversen (a neuropharmacologist/biochemist who had been sent to us by Julius Axelrod and Arnold Burgen) and with Paula Orkand (an anatomist), we had shown that a GABA uptake system existed in crustacean neuromuscular preparations. With no way to inhibit the uptake system, other than by omitting Na^+ from the bathing medium which would block conduction, any GABA collected by us only represented the overflow from the uptake system.

Dave Potter and I had made a few early attempts to demonstrate GABA release, but found ourselves searching for GABA at the limits of detection of the enzyme assay, even at its most sensitive. Masanori also made several attempts to demonstrate the release of GABA, using radioactive GABA that was taken up into muscles, but he too was working at the limits of detection of his method. We speculated that larger muscles containing greater numbers of nerve terminals would be required to bring us over the threshold of detection of GABA in saline superfusing muscle preparations. Dave and I were using the opener muscle of the dactyl (the moveable finger) of the walking leg for our early experiments (the same preparation used for bioassay), because these were easy to dissect with their innervation intact and because the surrounding exoskeleton formed a chamber suitable for superfusion with minimal volumes of saline. In the search for larger muscles, we went to the much larger opener muscles in the crusher claws of lobsters (we called them the "big openers"). By that time Dave and Steve had turned their attention elsewhere, leaving Masanori, Les, Zach Hall (my first graduate student), and myself the task of trying to complete the release experiments.

These were labor-intensive, long-lasting experiments in which we divided the many tasks involved between the four of us. First, there was a difficult dissection, requiring cutting through the tough exoskeleton surrounding the claw without damaging the muscle and cleaning the muscle surface of as much connective tissue and clotted hemolymph (lobster blood) as possible without damaging the nerves innervating the preparation. Next, the preparation had to be set up for superfusion, the excitatory and inhibitory nerves drawn into suction electrodes, and intracellular microelectrodes inserted into muscle fibers to record synaptic responses. The tissue had to be superfused with saline for 4 hr to lower a background washout of GABA to low and stable values. Then in 25-min time bins we stimulated excitatory and inhibitory nerves while superfusing muscle preparation with saline containing or lacking calcium (to block transmitter release). Even under these optimized conditions, the amounts of GABA released turned out to be very small. They were in the range of 10^{-10} mol of GABA for a 25-min period of continual stimulation of an inhibitory axon. An elaborate ion-exchange procedure quantitatively recovered these tiny amounts of GABA from a multimillion-fold excess of salts in the saline collected during the superfusion periods. Finally, the enzyme assay at its highest sensitivity was used to measure the amount of GABA in each sample. It was rare that everything worked in a single experiment, so we had to carry out enough of these difficult experiments to convince ourselves that GABA was indeed released by inhibitory nerve stimulation.

While my three colleagues literally were up in the air, I completed the experiment that unequivocally demonstrated the transmitter role of GABA. Masanori was on his way to Japan, Les was on his way to England, and Zach was on his way to California. The four of us began the experiment together, but Masanori, Les, and Zach left for the airport during the experiment, leaving me to complete the final analysis. Fortunately, the experiment worked. With no email, "snail mail" and phone calls announced the results: we now had in hand the final crucial piece of evidence required to show that GABA was a transmitter compound.

How Was Our "Discovery" Greeted?

Soon after that at the MBL, I gave my first major talk on GABA as a transmitter compound. The first person to stand up after the talk was David Nachmanson who said, "Well, we don't know what that little bit of an amino acid that you see being released is when you stimulate a nerve, but it certainly is not a chemical transmitter compound, because we all know that transmission is electrical." Les had a similar experience when he presented the results at a Royal Society Meeting, where someone in the audience took issue with him calling GABA a transmitter compound. It couldn't be a transmitter because it was released from a neuromuscular junction and not a synapse. Luckily, Steve came to my defense at the MBL and Bernard Katz to Les's defense in England. Even 20 years later, in May 1985 at the inaugural meeting of the Merck Sharpe and Dohme Neuroscience Center in England, we didn't fare much better. Les had asked Kresimer Krnjevic to give a history of GABA as a transmitter for the meeting. His history divided the story of GABA into various ages. The 1960s, when we thought we had shown that GABA was a transmitter, were considered the Dark Ages by Krnjevic. The Rennaissance, according to him, wasn't until the 1970s, when investigators finally began to believe that GABA might be an inhibitory transmitter compound in the vertebrate CNS. It was one of my first encounters with a higher vertebrate chauvinism, that unfortunately has come more and more to dominate neuroscience research *and neuroscience funding* in this country. Even today, it is difficult to find in most textbooks of neuroscience mention of the crustacean story demonstrating the transmitter role of GABA.

To complete the story of GABA as a transmitter compound, we sought an explanation for the selective accumulation of GABA in inhibitory neurons. We carried out these studies at about the same time as the release experiments. With Deric Bownds (a postdoctoral Fellow from the Wald laboratory), Perry Molinoff (a medical student), and Zach Hall, we worked out the pathway of GABA metabolism in crustacean tissues, characterized the lobster enzymes, scaled down our assays for these enzymes to the point where we could measure activity in single axons, and quantitatively measured the levels of enzymes and substrates for the GABA pathway in single excitatory and inhibitory axon extracts. Deric even ran microgel electrophoresis of the extracts of single axons to demonstrate that no decarboxylase activity was detectable in excitatory axon extracts. The results of the single axon experiments offered an explanation for the selective accumulation of GABA in inhibitory neurons and allowed a suggestion of why GABA accumulated to an 0.1 *M* concentration in inhibitory axons. The data showed that the synthetic enzyme glutamic decarboxylase was found only in inhibitory axons, but the degradative enzymes, the transaminase and dehydrogenase, were found in both excitatory and inhibitory axons. Without decarboxylase, excitatory axons could not accumulate GABA. The units of enzyme activity showed that inhibitory axons could synthesize more GABA than they could destroy, thereby allowing GABA to accumulate. At 0.1 *M* levels of GABA, however, product inhibition of the decarboxylase reduced the synthetic capability to the levels of the degradative capability. Thus, 0.1 *M* GABA, which was the final concentration in axons, represented a steady state in which synthesis was balanced by destruction.

Of course, some people did appreciate our work on GABA. With help from Jack Eccles and others, I was nominated for and became a tenured Professor at HMS only 9 years after my arrival as an Instructor. Les became the director of an MRC unit in Oxford, and Masanori became the youngest professor in Japan. Zach went on to a postdoctoral position at Stanford and to his own distinguished career.

Procion Yellow and Neuronal Geometry

The other major research story from our laboratory in the 1960s began when Tony Stretton (a postdoctoral Fellow sent to us by Sydney Brenner) and I began our studies of neuronal geometry. Tony and I were interested in whether identified cells in lobster ganglia always had the same geometrical shape. The question arose from Tony's background in molecular genetics and the two of us starting to ask questions such as "were the shapes of neurons genetically specified." The use of lobster central ganglia to address this question derived directly from Masanori Otsuka's maps showing that the cell bodies of identified neurons were in pretty much the same positions from ganglion to ganglion and from animal to animal. At the time, a method developed by Ed Furshpan and Jaime Alvarez (a postdoctoral Fellow from Argentina) seemed to offer an ideal tool with which to address the question. To try to determine where particular synaptic inputs were localized on Mauthner neurons in fish brains, Ed and Jaime attempted to localize their recording electrodes through the use of immobilized dyes. They had solved many technical problems around injecting dyes into neurons and in processing tissues in ways that allowed them to localize the sites of injection. In addition, they had accumulated an extensive collection of dyes in their search for the appropriate substance to inject into the Mauthner cells. They generously shared this knowledge with us and allowed us access to their dye collection. Among Ed and Jaime's dyes was a Procion dye, and this worked best of all the substances we tested. Still their dye did not fully stain the neuropil processes of the neurons we injected. A visit to Imperial Chemicals in Providence, RI, the manufacturer of Procion dyes that were used to stain fabrics, provided us with 120 Procion-related dyes. We tested all of these dyes by injection into lobster central ganglia. Only Procion Yellow showed the features we required. It was highly soluble, readily releasable from microelectrodes, completely filled cells and their processes, and survived fixation and dehydration. In addition, and most importantly, it was fluorescent, which enhanced our ability to detect the dye in the fine branches of neurons and in nerve terminals, thus allowing us to easily localize the dye in tissue sections. Using Procion Yellow, we injected over 100 physiologically identified neurons, processed and sectioned the ganglia containing these neurons, and reconstructed cell shapes from these injections.

I vividly remember Edith Maier (our superb research assistant) completing the first reconstructions of a pair of identical cells from different animals, with Tony and I hovering over her shoulder. As each data point from the photographs of the serial sections was hand drawn onto the reconstructions (no computer programs existed for reconstruction of neurons in those days), it became clearer and clearer that the two cells had close to the same morphological shape in the two animals. In great excitement, Tony and I ran down the hallway telling everyone the results. Our ardor was cooled, however, by the responses we received, ranging from "so what?" to what did you expect—after all, Purkinje cells all have pretty much the same shape too." At first, only Hubel and Wiesel recognized the potential of the method, and within days they were attempting to fill vertebrate CNS neurons with the dye. Procion Yellow had a short lifetime, being replaced within a few years by the much more fluorescent and easier to obtain Lucifer Yellow. However, Tony and I had the joy of developing a technology that we knew would allow investigators to unravel the morphology of complex synaptic regions, a task that Bullock and Horridge had declared to be impossible just a few years earlier in their monumental work "Structure and Function in the Nervous System of Invertebrates." Our colleagues from the Biochemistry Department wondered how two good biochemists like us could waste our time on such a mundane anatomical problem.

Creation: A Department of Neurobiology at HMS

The Neurophysiology Laboratory in the Department of Pharmacology at HMS

Though science was first and foremost in our lives at HMS during the early 1960s, there was much more. Steve was Dad to his "boys," and Thanksgiving dinners with him, Phyllis, and the Kuffler kids (Susy, Damien, Genie, and Julian) and regular Sunday morning phone calls were part of the routine of our lives. Steve never returned from a trip without greetings for each of us from colleagues. He was a notorious punster, and at one time was restricted to one pun a day (a rule he regularly broke). Probably the most chaotic time of the year, though, was the end of November, when the design for the annual Christmas card had to be created. All work stopped as we brainstormed the topical theme for the year, after which all activities in and around the photography lab stopped while photos were taken of everyone in the department, and the card was constructed, photographed, printed, addressed to colleagues all over the world, and sent out.

The Parties

The legendary Christmas parties began with a "social hour" and party games and continued with a huge sit-down meal cooked by Theresa (our lab assistant for many years) and her family in the jam-packed lunchroom. After dinner, there was the "suit joke" and the student skit satirizing the faculty. The suit joke is an action joke that I told over at least a 30-year period at Christmas parties and that had occasional performances at restaurants in San Francisco, at places where I gave seminars, and at international meetings in Norway and England. Steve and Roy Vagelos were great fans of the joke. It's hard to describe the joke other than to say that it was told in an ethnic (Jewish) dialect and involved extensive, rather ridiculous-looking body contortions around a new suit that didn't fit properly. The following of the suit joke was enormous. Children who grew up hearing it over the years at departmental Christmas parties would correct me if I changed even a single word. After the entertainment, the tables and chairs were removed from the lunchroom and the dancing started. Lab spring picnics and communal meals at Woods Hole in the summers complemented the "eating scene." Steve was a visible and active presence at these events, and almost all of our children were tumbled upside down over his shoulder at least a few times over the years. Once a month "evening meetings" were held at which lab groups took turns preparing dinner for the department and presenting their latest experiments in detail. While these ended in long evenings, it was an important way to keep abreast of what was happening in an ever-growing department. Almost daily seminars were held over lunch, and the week concluded with a departmental beer hour (with elaborate snacks) on Friday afternoons.

The Lunchtime Seminars

I don't remember when the scheduling of talks at lunchtime began. When we arrived at HMS, all medical school departmental seminars were held at 4:00 PM, usually with tea beforehand. Our seminars probably grew out of the elaborate, highly ritualized lunches we ate together in the Pharmacology

Department lunchroom (much to the amusement of the rest of Pharmacology). I suspect they started by our first asking guests to join in the repast and then asking them to tell us what they were doing. The logic of having seminars at lunchtime was "well you have to eat lunch anyhow, and we all eat together, so why not listen to talks at the same time." Sometimes, for days on end, we had lunchtime seminars. No notices were sent out announcing these seminars, and only rarely were they formally scheduled in advance. Instead, they were written on a calendar hanging on the lunchroom door, which therefore had to be checked daily to see whether there was a talk that day. Steve's wide circle of friends regarded a stop in Boston as an essential part of any trip. As each of us became prominent in our fields, we too had regular visitors. Essentially, all visitors were asked to tell us about their latest experiments over lunch. At first this caught visitors by surprise. Pleading that they had not brought slides, we said, "it's OK, just go to the board and tell us what you're doing—it's really very informal." On second visits though, friends showed up with sets of slides in their pockets and talks prepared, just in case.

The entire department turned out for seminars, cramming into the small lunchroom that was the hub of so many departmental activities. Great scurrying around preparing lunches preceded the talks, which started around 12:15 PM (the origin of the 12:15 start time of the much more formal departmental seminars today). The seminar speakers were introduced by their hosts and then the trial began. Speakers were lucky to show one or two slides (if they had brought slides) or to get through the introduction to their presentation before the questions started flying. At times, it seemed as if every detail of every slide was being questioned, which had to be frustrating for the speakers, but was exciting for us. We shared an overwhelming desire to really know and understand what was being done, why it was being done, and whether the results supported the conclusions. I don't believe it was arrogance on our part, although I suspect it bordered on rudeness. The discussions could go on for hours, until we, or the visitors, exhausted by the ordeal, called for closure. On one visit to the department, Paul Greengard, who had a biochemistry seminar scheduled for 4:00 PM was asked to deliver a lunchtime seminar. An exhausted Paul barely finished the session when it was time for him to deliver his biochemistry seminar (which we all attended, of course).

More often than not, the seminars were the highlights of our days, and they were exhilarating. It's the way we learned about the breadth of a newly emerging field. We were treated to Bernard Katz delivering a 3-hr Saturday morning discourse on synaptic transmission, and we were visited and lectured to by many past, present, and soon-to-be giants of the early days of neurobiology. A few of the large pool of visitors included Seymour Benzer, Sydney Brenner, Ted Bullock, Jose del Castillo, Francis Crick, Jack Eccles, W. Feldberg, TP Feng, Norm Geschwind, Paul Greengard, S. (Hagi)

Hagiwara, Eric Kandel, Vernon Mountcastle, Walle Nauta, Rami Rahami-moff, Miriam (Mica) Salpeter, Gordon Shepherd, Ladislav Tauc, Pat Wall, and Victor Whitaker.

Teaching

Under the leadership of Ed Furshpan and Dave Potter, our department always has had a serious, dedicated commitment to outstanding instruction. The neurobiology block of the medical school curriculum consistently received rave reviews from medical students. On occasion, this led to notice by the greater medical community as well. In the late1960s, we were visited by the President of the American Academy of Neurology wondering why so many young doctors from HMS were turning toward neurology. In the early years, Ed and Dave headed off to Woods Hole several weeks before the scheduled start of the neuro-block of teaching for medical students (Area III in those days) to prepare their lectures. The lectures were not memorized, but instead were an elegantly crafted, carefully thought through, and argued out system of presenting neurophysiology in a comprehensive and comprehendible manner, with each lecture building on an earlier one and leading logically to the next. To do this, Ed and Dave stood in front of and "rehearsed" each other, thrashing out the best ways to cover the material and examining the current literature to construct their lectures. The result was some of the clearest and best lectures ever presented at HMS and a system of teaching and learning that the medical students loved.

I joined Ed and Dave at Woods Hole for these rehearsals and added my few "biochemistry of synaptic transmission" lectures to their elegant set of neurophysiology lectures. A few well-placed "jokes" also were added to the lectures (probably because Jack Diamond, a visiting colleague from Canada, and I joined Ed and Dave in Woods Hole), and these too built on each other and showed up in multiple lectures. Presentations by Dave Hubel and Torsten Wiesel rounded out the Area III lecture set. Steve lectured for one or two of the early years, but was not invited to participate in future years because his presentations were not considered clear enough (we suspected that Steve did this on purpose). The popular Kuffler and Nicholls textbook *From Neuron to Brain* was heavily based on the spectacular teaching system originally devised by Ed and Dave. On top of all of that, Ed and Dave memorized the names of the medical students from the class photos sent to us each fall and surprised and delighted many a medical student of that era by calling them by their first names as they walked in the door for the first class sessions. My dedication to teaching, initially inspired by Ed and Dave, began in those early days and continued throughout my career with courses at Harvard for advanced undergraduates and graduate students in Synaptic Chemistry and the Neurobiology of Disease (which continues to the present) and with national courses such as the MBL Neurobiology Course and the Neurobiology of Disease Teaching Workshops at the Society for Neuroscience annual meeting.

A New Department and a New Direction for HMS

The Pharmacology and Physiology departments were without Chairs in 1966. Our Neurophysiology Laboratory based in the Department of Pharmacology was in full bloom under Steve's leadership, with major, fundamental research discoveries being made by all members of the original group. Thus, it was reasonable for Dean Bob Ebert to turn to Steve and ask which of the two departments he would like to take over. This began a round of discussions within our group, most of which bogged down on two issues. The first was that each of the existing departments already included substantial numbers of tenured and non-tenured faculty, some of whom were carrying out distinguished research, but others of whom were not. In joining either of the existing departments, there would be a major expansion of our group, and we would lose the coherence that was the hallmark of our department and its greatest strength. Steve's style of running the department as a family also would be lost, and we would become like all other Physiology and Pharmacology departments in the country. The second concern was that we would be responsible for the teaching of either Physiology and Pharmacology, and none of us had an interest in doing that. Teaching was a major part of our lives, but we were teaching in areas we were expert in, which undoubtedly contributed to the outstanding quality of the courses we offered. Finally, we all agreed. We wanted our own department and, after prolonged discussion, decided that "neurobiology" was the name we wanted assigned to the department. We recognized that we might run into substantial opposition in the faculty to this notion. Most departments in most medical schools in the country were based on a set of methodologies, such as biochemistry and biochemical methods, anatomy, pharmacology, physiology and their methods. We were requesting something different. What we proposed would create a department based on understanding how the brain functioned, using whatever methodologies were required to do that. Steve's view was that one used whatever tools were required to understand the nervous system. Hence, the new department would include neurophysiologists, biochemists, anatomists, and, eventually, molecular biologists and geneticists.

The issue came before the faculty on June 17, 1966. The Dean strongly supported the concept and had done so in a document that was sent to the faculty prior to the meeting. Then a most interesting discussion ensued, which was mostly a turf war. Jordi Folch-Pi, a well-known lipid biochemist who had built a Neurochemistry Unit at McClean Hospital, spoke out early in the meeting, clearly distressed that a group at the quadrangle was going to usurp the name Neurobiology and possibly claim the field as its own. Even as the matter was brought to a vote, Jordi made one last ditch effort to keep the name from the quadrangle group, but the Dean would not accept that. The neurologists and neurosurgeons also were divided in their support, with Derrick Denny-Brown and William (Bill) Sweet strongly in favor of the concept, while Ray Adams was opposed. Again, the opposition stemmed from concern that efforts to build clinically based research units would be jeopardized by forming a new department. After extended discussion, the matter was put to a vote and by a substantial majority, but not a unanimous vote, the Department of Neurobiology was formed.

Political Activism

The 1960s were filled with serious, non-academic events of great magnitude. The Vietnam War, blatant racism in our universities, and the assassinations of Jack and Robert Kennedy and Martin Luther King, Jr. weighed heavily on us, raising our social consciousness, dominating our existence for periods of time during the decade, and making social activists out of all of us. They too are an important part of my life as a scientist.

A Program to Significantly Increase the Numbers of Minority Medical Students at HMS

Three days after the April 4, 1968, assassination of the Reverend Dr. Martin Luther King, I received a phone call from Jonathan Beckwith, a colleague from the Microbiology Department at HMS. "We must do something about this at the medical school," said John. We agreed to convene a meeting the next evening in my house, with each of us inviting a few people who would be sympathetic to recruiting and training greater numbers of minority doctors. I invited my Neurobiology colleagues Ed Furshpan, Dave Potter, and Torsten Wiesel. John invited Luigi Gorini from microbiology, a fascinating man who had been a partisan in Italy during World War II, and who was responsible for saving thousands of Jewish youths from the death camps of the Nazis. Leon Eisenberg, Warren Gold, and Robert Buxbaum rounded out the group. That evening we drafted a proposal for the HMS faculty to substantially increase the number of minority students by establishing "fifteen suitably named scholarships per year" and by appointing a faculty committee to immediately implement the program. We wanted to name the scholarships after Reverend King. We recognized that with these proposals we were requesting a substantial change in the student population of HMS, which was predominantly white and male. In fact, HMS had averaged $\frac{3}{4}$ of a minority student per year in the 30 years prior to 1968.

The next morning we met with the Dean of the Medical School, Bob Ebert. He was sympathetic to our efforts and told us he would support us, but he also told us he could not do so publicly. We asked his advice on how to move this proposal along in order to have it approved at the next faculty meeting, which was three weeks away. Ebert said that to have any chance of getting this approved, we would have to enlist the support of the heads of all the clinical and preclinical departments. We rushed back to the Neurobiology Department conference room to figure out how to proceed in this daunting task. We didn't know most of the people in the clinical departments, so how on earth were we going to convince them to support our efforts? Still, we plunged forward. First, we generated a list of the departmental heads and assigned members of our group the task of contacting them to arrange a meeting. We agreed that more than one of us would show up at each meeting and that these meetings would be wherever and whenever the Chairs were willing to meet with us.

We knew that we had to do much fact finding before the faculty meeting to head off what we anticipated would be partially hostile, but not necessarily unreasonable questions. Was there a large enough pool of outstanding minority students to fill 15 places in our medical school class? The answer to this question was easy. Yes, there was a large enough group of minority students out there, but Harvard would have to go beyond the small group of mostly Ivy League colleges that were its traditional sources of medical students. In fact, we were certain that special recruitment efforts would be required on our part to convince students attending urban or traditional black colleges and universities, where there were large numbers of minority students, that this was a sincere effort on our part. Would we be lowering our admission standards in accepting this large group of minority students? This question was harder to address. Part of the reason was that to HMS admissions committees, an "A" grade at Harvard carried much greater weight than an A grade at less elite institutions. In this climate, would the committee consider accepting credentials other than grade point averages and medical college aptitude tests for admission to HMS? For example, would the committee consider the running of a program for 50,000 youths in New York City (as done by one of the first students admitted in this program) a worthy criterion for admission to HMS? Would remedial training be necessary for these students and how would we arrange for that training? We actually anticipated that remedial training might be required for some students and suggested that it be made available on a voluntary basis by faculty. That suggestion, however, never was implemented because existing minority students considered it demeaning. Who was to cover the tuition and other expenses involved in bringing these students to HMS? Here, we planned to suggest the establishment of a Martin Luther King Scholarship Program to help cover the costs of bringing this new group of students to HMS.

A Contentious Faculty Meeting—April 26, 1968

In the short time between our meeting with the Dean and the faculty meeting, we managed to gather the support of essentially all the departmental

Chairs. In addition, with help from a minority medical student, Noel Solomons, we identified, contacted, and gathered additional support from a group of key faculty whom he felt would be sympathetic to our cause. To present the petition to the faculty, we asked the help of some of the most highly respected members of the HMS faculty. We did this because we knew that if the petition came from a group of "radical" young faculty, we stood little chance of success with the conservative clinical faculty of that era. Elkan Blout introduced our resolution to add 15 minority students and to form a faculty committee to implement the program. Elkan was followed by Jon Beckwith, who, in explaining our selection of the number 15, also offered evidence that there should be little trouble finding qualified students from urban colleges and universities and via special programs that already existed, such as an "Intensive Summer Study Program" at Harvard and other leading universities. He also emphasized the importance of acting now. Members of the admissions committee also spoke up, including the highly respected Herman Blumgart, who documented the sad state of affairs then existing regarding minority enrollment at the medical school. Blumgart was concerned, however, about whether we would find suitable numbers of candidates. Other faculty also offered generally favorable remarks, but, then suddenly, things took a turn for the worse. Dr. Norman, a black Assistant Professor in one of the clinical departments, delivered what we sensed was a "we don't need your help, brother" speech. He commented that the Harvard admission standards were right where they should be and that they shouldn't be lowered to admit unqualified students of any ethnic group. He added that we would not have any difficulty finding qualified black students, but he was uncertain about the number 15. Then the floodgates opened, and many people spoke out against the number 15. Harold Amos tried in vain to stem the tide, but it was clear we were going to lose if we insisted on the number. After considerable rather chaotic discussion, the Dean asked Elkan Blout if the resolution could be modified to replace the number "fifteen," with "a substantial number." Elkan agreed and a vote carried the modified petition by a huge majority. Our group tried in vain to keep the discussion going regarding the number, since we felt that a substantial number might mean 3 rather than the $\frac{3}{4}$ of a student now in our medical classes. At that point, we actually were shouted off the floor by some of our clinical colleagues with cries of "sit down" and "shut up." The Dean, seeing the continuing confusion, called for a show of hands on including the number 15. Seeing that the faculty was seriously divided on the issue, he said that he would appoint a committee to look into the number. With that he ended the faculty meeting. The official minutes of the faculty meeting ended with the comment that we had made "a passage from the profane to the sacred during the course of the afternoon," since the first half of the meeting had been concerned with whether there should be a cap on clinical faculty salaries, leading to a huge turnout of the clinical faculty defending their rights not to have caps put on their salaries.

Our ad-hoc group gathered in the hallway outside the meeting room, furious about what had just transpired and feeling betrayed by the omission of the number. The Dean came over to us with a huge smile on his face and said, "What's wrong with you guys? Don't you know you've won? I said I would appoint a committee to look into the number and bring in a suggestion to the next faculty meeting, and *you* will be the committee!" Feeling somewhat sheepish, we quickly recognized that the Dean had successfully maneuvered our proposal through a reluctant faculty for what was to become an enormous and historic change in HMS and its student population. That change would implement what became and has remained the best program in the nation training minority physicians in a majority medical school. In the more than 30 years of existence of the program, close to 800 minority M.D.s have graduated from HMS, compared to about 25 in the previous 30 years.

A War in Vietnam and "Strikes" on College Campuses

With a notice sent by the deans of the Medical and Dental schools, an official day of mourning was announced "to mark the deaths of those students needlessly killed at Kent State University." The notice continued that "on Friday, May 8 (1970), the normal activities of Harvard Medical School will be suspended. All members of the medical community who do not have patient-care responsibilities are encouraged to devote that day to discussion and other constructive activities." This action was taken as part of a nationwide strike on college campuses to protest the latest horror of the most unpopular war in American history, the invasion of Cambodia, and in memory of the four students killed and nine wounded when the Ohio National Guard opened fire on unarmed students on the campus of Kent State University (May 4, 1970). It was the double horror of the expansion of the war and the invasion of our universities by the military that prompted the massive protests that followed.

My office was one of the Harvard Medical School Strike Centers, and I was the organizer of a teach-in that was scheduled for May 8. Our goal was to educate the clinical and basic science faculty and the student body about what was happening in Vietnam. With a small ad-hoc committee, and with very little time, we put together a program the likes of which had never been seen before on the Harvard Medical campus. We reserved and filled two amphitheaters for the event. Russell Johnson of the American Friends Service Committee described in graphic detail what actually was happening in Vietnam. Donna Howell of the Black Panther Party spoke next to explain what the Panthers were doing in the community that surrounded the medical school, including the running of a free medical clinic. Finally, Francis Moore, a highly respected neurosurgeon, who was not on the original program, requested and was granted time to talk about setting up a strike fund at the medical school. The formal lectures were followed by small group seminars on topics such as the legality of the war, American imperialism, chemical and biological warfare, repression of the Panthers, and health care delivery in minority communities. The day ended with a roundtable discussion centered on what we as a medical community could do both to improve the delivery of health care in the neighboring Roxbury community and to end the Vietnam War. One outcome of that discussion led to a scene that probably startled many Bostonians and shocked some of the clinical faculty: Dean Bob Ebert, in his white coat, manned a table on a downtown Boston street giving out postcards to be mailed to the President of the United States supporting an end to the war.

I also organized a petition signing at the Medical School calling for the impaneling of a Federal Grand Jury to investigate the Kent State massacre in response to a phone call from the Kent State Student Council. Later, I organized a benefit showing of the film "Z" to benefit the families of students slain at Jackson State College in Mississippi, participated in the march of 100,000 people to the Boston Common to protest the war, and signed countless petitions to end the war. While this was going on, we kept the research going too, as we started moving in new directions.

New Directions, Educational Enterprises, Special People (1970–1992)

New Directions: More Transmitters and Then Amines and the Modulation and Behavior

Glutamate as an excitatory transmitter compound at crustacean junctions. Following our success in identifying GABA as an inhibitory transmitter compound, we turned to the question of whether glutamate was the excitatory transmitter compound at the same crustacean neuromuscular junctions. Physiological and pharmacological studies suggested that glutamate acted just like the excitatory transmitter compound, but we ran into serious problems in trying to demonstrate its release. The most difficult was the high background release of glutamate from neuromuscular preparations, requiring many experiments for us to see any release whatsoever. Still, we did see a selective liberation of glutamate with excitatory but not inhibitory nerve stimulation and in amounts comparable to those we had seen earlier in the GABA released by inhibitory nerve stimulation. Unfortunately, it took us 39 experiments to reach statistical significance, and that made it difficult to do controls such as attempting to demonstrate a calcium dependence of the release. Still, when we added in further elegant experiments from the Takeuchis in Japan showing that areas of high glutamate sensitivity on muscle fibers overlapped with excitatory nerve endings and that they too saw a small release of glutamate with excitatory nerve stimulation, most investigators agreed that glutamate was the likely excitatory transmitter compound at crustacean junctions.

Thus, by the early 1970s, a definite transmitter role for GABA and a highly likely role for glutamate had been established using crustacean neuromuscular preparations. In vertebrate systems, by contrast, little progress had been made in demonstrating transmitter roles for these substances. Invertebrate preparations, however, had another huge advantage over vertebrate tissues in explorations of transmitter function. Lobster neurons were large, uniquely identifiable, and could be dissected as single cells free of contaminating neuronal tissues. Thus, in addition to clear-cut demonstrations of transmitter roles for proposed neurotransmitter candidates, single cell biochemical studies were possible that allowed us and other investigators to ask "just how different from each other were neurons using different substances as neurotransmitter compounds." Could transmitter function be changed by altering the levels of expression of key enzymes such as transmitter synthetic enzymes? Buoyed by our success with the amino acid transmitters, we asked whether we could identify other transmitter compounds in the lobster nervous system. If we could, would it be possible to explain transmitter accumulation in those neurons too by continuing the analysis of the levels of metabolic enzymes and substrates relating to that transmitter compound. Finally, by continuing that analysis would we be able to uncover general rules about how neurotransmitters accumulated in neurons? Would that give us any insight into the genomic regulation of transmitter accumulation in neurons?

The "hot zap". Before beginning our search for other transmitter compounds, we felt that a rapid method was needed to identify transmitter candidates. Thus, the affectionately named "hot zap" method was developed in the laboratory by myself, Dave Barker, John Hildebrand, and Ed Herbert (then on sabbatical with us in his first foray into neurobiology). In this method, we incubated tissue samples with high specific activity radioactive precursors of one or several of the known transmitter candidates. We followed the incubations by a single step, rapid separation of the precursors from products by high voltage electrophoresis (at 6000 V and 100 mamps of current—hence the name hot zap) and used the incorporation of radioactivity into a transmitter product to support a possible transmitter role in the tissue under examination. The method was sufficiently sensitive to detect synthesis of transmitter in single neurons. To illustrate the potential of the method, we used vertebrate sympathetic ganglia to demonstrate the synthesis of acetylcholine (ACh) and norepinephrine (leading to an elegant use of the method by Paul Patterson and his colleagues), small numbers of single leech Retzius cells to demonstrate a synthesis of serotonin (5HT), and lobster single cell bodies to demonstrate the synthesis of radioactive GABA in inhibitory neurons. We also tested the potential of the method to detect unknown transmitter candidates in tissues by using the full cocktail of precursors in lobster nerve roots that either did or did not contain sensory fibers. Radioactive ACh was found only in the roots containing sensory fibers. We followed up these studies by showing that crustacean stretch receptor preparations, which contained single sensory neurons and their inhibitory innervation, synthesized only ACh and GABA. The hot zap was widely used by other investigators for a time, but soon became obsolete because of the need for special, rather dangerous equipment and because other methods of transmitter identification, such as the use of antibodies to localize transmitter synthetic enzymes, were becoming acceptable in the field to define transmitter function.

Acetylcholine as the lobster sensory transmitter compound. The preliminary studies with the hot zap were followed by more detailed studies on the possible role of ACh as the lobster sensory transmitter compound. Although it was well known that large amounts of ACh were found in crustacean and insect nervous systems, it was equally well known that in contrast to vertebrate systems, invertebrate neuromuscular preparations were insensitive to ACh and to agonists and antagonists that affected cholinergic transmission. Florey and colleagues had proposed that ACh might be the sensory transmitter compound in crustaceans after their bioassay procedure showed that little or no ACh-like material was found in excitatory and inhibitory motor axons, while large quantities were found in sensory nerve bundles. To examine this possibility in greater detail, we used an enzyme assay for choline acetyltransferase (the ACh biosynthetic enzyme) to measure levels of ACh synthesis in tissue extracts and the hot zap to demonstrate ACh synthesis by intact tissues throughout the lobster nervous system. First, we demonstrated a dramatic decrease in ACh synthesis in sensory nerve bundles in which nerve fibers had been severed from their cell bodies. Next, we examined different kinds of sensory receptors, showing in all cases that they synthesized ACh. In physiological studies we demonstrated that the cell bodies of central motoneurons were sensitive to iontophoretically applied ACh and that this effect was blocked by curare and atropine and potentiated by acetylcholinesterase inhibitors. Finally, we examined the physiological responses of an identified CNS motoneuron to stimulation of identified peripheral sensory receptors and showed that the resultant excitatory responses were blocked by cholinergic receptor antagonists. When Jim Townsel joined the laboratory, we carried out one final set of experiments involving sensory neurons. As with the excitatory and inhibitory motoneurons, we asked whether an analysis of the enzymes and substrates of ACh biosynthesis and degradation would explain the selective accumulation of ACh in sensory neurons. Here again, we found that the biosynthetic enzyme was found exclusively in sensory neurons and, therefore, was the key to accumulation of the transmitter product. The degradative enzyme acetylcholinesterase was uniformly distributed between all neuron types, being mainly localized in the sheath surrounding peripheral axons.

Octopamine is the major amine synthesized from tyrosine in lobsters. We turned next to the amine neurotransmitters, focusing first on amines derived from tyrosine because a candidate neuron already was available. Ian Cooke's laboratory had shown, using histofluorescence techniques, that a single large neuron present in the relatively small circumesophageal ganglion probably contained dopamine. This neuron sent processes to the plexus of neurosecretory endings in the pericardial organs surrounding the heart. Using standard biochemical procedures for isolating and measuring catecholamines, Dave Barker found anticipated low levels of dopamine, but could not detect any other catecholamines. In scouring the literature for other amines that might possibly derive from tyrosine, we found that in 1952 Erspamer had reported high levels of octopamine, the phenolamine analogue of norepinephrine, in the posterior salivary glands of the octopus. Could it be that, in invertebrates, the phenolamine octopamine replaced the catecholamine norepinephrine as the major amine derived from tyrosine? Perry Molinoff, a former student, was in Julie Axelrod's laboratory at NIMH at the time Dave began his studies. There Perry had just developed a highly sensitive and specific enzymic assay for octopamine, which he used to demonstrate that low endogenous levels of octopamine were found in vertebrate tissues. Perry in Axelrod's laboratory and Irv Kopin and his colleagues had earlier postulated that octopamine functioned as a "false transmitter" in the vertebrate nervous system, since it accumulated in sympathetic ganglia in large amounts after treatment with monoamine oxidase inhibitors and since it was released from these tissues with stimulation. Perry's results suggested that octopamine might serve a normal role in vertebrates as well, but with the very low levels of amine present it was difficult to determine what that role might be. When contacted, Perry jumped at the opportunity to see whether lobster tissues contained octopamine. To our delight, he found that octopamine was present and in much larger amounts in lobster nervous tissues than in any vertebrate tissue examined thus far. Thus began about a decade's worth of experiments exploring the role of octopamine in the lobster nervous system.

Bruce Wallace picked up the studies where Dave Barker had left off, starting with partially purifying and characterizing the lobster enzyme that synthesized octopamine from tyramine, the tyramine-β-hydroxylase. In all respects, the enzyme resembled the vertebrate dopamine-β-hydroxylase. Bruce also devised a highly sensitive assay for the enzyme that involved monitoring the release of tritiated water from side chain labeled tritiated tyramine. Joined now by Peter Evans and Barbara Talamo and using Perry's assay for octopamine and Bruce's enzyme assay, we started searching for the sites of highest octopamine concentration and synthesis in the lobster nervous system. To our surprise, this turned out to be along thin nerve roots associated with thoracic ganglia, which we had ignored in our first screens for the amine. These regions contained many orders of magnitude higher concentrations of octopamine than any other place in the nervous system. Backfills of these roots with cobalt chloride demonstrated the presence of slender fusiform cells along the roots. Ann Stuart and Jim Hudspeth, who were in the department at that time, had accidentally discovered that the dye neutral red stained leech Retzius cells that contained serotonin. Thinking that this might be a general stain for amine neurons, we tried the dye on our roots and discovered the existence of about 120 of these cells in a bell-shaped distribution of numbers along all thoracic roots and the last several roots of the subesophageal ganglion. We were able to correlate the numbers of cells along a root with the content of and synthetic capability for octopamine. We showed further that octopamine could be released from the roots with depolarization by potassium, that dissected single cell bodies from the roots contained high levels of octopamine, and in physiological studies, that the cells were responsive to ACh. This set of results left us fairly certain that the root cells were octopamine neurons, and we suggested that these neurons, with their peripheral location, might be lobster homologues of the vertebrate sympathetic ganglia. It was not until almost eight years later, in studies carried out by Marge Livingstone and Sue Schaefer, that we fully realized how completely wrong we were.

For her thesis work with us, Marge had begun studies exploring the role of serotonin in the lobster nervous system. Marge noticed that not only were there high levels of octopamine along second thoracic roots, there also were high levels of serotonin at exactly the same locations. Working with Sue, who was an electron microscopist, they set out to localize the sites of serotonin and octopamine biosynthesis using combined electron microscopic autoradiography and biochemistry as their primary research tools. Their results demonstrated that four morphologically distinct categories of nerve terminals could be found close to the root cells, and of these, one was the site of serotonin synthesis and a second the site of octopamine synthesis. They found further that terminals of both these types surrounded the root cell bodies, making these cells different from all other lobster CNS neurons, in which no terminals were ever found close to cell bodies. These terminals would have contaminated the single cell samples examined, thereby misleading us to suggest that the cells themselves were octopaminergic. As soon as antibodies became available for octopamine (some developed by Barry Trimmer), the plexus of octopamine endings surrounding the cells were revealed in rich detail, and we recognized that the octopamine-containing cell bodies were found in central ganglia.

Almost 15 years later, Henning Schneider finally did map the octopamine neurons in lobsters when good antibodies became available, and even today, many of the roles served by these cells remain to be explored. While we were thinking that the root neurons were octopaminergic, however, Shiro Konishi and I carried out a detailed set of physiological studies on these interesting, but difficult to record from cells. We found that although the cells were widely distributed along nerve roots in the nervous system, they shared synaptic input and were electrically coupled to each other, meaning that they might operate as a unit. Very recently, we found that the root cells contain one or more of the crustacean hyperglycemic hormone family of peptides, which are believed to be the lobster stress hormones. With an octopaminergic and serotonergic innervation, the root cells offer an excellent system in which to examine interactions between neurohormonal systems that are important in behavior at an identified cell level. A present graduate student, Alo Basu, is engaged in such studies now. Finally, with Mary Kennedy's help, we were able to show that lobsters do not metabolize amines via the vertebrate pathways involving monoamine oxidase and catechol-*O*-methyl transferase. Instead, amines are metabolized to single or double conjugates in which a sulfate group is added to the ring hydroxyl group and the amino acid β-alanine is added to the amino group. Such metabolites are expensive to synthesize, and we suspect that they will yet be found to have interesting physiological actions of their own, perhaps, for example, in signaling between organisms.

Amines and modulation—we become neuroethologists. Marge Livingstone was only a little way into her studies on the role of serotonin in lobsters when she made a remarkable discovery. We had been using neuromuscular junction preparations to examine the actions of amines, and later peptides, as modulators of synaptic function. Some early studies of these types were carried out by the Floreys shortly after serotonin was characterized by Rapport and his colleagues in the late 1940s. About a decade later, Grundfest and Reuben and Josef Dudel independently showed that serotonin increased the release of transmitter from excitatory nerve terminals in crustacean neuromuscular preparations. No connection was made, however, between the physiological actions that these investigators reported and a normal role for serotonin in crustaceans. The effects were being treated more as a pharmacological oddity than as a normal physiological mechanism. Our studies showed that serotonin, octopamine, and the peptide proctolin, which Tom Schwarz and Kathie Siwicki had recently characterized in lobsters, all had actions on neuromuscular preparations, but their sites and mechanisms of action varied. Thus, serotonin had presynaptic actions on excitatory and inhibitory nerve endings, while all three substances had postsynaptic actions on muscle fibers as well. Michael Goy showed that cyclic AMP could account for some, but not all of the actions of serotonin, while the actions of proctolin involved completely different mechanisms. Marge reasoned that if these substances were naturally occurring modulators as we were hypothesizing, and if they were not synthesized or released at muscle junctions, which we knew to be correct, then they were in fact hormones. Perhaps then, she would see something interesting by injecting amines into lobsters. I was certain that nothing of interest would result, as I expected amines to have actions at many sites in lobsters, and any consequences of amine actions on so many targets would yield patterns of behavior too complex to interpret.

We were in Woods Hole during my tenure as Director of the Neurobiology Course when Marge rushed into the laboratory, took me by the hand, literally, and led me downstairs. There she showed me two lobsters, one standing tall, looking like a dominant animal, and the other standing in a lowered posture, looking like a subordinate. "What do you see?" she asked. I replied, "A dominant and subordinate lobster pair." "Wrong," she said and proceeded to explain what she had done. One of the animals, the one standing in the elevated posture, had been injected with serotonin, while the other, in the lowered stance, had received octopamine. These results immediately suggested an interesting possibility: perhaps as a consequence of animals interacting to establish a dominance relationship, serotonin–neuron function became more important in winners, while octopamine–neuron function became more important in losers. Subsequent to the interaction, longer term changes in the functioning of those neurons might reinforce the newly acquired behavioral patterns. Or putting it another way, social interactions might modify the function of amine neurons, and the modification of amine–neuron function might influence the outcome of future social interactions. That idea and exploring ways to test it have dominated our research interests to the present day.

Serotonin neurons. To ask whether changes in amine neuron function resulted from changes in social status, we devised the following research strategy: first, we had to find amine neurons in lobsters and learn to record from them; then we had to learn how they functioned; and finally, we had to ask if there were changes in function accompanying changes in social status. Our first task was to find the neurons. A talk in our department by Harvey Karten, in which he showed spectacular images of immunostaining for peptides in the vertebrate retina, prompted me to send Barb Beltz to Harvey to learn immunocytochemical methods. We knew that a good antibody was available from commercial sources for the detection of serotonin and anticipated that we would generate our own antibodies to octopamine. Using the commercially available antibody, Barb generated the first complete map of an invertebrate nervous system for serotonin. Her fluorescent images of serotonin immunostaining were so spectacular that we had trouble retrieving our original photographs from the editors of the *Journal of Neuroscience*, one of whom was using her figures as wall decorations. Barb's maps showed the existence of about 120 serotonin-immunostaining neurons in lobsters, which appeared to be organized in sets. Two pairs of these cells (one pair in the first abdominal, one in the fifth thoracic ganglion) were particularly prominent, sending processes from their ganglionic locations throughout the anterior part of the nervous system with ramifications of branches in every ganglion up to the subesophageal. These same cells send branches out all of the thoracic second roots that ended in varicosities close to the root neurons described above, with second sets of varicosities seen in the pericardial organs surrounding the heart. Thus, these cells were capable of communicating with central neurons through their ascending branches and with all tissues of the body through their two sets of peripheral endings.

Meanwhile, Ron Harris-Warrick and Marge had shown that injected amines triggered opposite postural stances by directing the readout of opposing motor programs from the ventral nerve cord. Serotonin caused the readout of a "flexed" program, in which increases were seen in the rate of firing of excitatory motoneurons to postural flexors and inhibitory neurons to the extensors, while at the same time decreases were seen in the rate of firing of excitatory neurons to extensors and inhibitory neurons to flexors. Octopamine caused the readout of an "extended" posture by triggering opposite patterns of firing of the same groups of motoneurons. The readout of complex programs of these types from crustacean central nervous systems can be elicited by the firing of so-called "command neurons." Dominant animals assuming an elevated stance when in proximity to subordinates are seen in many species of animals. Therefore, we were not surprised to see this in lobsters too. In trying to identify amine neurons that might be important in fighting behavior, we began looking for cells that could exert central actions on the readout of motor patterns and also have peripheral actions on the muscles that were the targets of the motor readout. The large cells Barb had found seemed ideal candidates for the "right cells" to be working on, since their multiple sets of endings seemed able to reach both central and peripheral targets of the amine.

Educational Enterprises: The MBL Neurobiology Course (1975–1979)

Along with the enormous growth of the field of Neurobiology through the 1960s and early 1970s, large numbers of investigators working on neuroscience research projects began filling summertime laboratories at the MBL. In 1954, 21 summer investigators identified themselves as neurobiologists; by 1970, the number had increased to 110. That represented 40% of the investigators in summer residence at the Institution. Major neuroscience discoveries had been made at the MBL, including Hartline's use of the eye of the horseshoe crab Limulus in the study of visual processing, and J. Z. Young's demonstration that the giant axon of the squid mantle was indeed a nerve fiber that could be used to investigate the mechanism of nerve conduction. Instruction in neurobiology began in the famous Physiology Course, whose origins dated back to the start of the MBL in 1888, and was continued in a highly successful Training Program in Neurobiology organized by Steve Kuffler, Dave Potter, and Ed Furshpan, which ran for 10 years (1957–1966). The Program included among its 74 "students" such luminaries as Seymour

Benzer, Larry Cohen, Don Pfaff, Denis Baylor, John Nichols, Jack Diamond, Pablo Rudomin, and Zach Hall. After a gap of several years, two new neurobiology courses were added to the MBL roster to replace the Training Program. One, an Excitable Membrane Biophysics and Physiology Training Program under the direction of Bill Adelman, began in 1969; the second, a Neurobiology Course under the leadership of John Dowling and Mike Bennett, began in 1970. During the summer of 1974, Jim Ebert, who was President of the MBL at the time, asked whether I would be interested in assuming the Directorship of the Neurobiology Course. He mentioned that the MBL would be discontinuing support for the Excitable Membrane Training Program the next year and wondered whether a new neurobiology course might cover some of the territory offered by that program as well. Basically, Ebert and the MBL Education Committee were dissatisfied with the educational value to the MBL of the Training Program and wanted it eliminated. I didn't realize the hornet's nest I was invading by taking on the latter challenge.

Before agreeing to become Director, I felt it important to line up a group of outstanding colleagues to help in the teaching of the course. First, I needed a Co-Director, and Tony Stretton was my first choice. Tony and I had rented a laboratory at the MBL that summer to search for dyes that could be used to optically monitor active neurons. That project grew mostly out of our looking for an excuse to work together again after the great fun we had in finding Procion Yellow a decade earlier. To my delight, Tony agreed, and together we generated a list of potential faculty to teach a course that would be divided into five blocks: Ed Furshpan and Dave Potter in neurophysiology; Tom Reese in neuroanatomy; Gerry Fischbach in cell culture; and Zach Hall (who then was back at Harvard) in receptor mechanisms. For the fifth block, Tony and I would add a biochemistry section. That group, we felt, would do an outstanding job of covering the area of cellular neurobiology. To our surprise, everyone was willing to teach with us, and with that we told Ebert we would give it a try. The Biophysics contingent was not happy with our choice as directors, let us know this, and withdrew funding for the new course from a private source of support they had acquired.

I have vivid memories of the evening before the first day of the course. It was Sunday, June 22, 1975. We were in a basement area in the Loeb building of the MBL, which was mostly a storage area and where part of the course was to be housed. A few rooms had been constructed in the basement for us by the MBL staff, one of which was designated as a course lecture room. None of the equipment in the laboratory was ready for the neurophysiology section, and we were convinced that there was no way we could get the course area ready in time for the students. A blackboard and screen had been placed in the lecture room, but the only illumination in the room was a few old ceiling fluorescent fixtures that left the blackboard dark. We solved the board lighting problem by rushing to a hardware store in Falmouth and purchasing several clip-on lights which we wired across the ceiling of the room. That created a problem though, because when we plugged in the board lights we could not use the slide projector since there were too few electrical outlets in the room. Tables and chairs for the students had been scavenged from the old Mess Hall at the MBL and were in terrible shape. While sitting around moaning about the disaster that was about to befall us, Dave Potter began sanding one of the old oak Mess Hall tables. Slowly, we all joined in, grabbing steel wool and sand paper. One of us rushed to Falmouth again to purchase a clear lacquer to coat the tables. We spent the next several hours "finishing" the old tables, ending up making them look better than new. No one said "let's do the tables." Somehow or other, it just happened. After that completely unnecessary break, everything fell into place, and the course began, as scheduled, the next morning. New laboratories eventually were built for us in the basement in time for the third year of the course. The area was named the Grass Laboratory in honor of Ellen and Albert Grass for their loyal financial support of the course since its inception.

The course truly was a special experience for everyone involved. During each block, mornings were dedicated to teaching lectures, and afternoons and evenings, often running to 1:00 AM or later, were dedicated to the laboratories. Labs were always staffed with faculty willing to stay as long as students were there. Two research seminars a week, special symposia featuring invited guests (on topics such as Membrane Biophysics, Animal Behavior, Neuronal Peptides, and Vertebrate Central Nervous System), and special open-ended seminars on Saturdays where invited guests could talk at length on their field of study, all complemented the total immersion of the students in neuroscience. Evening parties capped off the special symposia with music, dancing, and margaritas, leading to long evenings of fun and relaxation for all involved with the course. Softball too was an important part of the course activities, with Coach Fischbach driving his charges hard in practice sessions before the games with other MBL courses. It was easy to spot the somewhat older group of Neurobiology students on the MBL campus. They were the ones with bandaged legs and arms resulting from muscles pulled during the softball games. The job of Course Director ranged from ensuring the smooth running of each block of the instruction program to making sure that paper cups were available for the morning coffee breaks.

There was considerable rotation of our faculty over my five-year tenure as Course Director. Tony Stretton, feeling the pressure of trying to run a laboratory thousands of miles away in Wisconsin while in residence at the MBL, finally had to drop out as Co-Director after the third year. My good friend and constant partner in wild new ventures, John Hildebrand, succeeded Tony. John also shared the directorship of the course with Tom Reese for a second five-year cycle after I stepped down as Director. Paul O'Lague and his student, Sue Huttner, taught regularly in the neurophysiology section. Sue also was our course assistant for several years. In addition to being an excellent scientist, teaching in the neurophysiology block, and helping me organize all other blocks, Sue was the life of the course: she got the dancing going at all of the parties and made sure that students were out of the laboratory and on the field for softball practices and games. Gerry Fischbach's student, Ruth Siegel, also was a gem. She made sure the cell culture part of the course happened every summer, since, somehow or other, Gerry invariably had a hard time remembering things like ordering supplies for his section. Ruth taught in the cell culture section and also helped me generate an inventory of course supplies and equipment. Even more importantly though, Ruth kept me informed (to my amazement) about the complex social goings-on within the course every summer. John Heuser taught regularly in the anatomy section with Tom Reese, as did Philippa Claude, Story and Dennis Landis, and various students, postdocs, and former colleagues of Tom. Zach Hall taught for only one year and a receptor block was not reintroduced to the course until Jon Cohen joined our faculty in 1977. Finally, present and former postdoctoral associates and graduate students of mine and Tony's assisted in teaching the biochemistry part of the course.

The great joy of the summer was in teaching the exceptional students who took the course. With students like David Anderson, Mary Beth Hatten, Marge Livingstone, Jeff Corwin, Tim Ebner, Ben Peng, Jane Dodd, Jose Lemos, and Jose Garcia-Arraras, and more senior "students" like Hennig Stieve, Terry Sejnowski, Jerry Pine, Jerry Hurwitz, and Mike Zigmond, how could we miss? The pleasure of instructing this group was that they really wanted to know everything we could teach them, and they were insatiable in their quest for more. They were tired at the end of the summer, but felt invincible. There was nothing they could not do. Of course, reality set in when they returned to their home laboratories at the end of the summer. Still, all of us involved with the course felt a wonderful sense of accomplishment at the end of every summer. When my tenure as Director ended, the students threw a special party for me at which they unveiled a movie they had made over the entire summer, without my knowing anything about it. What was most embarrassing about my blissful ignorance was that son James was the cameraman for a script put together by David Anderson and Mark Noble. It was called "Abnormal Morphogenetic Movements" and featured, among other things, the famous nose/lobster claw transplant experiments. At the end of these five intensive years, I was at a bit of loss about what to do next, besides research that is, to enrich my life. I didn't have to wait long though as The Neurobiology of Disease Teaching Workshops, joining the Hereditary Disease (HD) Foundation Board, starting Neuroscience Commentaries, and beginning the Harvard Program in Neuroscience soon filled whatever void I might have been feeling.

Special People: The Wexlers, Marjorie Guthrie, The HD Foundation, and The Neurobiology of Disease

First Meeting

I first met Nancy Wexler and Marjorie Guthrie (second wife of Woody Guthrie and mother of Arlo) at an NINCDS-sponsored Long-Term Strategies Planning Panel on Inflammatory, Demyelinating and Degenerative Diseases, held in Williamsburg, VA, in May 1978. Nancy, a Health Scientist Administrator at NINCDS, was an observer at the meeting, and Marjorie, the President of the New York-based Committee to Combat Huntington's Disease, was there to speak about Huntington's Disease. Nancy, Marjorie, and Milton Wexler (Nancy's dad) had in 1977 worked together as members of a congressionally mandated commission for the Control of Huntington's Disease: Marjorie was the Chairperson, Milton was the Vice Chairperson, and Nancy was the Executive Director of the Commission. As an observer at the Planning Panel, Nancy was supposed to sit quietly in the background and take notes. Being Nancy, of course, she'd have none of that and was outspoken on many issues relating to disease-related science, contributing intelligent, thoughtful, and provocative comments to much of the discussion that followed the formal presentations. Marjorie described the commission report and delivered a stirring presentation on the role of Health Voluntary organizations in the battle against degenerative diseases.

Without doubt, Nancy and Marjorie were the most lively participants at the panel meeting. They spoke about neurological diseases with such passion that I went out of my way to meet both of them and to invite them to speak at the MBL Neurobiology Course that summer. It was their presentations at the panel meeting that made me recognize that we never mentioned neurological diseases and disorders in our course. As far as our students were concerned, and as far as we were teaching them, the nervous system always functioned properly. That summer and the next, Nancy and Marjorie visited and lectured in the course. Their inspiring presentations excited the students and kindled in me the desire to do something about trying to interest next generation scientists in the poorly understood and mostly untreatable neurological and psychiatric diseases and disorders that afflicted countless millions of people throughout the world. It was over lunch at the Fishmonger Restaurant in Woods Hole during Nancy's second visit to the MBL in 1979 that five of us, Nancy, Alan Pearlman, Michael Zigmond, Dennis Landis, and myself, formulated the outline for a national course to teach young people about disease (The Neurobiology of Disease Workshops and the Harvard course that followed).

The Hereditary Disease (HD) Foundation

My ties to Nancy, Alice (Nancy's sister), and Milton Wexler and their Foundation began when Allan Tobin, who was the Scientific Director of the Foundation, invited me to attend an International HD Meeting and a Foundation workshop at the Hotel del Coronado on Coronado Island near San Diego in October 1978. The invitation likely derived from our earlier work on GABA neurons, which are the first to die in the brains of patients with HD, and from my interactions with Nancy at the MBL course. A letter to Milton summarizing my impressions about the research presented at the meeting and workshop ended with "I hope I can assist you in other ways in the future. One cannot help but become involved when one is confronted with people like you and Nancy (in particular), Jennifer Jones Selznick and your crew of young enthusiasts and your devotion to this cause." Allan invited me to join the Scientific Advisory Board of the HD Foundation in December 1979, and I was elected to the Board in January 1980.

When I first joined the Board I was impressed with the dedication and enthusiasm of the members, most of who had been with the Foundation from its inception. I was disappointed though at the quality of much of the research they were supporting. Part of the problem was that grants were going to Board members, some of whom were not doing forefront research, but a more important part dealt with the quality of the applications the Foundation was receiving. At one of the first meetings I went to, there were two applications investigating whether membrane defects existed in fibroblasts in patients with HD. Both of these laboratories were supported by the Foundation, and they continually reported opposite results in their studies. Instead of continuing to support both groups, I suggested that a single grant be given to the investigators involved, with the requirement that they work together on the project. Unfortunately, or perhaps fortunately, that put an end to Foundation support for those studies, since neither of the principal investigators was willing to meet the required condition. In March of 1980, before my official Board duties had begun, I organized a workshop for the Foundation on "Cell Death." I was surprised that this was not a dominant theme in earlier workshops. As I saw it, two striking facts defined HD, and these I believed should become the focus of the Foundation's research efforts: one was that HD was an autosomal dominant disorder, and hence, a search for the gene should be undertaken; the other was that neurons died in the brains of Huntington's patients, and hence, understanding how, why, and where neurons died should become a central research theme.

If I had to evaluate my time on the Board, I would say I played a role in several major changes in the directions of the Foundation. One was in my very strong support for David Housman's initiative to use restriction fragment length polymorphisms (RFLPs) to try to find the mutated gene. Here is what I said about this in a letter to Milton Wexler reporting on the January 1980 workshop. "What seemed to me by far the most useful and far-reaching technology in relation to disease that we heard about, however, was the work David Housman described on the attempted cloning of human genes. There seems to be little doubt that this will work. All of the techniques that are needed now are available to the molecular biologists and while I am certain that problems will arise . . . this seems to be a most promising avenue to a pre-natal diagnosis of human disease. I agree entirely with Bill Dreyer (who was on the Board) that within the decade this will be done (and should be strongly supported financially), but I don't agree that we will understand all about genetic diseases of the nervous system. One still has to know what the mutant gene is producing and where it fits into an animal's behavior to produce the disease." In a way, my comments were prophetic. Everyone was very surprised at how quickly a linkage to HD was found by Jim Gusella (who had started out with David Housman on the project) in 1983, leading to the isolation of the mutant gene Huntingtin 10 years later. But, 22 years later, one still does not know how the gene functions in producing the disease. With the development of excellent animal models of HD and other degenerative diseases of the nervous system, however, investigators are coming closer and closer to understanding the disease process. Hopefully, this also will lead to new therapies.

Another important role I played on the Foundation Board was in pushing to move in the direction of understanding the mechanism of neuronal cell death. I felt even if one did not succeed in the genetic approach to understanding HD, if you knew how neurons died and if there was a final common pathway of neuronal cell death, it might be possible to slow the death process and thereby reduce the ravages of the disease. I introduced Bob Horvitz to the Foundation at the Cell Death Workshop I organized, and he soon joined the Board and became one of its strongest and wisest supporters over the years. Bob has just shared the Nobel Prize for Physiology and Medicine for his and Junying Yuan's original work in *Caenorhabditis elegans* on cell death.

As one of my last contributions, Steve Matthysse and I originated the concept of "Collaborative Research Agreements," which invited outstanding researchers to work in HD-related research by offering them partial funding for directed studies. Unfortunately, our first venture in these directions was not well treated by the Board. As the first candidate for this award, we selected an HMS researcher who had developed excellent new methods to generate monoclonal antibodies that were highly selective for nervous tissue of different types. Steve and I felt that this investigator actually might be able to generate specific antibodies to HD-diseased tissue, and hence, our support for the project. Unfortunately, we were accused of nepotism for having selected an HMS investigator. We still felt the Collaborative Research Agreements were a good idea, and ultimately, a more mature form of these agreements was awarded to a collaborative that included some of the best research groups in the world working on human disease-related genes. That was, in fact, the group that isolated the mutant Huntington's disease gene.

Although my membership on the HD Foundation Scientific Advisory Board lasted only 4 years (I stepped down, deciding not to serve for a second term), this was a most fulfilling adventure for me, opening new horizons and new dimensions in my life. It also allowed me to form long-lasting close friendships with the amazing Wexlers, Milton, Nancy, and Alice and to interact with their dazzling array of celebrity friends.

The Neurobiology of Disease

A National Course—The Neurobiology of Disease Teaching Workshop

After Nancy's second visit to the MBL in 1979, we formulated a plan for a national workshop whose goal would be educating young scientists about the diseases and disorders of the nervous system. The plan incorporated what I believed were the best elements of the HD Foundation workshops, the ways that Ed Furspan and Dave Potter taught medical students, and the way I taught graduate courses at Harvard and at the MBL. Even today, I feel that this is the most creative educational enterprise I ever have been involved in.

To attract an audience for these national workshops, we felt it important to link them to the Annual Society for Neuroscience Meeting. Therefore, during the fall of 1979, Nancy and I met with Sol Snyder, who was President of the Society for Neuroscience at the time, to get approval for this affiliation. Sol liked the idea a lot, gave us a go ahead to carry out a first workshop on a trial basis at the Society Meeting in 1980, promised us administrative support from the Society, but said that the Society would not offer financial support for the enterprise. Thus, the bottom line once again was that we would have to raise all the money required for the workshop ourselves from foundations or federal sources. This was not an easy task. Even the HD Foundation was not enthusiastic about the idea at first, awarding us only a small sum of money that covered only a fraction of the anticipated expenses. The Head of the National Multiple Sclerosis Foundation (M.S. was one of the diseases we planned to cover the first year) wondered how we could possibly cover their disease in one 3-hr session. He patiently listened to my description of our concept and then carefully explained how they organized meetings that went for many days covering only small areas relating to their disease. I felt like saying, but didn't since we hoped to get some money from them, that I didn't really need 3 hr to teach students all that was *really* known about M.S. I could do that in 30 min. The M.S. Foundation gave us nothing the first year. Somehow or other, I did piece together the needed funds, going to friends such as the Bay Foundation (Bob Ashton), Merck Sharp and Dohme (Roy Vagelos), and the Klingenstein Fund. Even NINCDS officials like Katherine (Kit) Bick, who really liked the concept of the workshops, did not support us until the third year of the workshops.

Our plan for the workshops was that they would last two days, and we would cover different diseases on each day. Both days would begin with a patient presentation followed by core clinical and basic science lectures. Nancy, Allan Pearlman, and I traveled the country searching for outstanding teachers to deliver the core lectures. We emphasized that we wanted real teaching lectures and not research seminars. Our aim was to build a base of knowledge for our students about where research was in the field and where it might go in the future. Even more, we wanted students to begin to think about how their own research might fit in—how it might be relevant. To ensure that the core lectures really would be cores of knowledge, we required that faculty delivering these lectures "practice" and refine them at a premeeting held several weeks before the actual workshop. The audience for these rehearsals would be the organizing committee and other faculty participating in the workshop. We figured that if we as a group could not understand the lectures, there would be no way that students unfamiliar with the topic would understand them. These turned out to be amazing, fun, and intellectually satisfying sessions with a distinguished faculty from all over the country arguing about what the core facts were and how best to present them. Some faculty even admitted that after these sessions they delivered the best lectures they ever had presented. At the workshops, core lectures were followed by small group discussions in which students were encouraged to talk about what they had just heard and to speculate on how research might "solve" these difficult, intellectually challenging problems. Each day ended with special workshops in which investigators expert in new technologies would brainstorm with students about how their technology might be applied in the battle to conquer disease. In the evening, a banquet was held featuring a speaker from a health voluntary organization talking about the human side of disease—how these tragic diseases impacted of families. The workshop ended on the second day with a presentation by Nancy about how to apply for funding from the NIH. Our goals were to totally immerse students in these diseases for the two days of the workshop and, of course, to hope that some of them actually would begin to work in these areas as well.

The first workshop was held at The University of Cincinnati Medical Center under the sponsorship of their Neurology Department on November 8 and 9, 1980. The themes were autoimmune diseases—myasthenia gravis and multiple sclerosis—on the first day and degenerative disorders—Parkinson's and Huntington's Diseases—on the second day. Jon Lindstrom delivered our lead-off talk with his research showing that myasthenia gravis was an autoimmune disease in which patients developed antibodies to their own ACh receptors. We felt that Jon's work was the model of what the workshops were all about—how basic science could make a fundamental contribution to an understanding of a neurological disease. Marjorie Guthrie gave the evening lecture on her "Personal Experiences with Huntington's Disease." One student gave Marjorie's talk a rating of 10,000 on a scale of 1–10. Another student commented that he "would steal hubcaps" to attend the next year's meeting. I have vivid memories of Nancy and I running around the halls of the medical school at the end of the workshop locking the doors of rooms used during the small group discussions, thoroughly thrilled that we actually had pulled it off: the workshop had happened and had been an enormous success. Twenty-three years later, the Neurobiology of Disease Workshops still are going strong. They now are reduced to a single day before the Society Annual Meeting, but still have NINCDS support and present the ever-growing base of scientific information to enthusiastic audiences of young investigators interested in going out and doing something to effect a cure for these diseases.

The Neurobiology of Disease Course at Harvard

With the national course off to a terrific start, I felt it important to have a Harvard version of the course too. Joe Martin agreed to be Co-Director and we offered the first cycle of the course during the fall semester of 1983. Joe and I generated a list of diseases and disorders that we planned to cover over the semester and selected faculty teaching teams who we felt were good teachers and experts in the clinical or basic science aspects of each topic. Occasionally, we found one investigator who could do both. In designing the course we kept as many of the features of the workshops as possible. Thus, we included patient presentations, teaching lectures as opposed to research seminars, and a survey of the current literature in the field. The emphasis was to be on what was and what was not known about the disease and how basic science might contribute to understanding the disease and help in the development of new therapies. Each week we presented a major disease or disorder, had patient presentations and core clinical and basic science lectures, had student presentations of current literature, and extended free-form discussions of the topic. Topics the first year included myasthenia gravis; the muscular dystrophies; Alzheimer's, Huntington's, and Parkinson's diseases; affective disorders; pain; and others.

As with the national disease workshops, I offered to rehearse faculty prior to their presentations, but none of my Harvard colleagues took me up on the offer. Still, faculty really did enjoy their involvement with the course. Marcel Mesulam wrote: "I have taught in more courses than I care to count. However, I would like you to know that the two sessions in your course on the Neurobiology of Disease have been just about the most enjoyable teaching experiences I have had." Gerry Klerman added, "This experience convinced me that we need to do more teaching about the pathophysiology and neurobiology of psychiatric disorders." The students gave us the highest ratings of all the graduate courses offered at the Medical School. Faculty and former students who participated in the early years of the course have come back year after year to teach with us. This has been particularly rewarding for me because we ask a lot of our faculty and do not offer any recompense for their efforts.

Actually, it was hard to miss having an outstanding course when the first students included Ben (then Barbara) Barres, Peggy Mason, Junying Yuan, and Tony Monaco, all of whom have gone on to distinguished research careers working at the clinical/basic science interface. Tony's thesis was concerned with cloning the defective gene for muscular dystrophy. He was in his first year of study, when Lou Kunkel, teaching in the disease course, outlined a strategy for cloning the defective gene in Muscular Dystrophy. Excited by the lecture, Tony went to see Lou the next morning and said he wanted to work on the project. Early the next week, the work began. The result is history. That outcome represented much of what the Program in Neuroscience and the Neurobiology of Disease National Workshops and Harvard course were all about for me. Finally, we were starting to see progress in understanding the diseases that so touched me as a camp counselor so many years ago. Possibly, just possibly, I had played some role in facilitating that progress.

Neuroscience Commentaries—A short Lifetime for an Exciting Adventure (1981–1984)

When Eric Kandel, the President of the Society for Neuroscience, first asked me to edit a new section for the Neuroscience Newsletter, I turned him down. Eric felt that the newsletter was boring, containing almost exclusively Society business, job postings, and meeting announcements. He recognized the great excitement that neuroscience research was generating, that the field was growing at an enormous rate, and that the Society should be doing a better job of informing the membership of what was happening in the field. The model that Eric had in mind was a "News and Views" section like the one that existed in the journal *Nature*. Even though I said no, I was intrigued by the concept of playing a central role in keeping the membership of the Society informed about current trends in neuroscience. Later, at the same Society meeting, in brainstorming sessions with two of my favorite people, Nancy Wexler and John Hildebrand, we began discussing the kind of vehicle that might be launched to explain the field in an exciting and useful way. We felt it important to not only reach the membership of the Society with whatever we offered, but to go farther—to the press, the public, and Congress, who, after all, were going to fund the science and should know what we, as a field, were doing. With my and Nancy's heavy involvement in disease-related issues at the time, we also felt it important to aim whatever basic science we presented toward the solution of clinical problems. Together, Nancy, John, and I formulated and presented Eric with the idea of a new mini-journal called "Neuroscience Commentaries." He immediately liked the concept and encouraged us to assemble a first issue to be enclosed within the *Neuroscience Newsletter* and sent gratis to the membership of the Society. Eric already had acquired a $5000 grant from the Klingenstein Foundation (and our good friend Bob Ebert) to begin the venture, and together, he and I acquired a second grant of $10,000 from the same foundation to continue publication after the first issue came out. John, Nancy, and I agreed to serve as Interim Editors to get *Commentaries* off the ground.

Our plan was to publish three or four issues of *Neuroscience Commentaries* a year that would include "clusters of essays, loosely organized around a common theme, that would consider the historical perspective, the methodology, and the recent advances of key research groups in the thematic area; brief summaries of these essays aimed at nonscientists; articles examining issues arising at the interface between the neuroscience community, the government and the press; and reports of services available to neuroscientists such as brain banks, cell culture facilities, and sources of research materials, including antibodies, enzymes, drugs, and experimental animals" (from an editorial appearing with the first issue). The first lay translation was included with the second issue and was brilliantly done by Julie Miller, who had received a Ph.D. from the Harvard Department of Neurobiology some years before and who later went on to found her own journal, *Bioscience*. We also received outstanding editorial help from Gerry Gurvitch in the offices of the Society for Neuroscience, who with great skill, good humor, incredible patience, and occasional poems kept us on target in getting issues of *Commentaries* published and sent out to the membership. Gerry was our Managing Editor. All of the work involved in getting *Commentaries* off the ground was done without remuneration to John, Nancy, or myself. One difference between *Commentaries* and other review journals of the day was that the three of us did extensive rewrites of the articles, something our authors were not used to. The quality of the final product, however, was well worth it, as all the articles ended up eminently readable. Eric remained our strongest supporter, continually applauding our efforts, trying through all his varied connections to get us funding for the journal, and arguing with the powers that be within the Society for allowing us to maintain the free-ranging and unfettered style with which we were operating.

Three issues of *Commentaries* appeared before its demise: the first, in September 1981, was on "Peptides in the Nervous System"; the second, a year later, was on "Neuronal Cell Death"; and the final issue, published in December 1983, focused on the ACh receptor as the prototype for the mediation of fast synaptic responses. A survey of the membership showed an overwhelmingly favorable response to *Commentaries* from the 500 or so members who responded. In addition to Eric's support, the Chair of the Publications Committee, Sam Barondes, and the Editor of the *Journal of Neuroscience*, Max Cowan, also were full of praise for our enterprise. So what killed *Neuroscience Commentaries*? Actually, it was a combination of several factors. Despite multiple applications, including one to NIMH, neither Eric nor I could get any long-term funding for *Commentaries*. We did receive a $20,000 grant from the Sloan Foundation that required matching support, but none was forthcoming from the Council of the Society for Neuroscience or from any other sources. We also felt that many members of the Council were lukewarm in their support for *Commentaries* and didn't see anything unique in what we were trying to do. One suggestion was to fold *Commentaries* into the *Journal of Neuroscience*, but we felt that Max Cowan was not very enthusiastic about that possibility. Max liked *Commentaries*, but did not want an independent venture as part of "his" journal. Finally, after much discussion, a complete submersion of *Commentaries* within the journal was the option offered us by Gerry Fischbach, who was then President of the Society. The terms outlined for this were not satisfactory to any of us involved with *Commentaries*. The three of us resigned, hoping that the Society for Neuroscience would try to keep the concept alive, but along with us and the three issues that were published, *Neuroscience Commentaries* disappeared into the proverbial sunset.

Colon Cancer (1982)

I wish I had the voice of Homer
To sing of rectal carcinoma,
Which kills a lot more chaps, in fact,
Than were bumped off when Troy was sacked.

So now I am like two-faced Janus
The only god who sees his anus.
I'll swear, without the risk of perjury,
It was a snappy bit of surgery.

Excerpts from "Cancer's a Funny Thing," a poem by J.B.S. Haldane

Someplace in the middle of all of this, I was diagnosed with colon cancer. Therefore, this section is placed someplace in the middle of all the other sections covering this period of my life. The statistics on survival with colon cancer were that 50% of people with the disease would die within one year of diagnosis. I decided that I would be in the other 50%. I really wasn't ready to die, and that was that! There were many things that had to be done in a very short period of time though, just in case things didn't work out the way

I expected. First and foremost, my family had to be protected. Kathryn and I had not drawn up a will, which therefore had to be done immediately. Then, who was I to tell about the upcoming surgery? My family had to know, the lab group had to know, and a few special friends had to know. I decided that was as far as I would go. I also felt it was essential for someone to be in the operating room during the surgery to take a piece of my tumor. This too was just in case the prognosis for the future was not as rosy as I anticipated. My plans were to make monoclonal antibodies to my tumor, attach a toxin to the antibodies, and inject them into myself to try to destroy the tumor. After all, I was a scientist, and I was not going to die without battling every inch of the way with whatever special skills I could muster as a scientist. I also had read that human tumors could be placed in cell culture in order to devise a rational strategy for chemotherapy. For this too, I needed a fragment of my tumor.

A few days before surgery, the members of the lab group asked to meet with me. Tom Schwarz said, "Ed, we can't understand how you can be so calm about this." My response was, "I have an awful lot to do in a very short period of time to protect my family, myself and all of you, and if it helped to be hysterical, you can be sure that I would be hysterical." Michael Goy generously agreed to continue teaching my course for me, and with everything as well in hand as possible, I went off to have my colon removed. Part of the anesthetic involved an injection of morphine into my spinal cord, and the resident who was doing the injection was a former medical student of ours. She remembered me, was a bit nervous, and then missed getting into the spinal cord on the first try. I was thinking at the time that I wish she didn't remember me. With help from Art Pardee, Dr. Howard Fingert was in the operating room to take a fragment of my tumor for research purposes. Luckily, it wasn't needed. When I awoke from anesthesia in the recovery room, John Brooks, my surgeon, was standing over me. He said, "We have a cure!" What a relief those words were. The first two people to visit me when I awoke in my hospital room were Dan Tosteson, who was the Dean at the time, and Nelson Kiang, a colleague and friend. Both came in to see me with big smiles on their faces and with books for me to read. I have no idea how they found out about my surgery.

The Program in Neuroscience (1982–1990)

In 1981, a university-wide graduate Program in Neuroscience was established by the Harvard University Committee of Biological Sciences. I was offered, and accepted, the Directorship of this Program. With the enormous growth of the neurosciences in the nation, and with more and more hiring of neuroscientists by HMS, Harvard College, School of Public Health, and Harvard-affiliated hospital departments, the time was ripe to form a broadly based new program. The goals of the Program, as I viewed them, were (1) to bring together basic science and clinical faculty engaged in neuroscience research throughout the University and (2) to attract the best graduate students in the nation to this emerging and rapidly growing field of study. I managed to negotiate a budget from the Medical School for a student office, a Program Coordinator, and an Associate Director to run the Program, which may have been the first time that a cross-university program of this sort had its own budget. Before accepting our first students though, I had to build a faculty and establish an academic teaching program. To do this, I had to convince investigators engaged in neuroscience research throughout the University that we were going to make a serious effort to build a focused research community out of what was a widely scattered assortment of investigators. One reason for skepticism about the seriousness of my intent was that the Neurobiology Department did not allow faculty appointments outside the physical confines of our quadrangle-based department. This policy had earned the department the reputation of being elitist, but the policy of exclusion had its purpose. Steve desired to maintain a strong, coherent, manageably sized unit that could be run more like a family (as was Steve's style) than like the corporate entities typical of other medical school departments of the day.

Personal visits to other centers of concentration of neuroscientists, permission from the Medical School to make appointments in the Program in Neuroscience (another first), a firm commitment from me that graduate students would be shared among all faculty, and a guarantee that affiliates would play roles in the planning and running of the Program soon led to applications by many faculty members to join us and wide representation of many departments throughout Harvard and its affiliated hospitals in the Program in Neuroscience. In meeting my promise of faculty involvement, I established two administrative committees that ran the Program: an "Executive Committee" of senior neuroscientists and administrators that was responsible for overview of the Program and approval of faculty affiliate appointments and a "Working Committee" of younger faculty that actually ran the Program. Quite early in these efforts, I had the good fortune to have Tom Fox join me as Associate Director.

From the start to the finish of my tenure as Director (1982–1990), the Program in Neuroscience was student oriented. We did attract the truly outstanding students we were looking for. Included in our early classes were Ben Barres, Tony Monaco, Peggy Mason, and Junying Yuan (who started out in Neurobiology, but transferred to the Program after 1 year), among others. Starting with five accepted students in 1982, the Program grew by 1988 to 34 students (15 Ph.D., 10 M.D./Ph.D., and 9 M.D. returning for their Ph.D.) and 90 affiliated faculty representing 12 different research centers. Tom and I felt strongly that the center of the Program in Neuroscience was our students. Therefore, we did all we could to enrich the quality of their lives. Excellence in scientific training and research was stressed, of course, but an intimate involvement of the students in running the Program and in having fun were not forgotten. Potluck dinners, open office hours, two annual retreats on Cape Cod (one for students only, the other for faculty and students for symposia in which the students selected and hosted the speakers), and a revival of BANG (the Boston Area Neuroscience Group) all were for our students. We involved them in organizing and running as many of these events as possible. Tom and I usually were invited to the student's Fall Retreat, but we suspected that was mainly to make margaritas and start the dancing. The two of us served a similar role in the much larger Spring Retreats (dancing and margaritas), which also featured occasional dips in chilly swimming pools by students and faculty who will remain nameless. Tom and I also began ethics discussion groups for our students, many years before they were an NIH requirement, to deal with issues that surfaced in interstudent relationships.

One nice benefit of the ability to grant titles to faculty outside the Department of Neurobiology was the good will that was generated between quadrangle- and hospital-based faculty. Very shortly after Seymour Kety was appointed Professor of Neuroscience in the Department of Psychiatry (February 1983), he wrote me a lovely note about the title stating, "I am very pleased with my new title and, in a meeting last week at which I was identified by that title, my colleagues at the conference seemed pleased as well." Clearly, the granting of titles identifying colleagues based in clinical settings as belonging to a quadrangle-based program was important in helping to build the community of scholars envisioned in the formation of programs of this sort by the University Committee of Biological Sciences. When Gerry Fischbach came to HMS to Chair the Department of Neurobiology in 1990, I stepped down as Director of the Program in Neuroscience, feeling that the Program was a success and that a new Chair should have a free hand to pick new leadership for the graduate program.

Life as a Neuroethologist, Honors, Family (1992–Present)

Life as a Neuroethologist

Serotonin neurons, quantifying behavior, and changes in neuronal function with changes in status. In what follows, I present a few highlights from this decade of my life as a scientist. I limit my description here because I believe that the story of my accomplishments as a neuroethologist is in its infancy. The problem is that attempting to understand complex social behavior at the level of neuronal function is an enormous challenge, one that we still find ourselves learning how best to address. Mind you, I believe we have made interesting contributions to the scientific literature during this decade, but we still do not know how, or even if, serotonergic neurons function during fighting behavior. Moreover, we have only the faintest outlines of notions about how a behavior such as aggression is assembled in nervous systems.

The "gain-setter" role. Barb Beltz had done a great job in finding the amine neurosecretory cells and in elaborating methods to routinely record from these neurons. She also carried out the first experiments that described the "gain-setter" role served by these neurons. Pokay Ma picked up on this theme and in a monster set of experiments elaborated the gain-setter story. His and Barb's results showed that serotonergic neurosecretory cells were part of the motor command circuitry, as expected, but in a much more interesting way than anticipated. First, the cells were not concerned with point-to-point wiring in the lobster nervous system. Stimulating cells through intracellular electrodes did not produce motor output from the ventral nerve cord, as had been seen with bath application of amines. Instead, when flexor command neurons were activated, in addition to turning on flexor motor programs, they increased the firing of serotonergic neurons, which in turn enhanced the output of the command. If extensor commands were activated, the serotonergic neurons were inhibited. If serotonergic neurons were forced to fire with an intracellular electrode when extensor commands were activated, however, the output of these commands too would be enhanced. Thus, the circuitry determined whether the serotonergic cells would show increased or decreased firing after activation of motor commands, and the serotonergic neurons would function as general gain-setters whose activation enhanced the output of motor circuitry.

Autoinhibition. It had been long known from studies in vertebrate systems that serotonin neurons showed autoinhibition, the property of turning themselves off after high-frequency stimulation. This was believed to be due to released serotonin having actions both on postsynaptic targets and on terminals that had released the amine to reduce further release. Therefore, we were not surprised when we found that after a period of high-frequency firing of A1-5HT neurons, there was a pause in the firing of the cells. Studies of this type were begun by Michael Horner, Don Edwards, and myself while at the MBL in Woods Hole the summer of 1997. They were elegantly continued by Ralf Heinrich at Harvard on our return from Woods Hole, with Stuart Cromarty joining in on some of the experiments.

There were two very interesting outcomes of these studies. One was that the autoinhibition seen in lobster serotonergic neurons did not result from the actions of released serotonin. What convinced us of this was (1) that the inhibition was seen in A1-5HT neurons from animals that had been treated with 5,7-dihydroxytryptamine, which depletes the A1-5HT cells of 5HT, and (2) that autoinhibition still was observed in the absence of extracellular calcium, which would prevent the release of the transmitter. Thus, "autoinhibition" appeared to be an endogenous property of these neurons: when forced to fire at high frequencies, they turned themselves off. In the original description of autoinhibition by Aghajanian, such a possibility was discussed, but that notion disappeared from the literature. Possibly of greater interest, though, was that the duration of the autoinhibition was inversely related to the initial firing rate of the cells. Cells that fired spontaneously at low frequencies showed sustained periods of autoinhibition, while those that fired initially at higher rates showed little or no pause in their firing after high-frequency stimulation. Here was a surprising finding, for we had been paying little attention to whether A1-5HT cells fired at 1 or 2 or 3 Hz. Now we recognized that, within this narrow range, the initial firing rates of cells were important determinants of how the neurons functioned after high-frequency activation. Therefore, questions such as what set the firing rates of cells became issues we had to start thinking about. This might represent, in fact, a cellular mechanism whereby the way cells were used in the past influenced how they would be used in the future.

A quantitative analysis of lobster fighting behavior. I had been trying for years to interest a behaviorist in working with us to quantify lobster fighting behavior. I felt that this was important to do, because how else could we interpret pharmacological experiments we were planning to carry out involving changing amine levels in lobsters to search for effects on fighting behavior. If we didn't know what normal lobster fights looked like, how could we possibly interpret anything we saw with amine level manipulation. Jean Fraser, a behaviorist, worked with us for a while, and although she carried out some interesting learning experiments with lobsters, I couldn't convince her to analyze the behavior. We shared an NIH Program Project Grant with Jelle Atema for a while, and he too didn't seem particularly interested in performing the analysis (although a few years later members of his lab group did analyze fighting behavior in adult lobsters). Finally, on a trip to Texas Tech University to deliver a seminar, I met Robert Huber, who was finishing his graduate studies at the time. After my talk, Robert and I discussed the prospect of his coming to the laboratory to do the analysis that I had been so anxious to have done for so many years.

Robert was Konrad Lorenz's last student, and as such, he was a classically trained ethologist. However, he also was trained in evolutionary biology and in the use of computers for analyzing complex situations such as behavior. Thus, he appeared perfect for these studies. We thought it best to use young, socially naive animals that had never seen or fought with another lobster before to examine the elements that comprised the fundamental patterns of fighting behavior in lobsters. For this purpose, we used animals raised at the New England Aquarium that had not seen another lobster since the fourth larval stage when they began their benthic existence. The animals were between one and two years old (several inches in length), and to our great surprise, they knew all the rules of fighting behavior. Fights involved displays in which lobsters stood as tall as they could, showing their major weapons, the claws; limited aggression in which they held onto each other with the claws and tried to turn each other over; and high-level aggression in which they grabbed onto each other with their claws and used short upward tail flips in an attempt to tear limbs off the opponent. Decisions could be made at any time during a fight, and once a decision was made, the behavior of both animals was changed. Recently, Rachel Rutishauser in my laboratory found that the changes in behavior can be detected as long as a week after initial decisions are made, demonstrating that long-term changes in behavior result from winning or losing fights. Robert showed further that lobster fights fit well with models of "game theory" in terms of their progression, the decision to retreat, and when they display and use their weapons.

One other line of investigation begun by Robert involved the pharmacological manipulation of amine levels in living, behaving lobsters. In the early 1980s, Marge Livingstone had shown that amines injected into lobsters triggered postural changes, but we hadn't followed up on her original studies to ask whether there were any other consequences of amine injections. Since a main theme in the laboratory was that serotonergic function might be enhanced in winning lobsters, Robert decided to inject serotonin into losing animals immediately after a fight to search for actions of the injected amine. He waited for the postural changes to decay away before pairing the now serotonin-injected losers with their former opponents. Once again, we got a surprise. The former losers now advanced on the winners, engaging them in fights, and fighting at intensity levels and for periods of time comparable to those seen at the start of the original fights. Robert got so excited at this result that he immediately paired the injected loser with a much larger animal, which promptly cut off the claws of the advancing smaller animal and killed it (the first and only time we saw a behavioral reversal in studies of these types). Our follow-up studies suggested that the observed effect was likely due to the uptake of the injected serotonin into serotonergic or other kinds of neurons and its subsequent release. We used Prozac-injections to determine that this was the likely scenario, which got us into Dave Berry's nationally syndicated column. We believed this behavioral reversal to be a motivational effect of the injected amine, although other possible explanations of the effect also were possible.

Robert's initial observations have been followed up by us, by him, and by other investigators using a variety of pharmacological reagents that raise or lower serotonin levels or effectiveness in lobsters and other crustacean species. The results of these studies, including our most recent ones, suggest that no simple relationship can be demonstrated between serotonin levels in crustaceans and agonistic behavior, at least not by using pharmacological manipulations that change amine levels or amine effectiveness in entire organisms. We still believe that serotonin is involved in aggression. It may be, however, that serotonin has to be released in appropriate amounts at the correct time, and in the correct place in the nervous system, to function in complex patterns of behavior such as aggression. The relatively gross pharmacological procedures we have been using up to now may not offer the precision needed to influence behavior in a meaningful way.

Fighting flies. Lobsters seemed to be an excellent model system for studies on aggression. It was easy to get the animals to fight, and the patterns of behavior appeared to be prewired in the nervous system and modifiable by behavior. Anatomical and physiological studies could bring us to some of the neurons likely to serve important roles in the behavior and would allow us and other investigators to ask whether neuronal function changed as a consequence of winning or losing fights. Recently, our colleague Don Edwards showed changes in the serotonergic modulation of particular synaptic regions in crayfish as a consequence of changes in social status. Gene cloning and other kinds of molecular experiments also are possible with lobsters. So why stop working on a system that has yielded so much valuable information at this point in my career? The problem was that I felt we were at an impasse at ever getting closer to understanding how serotonergic neurons functioned in aggression or, in more general terms, at understanding how behaviors like aggression are assembled in nervous systems. Moreover, we were guessing at the neurons that were important in the behavior. It was an informed guess, of course, since serotonergic neurons appear to be important in aggression in all species of animals. But how would we ever discover new neurons or new pathways important in the behavior using a lobster model? The answers I felt might lie with an organism where the genetics already were well worked out, where the genome was available, and where a wealth of genetic methods were available for the asking—hence, the Fruit Fly Fight Club.

Sturtevant first reported that flies fight in 1915 in a paper on mating behavior in flies. There were more recent papers too, some dating to the 1980s, but even some of the world's greatest experts on flies, such as Seymour Benzer, didn't know that flies fight. The question was how to get them to do it in a simple enough experimental situation that the behavior could be quantified and that genetic approaches could be applied easily. Three excellent Harvard undergraduate students, Nina Bowens, Selby Chen, and Ann Lee, undertook the task of getting flies to fight in the laboratory. Our goal was to have just two males fight, so that eventually we might have a normal fly fighting versus a mutant to ask what effect the mutation would have on the behavior. As we learned more about the kinds of genetic methods that were available in flies, we realized that there were experiments we could do that were infinitely more elegant and more sophisticated than just making mutations.

We reasoned that flies would fight over the same sorts of resources that other animals fought over: territory, mates, and food. After much experimentation, we designed our fly fighting chamber which we affectionately called The Colosseum. It included glass walls made out of two standard microscope slides that were cut in half and glued together at the ends, which were then placed on an agarose surface to supply humidity. A small 1-cm food cup was placed in the middle of the chamber, and a headless mated female was placed on the surface of the food. Mated so she was not as attractive to the males as a virgin female, and headless so she wouldn't fly off the food surface while the males were fighting. The males didn't care whether the female had a head or not. A petri dish with holes for ventilation served as the lid of the chamber, and a piece of dark filter paper restricted the light to the food surface. It was simple, but, more importantly, it worked. Within minutes of being placed in the chamber, males ended up on the food surface, and shortly after that, they began to fight. The fights were quite funny, including "wings-up" displays; fast and slow charges; pushing off with legs; grabbing; tussling; and my favorite, "boxing," where the two flies stand on their hind legs and duke it out. Of course, decisions are made in these fights, with winners and losers emerging as in other species of animals. To analyze the behavior, Selby and Ann carried out 75 fights, involving over 2000 meetings between the flies and more than 9000 behavioral transitions during those meeting. All these data were entered on computer spread sheets, and with Robert Huber's help again, we carried out a quantitative analysis of the behavior. With that in hand, the mutant studies now became possible.

These are in their infancy, and so will not be described in detail here. Our readings of the fly literature led us to the discovery of the powerful GAL4/UAS method originally described by Brand and Perrimon at Harvard Medical School about a decade ago. What this method will allow us to do when we have it fully operational in our laboratory is to essentially reach into the brain of a fly and reversibly turn on or off the function of any neuron types we are interested in, while the flies are fighting. It's like a dream behavioral experiment, and we are in the midst of carrying out these experiments as I write these words. We also will be able to ask whether changes in gene expression accompany changes in social status in flies, and using gene chips or other methods of analysis, we can quickly identify the genes that are changing and localize them in fly brains. Such studies will be carried out with Heinrich Reichert and Ronny Leemans of Basel, Switzerland, in the next few months. Hopefully, these lines of experimentation will allow us to get closer to the questions that have been driving my research efforts for the last two decades. Even if they don't, however, we are having fun thinking that they will.

Honors and Awards

Honors are not why we do science. Still, recognition by peers is nice, and it certainly made my parents happy when they could read about "my son, the doctor" in announcements in New York newspapers. This article begins with a partial listing of my honors, so they will not be listed here. Comments on a few of the honors might be worthwhile though. One of the more interesting happenings was that I almost turned down the invitation to become a member of the Institute of Medicine (IOM) because I knew nothing about the organization prior to 1986. I thought the letter was a ploy to get me to contribute money to a vanity organization. Luckily, I made inquiries and felt appropriately honored after I found out that they were medicine's equivalent of the NAS. Shortly after becoming a member, I served on the IOM Council (1991–1993) under two presidents, Sam Thier and Ken Shine. Shine was much more fun to serve under, as he was less of an autocrat than Thier. I don't remember that I was a particular success as a Council member though, as I had little practical experience working at the interface between medicine and politics. I suspect that I was there to represent the viewpoint of a basic scientist, since relatively few members of the IOM at the time were practicing scientists. Luckily, now large numbers of basic scientists are members who can be called to serve on the IOM Council. I am particularly proud of two awards on my list. One is a Lifetime Achievement in Mentoring Award, presented to me on December 2, 1998, as part of the A. Clifford Barger Excellence in Mentoring Awards ceremony at Harvard Medical School. This award comes via nomination from former students, and I am truly honored that my students went to this effort for me. The second is the Education Award from the Association of Neuroscience Departments and Programs that I shared with my colleagues Ed Furshpan and Dave Potter. That was presented at the Society for Neuroscience Meeting in San Diego on November 10, 2001. Since teaching has been such an important part of my life, I was greatly pleased to have this acknowledged by the organization representing neuroscience programs throughout the United States.

Family

I have already talked some about my wife of close to 45 years, Kathryn. She has been my constant companion, best friend, and the supporting and guiding hand in the raising of our two wonderful children. Along the way, she also has been a historian, a map maker, a social worker, and now a bible scholar. In fact, she has more degrees than anyone I know. Her latest, which took 14 years to complete from beginning to end, was a Ph.D. from Brandeis University in Near Eastern and Judaic studies on trophy taking in the ancient world. She therefore is a whiz in the bible category in Trivial Pursuit and is one of the very few people I've ever known who has taught Akkadian and who can read and understand Ugaritic, Aramaic, and ancient Hebrew. I've noticed that despite substantial differences in our upbringing, when we go to a synogogue for a wedding or bar mitzvah, I am reading the English translation or transliteration of the text, while Kathryn is reading, and understanding, the original Hebrew. Kathryn is extraordinarily well read, and somehow or other, even after 45 years together, we still find much of interest to talk to each other about. That alone says a lot about our relationship.

Our son Dave was born February 21, 1964, and our son Jamie was born on May 14, 1966. Their childhood was, I expect, a fairly normal one, although we always felt it was special. The arts have been an important part of all of our lives, but more so in a professional way for the boys who make their living in these fields. Dave began singing and Jamie began making movies while both were in high school. Dave graduated from Swarthmore with majors in both music and science, while Jamie graduated from the honors program at the University of Michigan in film and video studies.

After college, Dave returned to the Boston area to attend the New England Conservatory in their opera program. Then he taught math, science, and Spanish for a while at the Commonwealth School, his high school alma mater. During that period, while singing for pay in a church choir, he met his wife to be, Majie Zeller. Majie, a lovely woman with a beautiful voice, also works as a project manager for the Lotus Corporation. Together, they moved to Ann Arbor where Dave got a law degree. This was followed by a clerkship in Boston with the soon-to-be Supreme Court Justice Breyer and then a second clerkship one year later with Justice Sandra Day O'Conner at the Supreme Court. All this high-profile law led to a position with a major law firm that left Dave no time for singing, a subsequent position as legal counsel with the Governor of Massachusetts, and now, a career doing legal writing at home so that he can have adequate time for his singing. Dave, a lyric baritone, and Majie, a mezzo soprano, fill our weekends with glorious music singing in Boston with the Cantata Singers, Emmanuel Music, and various local and regional opera companies. Of course, we wait anxiously with Dave and Majie to read the reviews of their performances and are delighted when reviews like this from "Opera News" show up: "The unequivocal show-stealer was baritone David Kravitz as Leporello. A natural crowd-pleaser, Kravitz sang with resonance and fluency, and he acted with an ease and expressiveness that far outshone the rest."

Jamie returned to the Boston area after leaving Ann Arbor and worked for the Cambridge Community Access Television station. He then moved to Los Angeles, where he set up the West Hollywood Community Access cable television station, initially teaching all their courses and beginning the station's regular schedule of cable casting. For a short while, he danced professionally with Naomi Goldberg's L.A. Modern Dance and Ballet troupe and the Rudy Perez Dance Theatre, culminating in performances in the 1993 Dance Kaleidoscope and L.A. Festival. His dance interests began in high school and continued at the University of Michigan, where he performed in and served as Co-Artistic Director of a modern/jazz dance group. Jamie met his partner, Sebastian (Bas) Uijtdehaage, an Assistant Professor at UCLA specializing in media and education, during this period. After stepping down as the Director of the community access channel, Jamie moved to a dot com company for a while. More recently, while in transition between positions, Jamie made an award winning documentary called "Into the Streets" for the City of West Hollywood. This powerful, beautifully paced video documents the refusal in 1991 of Governor Pete Wilson of California to sign AB101, a moderate gay rights bill, and the stirring demonstrations that followed that refusal. It has been shown to acclaim at numerous film festivals.

I am delighted that both our sons are in the arts, that they are so intensely creative, and that they maintain the outspoken liberal beliefs that Kathryn and I so firmly hold to. The family was very proud to attend Kathryn's graduation ceremony, and Dave and Majie gave Kathryn a highly appropriate gift to celebrate the event afterwards at an elegant Cambridge restaurant. "Gave" is actually the wrong word. Since her thesis was on "trophy taking," she was shown one of those large cups given to athletes who win national championships, which she then had to wrestle away (take the trophy) from Dave and Majie in the restaurant. In a way that tells a lot about my wonderful family. We are, and always have been, very close, warm, and affectionate toward each other. We maintain a sense of humor and a sense of perspective in and about everything we do. We take pride in each others accomplishments and share in their celebration. We honor, respect, and support each other. Who can ask for anything more!

Epilogue

Steve Kuffler used to say "the good old days are now." He meant that in the best sense, which was don't look back with nostalgia at what used to be. It's a philosophy I agree with, and this autobiography, therefore, is not an attempt to offer a sentimental view of my good old days. The first decades of Neurobiology were unique and were an exciting time for all of us. But the progress being made today in the human genome, in our understanding of how the nervous system works, and in unraveling the mysteries of neurological and neuropsychiatric disorders dwarfs many of the accomplishments of those early years. Society too has made remarkable progress, with women and minorities now making up large portions of our student and post-doctoral populations and increasingly occupying prominent academic positions as well. The grant scene could be better of course, and there are serious challenges to academic excellence being promulgated by grant-dollar counting administrators. Such nuisances can and should be dealt with though, and I plan to continue to do so as long as I maintain my active academic career. I have learned much from my colleagues and mentors. Throughout my career I have tried to emulate Steve and run my laboratory as a "family"; to follow my colleagues Ed Furshpan and Dave Potter and maintain a commitment to excellence in teaching; to give back through service to a field that has given me so much; and to nurture and support our next generations trying to instill in them the same values that I hold to so dearly. Science was fun in the decades of the 1960s, 1970s, and 1980s, and I suspect we could keep it fun for future decades as well with some serious attention to that aspect of academic life by all of us. Overall though, the good old days are now still seems to ring true to me.

Selected Bibliography

Barker DL, Herbert E, Hildebrand JG, Kravitz EA. Acetylcholine and lobster sensory neurons. *J Physiol* 1972;226:205–229.

Battelle BA, Kravitz EA. Targets of octopamine action in the lobster: Cyclic nucleotide changes and physiological effects in haemolymph, heart and exoskeletal muscle. *J Pharmacol Exp Ther* 1978;205:438–448.

Beltz BS, Kravitz EA. Mapping of serotonin-like immunoreactivity in the lobster nervous system. *J Neurosci* 1983;3:585–602.

Beltz BJ, Kravitz EA. Physiological identification, morphological analysis and development of identified serotonin-proctolin containing neurons in the lobster ventral nerve cord. *J Neurosci* 1987;7:533–546.

Chen S, Lee AY, Bowens N, Huber R, Kravitz EA. Fighting fruit flies: A model system for the study of aggression. *Proc Natl Acad Sci USA* 2002;99:5664–5668.

Doernberg SB, Cromarty SI, Heinrich R, Beltz BS, Kravitz EA. Agonistic behavior in naive juvenile lobsters depleted of serotonin by 5,7-dihydroxytryptamine. *J Comp Physiol A* 2001;187:91–103.

Edwards DH, Kravitz EA. Serotonin, social status and aggression. *Curr Opin Neurobiol* 1997;7:812–819.

Evans PD, Kravitz EA, Talamo BR. Octopamine release at two points along lobster nerve trunks. *J Physiol* 1976;262:71–89.

Evans PD, Kravitz EA, Talamo BR, Wallace BG. The association of octopamine with specific neurons along lobster nerve trunks. *J Physiol* 1976;262:51–70.

Glusman S, Kravitz EA. The action of serotonin on excitatory nerve terminals in lobster nerve-muscle preparations. *J Physiol* 1982;325:223–241.

Goy MF, Kravitz EA. Cyclic AMP only partially mediates the actions of serotonin at lobster neuromuscular junctions. *J Neurosci* 1989;9:369–379.

Goy MF, Schwarz TL, Kravitz EA. Serotonin-induced protein phosphorylation in a lobster neuromuscular preparation. *J Neurosci* 1984;4:611–626.

Hall ZW, Bownds MD, Kravitz EA. The metabolism of gamma-aminobutyric acid (GABA) in the lobster nervous system—enzymes in single excitatory and inhibitory axons. *J Cell Biol* 1970;46:290–299.

Harris-Warrick RM, Kravitz EA. Cellular mechanisms for modulation of posture by octopamine and serotonin in the lobster. *J Neurosci* 1984;4:1976–1993.

Heinrich R, Bräunig P, Walter I, Schneider H, Kravitz EA. Aminergic neuron systems of lobsters: Morphology and electrophysiology of octopamine-containing neurosecretory cells. *J Comp Physiol A* 2000;186:617–629.

Heinrich R, Cromarty SI, Hörner M, Edwards DH, Kravitz EA. Autoinhibition of serotonin cells: An intrinsic regulatory mechanism sensitive to the pattern of usage of the cells. *Proc Natl Acad Sci USA* 1999;96:2473–2478.

Hildebrand JG, Barker DL, Herbert E, Kravitz EA. Screening for neurotransmitters: A rapid radiochemical procedure. *J Neurobiol* 1971;2:231–246.

Hildebrand JG, Townsel JG, Kravitz EA. Distribution of acetylcholine, choline, choline acetyltransferase and acetylcholinesterase in regions and single identified axons of the lobster nervous system. *J Neurochem* 1974;23:951–963.

Hörner M, Weiger WA, Edwards DH, Kravitz EA. Excitation of identified serotonergic neurons by escape command neurons in lobsters. *J Exp Biol* 1997;200:2017–2033.

Huber R, Kravitz EA. A quantitative analysis of agonistic behavior in juvenile American lobsters (*Homarus americanus* L.). *Brain Behav Evol* 1995;46:72–83.

Huber R, Smith K, Delago A, Isaksson K, Kravitz EA. Serotonin and aggressive motivation in crustaceans: Altering the decision to retreat. *Proc Natl Acad Sci USA* 1997;94:5939–5942.

Iversen LL, Kravitz EA. The metabolism of gamma-aminobutyric acid (GABA) in the lobster nervous system—uptake of GABA in nerve muscle preparations. *J Neurochem* 1968;15:609–620.

Kravitz EA. Enzymic formation of gamma-aminobutyric acid in the peripheral and central nervous system of lobsters. *J Neurochem* 1962;9:363–369.

Kravitz EA. Hormonal control of behavior: Amines as gain-setting elements that bias behavioral output in lobsters. *Science* 1988;241:1775–1781.

Kravitz EA. Serotonin and aggression: Insights gained from a lobster model system and speculations on the role of amine neurons in a complex behavior like aggression. *J Comp Physiol A* 2000;186:221–238.

Kravitz EA, Kuffler SW, Potter DD. Gamma-aminobutyric acid and other blocking compounds in Crustacea. III. Their relative concentrations in separated motor and inhibitory axons. *J Neurophysiol* 1963;26:739–751.

Kravitz EA, Molinoff PB, Hall ZW. A comparison of the enzymes and substrates of gamma-aminobutyric acid metabolism in lobster excitatory and inhibitory axons. *Proc Natl Acad Sci USA* 1965;54:778–782.

Kravitz EA, Potter DD. A further study of the distribution of gamma-aminobutyric acid between excitatory and inhibitory axons of the lobster. *J Neurochem* 1965;12:323–328.

Kravitz EA, Potter DD, van Gelder NM. Gamma-aminobutyric acid distribution in the lobster nervous system: CNS, peripheral nerves and isolated motor and inhibitory axons. *Biochem Biophys Res Commun* 1962;7:231–236.

Kravitz EA, Slater CR, Takahashi K, Bownds MD, Grossfeld RM. Excitatory transmission in invertebrates—glutamate as a potential neuromuscular transmitter compound. In Anderson P, Jansen JKS, eds. *Excitatory synaptic mechanisms.* Oslo: Universitetesforlaget, 1970;85–93.

Livingstone MS, Harris-Warrick RM, Kravitz EA. Serotonin and octopamine produce opposite postures in lobsters. *Science* 1980;208:76–79.

Livingstone MS, Schaeffer SF, Kravitz EA. Biochemistry and ultrastructure of serotonergic nerve endings in the lobster: Serotonin and octopamine are contained in different nerve endings. *J Neurobiol* 1981;12:27–54.

Ma PM, Beltz BS, Kravitz EA. Serotonin-containing neurons in lobsters: Their role as "gain-setters" in postural control mechanisms. *J Neurophysiol* 1992;68:36–54.

Orkand PM, Kravitz EA. Localization of the sites of gamma-aminobutyric acid (GABA) uptake in lobster nerve-muscle preparations. *J Cell Biol* 1971;49:75–89.

Otsuka M, Iversen LL, Hall ZW, Kravitz EA. Release of gamma-aminobutyric acid from inhibitory nerves of lobster. *Proc Natl Acad Sci USA* 1966;56:1110–1115.

Otsuka M, Kravitz EA, Potter DD. The physiological and chemical architecture of a lobster ganglion with particular reference to gamma-aminobutyrate and glutamate. *J Neurophysiol* 1967;30:725–752.

Schneider H, Budhiraja P, Walter I, Beltz BS, Peckol E, Kravitz EA. Developmental expression of the octopamine phenotype in lobsters. *J Comp Neurol* 1996;371:3–14.

Schneider H, Trimmer BA, Rapus J, Eckert M, Valentine DE, Kravitz EA. Mapping of octopamine-immunoreactive neurons in the central nervous system of the lobster. *J Comp Neurol* 1993;329:129–142.

Schwarz TL, Harris-Warrick RM, Glusman S, Kravitz EA. A peptide action in a lobster neuromuscular preparation. *J Neurobiol* 1980;11:623–628.

Schwarz TL, Lee GM-H, Siwicki KK, Standaert DG, Kravitz EA. Proctolin in the lobster: The distribution, release and chemical characterization of a likely neurohormone. *J Neurosci* 1984;4:1300–1311.

Siwicki KK, Beltz BS, Kravitz EA. Proctolin in identified serotonergic, dopaminergic and cholinergic neurons in the lobster, Homarus Americanus. *J Neurosci* 1987;7:522–532.

Stretton AOW, Kravitz EA. Neuronal geometry: Determination with a technique of intracellular dye injection. *Science* 1968;162:132–134.

Stretton AOW, Kravitz EA. Intracellular dye injection: The selection of Procion Yellow and its application in preliminary studies of neuronal geometry in the lobster nervous system. In Kater SB, Nicholson C, eds. *Intracellular staining in neurobiology*. New York: Springer-Verlag, 1973;21–40.

Wallace BG, Talamo BR, Evans PD, Kravitz EA. Octopamine: Selective association with specific neurons in the lobster nervous system. *Brain Res* 1974;74:349–355.

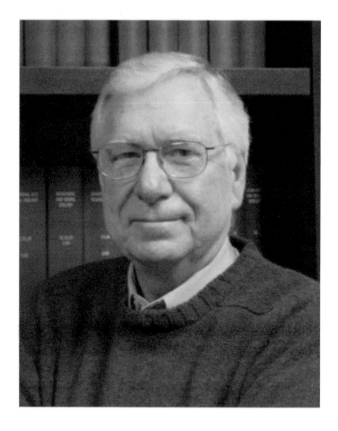

James L. McGaugh

BORN:
Long Beach, California
December 17, 1931

EDUCATION:
San Jose State University, B.A. (Psychology, 1953)
University of California, Berkeley, Ph.D. (Psychology, 1959)
Instituto Superiore di Sanita, Rome (Postdoctoral Study, 1961)

APPOINTMENTS:
San Jose State University (1957)
University of Oregon (1962)
University of California, Irvine (1964)
Founding Chair, Department of Neurobiology and
    Behavior (1964)
Founding Director, Center for the Neurobiology of Learning
    and Memory (1983)

HONORS AND AWARDS (SELECTED):
Distinguished Scientific Contribution Award, American
    Psychological Association (1981)
National Academy of Sciences, USA (1989)
President, American Psychological Society (1989)
William James Fellow, American Psychological Society (1989)
Society of Experimental Psychologists (1991)
American Academy of Arts and Sciences (1992)
UCI Medal, University of California, Irvine (1992)
Foreign Member, Brazilian Academy of Sciences (1994)
John P. McGovern Award, American Association for the
    Advancement of Science (1996)
Mexican Academy of Sciences (2000)
Laurea Honoris Causa, University of L'Aquila, Italy (2001)

James McGaugh pioneered research investigating brain systems mediating the effects of drugs and stress hormones on memory consolidation. He was the first to use posttraining treatments to distinguish between learning and performance effects in studies of drug enhancement of memory. He is also recognized for revealing the role of the amygdala in regulating memory processes in efferent brain regions. He founded the first Department of Neurobiology and Behavior and the first Center for the Neurobiology of Learning and Memory.

James L. McGaugh

I assume that those who discover this chapter, either by chance or on purpose, will, or should, expect to learn about my origins, family background, early experiences, family life, jobs and hobbies, education, friendships, and other kinds of direct or accidental influences that ultimately guided my academic and research career in neuroscience. Much of my story is, of course, based on memory. But, as remembering is a creative act, the story I tell cannot be accurate in all details. Certainly, making retrospective judgments about the causes of critical choices, decisions, and actions that shaped my career is, at best, risky. I will try to tell the truth and most of the truth, but I cannot guarantee that it will be nothing but the truth.

Immigrant Origins

My father, William McGaugh, was a fifth-generation McGaugh in this country. The first William McGaugh, a transplanted Scot from Northern Ireland, arrived in Virginia in the mid-18th century to work on a plantation. We believe that his wife came here as an indentured servant. In 1755 he enlisted in the Virginia Rangers and was then a private in the Revolutionary War. As a veteran, he received a land grant and was one of the first 100 settlers in the area of Nashville, TN. I have wondered about his role in the war as it is well documented that the Scotch-Irish were not fond of their English employers and frequently fought with the British at night and with the Colonists by day. Perhaps it was best that he soon departed for Tennessee. On the move to Tennessee, one of his daughters was killed by Indians near Hickman's Station. My grandfather, Dee Lafayette McGaugh (named after the French General de Lafayette who fought with the Colonies in the Revolutionary War, and the source of my middle name), was a cowboy-rancher-farmer in Texas, Arizona, and California, in that order. When he was young he rode cattle drives on the "Chisholm Trail" several times. I met him a few times when I was young, but did not really know him or know much, if anything, about him at that time. I remember him as a rather distant and forbidding figure. His wife, Nancy Callie Lawrence, was born in Parker County, Texas (a county named after my maternal great-grandfather) in 1873 and died in childbirth when my father was 7 years old.

My mother, Daphne Hermes, was a third-generation immigrant from Germany. Her grandfather, Emil Hermes, emigrated from Prussia to South

Texas in the mid-19th century in order to avoid military conscription. But, perhaps to his surprise, on arrival here he was not able to avoid military service. He fought in the Civil War and is buried in the Civil War Veteran's Cemetery in Austin, TX. There were, of course, many other German emigrants in Texas. At that time, and up to the latter part of the 19th century, German was the most commonly spoken language in the region of San Antonio. My maternal grandfather, James Hermes (source of my first name), was a middle-class, or perhaps upper-middle-class merchant in Beeville, TX. He had a "drayage," or transportation company, that provided taxi and hauling services.

My maternal grandmother was Mattie Parker Hermes. Although the record is unclear, we believe that her family was of English origins. The early to mid-19th century was a very dangerous period in Texas history. In 1836 her 9-year-old second cousin, Cynthia Ann Parker, moved from Illinois to Texas and was abducted by Comanche Indians from a Texas Rangers' settlement now known as Fort Parker. She was raised as a Comanche and eventually married a Comanche chief and had three children. In 1860 Cynthia was discovered and captured by Texas Rangers and was never allowed to return to her Comanche life. She died in captivity in 1870. One of her sons, Chief Quanah Parker, is now one of the most highly recognized of the Indian chiefs of that era. Sadly, he spent most of his life searching for his mother, only to discover her grave. This story is the source of many books and is a well-known part of Texas history. Fort Parker is now a Texas State Park. Yes, the West was wild and my family was part of that wild West history. There is yet more.

My Family

My mother, Daphne Hermes, was born two weeks before the beginning of the 20th century, on the 100th anniversary of the death of George Washington. Her family was sufficiently prosperous to send her to college at what is now Texas Woman's University (TWU) in Denton, TX. I found this to be of special interest only after I learned that at that time only approximately 56,000 women out of a U.S. population of approximately 92 million people attended college. When I was invited to lecture at TWU a number of years ago, they gave me a copy of her college transcript. She should have devoted more study time to her chemistry course. When she was a senior in high school, her father, James Hermes, was murdered. He had received a contract for hauling materials required for the construction of a new post office. The supervisor of the excavation project, R.B. Brown, confronted him at the construction site and shot and killed him. Although his killer was convicted of murder, the conviction was overturned by the U.S. Supreme Court in a decision written by Justice Oliver Wendell Holmes (*Brown* v. *United States*, May 16, 1921, pp. 501–502). The following was part of the court record: "The

Supreme Court... cannot disregard the considerable body of evidence that the shooting was in self-defense, though there was evidence that the last shot was fired after the deceased was down" (p. 501). It seems that the fact that my grandfather carried a knife made the case for murder less clear-cut—more wild West.

My father was born in Azle, TX, near Ft. Worth. He attended Wesley College for three years, but his studies were interrupted by an "illness." During World War I he was deferred because of his illness and went to Arizona where he worked on the Porter Ranch (the largest in Arizona) where my mother's uncle (twin brother of her mother) was the ranch foreman. There in discussions with her uncle, he learned about my mother and wrote to her when she was a college student. They continued their correspondence after she returned home and got a job as a Spanish teacher in Skidmore, TX. My father then started a bakery (Blue Ribbon Bakery) in Wickenburg, AZ, and then, or soon after, became a Methodist minister. My parents were married in 1920, and for the next 20 years they moved to a series of small towns in Arizona as my father was transferred by the church organization. The hazards in those days included pistols that my father required the churchgoers to deposit at the entrance to the church and occasional bank robberies committed by riders on horseback.

I was born in Long Beach, CA, in 1931, the youngest of four children (two brothers and a sister) at the dawning of the Great Economic Depression. At Long Beach, my father was on a leave of absence from his church position because of yet another illness. The next year our family returned to Arizona, where we lived for several years in Claypool, a small copper mining town in the mountains east of Phoenix. As the mines were closed because of the economic depression, there was no employment. We survived on barter of milk, eggs, and vegetables, as well as a very small salary from the church organization. My first memories are of events that occurred during those years. We then moved to Nogales, AZ, a small town on the border of Mexico. Our home was perhaps a few hundred yards from the border. Reading was highly valued by my family, so we had a home full of books. Also, the city library was directly across the street from our home.

When I was seven years old I became ill with brucellosis (also called "undulant fever" or "Malta fever"), a serious infectious disease that I probably got from drinking unpasteurized milk. As I was confined to a bed and thus unable to go to school (the second grade), my mother became my teacher. It was there that her Prussian heritage emerged. Unceasingly and mercilessly, I was drilled daily on spelling, arithmetic, and reading. Also, as I had nothing else to do, I read whenever I was not being given my lessons. I must have read dozens of books, mainly Western adventure stories. I dreamed of being a cowboy and acquired toy pistols and rifles as birthday and Christmas gifts. I also learned Spanish from our Mexican maid who spoke no English but spent much time with me. In many ways it was a horrible time in my life.

I was alone much of the time, had no playmates, and was constantly confined to my bed. My only contact with the outside world was the view from the front window. My parents placed my bed there so I could at least see something of the outside. My worst memories were those of watching neighbor children play outside in the snow (yes, it snows in southern Arizona). But, it was not a wasted time. It taught me something about personal adversity and challenge. It also prepared me academically for many subsequent years of school. After I was ill for about a year, the world's first miracle drug, a sulfa drug, became available. I was told that I was a subject in an early clinical trial. If that is true, then I certainly was not in the placebo group. My illness vanished, and I returned to school within weeks of receiving the drug. I skipped the second grade and joined the third grade class. Daniel Bovet, a Swiss pharmacologist who was then at the Pasteur Institute, received the Nobel Prize in 1957 for the discovery of sulfa drugs (as well as antihistamines and muscle relaxants). There is more to this story below.

There were also many happy and interesting times in Nogales. Much of our family life centered on church activities. Our summer "vacations" were church camps located at closed and abandoned copper mining company facilities in nearby mountains. In Nogales, our next-door neighbor was the head of the German Consulate. As Nogales was a major commercial inland port of entry, he was responsible for visas and other matters of international German commerce. He and his family organized magnificent fireworks displays on the Fourth of July, and their home was warmly and beautifully decorated at Christmas time. Unfortunately, as we learned only much later, he was also the head of the German spy network for all of Arizona and California during World War II. Our highly respected Japanese dentist was the head of the Japanese spy network for the same area.

In 1940 my father was transferred to Arlington, CA, which is now part of the city of Riverside. It was a major promotion. My oldest brother, Bill (yet another William McGaugh), was in college. My other brother, Dana, was completing high school at the age of 15, having skipped two grades of school because of his extraordinarily precocious intellectual ability. My sister, Daphne, was also an outstanding student. She was the class valedictorian at one of her graduation ceremonies. Thus, my siblings set high (perhaps excessively high) standards for me. But, I was also an excellent student for a number of years, perhaps at least partly because of the "Prussian" education I had received from my mother. School was very easy for me. Later on when I was in high school, I found that it had been much too easy, as I had formed no consistent study habits.

One year after moving to California my father became seriously ill again. This time, he was *very seriously* ill. In the fall of 1941 he committed suicide. The illness that he suffered from on and off for so many years was no doubt bipolar depression, but nothing was known about depression at that time. His suicide was a catastrophic event for our family. There was huge emotional loss, public (and personal) shame of a suicide of a very prominent member of the community, and an abrupt family financial crisis. Our home and income had always been provided by the church. We were quickly evicted. We had no savings and no source of income. My mother's Texas teaching credentials were not honored in California. I was sent to live on a ranch with relatives until my mother managed to get some temporary financial help and found a house to rent. I then quickly became an entrepreneur. I became a shoeshine boy and sold newspapers on a street corner. The outbreak of World War II (four months after my father's death) was especially good for my business. I received a penny for each paper and sold more than 100 papers when Pearl Harbor was bombed—my first dollar. For me, at the age of 10, war was not Hell. It provided economic salvation.

Within a few months, the nearby countryside foothills were filled with temporary army camps crowded with soldiers confined to tents before they were shipped off to the Pacific war areas. It was a perfect condition for a small-time (and small) war profiteer. I bought needles, thread, matches, candles, candy bars, and other items prized by the soldiers and sold them at a large but acceptable markup. After all, money would be of no use to them where they were headed. More formal and permanent army bases were also established nearby, and my mother was soon able to get a job as a secretary at one close to our home. I also raised and sold rabbits, as meat was rationed during the war. Thus, World War II not only brought an end to the Great Depression, it provided a solution to our family's personal economic crisis. I then got a somewhat more secure job as a newspaper delivery boy and made the daily bicycle trips, a 17-mile route, on dirt roads. It was not much fun during the winter rainy season.

Although my life was difficult during the first several years after my father's death, I think that I learned important lasting lessons. I learned that difficulty does not mean disaster. I also learned that good things did not come my way by chance. My personal initiative was critical. It still is, of course.

Because I was raised in a religious family, I should perhaps mention, at least briefly, the role of religion in my life. I don't recall any deep theological influences. If there were, they were from the Protestant New Testament of the Bible—no hellfire and brimstone. I think I simply learned from my family and my experience in church programs that it is very important to help others, particularly those in need, and to try to make the world a better and more decent place. *"Do unto others as ye would have them do unto you,"* was the minimal condition. The other influences were simply matters of custom. I attended church by requirement when I was young and then by habit, until my agnostic view developed gradually and crystallized in my early years of college. It seemed to me very highly unlikely that an Almighty unwilling or unable to prevent my grandfather's murder and my father's suicide, not to mention World War II and other catastrophic world events, would or should have any influence on the more minor and routine matters of daily life. Perhaps the tasks of managing the physical universe and guiding evolution preclude any attention to other more minor matters. In any case, I decided that I would look elsewhere for the causes of and solutions to life's challenges and mysteries.

Early Education and Interests

So far, I have not mentioned science, and certainly not neuroscience. No one in my family had any interest in or (as far as I know) knowledge of science. Science was not taught (as I recall) in my primary or middle school. In high school I took the courses in mathematics, chemistry, and physics required for college admission. But, the courses were dull and uninspiring. They were mainly demonstration and drill. There was certainly no spirit of inquiry or wonderment. In school, my main interests were in drama, literature, and music. The teachers who had the greatest influence on me were my drama teacher, Mr. Chester Hess, and my band and orchestra teacher, Mr. Lester Oakes. I was in many school plays (as well as community theatre) and played clarinet and bass clarinet in the school concert band, marching band, and orchestra (that was also the community opera orchestra). In my senior year I was the band commander and Captain of the ROTC band and was a member of the All Southern California Concert Band.

My other major interest was in bicycle and automobile mechanics. Out of financial necessity, I created working bicycles out of broken ones. I made a "motor-bike" when I found a gasoline washing machine engine and attached it to my bike. It was probably the most dangerous 40 mile per hour vehicle in the history of motor-propelled vehicles. When I was in high school my brother Bill was an office manager in a small manufacturing plant and managed to get me an after-school job there. A very kind machinist in the plant loaned me some money to buy a better engine, taught me how to weld, and helped me modify my bicycle so that it looked and drove like a motorcycle. It was modestly less dangerous than the first model. I then found an old rusted car (1929 Nash coupe) that I bought for $40 and nursed to semi-health. A previous owner had painted "Bonnie Blue Eyes" on the visor above the windshield. Bonnie Blue Eyes was my chariot for several years. Keeping it running in semi-health required that I learn how to repair and replace transmissions and engines and learn about carburetors, generators, etc. In the process I also acquired several other cars that I repaired and sold or pirated for parts. My family was absolutely convinced that I would become an automobile mechanic. I probably thought that as well. Certainly, it never crossed their minds or my mind that I would eventually choose a career in science. There were no signs in my early education, experiences, or interests that pointed in that direction.

College Education

When I was in high school I didn't think much about college. One of the great advantages of living in California was that the highest quality college education was provided free to all qualified resident applicants. The thought of applying to a private college or university never entered my mind. If it had, it certainly would not have remained there for long, as the only money that I had available was what I earned each previous week or month from my part-time jobs. My brother Dana and my sister had both attended the University of California, Berkeley. In 1949 I applied to and was admitted to Berkeley, but decided to go to San Jose State College (now a University) primarily because it had a highly recognized drama department and a good music department. I don't recall it being a difficult decision to make. I guess I simply wanted to continue studying in the areas that interested me most in high school. So, I took a bus to San Jose and enrolled as a drama major and music minor. I found a part-time job loading soft-drink trucks each evening and rented a room. There was, as I noted above, no tuition and there were no fees, so my only expenses were living expenses. Because play auditions, rehearsals, and performances were in the afternoons and evenings, I had to get a different job. So, I worked in a bakery, starting at 3:00 AM daily. I was in plays, played in the concert band, and sang in the chorale. I studied opera and conducting and was elected to the music honor society. My interest in drama, however, waned. The department was production oriented and gave little attention to the literature of drama, which was my major interest. So, I sampled other areas, including cultural anthropology, sociology, and biology. Biology was descriptive, dull, and disappointing. During my sophomore year I discovered psychology, and it seemed like a good fit for my interests. I kept drama, speech, and music as minor areas.

During my first few weeks in San Jose I met a beautiful and charming young woman named Carol Becker at a church youth group. Becky (her nickname) and I dated for several years and were married in 1952. My name changed from "James," the name I had always used, to "Jim," as Becky said I was Jim and who was I to argue with her about a trivial thing such as a name change? I also fell in love with Becky's parents, Ruth and George Becker, two of the kindest, most decent, understanding, and supportive people I have ever known. They were ideal "in-laws" and, eventually, absolutely wonderful grandparents.

Shortly before I started college, a close friend of our family who knew me well warned me that my high school study habits (or lack thereof) would get me flunked out of college in one term. So, with that severe warning, I studied hard and got excellent grades during my first year. In addition to studying, working, and dating, I managed to buy an old abandoned car that needed serious repairs and put it in running order. At the end of the first year, in June, I drove my car down the Pacific Coast Highway on my way home to Riverside to visit my family. The highway was jammed with a series of military convoys. As I had no radio in the car, it was only later that night that I learned that the Korean War had started. Very soon I was issued a draft card and learned that although I could get a student deferment, the draft boards were drafting students into the army on the basis of their college grades—the poorer the grades, the greater the chance of being drafted. I did not neglect this important bit of information. I decided immediately that I had to receive only "A's" in my classes from then on. I did, and graduated three years later at the top of my class with highest honors.

One can certainly question the social policy underlying the decision to have college grades influence eligibility for the draft. But, it is not clear to me what policy is best for selecting 18-year-old boys and girls/men and women to fight in our wars. The Korean War is often referred to as "the forgotten war." For those who have seen either the movie or television episodes of "MASH," it would be easy to get the impression that the Korean War might have been some fun mixed in with some occasional battle casualties. At least 52,000 U.S. soldiers were killed in that war and thousands more were seriously wounded. For many of us of military age at that time, the case for U.S. involvement in the Korean War was considerably less convincing than was the case for our prior involvement in World War II. I was certainly not alone in wishing to avoid being sent to Korea as a ground soldier. But the fact that I was not drafted into the military made the issue moot.

When I changed my major from drama, I quit my early morning job in the bakery and then had a series of unpleasant part-time afternoon jobs. I eventually got a job on a chicken ranch just outside of town and worked there for a year. I ate a lot of chicken and eggs that year. I also got a job as a church choir director to provide some additional, much-needed income. Becky's dad did commercial grain harvesting each summer, and for two summers I worked for him. On some days I worked on the self-propelled harvester, sewing the sacks after each was filled with freshly harvested grain, and on other days I drove a truck alongside the harvester, making every effort to make sure that the grain spewed into the back of the truck and not on to the ground. Eventually, I was able to get a full-time job as a psychiatric technician at Palo Alto Veteran's Hospital. These were the final years *before* the introduction of the first antipsychotic drugs (reserpine and thorazine). So, I interacted with very ill, unmedicated mental patients on a daily basis. Rather, it was on a nightly basis, as I worked the graveyard shift from midnight to 8:00 AM. There were also many prefrontal lobotomy patients there, as the popularizer of prefrontal lobotomies, Walter Jackson Freeman, was still performing those highly questionable operations there at that hospital.

Some years later I was able to draw on my experiences at that hospital in my classroom teaching. That experience also helped forge my scientific interest in the biological bases of behavior. It seemed very clear to me that those patients had serious brain problems that could not be cured by the "talk" therapies popular at that time. It was also clear that prefrontal lobotomies provided no cure. The psychiatric technician position was a perfect job for me because it fit well with my psychology major and allowed me at least 6 hr each night for studying. I don't recall clearly how I managed to find time to attend classes, sleep sometime during the day, and hold evening choir practices, but I also don't recall it being a critical or difficult problem. Besides, there was the omnipresent Draft Board to think of.

When I discovered psychology it was, for me, much like the change from black and white to Technicolor in the film "The Wizard of Oz"—a world of wonderment. It was in psychology classes that I first learned about the excitement and challenge of science and found my academic home. In classes on experimental psychology, I learned about developing hypotheses and selecting appropriate methods of inquiry. I learned that hypotheses, however clever and integrative, must, ultimately, be potentially falsifiable. A course in philosophy helped. The required two years of statistics significantly aided that understanding. I learned about the fundamental difference between correlation and causation. Also, I learned a lot of what was known about brain and behavior in courses in physiological psychology, as well as required courses in anatomy and physiology. Robert S. Woodworth's *Experimental Psychology* (1938) and Ernest Gardner's *Fundamentals of Neurology* (1948) became my "bibles." Although Woodworth's book was published in 1938, it was only 12 years old when I first got a copy, and four of those years were the years of World War II when the most prominent and productive experimental psychologists worked exclusively on studies related to the war effort. Thus, it was still the most up-to-date and comprehensive summary of research in experimental psychology.

As I also served (for very modest pay) as a teaching assistant in several courses, including Experimental Psychology and Statistics, I had to know the content of those classes well in order to prepare and grade examinations. Edward Minium was my most demanding and inspiring teacher. Edward Chace Tolman was his Ph.D. thesis advisor when Minium was a graduate student at UC Berkeley. Recently, Minium endowed a lectureship at Berkeley in honor of another one of his professors, Ed Ghiselli. I was honored to be invited to give the inaugural Ghiselli lecture and was further honored to have my undergraduate teacher, Edward Minium, who had long been retired, attend my lecture.

Joseph Cooper was another very influential teacher. His course in "Theories of Learning" firmly established my interest in this area. I also took courses in theories of personality and theories of abnormal psychology. In all of these courses, the various views were presented as equally valid alternatives. That bothered me. As the various theories were at odds with each other on many issues, why weren't the issues resolved? In the area of learning theory, certainly Thorndike, Guthrie, Tolman, and Hilgard had very different views about the causes and nature of learning. Which ones were the correct ones? Better still, which *one* was the correct *one*? I wanted to know that. The textbooks all adopted ecumenical positions, leaving the impressions that the different views were equally valid. In the area of personality and abnormal psychology, I readily dismissed the then enormously popular Freudian theory simply because there was no experimental evidence to support it. The beauty of Freud's ideas, I decided, was also their fatal flaw: no matter the finding, there was always an alternative explanation within the theory. I did not, and do not, share the commonly held belief that Freud's ideas were among the most important scientific ideas of the 20th century. In fact, as I indicated, I don't think they should even be regarded as scientific ideas. They may have been good ideas for bad novels, but they were bad ideas for good science.

At the end of my third year at San Jose it was clear that I would plan to go to graduate school and aim for an academic career in experimental psychology. I wanted to help discover answers to important and as yet unanswered questions concerning the nature and bases of behavior. I did not think at that time that there might also be many important, but not yet asked, questions. Stanford University is about 20 miles from San Jose and Berkeley is about is 45 miles. In the fall of 1952 I applied to both of their graduate programs in psychology and was admitted to both. I chose Berkeley because I was offered a teaching assistantship there. Also, I think my prior admission as an undergraduate as well as the fact that my brother and sister had attended Berkeley probably influenced my decision. I knew that both departments had very distinguished faculty, but did not know enough to make a judgment about which department would be best for my background and interests. Whatever the reasons for my choice, I chose well.

In the spring of 1953, just before I was to graduate, I learned that my student deferment from the military draft ended with my graduation. There was to be no extension of my deferment to allow continued study in graduate school. I also learned that I could join the Air Force as an officer (for an additional year's commitment) as an alternative. So, I enlisted in the Air Force. I had my physical examination at a local Air Force base and prepared to become a second lieutenant in the Air Force that summer. Events in late spring and summer altered those plans. On July 27, 1953, a cease-fire agreement was signed in Korea and the Korean War ended. I received a letter from the Air Force telling me that my enlistment was terminated without any military benefits. I was, of course, very happy with the alternative benefits of going to graduate school.

Graduate Studies at the University of California, Berkeley

Becky and I moved to Berkeley in the fall of 1953. She got a position at the Radiation Laboratory (now the Lawrence Laboratory), located in the hills above the campus, and I started graduate studies and began to serve as a teaching assistant. The graduate program consisted of a "proseminar," a first-year seminar that seemed to be designed only to eliminate weak graduate students; "Prelims," a two-day set of comprehensive exams on *all* areas of psychology given in the second or third year; submission of a Ph.D. thesis; and a final oral exam. The program was very clearly designed, either by plan or by accident, for the highly self-motivated student. When I arrived there many of the graduate students were World War II veterans who enjoyed graduate student life and were in no hurry to complete their degrees. The average number of years for completing a Ph.D. at that time was about eight or nine years. I immediately decided that I was on a four-year program.

My first teaching assistant assignments were to work with David Krech and Edward Tolman. Krech, who later became one of my most supportive graduate advisors and had a very significant influence on my career, was, on my arrival at Berkeley, a crusty, intimidating grouch. So, I initially avoided him whenever possible. So did most of the other graduate students. When I approached Tolman for the first time, he invited me to go off campus for a cup of coffee to get acquainted. As he was without doubt one of the most important and influential psychologists of that era, I was enormously honored just to meet him.

Tolman had just returned to Berkeley after four years of exile at the University of Chicago and Harvard. On June 14, 1949, the Regents of the University of California mandated that all faculty were to sign a loyalty oath. Tolman refused to sign, became a leader of the University of California faculty non-signers, and was fired. He also encouraged younger faculty to sign and keep their jobs. He was able to return to Berkeley in 1953 after the special loyalty oath was declared unconstitutional. Tolman and all of the University of California faculty members who had refused to sign the Regents' loyalty oath were reinstated with full back pay.

On the first day of the undergraduate class he was teaching, and for which I was his teaching assistant, Tolman asked me to walk to class with him and said that he had a special favor to ask of me. It was a great moment in my personal history. The great Tolman himself asked me for a favor! He then handed me his pack of cigarettes and asked me to take them and sit in the back of the class, as he was trying to quit smoking. He said that at some time during the class he would probably walk up the aisle to me and ask me to give him a cigarette. My assignment was to tell him, "No." We played out that ritual during each class, and, of course, each time he asked I meekly handed him his cigarette.

Tolman was an interesting (to me), but rather unsystematic lecturer. But his research and writings influenced me enormously. In his book *Purposive Behavior in Animals and Men* (Tolman, 1932) and in many theoretical and experimental papers, he made what seemed (and still seem) to me to be three fundamental observations. First, behavior consists of acts and sequences of acts, not *merely* muscle movements and glandular secretions. Second, learning consists of acquiring cognitive information about "what-leads-to what," enabling us to adapt to changes in experiences. Responses are "docile," that is, changeable according to the specific circumstances. Third, although rewards (reinforcements) influence what we do and thus, indirectly, what information we acquire, rewards are not essential for learning. These observations were supported by evidence from a variety of original and clever studies of "latent learning" (learning by experiences without explicit rewards) and "place vs. response." Underlying all of these conclusions was his fundamental distinction between learning and performance. Tolman was the first to emphasize that learning is not directly observed, but is *inferred* from performance. As a great many factors can influence performance, the difficult but necessary task is that of determining the contribution of learning to the changes observed in performance. Tolman's observations and inferences profoundly influenced my thinking at the time and have explicitly and consistently guided my own research and my interpretations of research findings. Despite his confrontation with the Regents of the University of California, he received an honorary degree from Berkeley in 1959, a few months before his death. Three years later the psychology building was named "Tolman Hall" in his honor.

Although all of Tolman's findings and interpretations were readily available from his writings as well as from many textbooks, my understanding of it was increased by participating, each term, in Tolman's "Animal Seminar." This was a weekly evening seminar attended by many faculty, including David Krech, Mark Rosenzweig, Al (Donald) Riley, and Leo Postman, as well as visiting faculty, including, in different years, Jeff Bitterman, Harry Harlow, Wolfgang Köhler, and Donald Hebb. A few students (usually three or four) also attended. It was a heady experience listening to the intense, heated, and complex discussions of the latest theoretical and experimental controversies. For me it was, during the first few months, like being transported to a foreign country without knowledge of the language. But, I gradually learned the language and eventually came to regard participation in this seminar as one of the most important opportunities of my graduate experience. The graduate students at Berkeley at that time included, among others, John Garcia, Robert Bolles, and Lewis Petrinovich. It was an outstanding group of bright, original, and industrious graduate students who subsequently made very significant contributions to our understanding of the nature and bases of behavior. As they were slightly older (and very much wiser) graduate students, I turned to them for advice, support, and, as I discuss below, research collaboration.

For the graduate students, one of the most important events of each year was the big party at which we presented a musical comedy. Petrinovich and I wrote, produced, directed, acted, and sang in those ribald reviews. All graduate students attended and many performed. Although most of faculty usually attended, many of them thought that our musical sketches poking fun at the faculty and the graduate program (and, sometimes, the graduate students) were in bad taste. We thought that the faculty were sometimes too "thin-skinned." On reflection, I think we were both correct.

In my second year at Berkeley, Krech and Rosenzweig, together with Edward Bennett, a young biochemist working in Melvin Calvin's laboratory, initiated a "Brain Chemistry and Behavior" research project. The research focused on the role of acetylcholine in behavior using acetylcholinesterase as the index of cholinergic activity. I was fortunate to be asked to work on the project and eventually to investigate, as part of my Ph.D. thesis, the relationship between acetylcholinesterase activity and maze learning in rats. I did the biochemical assays (using a newly invented and only marginally cooperative automatic pH recorder) in Bennett's facilities in Calvin's laboratory and participated in Calvin's weekly lab seminar. I was also fortunate to get a very well-paying research assistantship. As the work of Calvin's lab focused on photosynthesis, I understood only my own presentations in that seminar. A few years later Calvin received the Nobel Prize for his work on photosynthesis.

Although my graduate work was very exciting and satisfying, another much more important and exciting event occurred in my second year at Berkeley. Our son, Douglas, was born.

Krech, Rosenzweig, and Bennett also held a weekly seminar on brain chemistry and behavior. As a project for the seminar, my graduate student colleague Lew Petrinovich and I decided to do a comprehensive review of all published studies of drug effects on learning. It was difficult detective work because there was, of course, no Internet, no PubMed or any other bibliographic aid, and no copying machines. We found a total of approximately 100 references, including many reporting the effects of vitamins. After presenting our findings at the seminar, we continued to revise and update our review and finally published it a decade later when we decided, quite arbitrarily, that it either was or it soon would be impossible to summarize the findings in this very rapidly growing research area in a single review paper (McGaugh and Petrinovich, 1965).

In searching through old journals, we discovered a paper by Karl Lashley (1917) reporting that strychnine administered to rats before daily training trials improved rats' maze learning. This was of particular interest because it was the only report of drug enhancement of learning. Additionally, we found some evidence suggesting that strychnine inhibited acetylcholinesterase activity. So, we decided to replicate Lashley's study. We built the maze, acquired rats from the vivarium, and conducted the study. We were delighted to find that we replicated Lashley's results. Harry Harlow, the Editor of the *Journal of Comparative and Physiological Psychology*, was not delighted. He rejected the paper in a multipaged letter that included, among other things, the advice that publication of these findings might adversely affect our research careers. But, the main reason given for the rejection was that he did not believe the findings. As Harlow put it, "The results of your paper upset a fundamental pharmacological assumption that no drug improves behavior." We eventually published the paper in a different journal (McGaugh and Petrinovich, 1959).

Our paper was rejected for the wrong reason. In it we suggested that strychnine "...*facilitates learning by increasing the efficiency of transmission in the central nervous system*" (p. 102). But, our findings, as well as those of Lashley, only indicated that maze *performance* was improved. And, as Tolman taught us, learning is not observed, but is inferred from performance. As strychnine might influence rats' maze performance by affecting processes other than those underlying learning, our interpretation of the findings was, at best, only speculation. I decided to pursue this problem further as part of my Ph.D. thesis research. More specifically, I decided to tackle the learning-performance problem. The major clues came from an experiment by Carl Duncan and a book by Donald Hebb, both published in 1949. Duncan (1949) reported that electroconvulsive shock administered to rats after training produces retrograde amnesia. These findings supported Müller and Pilzecker's "Perseveration-Consolidation Hypothesis" proposed a half-century earlier (1900), which was largely ignored. In his now well-known book, *The Organization of Behavior*, Hebb (1949) proposed that reverberatory neural activity initiated by training was essential for establishing synaptic connections underlying learning. These findings and theoretical speculation suggested, to me, the possibility that a drug might facilitate learning by acting on posttraining neural activity initiated by training. Thus, I reasoned, it should be possible to enhance learning with a drug administered *after* training, during the postlearning period of memory consolidation. This procedure, if effective, would solve the learning-performance problem, as the "enhancing" drug would not be in the animals either during the training or the subsequent testing for memory of the training. I decided to test this hypothesis.

With enormous excitement (and an equal amount of anxiety), I told Krech of my reasoning and my plans to study the effect of posttraining drug injections. He responded with less enthusiasm than Harlow had expressed for our rejected strychnine paper. Fortunately, Krech soon went off to Norway for a sabbatical leave and my other research advisor, Rosenzweig, was more enthusiastic. So, as soon as I could get some rats, I repeated the previous experiments investigating the effects of strychnine on maze learning, but gave the strychnine (or saline) injections *after* each daily training trial. The drugs were coded so that I did not know which animals received the drug and which received saline injections. When I broke the code after the experiment was completed, I was astounded, delighted, and extremely elated to find that the post-trial strychnine injections enhanced the rats' maze learning. It was clearly one of the most euphoric moments in my entire scientific career. The drug-effect learning-performance problem appeared to be solved.

San Jose State College Reprise

It was at about this time that my self-imposed, four-year Ph.D. plan required urgent action. I informed my advisors that I would be completing my thesis at the end of the year and would like to have a university position. In those days, all faculty recruiting was in solid secrecy. Jobs at the best universities were not advertised. Thus, I was simply informed that I would receive offers of assistant professor positions from Cornell University and Ohio State University. I received the offers: $5000 salary plus $500 moving expenses. There were no invitations for interviews or visits. Although those were excellent universities with outstanding departments of psychology, they were in the wrong part of the country. My roots, as well as Becky's, were firmly in the West. As I was not offered any positions in the West, I contacted faculty friends at San Jose State and asked if there might be a position for me there. There was. So, Becky, Douglas, and I moved to the San Jose area in 1957, and I was appointed to my first faculty position; Assistant Professor of Psychology at a higher salary ($5700) than that offered by the other universities. There was, however, one small immediate problem. Completion of my thesis research was delayed because of a problem in the rat colony at Berkeley. As all of the rats in my experiments were bred in that colony, I had to wait several months in order to have the rats needed to complete my thesis research. I completed the research during the summer after moving to San Jose, wrote the thesis during that year, and handed in the thesis in June 1958, one day after the deadline for receiving my Ph.D. that year.

San Jose State College emphasized teaching, almost exclusively. Research was optional, but not encouraged or supported. I was assigned to teach introductory psychology, social psychology, and a graduate course in perception. I was never given a chance to teach courses in learning or physiological psychology. To compensate for this restraint, I developed an undergraduate honors seminar and started an undergraduate research opportunity program that has continued for over four decades. The teaching "load" was four courses per term. After several years I was able to get the honors seminar included as one of the four courses. The main consequence of the seminar was that I was able to find the very best students and invite them to help me in my research program.

At San Jose, I first built a laboratory in the garage at our new home and then moved it to a storeroom where the department kept its office supplies. That caused many well-justified complaints, as that room was not air conditioned, had no windows, and was across the hallway from departmental and faculty offices. After a lot of searching, I found two large abandoned basement rooms in the oldest building on the campus (San Jose State was established in 1857) and turned them into a laboratory. I moved several mazes from Berkeley and made many more. As a graduate student I had acquired a lot of carpentry experience by making mazes and other equipment. We made animal cages out of wire and used aluminum baking pans for the cage bottoms. All of these activities were fun, rather than work, because I enjoyed building the laboratory equipment. I obtained unused rats from Berkeley and talked my department into buying food for the rats. I then started a very active research program investigating further the effects of posttraining drug injections on memory for different kinds of training. A first study found that, like strychnine, the GABAergic antagonist picrotoxin enhanced memory consolidation (Breen and McGaugh, 1961). We also found that posttraining injections of a strychnine-like compound obtained from a lab in Italy enhanced "latent learning" (Westbrook and McGaugh, 1964). Rats given posttraining injections after each non-rewarded trial made fewer errors than saline controls when a reward was subsequently introduced. This finding remains as the strongest evidence that a drug can enhance learning without directly affecting performance. So, these findings confirmed and extended my initial report that posttraining drug injections can enhance memory and strengthened the conclusion that the effects were due to facilitation of memory consolidation. But, the evidence for memory consolidation based on ECS came under attack from several sources. One suggestion (Coons and Miller, 1960) was that the treatment was simply a punishment. A simple experiment using what we now call "inhibitory avoidance" in our lab challenged that interpretation (Madsen and McGaugh, 1961). Animals given foot-shock punishment on stepping from a platform to the floor of a cage showed good retention of the shock the next day by remaining on the platform. Rats given the foot shock followed by an ECS treatment readily stepped off of the platform on the subsequent test trial. Clearly, the ECS treatment did not provide additional punishment. Because of the initial rejection of the first strychnine paper, I prepared manuscripts based on all of these findings, but did not immediately submit them for publication. I'll return to that issue below.

The research environment at San Jose State (or lack thereof) was abysmal. As the course in social psychology remained my primary teaching responsibility, I accepted an invitation to co-author a textbook in social psychology with my former undergraduate teacher, Joseph Cooper. However, my main interactions were with Karl Pribram and Tony Deutsch at Stanford. Both were very interested in my research findings and very supportive of my research program. We had a great many meetings and discussions. I owe a great deal to them for keeping my morale up under my less than optimal conditions. During those years I kept an active research program and received an NIMH research grant, the first research grant ever awarded to anyone at San Jose State College. Because of this achievement I was interviewed on the local television station—my first television appearance. The total amount (direct costs) for three years was $29,500 and included funds for a summer salary. The other very good news for Becky and me was the birth of our daughter, Janice, in 1959.

At the beginning of my fourth year at San Jose, Krech and others at Berkeley nominated me for a National Academy of Sciences-National Research Council (NAS-NRC) Senior Postdoctoral Fellowship. I was very excited to learn this. I decided that if I received the fellowship I would ask Daniel Bovet if I could work with him in the Istituto Superiore di Sanitá in Rome, Italy. Krech had told Bovet of my work and he had sent me the strychnine-like drug that we used for our latent learning experiment. Bovet had developed a research program investigating the effects, on learning and memory, of drugs newly synthesized at the Istituto. As I noted above, Bovet received a Nobel Prize in 1957 for his prior work at the Pasteur Institute where he pioneered the discovery of many important drugs, including the miracle sulfa drug that cured my brucellosis when I was a child.

I was invited to be interviewed for the fellowship, but was dismayed to learn that Harry Harlow was to interview me. I had hoped that one of the other members of the committee, Karl Pribram or Frank Beach, would do the interview. When I met with Harlow I took along several of my unsubmitted manuscripts. Although he was tough and grumpy, he liked my recent findings, the interview went well, and Harlow recommended me for the NAS-NRC fellowship, which I was granted. He also accepted the papers for publication in the *Journal of Comparative and Physiological Psychology.* Also, 20 years later, Harlow and I co-authored a textbook in psychology (with Richard Thompson; Harlow, McGaugh, and Thompson, 1971). As soon as I learned that I had received the fellowship, I wrote to Bovet to ask if I might come there for postdoctoral study. His response appeared to be written in French, but, although I could read some French (I had had to pass French and German language exams as part of the requirement for my Ph.D.), I couldn't understand whether he had said "yes" or "no" to my request. So, I took a chance and wrote to him to thank him for inviting me to come to his Institute for postdoctoral study. Later, when I was working with him, I found out that he routinely and liberally mixed French with Italian in both his speaking and writing. I noticed that no one ever brought that to his attention.

Rome, Italy

In September 1961, Becky, Doug, Jan, and I took a plane from San Francisco to New York, where I was a speaker in a symposium on memory. While we were there, Becky and I spent most of our time deciding whether I should return to San Jose after the year in Italy or accept one of three offers I had recently received from other institutions (two universities and a research institute). Just before we left New York, I sent a telegram to Robert Leeper and Fred Attneave at the University of Oregon, accepting their offer of a position there in the Department of Psychology. We then boarded the new ship, the *Leonardo da Vinci* (sister ship of the "unsinkable" *Andrea Doria* that sunk near the island of Nantucket in 1956) for an 11-day cabin class trip to Genoa. We picked up a new Volkswagon bug and drove south to Rome. All of these experiences were highly novel and very exciting for a family from the far West.

My postdoctoral fellowship provided my university salary, all family travel expenses, private school tuition for Doug, and travel expenses for me to visit European research laboratories. It did not pay for our family dog's flight to Rome. We had left our dog, Cisco, with friends, but as they informed us that he was despondent and had stopped eating we decided to send for him. In addition to his airfare, we had to pay for his breakfast in London on the way to Rome. At the institute in Rome, Bovet very graciously provided me with a laboratory, a large corner office, and a technician. As I knew no Italian, except for some Italian arias that I learned in college and two or three phrases that I memorized from listening to language records, I had to learn some Italian quickly. That effort was greatly aided by the technician who did not understand or speak any English. Bovet very warmly welcomed me to his laboratory and arranged for us to meet frequently. He was very interested in my use of posttraining drug injections for studying memory enhancement so that procedure was added to their experimental program. I collaborated with Enzo Longo in studies of the effects of drugs on behavior and EEG activity in rabbits, and I had many discussions about drug influences on avoidance conditioning with Giorgio Bignami, whose laboratory was next to mine. I also attended Bovet's weekly seminar, listened in my slowly improving Italian, but spoke mostly in English. The fact that all of the scientists in the laboratory spoke English certainly did not aid my efforts to learn Italian. During the year I took trips to visit the laboratories of Holgar Hyden in Sweden, Larry Weiskrantz in Cambridge, and Aubrey Manning in Edinburgh. At Rome, I also met many well-known scientists who came to visit with Bovet. I met Lucio Bini who, in 1938 with Ugo Cerletti, was the first to administer electroconvulsive shock to a human subject (Cerletti and Bini, 1938). I regret that I did not take advantage of that opportunity to discuss that historic event with him. I also enjoyed many discussions with Bovet's wife, Filomina Bovet-Nitti. She was the daughter of the last premier of Italy before Mussolini.

It was also a year of adventure for our family. We learned a lot about Rome and traveled extensively in Italy, as well as Switzerland and France, on holidays. We, including Cisco, climbed to the top of Mt. Vesuvius, looked down at the crater, and found it to look rather disappointingly benign. We took a spring vacation on the island of Ischia. We visited the newly excavated city of Ercolano (Herculaneum) that was buried by the same eruption of Vesuvius that buried Pompei in AD 79. We all learned to love the food, and Becky and I also learned to love the wine and espresso. We still do.

During that year we established lasting friendships with Italian colleagues and subsequently visited with them both in Italy and in the United States. I also established continuing research collaborations. My visibility there resulted in my subsequently being invited to speak at many international scientific meetings. Thus, the year with Bovet had an enormous influence on my academic research career. In the summer of 1962 we drove to Calais, crossed the English channel, visited London, and then boarded the Staatendam for the ocean voyage back to New York. We drove across the country in our VW bug to San Jose before moving to Eugene, OR, in September 1962. Shortly after our arrival, a huge storm hit Eugene and the "Pioneer Grove" of trees on the campus was destroyed. The Cuban missile crisis occurred the following month. It was clearly a month to remember.

The University of Oregon

My new position as Associate Professor of Psychology at Oregon offered everything that I had hoped for. I was given a recently constructed laboratory and was asked to teach graduate and undergraduate courses and seminars in learning and physiological psychology. The teaching responsibilities were very modest compared to my experiences at San Jose. I attracted excellent graduate students into my laboratory. I also had some very bright and industrious undergraduate students, including Bill Greenough and Ron Racine. I received new NIMH research grants and started new studies of drug effects on memory consolidation. My faculty colleagues were highly interesting, collegial, and supportive. Fred Attneave had a Dixieland band that needed a clarinet player so I was asked to join the group. We played badly, but frequently, at many departmental occasions.

In 1963, Karl Pribram invited me to participate in a conference on "The Anatomy of Memory" held in September at Princeton. The meeting was organized by Pribram and co-organized by Frank Fremont-Smith of the New York Academy of Sciences. The speakers at the conference included, among others, Sir John Eccles, Larry Kruger, Holgar Hyden, Albert Uttley, Heinz Von Foerster, and me. Other participants at that conference included Jan Bures, Robert Hinde, E. Roy John, Seymour (Gig) Levine, James McConnell, Neal Miller, David Rioch, Eugene Roberts, Roger Sperry, Hans-Lukas Teuber, and Larry Weiskrantz. It was my first presentation at a conference devoted solely to brain, learning, and memory. It was a heady experience for me to discuss my research with such an august group of distinguished scientists. Pribram included me as part of the core group that subsequently participated in meetings in Princeton each year for the next several years. At those meetings I had the opportunity to meet with most of the world's major researchers in brain and memory. This was another important way in which Karl Pribram greatly influenced my research career. The proceedings of the conferences were edited by Dan Kimble, my colleague at Oregon who had studied with Pribram as a postdoctoral fellow.

Family life was wonderful in Eugene. Becky and I found a wooded lot with a panoramic view of the city and built our dream home. We were there to stay, we thought. But our time in Eugene, though sweet, was short. Late in the fall term of my second year at Eugene, Krech told me that he had nominated me for a position at the yet-to-be established University of California, Irvine (UCI) located near Newport Beach in Southern California. I thought little about that until I received a telephone call from Edward Steinhaus, Dean of the School of Biological Sciences at UCI asking me to come to UCI for an interview. Steinhaus and Ralph Gerard (one of the subsequent founders of the Society for Neuroscience six years later, in 1970) met the helicopter that took me to Newport Beach from Los Angeles for the interview. As the UCI campus was in its very early stages of construction, we met in temporary metal buildings located about a mile from what was to become the campus. Almost four decades later, these temporary buildings are, of course, still in use. In the discussions with Steinhaus I learned that a Department of Psychobiology was to be one of four departments in the School of Biological Sciences and that I was being considered as a candidate for the founding chair of that department. I was the final potential candidate interviewed for the position. Although I did not like the thought of leaving a very good and highly supportive department at Oregon, the possibility of building an entire department devoted to brain and behavior, the first of its kind in the world, was simply too attractive and exciting to ignore. So, on the flight back to Eugene I decided that if the position were offered to me, I would accept, pending Becky's approval. She approved. The next day I received a call from Steinhaus offering me the position and I accepted it. So, with much sadness, but little regret, Becky, Doug, Janice, Cisco, and I moved to Newport Beach in June 1964. We couldn't move to Irvine as the city of Irvine was not established until 1971.

Department of Psychobiology at the University of California, Irvine

The move to UCI was complicated by a commitment I had made to teach in a Summer Institute on Behavioral Genetics run by Gerald McClearn at UC Berkeley. So, Becky and I settled our family in a new home and I commuted to Berkeley each week. Participating in that Institute gave me a chance to learn about the behavior of different strains of mice, and I subsequently introduced genetic strains of mice into my own research program. At Berkeley, I also met Fred Elmadjian who was responsible for interdisciplinary training programs in brain and behavior at NIMH. As I discuss briefly below, meeting Elmadjian had significant consequences for the development of our new Department of Psychobiology at UCI.

Two important events occurred in the spring before the move to UCI. First, I met, interviewed, and recruited Norm Weinberger to the yet-to-be-established Department of Psychobiology. He joined me in January 1965 as a founding faculty member of UCI. Second, Steinhaus called me to tell me that the Dean of the School of Social Sciences at UCI had the opportunity to recruit several very well-known psychologists, including Kenneth Spence, Gardner Lindzey, and Leon Festinger to UCI, but that they would come only if Psychobiology were integrated within a Department of Psychology in the School of Social Sciences. I was asked to meet with Lindzey at Stanford and then send a report to Steinhaus. Steinhaus then informed the Chancellor of UCI, Daniel G. Aldrich Jr., that if the Department of Psychobiology did not remain in the School of Biological Sciences he would resign from UCI and return to his position at UC Berkeley where he had not yet sold his home. As Steinhaus was very clearly a very distinguished "dean of deans" (the following year he was elected to the National Academy of Sciences), it was an easy decision for the Chancellor. Psychobiology remained as a Department in the School of Biological Sciences. I was very happy to learn of that critical decision as I had already resigned from my position at Oregon, sold our home, and bought a new home in Newport Beach. I didn't have Steinhaus' options.

For the third position allocated to our Department (the minimum required for department status), we recruited Richard Whalen from UCLA. My graduate student at Oregon, Marvin Luttges, joined me at UCI and became the very *first* UCI student. As there was, as yet, no admissions office at UCI, he was registered as a UCLA student during his first year at UCI. We quickly attracted many other outstanding graduate students, including Phil Landfield, Steve Zornetzer, Len Kitzes, Ossie Steward, and Rick Robertson, among others. For our first few years at UCI the number of applicants for our graduate program exceeded the total number of applicants for all other graduate programs at UCI. In the next several years, we recruited Marcel Verzeano from UCLA, Richard Thompson from Oregon, and Carl Cotman from Indiana. Those were exciting, roller-coaster-like days. We had launched the first Department of Brain and Behavior and had done so with great success in recruiting faculty and students and in developing our research programs. Steinhaus had told me on my arrival at UCI that I had three years to convince him that the Department was viable. He was convinced. So was Fred Elmadjian at NIMH. We received the only NIMH brain and behavior interdisciplinary training grant awarded to a graduate program located *within* a single department.

Three years later Steinhaus asked me to serve as acting dean of the school so that he could take a sabbatical leave. I agreed to do that and he subsequently resigned because of illness. I was named dean of the school and served for two more years until I was able to recruit Howard Schneiderman, a developmental biologist from Case Western University, and convince him to replace me as dean. I returned to the department and once again served as chair. I was beginning to become one of the more experienced administrators at this very young campus. In 1974 Chancellor Aldrich asked me to become the Academic Vice Chancellor. After first declining, I agreed and served in that position and, subsequently, as Executive Vice Chancellor (the position of provost at most universities) until the fall of 1982. I then founded, with Norm Weinberger and several other faculty, the Center for the Neurobiology of Learning and Memory (CNLM) and have continued to serve as Director for over two decades. I also served one more term as department chair. In these several roles I have had extensive opportunity to influence the development of UCI. However interesting they were, however, those various administrative responsibilities certainly did not aid my research career. It is now obvious to me that the administrative and academic aspects of my career probably occurred in the wrong order. Usually one assumes administrative responsibilities later in one's career, *after* firmly establishing an academic career. Perhaps someone should have informed me about that.

Consolidating Consolidation

When I arrived at UCI, I quickly set up a laboratory in a building adjacent to the one in which I had been interviewed and, with the help of graduate students and postdocs, continued to investigate drug effects on memory consolidation. Science is a skeptical enterprise. New findings and new ideas are generally not warmly welcomed. Harlow was not the only one to be skeptical about my findings suggesting that posttraining injections of stimulant drugs can enhance memory consolidation. As the consolidation hypothesis had been largely ignored for half a century before Duncan's (1949) findings of ECS-induced retrograde amnesia, it was not a popular idea. Also, as I indicated above, alternative interpretations of Duncan's findings were offered. Although Petrinovich and I countered the criticisms and alternative hypotheses of post training treatment effects in review commentaries, it was clear that what was required was more and stronger experimental evidence. So, the aim of my initial research program at UCI was to obtain that evidence. We conducted an extensive series of experiments examining the effects of posttraining injections of many CNS stimulants. We examined such effects in many kinds of training tasks, including appetitive as well as aversively motivated training tasks. The findings provided strong and consistent evidence that stimulant drugs administered after training can enhance memory for different kinds of information. In all experiments the effects were dose dependent and time dependent. Drug injections administered several hours after training were ineffective. Thus, the findings provided strong support for the hypothesis that the drugs improved retention by enhancing memory consolidation (McGaugh and Herz, 1972). Although those findings seemed to me to provide the needed evidence, my effort to counter the skepticism required booster shots a couple of decades later (McGaugh, 1989). My laboratory also initiated a series of studies investigating the retrograde amnesia induced by ECS in order to confirm that the impaired performance was due to disruption of memory consolidation. We also investigated the neural bases of ECS-induced retrograde amnesia.

As our evidence began to accumulate, Neal Miller, who was on the editorial board of *Science*, (and whom I had met at Pribram's 1963 conference in Princeton), invited me to write a review for *Science*. My paper, "Time-Dependent Processes in Memory Storage" (McGaugh, 1966), summarized our basic findings of drug and ECS effects on memory consolidation. Publication of that paper probably gained more recognition for my findings from studies of treatments influencing memory consolidation than any other paper I have published. It is still cited frequently, but, it is probably read *in*frequently. The following year, Bovet invited me to participate in and serve as co-organizer of an international conference sponsored by the Accademia Nazionale Dei Lincei and held in Sardinia and Rome (Bovet, Bovet-Nitti, and Oliverio, 1968). The other participants included E.A. Asratyan (a student of Pavlov), Harry Harlow, Mark Rosenzweig, Alberto Oliverio, and Jean Piaget. On a historical note, Piaget held the professorship previously held by Bovet's father, Pierre Bovet. In my presentation at that conference I suggested that the experimental findings supporting either a single-trace (e.g., Müller and Pilzecker, 1900) or dual-trace (e.g., Hebb, 1949) hypothesis of memory consolidation were equally compatible with the possibility that an experience initiates several independent memory traces that have different durations (McGaugh, 1968). I suggested that experiences may initiate short-term, intermediate-term, and long-term memory traces that are not sequentially linked. I did not pursue this idea because I couldn't think of any way or ways to test it. Recent findings from the laboratories of Tom Carew and Ivan Izquierdo have now provided critical evidence. In *Aplysia*, short-term synaptic facilitation and long-term facilitation are not sequentially linked (Emptage and Carew, 1993). In rats, drugs infused into the hippocampus or entorhinal cortex posttraining can block short-term memory without blocking long-term memory (Izquierdo et al., 1998; Barros et al., 2002).

The most important event at that time, however, had nothing to do with science. Our third child, Linda, was born in 1967 in Newport Beach.

Modulation of Memory Consolidation

Most of the research in my laboratory was focused on the effects of various stimulant drugs on memory consolidation. But, the original purpose of the research was to use drugs as tools to investigate the neural processes underlying memory formation. Unfortunately, the actions of most of the drugs that we used were poorly understood. At the time that we first studied the effects of picrotoxin, for example, it was not known that this drug acts by blocking GABA receptors. Amphetamine was one of the drugs that we (and others) found to enhance memory consolidation. As amphetamine was known to act via catecholamines, I decided to focus the subsequent experiments on the involvement of catecholamines, especially norepinephrine (NE), in memory consolidation. I also decided to use one-trial inhibitory avoidance training tasks for these experiments as we had used them productively for studies of ECS effects on memory. We adopted (and adapted) these tasks from ones originally developed by Murray Jarvik. Interestingly, Jarvik had adapted them from training procedures originally developed by Bradford Hudson in Tolman's laboratory. Using these procedures and this strategy we found that posttraining intracerebral ventricular (icv) injections of NE or dopamine enhanced memory. Norepinephrine injected icv posttraining also blocked the memory-impairing effects of a dopamine beta hydroxylase inhibitor that blocked the synthesis of NE. Thus, as Seymour Kety had suggested (1972), NE seemed to be involved in some way or ways in memory consolidation.

We also continued our studies of the effects of posttrial electrical stimulation of the brain on memory consolidation. The most commonly accepted hypothesis concerning the basis of the effects was that the stimulation created an "electrical storm" that disorganized brain activity as reflected in brain seizures. When Paul Gold came to my lab as a postdoc in the early 1970s, he continued studies of ECS that he had initiated during his graduate studies at the University of North Carolina and found that the effect of the electrical stimulation on memory varied with the locus of stimulation of the cortex, suggesting that brain seizures play no critical role in inducing amnesia. The additional finding that subseizure electrical stimulation of the amygdala administered after training induced retrograde amnesia confirmed Goddard's original report (Goddard, 1964) that amygdala stimulation induces retrograde amnesia and added the critical evidence that the induction of brain seizures played no role.

Two findings of these studies, the effects of NE and the effects of amygdala stimulation, set the stage for much of the subsequent research in my laboratory. Although these two lines of research were initiated as independent projects, as I discuss below, they converged and led to the development of an integrated hypothesis of the role of NE within the amygdala in memory consolidation. But I first need to discuss additional findings that led to that development.

It seemed very clear from all of our findings, as well as those from other laboratories, that memory consolidation can be enhanced as well as impaired by treatments administered shortly after training. In discussing these many findings, and focusing on the evidence of memory enhancement, Gold and I wondered what adaptive purpose would be served by enabling post-learning enhancement. An obvious (to us) possibility was that some endogenous process activated by learning might serve to select important information for memory. Further, as the importance of an experience is known only at the time of the experience, the endogenous process must, we thought, act after the experience during the early posttraining period when memory consolidation is initiated. Thus, some endogenous process or processes, such as our experimental treatments, may modulate memory consolidation to provide selective storage of important experiences (Gold and McGaugh, 1975). One possibility was that epinephrine released by the foot-shock training experience may play a role in modulating memory consolidation. Gold and Rod van Buskirk, a graduate student in my laboratory, investigated this possibility and found strongly confirming evidence. Epinephrine injected after inhibitory avoidance training produced dose- and time-dependent enhancement of memory (Gold and van Buskirk, 1975). Subsequently, and very importantly, Gold and van Buskirk also found evidence suggesting that epinephrine induces the release of forebrain NE (Gold and van Buskirk, 1978). Many subsequent studies provided extensive evidence that epinephrine and NE play a role in modulating memory consolidation (McGaugh, 1983).

Epinephrine, Norepinephrine, and the Role of the Amygdala in Modulating Memory Consolidation

In a chapter discussing "The Fixation of Experience," Ralph Gerard (1961) discussed my early findings, as reported to him by David Krech.

> Strychnine, according to an informal communication from Dr. Krech, shortens the fixation time.... The above facts fit well into a theory of continued activity in the nervous system... in the course of which a dynamic memory is fixed as a structural one.... Any change that would enhance the extent or intensity of reverberation should hasten the fixation process.... A fall in the threshold of cortical neurons, or an increase in impulse bombardment, should hasten fixation. Since epinephrine lowers thresholds, and is released in vivid emotional experiences, such an intense adventure should be highly memorable.

In that same paper Gerard also suggested that activation of "...the amygdala...could easily modify the ease and completeness of experience fixation *even if the nuclei were not themselves the loci of engrams* (italics mine)." Although I knew Gerard and interacted with him considerably here at UCI, he did not refer me to this chapter or discuss its implications with me. I discovered it only a couple of years ago. Had I discovered it in 1961, or even a decade later, it might have accelerated my research program. I cite Gerard's comments only as significant and prescient, but neglected suggestions.

The problem with epinephrine as a modulator of memory process in the brain is that it passes the blood–brain barrier either poorly or not at all. But, we knew from Gold and van Buskirk's work that it influenced the release of brain NE. We also knew from our concurrent studies that electrical stimulation of the amygdala could enhance, as well as impair, memory consolidation. Thus, we began to think of the amygdala and NE release in the amygdala as possibly playing roles in epinephrine influences on memory. Findings reported by Michela Gallagher and Bruce Kapp and their colleagues (Gallagher et al., 1977, 1981) greatly influenced our thinking about this possibility. They reported that posttraining infusions of the β-adrenoceptor antagonist propranolol impaired inhibitory avoidance retention and that concurrent infusions of NE blocked the impairment. A series of experiments conducted by two graduate students in my laboratory, Keng-Chen Liang and Cate Bennett, provided critical evidence linking epinephrine effects with amygdala activation. Posttraining electrical stimulation of the amygdala, which produced amnesia in controls, *enhanced* memory in adrenal demedullated animals (i.e., animals unable to secrete epinephrine). But, importantly, the amygdala stimulation produced amnesia in demedullated rats that were given epinephrine before the stimulation. The additional finding that propranolol infused into the amygdala blocked the memory-enhancing effects of posttrial injections of epinephrine provided compelling evidence that epinephrine affects memory consolidation by influencing activation of adrenoceptors in the amygdala. Evidence that NE infused into the amygdala posttraining enhances memory consolidation provided additional essential support for this hypothesis (Liang, Juler, and McGaugh, 1986). This set of findings suggested an integrating hypothesis concerning the central role of the amygdala in regulating the consolidation of memory for emotionally arousing experiences that has guided most of the subsequent research in my laboratory.

Integrating Neuromodulatory Influences on Memory Consolidation

Our findings, as summarized above, indicated that epinephrine released from the adrenal medulla influences memory by altering the release of NE in the amygdala. The findings of Cedric Williams and Rob Jensen indicate that the effect is mediated by activation of the ascending vagal projections to the nucleus of the solitary tract (NTS) that, in turn, sends noradrenergic projections to the amygdala (Jensen, 2001; Williams and Clayton, 2001). Some of the critical experiments were conducted when Williams was a postdoc in my lab, but the studies were initiated previously when Williams was a graduate student in Jensen's lab. However, as Jensen was a postdoc in my lab in an earlier decade, I suppose I could at least claim to have had some indirect influence on their studies of the involvement of the NTS.

Many drugs that influence memory consolidation readily enter the brain and, thus, don't need to use the vagal-NTS connection. But do any of the drugs also influence memory by altering NE functioning in the amygdala? That question motivated the next series of studies in my laboratory. To address this question we returned to two classes of drugs that we had studied extensively in our previous research: drugs that affect GABA receptors such as picrotoxin, a GABA receptor antagonist and one of the first drugs that I had studied several decades earlier, and drugs that affect opiate receptors such as naxolone, an opiate receptor antagonist. The findings of a series of experiments were unambiguous. Propranolol and other adrenoceptor antagonists infused into the amygdala blocked the memory-enhancing effects of GABA and opiate receptor antagonists administered either peripherally or directly into the amygdala posttraining. Two postdocs in my lab, Ines Introini-Collison and Jorge Brioni, both from Argentina, were responsible for conducting most of those experiments. In another, more recent series of experiments in my laboratory using *in vivo* microdialysis and HPLC, we found that naxolone and picrotoxin increase NE release in the amygdala. We also found that inhibitory avoidance training induces NE release in the amygdala, and the magnitude of the increase correlates very highly with subsequent retention performance.

Our evidence very strongly suggests that the interaction of neuromodulatory influences of drugs and hormones affecting memory consolidation is integrated via common actions on NE functioning within the amygdala. In an extensive series of studies conducted by Benno Roozendaal, a research colleague in my lab, we found that the adrenal stress hormone corticosterone (in the rat), like the adrenal stress hormone epinephrine, modulates memory consolidation via influences on noradrenergic receptors within the amygdala (Roozendaal, 2000). Other findings indicated that muscarinic cholinergic influences on memory consolidation also involve the amygdala, but may act "downstream" from the noradrenergic effects. Finally, but importantly, experiments using selective lesions of amygdala nuclei and selective drug infusions into specific amygdala nuclei determined that the basolateral nucleus (BLA) is the critical region of the amygdala mediating the modulatory influences on memory consolidation (McGaugh, 2002; McGaugh and Roozendaal, 2002).

Amygdala Interactions with Other Brain Systems in Consolidating Memories

The studies summarized briefly above provided no compelling clues to the locus of the neural changes underlying memory consolidation. It is theoretically possible, of course, that the amygdala might be a locus of the changes or part of a circuit involving other brain regions as well. These possibilities are strongly advocated by other laboratories studying the role of the amygdala in learning and memory (LeDoux, 2000; Davis, 2000). Although these possibilities cannot be excluded, our evidence provides no support for them. Or, at least, our evidence indicates that an intact amygdala is not *critical* for learning and retaining information. Complete lesions of the amygdala or complete lesions of the BLA do not prevent the learning of the many kinds of tasks we have used in our experiments (e.g., Cahill, Vazdarjanova, and Setlow, 2000; Lehmann, Treit, and Parent, 2000). Such lesions do, however, prevent the memory-modulatory influences of the drugs and hormones that we have investigated.

So, where does the amygdala act to influence memory consolidation? As the amygdala is richly interconnected with many brain regions (Young, 1993), it no doubt influences memory processing in many brain regions. When they were postdocs in my lab, Mark Packard (who did his graduate work with Norm White) and Larry Cahill found that the answer to that question depends on the training task used or, more specifically, the kind of information learned. Posttraining drug (amphetamine) infusions administered into the amygdala enhance spatial learning in a water maze, a task known to involve the hippocampus, as well as visually cued learning in a water maze, a task known to involve the caudate nucleus (Packard, Cahill, and McGaugh, 1994). In an extensive series of experiments, we subsequently found that lesions of the BLA or infusions of β-adrenoceptor antagonists selectively into the BLA block the memory-enhancing effects of hormones and drugs infused into the hippocampus or entorhinal cortex after inhibitory avoidance training. Conversely, lesions of the basal forebrain that provides cholinergic innervation of the cortex block the memory-enhancing effects of NE infused into the BLA posttraining (McGaugh, 2002).

Findings from Larry Cahill's studies of memory in human subjects, while he was in my laboratory, provide strong evidence implicating the amygdala in the consolidation of emotionally significant memory. Amygdala activity assessed by PET scanning during subjects' encoding of emotionally arousing material correlated very highly with memory of the material tested several weeks later (Cahill et al., 1996). This finding has been replicated and extended in other laboratories in studies using different emotional material and brain imagining techniques (Canli et al., 2000; Hamann et al., 1999). As these studies examined explicit or declarative memory, which is known to involve the hippocampus, these findings fit well with the findings of our studies with rats discussed above in suggesting that amygdala interactions with other brain regions are critical for its memory-modulating influences (McGaugh, Cahill, and Roozendaal, 1996). Cahill's finding that adrenergic activation is critical for the effects of emotional arousal on memory in human subjects (Cahill et al., 1994) also fits well with the extensive evidence from our experiments with rats.

Perhaps the best overall conclusion offered by our findings is that Gerard was correct. Epinephrine does have effects on memory like those of strychnine, and the amygdala does appear to " . . . modify the ease and completeness of experience fixation," even if it may not be the locus of engrams. But, it took my laboratory almost half a century to obtain the confirming evidence. But, of course, our findings are considerably more complex (McGaugh, 2000, 2002). Beyond that, our findings constitute only the very beginning of the next phases of research. We need to understand the specific actions of the amygdala that influence memory consolidation elsewhere in the brain and the changes at those sites that enable memory. My view is that most memories are not based on simple circuits. It seems much more likely to me that memories are enabled by the actions of highly complex, widely distributed circuitry capable of complex computations required for integrating representations of past experiences as they are activated by our ongoing experiences. How neuromodulatory systems and the amygdala act to regulate the formation of such circuitry remains to be investigated and understood. I presume that my present and former graduate students and postdoctoral researchers, or perhaps their students or the students of their students, will eventually find the answers to these questions.

Other Significant Influences

As I discussed above, scientific conferences, particularly small conferences, have very significantly influenced my research career. About the time that I began the series of experiments investigating epinephrine and amygdala influences on memory consolidation, Aryeh Routtenberg, Ray Kesner, Larry Squire, and I thought it would be useful to establish a small (i.e., fewer than 100 participants) annual meeting to enable us to meet and discuss our findings concerning these and other topics in the neurobiology of learning and memory in an informal setting. So, we organized the Winter Conference on the Neurobiology of Learning and Memory and held the first meeting in January 1976. The sessions at this annual conference held in Park City, UT, enabled me, as well as graduate students and postdocs in my laboratory, to present the findings from my laboratory and discuss them with other investigators, including Ray Kesner, Paul Gold, Michela Gallagher, Bruce Kapp, and Norm White, among others, who were investigating the effects of drugs and electrical stimulation of the amygdala on memory consolidation. Our discussions at this conference very significantly influenced all of our research programs. Of course, the program also included discussions of many other problems and issues in the neurobiology of learning and memory—a different set each year. Most neuroscientists studying learning and memory have attended at least several of the conferences. We celebrated the 25th anniversary of the founding of the conference at our meeting in January 2001.

I also participated in many conferences in Mexico, Argentina, and Brazil. These interactions created collaborations and lasting friendships with many colleagues, including Ivan Izquierdo, Rene Drucker-Colin, Federico Bermudez-Rattoni, and Roberto Prado Alcalá, each of whom have spent many months working on collaborative research in my laboratory. Many of my postdocs received their graduate training in the laboratories of these colleagues. During the "Cold War" days I also participated in a series of conferences organized by Hans Matthies in Magdeburg, East Germany. At those meetings, those of us from the West (including Steven Rose, Aryeh Routtenberg, Paul Gold, Bela Bohus, and Ivan Izquierdo, among others) were able to learn about neuroscience research on memory being conducted in Eastern European countries. There I had many discussions with Jan Bures, one of the pioneers in memory consolidation research, and later, after the Berlin Wall came down, invited him to come to UCI as a visiting Professor.

In 1982 our Center for the Neurobiology of Learning and Memory (CNLM) at UCI organized the first of a series of conferences on brain and memory, each attracting several hundred speakers and participants from the international community of neuroscientists. These conferences, held every two to four years, provided additional important opportunities for interactions with researchers investigating brain processes mediating memory and have served as "family reunions" for graduate students and postdocs who have worked in my laboratory. We held our seventh conference in 2001. The informal interchanges at these many conferences significantly shaped my thinking and my research. A few years ago I was extremely honored when Paul Gold and Bill Greenough organized a conference in my honor and subsequently edited a Festschrift based on the papers presented by my friends and former students (Gold and Greenough, 2001). Discussions of memory and many other matters at these many meetings created many new ideas and good memories, renewed old friendships, and established new lasting friendships.

I also made many friends and learned a great deal when I served on training grant and research grant review committees (then called "study sections") at the NIMH and, later, as a member of the NIMH National Advisory Council. I also played an active role in the founding of the American Psychological Society and served a two-year term as the first elected President of that Society. My role as founding Editor of the journal *Neurobiology of Learning and Memory* also provided many opportunities for interactions with international colleagues. But, the role of editor is not always a happy one, for authors of submitted papers are not always pleased with editorial actions. The general rule appears to be that if a paper is accepted it is because the authors are creative and if a paper is rejected it is because the editor is mentally deficient. Nonetheless, I managed to enjoy the role of journal editor *most* of the time during the several decades that I served in that role.

The CNLM has given me the opportunity to work closely, for many years, with colleagues, students, and visiting researchers who share a common interest in understanding the neural bases of memory. Over the years we have managed to raise funds from generous donors to enable the construction of beautiful and wonderfully functional research, office, and conference facilities. The CNLM has also adopted outreach to the public as part of its mission. We have organized the "Distinguished Lecture Series on Brain, Learning and Memory," a very well-attended public lecture series, each year for the past decade. This lecture series, as well as tours of the CNLM laboratories offered to school children, allow us to share with the public the excitement and importance of research investigating brain and memory.

Retrospection

Memories are good things to have, generally. As my research quest has emphasized, it is good that we have brains that sort out our experiences so that the most important ones are saved. Memories of significant experiences help us prepare for future experiences. But they also make us who we are. I have tried to use the memories I have preserved to summarize some of the major influences in my life and, in particular, the critical influences that aided my academic research career. I have had a very rewarding career in the Department of Neurobiology and Behavior (originally, as discussed above, called Psychobiology) and the Center for the Neurobiology of Learning and Memory at UCI. I was extremely honored to have my Department establish the McGaugh Award for Excellence in Research (awarded each year to a graduate student) and to have the School of Biological Sciences at UCI name a biology building McGaugh Hall.

My efforts over the half-century since I entered graduate school have been aided by inspiring and supportive mentors, superb graduate students and postdoctoral researchers, visiting researchers from other institutions, and creative and collegial colleagues. Norm Weinberger and I have been close colleagues for almost four decades. I have also been very fortunate to have the assistance of outstanding administrative staff. Nancy Collett has been an exceptionally supportive assistant for over a quarter of a century. Lynn Brown has been a highly creative and effective Assistant Director of the CNLM since its founding. Their superb and sustained assistance and guidance enabled me to focus my efforts on research and teaching.

But, much is missing in my report. It does not even begin to capture the uncountable subtle influences of many teachers, students, staff assistants, colleagues, and friends—including those unrelated to my academic life. Nor does this report say much about my life apart from the university. When I am not thinking and writing on the research topics discussed above, I enjoy my hobbies of making toys and furniture in my woodshop and playing clarinet and alto sax in jazz groups. Dave Schetter, a good friend and great jazz sax musician at UCI, is responsible for seeing that I get ready for wedding receptions (including Jan's, Linda's and Doug's), dinner dances, and other "gigs" with the *Butler Street Blues Band*. Science and jazz get mixed when I play with the *Synaptic Plasticity Band* whose members include my good friends, for many decades, Aryeh Routtenberg, Len Jarrard, and Mike Gabriel.

I enjoy skiing on fresh powder on sunny days, hikes in the mountains near our family cabin at Big Bear Lake, and walks in the nature preserve at the bay near our Newport Beach home. Family barbecues with swimming during the summer months provide special pleasures. Becky and I recently celebrated our 50th wedding anniversary. Doug, Jan, and Linda and their spouses helped with the celebration, as did our grandchildren, Billy, Scotty, Kaitlin, Kirby, Addie, Tristan, and Phoebe. My family has been superbly and consistently supportive of my academic career and highly proficient in providing experiences that make good and lasting memories—the kinds that are clearly worth preserving.

Acknowledgments

I would like to thank my sister, Daphne Kimbell, and my brother, William McGaugh, for providing information about our family's history and for jogging my memory about my own. Audrey Schneiderman's encouraging comments helped me shape the early sections. Larry Cahill, Norman Weinberger, and Adam Bristol reviewed an earlier draft of this chapter and provided many very helpful comments. Credit and thanks to Dan Berlau for the photo. I thank Nancy Collett for her pleasant diligence in reviewing drafts of the manuscript, providing comments and suggestions, and assisting in its preparation. I want to acknowledge and thank my wife, Becky, for her encouragement as she patiently reviewed each section of this autobiography as it emerged from my memories.

Selected Bibliography

Bermudez-Rattoni F, Introini-Collison IB, McGaugh JL. Reversible inactivation of the insular cortex by tetrodotoxin produce retrograde and anterograde amnesia for inhibitory avoidance and spatial learning. *Proc Natl Acad Sci USA* 1991;88:5379–5382.

Bovet D, McGaugh JL, Oliverio A. Effects of posttrial administration of drugs on avoidance learning of mice. *Life Sci* 1966;5:1309–1315.

Breen RA, McGaugh JL. Facilitation of maze learning with posttrial injections of picrotoxin. *J Comp Physiol Psychol* 1961;54:498–501.

Brioni JD, Nagahara AH, McGaugh JL. Involvement of the amygdala GABAergic system in the modulation of memory storage. *Brain Res* 1989;487:105–112.

Cahill L, Haier RJ, Fallon J, Alkire M, Tang C, Keator D, Wu J, McGaugh JL. Amygdala activity at encoding correlated with long–term, free recall of emotional information. *Proc Natl Acad Sci USA* 1996;93:8016–8021.

Cahill L, McGaugh JL. Mechanisms of emotional arousal and lasting declarative memory. *Trends Neurosci* 1998;21:294–299.

Cahill L, Prins B, Weber M, McGaugh JL. β-adrenergic activation and memory for emotional events. *Nature* 1994;371:702–704.

Cooper JB, McGaugh JL. *Integrating principles of social psychology*. Cambridge, MA: Schenkman Publishing Company, 1963;1–320.

Cotman C, Banker G, Zornetzer S, McGaugh JL. Electroshock effects on brain protein synthesis: Relation to brain seizures and retrograde amnesia. *Science* 1971;173:454–456.

Dawson RG, McGaugh JL. Electroconvulsive shock effects on a reactivated memory trace: Further examination. *Science* 1969;166:525–527.

deQuervain DJ-F, Roozendaal B, McGaugh JL. Stress and glucocorticoids impair retrieval of long-term spatial memory. *Nature* 1998;394:787–790.

Gold PE, Hankins L, Edwards RM, Chester J, McGaugh JL. Memory interference and facilitation with posttrial amygdala stimulation: Effect on memory varies with footshock level. *Brain Res* 1975;86:509–513.

Gold PE, Macri J, McGaugh JL. Retrograde amnesia gradients: Effects of direct cortical stimulation. *Science* 1973;179:1343–1345.

Gold PE, McGaugh JL. A single-trace, two-process view of memory storage processes. In Deutsch D, Deutsch JA, eds. *Short-term memory*. New York: Academic Press, 1975;355–378.

Guzowski JF, McGaugh JL. Antisense oligodeoxynucleotide-mediated disruption of hippocampal CREB protein levels impairs memory of a spatial task. *Proc Natl Acad Sci USA* 1997;94:2693–2698.

Guzowski JF, Setlow B, Wagner EK, McGaugh JL. Experience-dependent gene expression in the rat hippocampus following spatial learning: A comparison of the immediate-early genes, *Arc, c-fos* and *zif268*. *J Neurosci* 2001;21:5089–5098.

Harlow HF, McGaugh JL, Thompson RF. *Psychology*. San Francisco: Albion Publishing Company, 1971;1–496.

Haycock JW, van Buskirk R, Ryan JR, McGaugh JL. Enhancement of retention with centrally administered catecholamines. *Exp Neurol* 1977;54:199–208.

Introini-Collison IB, Dalmaz C, McGaugh JL. Amygdala β-noradrenergic influences on memory storage involve cholinergic activation. *Neurobiol Learn Mem* 1996;65:57–64.

Krivanek J, McGaugh JL. Effects of pentylenetetrazol on memory storage in mice. *Psychopharmacologia* 1968;12:303–321.

Landfield PW, McGaugh JL, Tusa RJ. Theta rhythm: A temporal correlate of memory storage processes in the rat. *Science* 1972;175:87–89.

Liang KC, Bennett C, McGaugh JL. Peripheral epinephrine modulates the effects of posttraining amygdala stimulation on memory. *Behav Brain Res* 1985;15:93–100.

Liang KC, Juler RG, McGaugh JL. Modulating effects of post-training epinephrine on memory: Involvement of the amygdala noradrenergic system. *Brain Res* 1986;368:125–133.

Liang KC, McGaugh JL, Yao H-Y. Involvement of amygdala pathways in the influence of posttraining amygdala norepinephrine and peripheral epinephrine on memory storage. *Brain Res* 1990;508:225–233.

Madsen MC, McGaugh JL. The effect of ECS on one-trial avoidance learning. *J Comp Physiol Psychol* 1961;54:522–523.

McGaugh JL. Facilitation and impairment of memory storage processes. In Kimble DP, ed. *The anatomy of memory*. Palo Alto: Science and Behavior Books, 1965;240–292.

McGaugh JL. Time-dependent processes in memory storage. *Science* 1966;153:1351–1358.

McGaugh JL. A multi-trace view of memory storage. In Bovet D, Bovet-Nitti F, Oliverio A, eds. *Recent advances in learning and retention*. Roma Accademia Nazionale Dei Lincei, Quaderno N. 109 Anno CCLXV 1968;13–24.

McGaugh JL. Drug facilitation of learning and memory. *Annu Rev Pharmacol* 1973;13:229–241.

McGaugh JL. Hormonal influences on memory. *Annu Rev Psychol* 1983;34:297–323.

McGaugh JL. Modulation of memory storage processes. In Solomon PR, Goethals GR, Kelley CM, Stephens BR, eds. *Memory: Interdisciplinary approaches*. New York: Springer-Verlag, 1989;33–64.

McGaugh JL. Involvement of hormonal and neuromodulatory systems in the regulation of memory storage. *Annu Rev Neurosci* 1989;12:255–287.

McGaugh JL. Dissociating learning and performance: Drug and hormone enhancement of memory storage. *Brain Res Bull* 1989;23:339–345.

McGaugh JL. Significance and remembrance: The role of neuromodulatory systems. *Psychol Sci* 1990;1:15–25.

McGaugh JL. Emotional activation, neuromodulatory systems and memory strength. In Schacter DL, Coyle JT, Mesulam M-M, Sullivan LE, eds. *Memory distortion: How minds, brains, and societies reconstruct the past*. Cambridge, MA: Harvard University Press, 1995;255–273.

McGaugh JL. Memory: A century of consolidation. *Science* 2000;287:248–251.

McGaugh JL. Memory consolidation and the amygdala: A systems perspective. *TINS* 2002;25:456–461.

McGaugh JL. *Memory and Emotion: The Making of Lasting Memories*. London: Weidenfeld and Nicolson, The Orion House Publishing Group Ltd. and New York: Columbia University Press, 2003.

McGaugh JL, Alpern HP. Effects of electroshock on memory: Amnesia without convulsions. *Science* 1966;152:665–666.

McGaugh JL, Cahill L, Ferry B, Roozendaal R. Brain systems and the regulation of memory consolidation. In Bolhuis JJ, ed. *Brain, perception, memory: Advances in cognitive neuroscience*. London: Oxford University Press, 2000;233–251.

McGaugh JL, Cahill L, Roozendaal B. Involvement of the amygdala in memory storage: Interaction with other brain systems. *Proc Natl Acad Sci USA* 1996;93:13508–13514.

McGaugh JL, Castellano C, Brioni JD. Picrotoxin enhances latent extinction of conditioned fear. *Behav Neurosci* 1990;104:262–265.

McGaugh JL, DeBaran L, Longo VG. Electroencephalographic and behavioral analysis of drug effects on an instrumental reward discrimination in rabbits. *Psychopharmacologia* 1963;4:126–138.

McGaugh JL, Ferry B, Vazdarjanova A, Roozendaal B. Amygdala: Role in modulation of memory storage. In Aggleton JP, ed. *The amygdala: A functional analysis.* London: Oxford University Press, 2000;391–423.

McGaugh JL, Gold PE. Modulation of memory by electrical stimulation of the brain. In Rosenzweig MR, Bennett EL, eds. *Neural mechanisms of learning and memory.* Cambridge, MA: MIT Press, 1976;549–560.

McGaugh JL, Herz MJ. *Memory consolidation.* San Francisco: Albion Publishing Company, 1972;1–204.

McGaugh JL, Introini-Collison IB, Cahill L, Kim M, Liang KC. Involvement of the amygdala in neuromodulatory influences on memory storage. In Aggleton J, ed. *The amygdala.* New York: John Wiley and Sons, 1992;431–451.

McGaugh JL, Introini-Collison IB, Nagahara AH. Memory-enhancing effects of post-training naloxone: Involvement of β-noradrenergic influences in the amygdaloid complex. *Brain Res* 1988;446:37–49.

McGaugh JL, Introini-Collison IB, Nagahara AH, Cahill L, Brioni JD, Castellano C. Involvement of the amygdaloid complex in neuromodulatory influences on memory storage. *Neurosci Biobehav Rev* 1990;14:425–431.

McGaugh JL, Martinez Jr. JL, Jensen RA, Hannan TJ, Vasquez BJ, Messing RB, Liang KC, Brewton CB, Spiehler VR. Modulation of memory storage by treatments affecting peripheral catecholamines. In Marsan CA, Matthies H, eds. *Neuronal plasticity and memory formation.* New York: Raven Press, 1982;311–325.

McGaugh JL, Petrinovich L. The effect of strychnine sulphate on maze-learning. *Am J Psychol* 1959;72:99–102.

McGaugh JL, Petrinovich LF. Effects of drugs on learning and memory. *Int Rev Neurobiol* 1965;8:139–196.

McGaugh JL, Petrinovich LF. Neural consolidation and electro-convulsive shock re-examined. *Psychol Rev* 1966;73:382–387.

McGaugh JL, Roozendaal B. Role of adrenal stress hormones in forming lasting memories in the brain. *Curr Opin Neurobiol* 2002;12:205–210.

McIntyre CK, Hatfield T, McGaugh JL. Amygdala norepinephrine levels following learning predict long-term memory. *Euro J Neurosci.*

Packard MG, Cahill L, McGaugh JL. Amygdala modulation of hippocampal-dependent and caudate nucleus-dependent memory processes. *Proc Natl Acad Sci USA* 1994;91:8477–8481.

Packard MG, Introini-Collison I, McGaugh JL. Stria terminalis lesions attenuate memory enhancement produced by intra-caudate nucleus injections of oxotremorine. *Neurobiol Learn Mem* 1996;65:278–282.

Packard MG, McGaugh JL. Inactivation of hippocampus or caudate nucleus with lidocaine differentially affects expression of place and response learning. *Neurobiol Learn Mem* 1996;65:65–72.

Parent MB, Quirarte GL, Cahill L, McGaugh JL. Spared retention of inhibitory avoidance learning following posttraining amygdala lesions. *Behav Neurosci* 1995;109:803–807.

Power AE, Thal LJ, McGaugh JL. Lesions of the nucleus basalis magnocellularis induced by 192 IgG-saporin block memory enhancement with posttraining norepinephrine in the basolateral amygdala. *Proc Natl Acad Sci USA* 2002;99:2315–2319.

Quirarte GL, Galvez R, Roozendaal B, McGaugh JL. Norepinephrine release in the amygdala in response to footshock and opioid peptidergic drugs. *Brain Res* 1998;808:134–140.

Quirarte GL, Roozendaal B, McGaugh JL. Glucocorticoid enhancement of memory storage involves noradrenergic activation in the basolateral amygdala. *Proc Natl Acad Sci USA* 1997;94:14048–14053.

Roesler R, Roozendaal B, McGaugh JL. Basolateral amygdala lesions block the memory-enhancing effect of 8-Br-cAMP infused into the entorhinal cortex of rats after training. *Eur J Neurosci* 2002;15:905–910.

Roozendaal B, Carmi O, McGaugh JL. Adrenocortical suppression blocks the memory-enhancing effects of amphetamine and epinephrine. *Proc Natl Acad Sci USA* 1996;93:1429–1433.

Roozendaal B, de Quervain J-F, Ferry B, Setlow B, McGaugh JL. Basolateral amygdala-nucleus interactions in mediating glucocorticoid effects on memory consolidation. *J Neurosci* 2001;21:2518–2525.

Roozendaal B, Holloway BL, Brunson KL, Baram TZ, McGaugh JL. Involvement of stress-released corticotropin-releasing hormone in the basolateral amygdala in regulating memory consolidation. *Proc Natl Acad Sci USA* 2002;99:13908–13913.

Roozendaal B, McGaugh JL. Amygdaloid nuclei lesions differentially affect glucocorticoid-induced memory enhancement in an inhibitory avoidance task. *Neurobiol Learn Mem* 1996;65:1–8.

Roozendaal B, McGaugh JL. Basolateral amygdala lesions block the memory-enhancing effect of glucocorticoid administration in the dorsal hippocampus of rats. *Eur J Neurosci* 1997;9:76–83.

Roozendaal B, Nguyen BT, Power A, McGaugh JL. Basolateral amygdala noradrenergic influence enables enhancement of memory consolidation induced by hippocampal glucocorticoid receptor activation. *Proc Natl Acad Sci USA* 1999;96:11642–11647.

Roozendaal B, Phillips RG, Power AE, Brooke SM, Sapolsky RM, McGaugh JL. Memory retrieval impairment induced by hippocampal CA3 lesions is blocked by adrenocortical suppression with metyrapone. *Nature Neurosci* 2001;4:1169–1171.

Roozendaal B, Quirarte GL, McGaugh JL. Glucocorticoids interact with the basolateral amygdala β-adrenoceptor-cAMP/PKA system in influence memory consolidation. *Eur J Neurosci* 2002;15:553–560.

Salinas JA, Introini-Collison IB, Dalmaz C, McGaugh JL. Posttraining intra-amygdala infusion of oxotremorine and propranolol modulate storage of memory for reductions in reward magnitude. *Neurobiol Learn Mem* 1997;68: 51–59.

Setlow B, Roozendaal B, McGaugh JL. Involvement of a basolateral amygdala complex—nucleus accumbens pathway in glucocorticoid-induced modulation of memory storage. *Eur J Neurosci* 2000;12:367–375.

Tomaz C, Dickinson-Anson H, McGaugh JL. Basolateral amygdala lesions block diazepam-induced anterograde amnesia in an inhibitory avoidance task. *Proc Natl Acad Sci USA* 1992;89:3615–3619.

Vazdarjanova A, McGaugh JL. Basolateral amygdala is not critical for cognitive memory of contextual fear conditioning. *Proc Natl Acad Sci USA* 1998;95:15003–15007.

Vazdarjanova A, McGaugh JL. Basolateral amygdala is involved in modulating consolidation of memory for classical fear conditioning. *J Neurosci* 1999;19:6615–6622.

Vianna MRM, Szapiro G, McGaugh JL, Medina JH, Izquierdo I. Retrieval of memory for fear-motivated training initiates extinction requiring protein synthesis in the rat hippocampus. *Proc Natl Acad Sci USA* 2001;98:12251–12254.

Westbrook WH, McGaugh JL. Drug facilitation of latent learning. *Psychopharmacologia* 1964;5:440–446.

Williams CL, McGaugh JL. Reversible lesions of the nucleus of the solitary tract attenuate the memory-modulating effects of posttraining epinephrine. *Behav Neurosci* 1993;107:1–8.

Additional Publications

Barros DM, Pereira P, Medina JH, Izquierdo I. Modulation of working memory and of long- but not short-term memory by cholinergic mechanisms in the basolateral amygdala. *Behav Pharmacol* 2002;13:1–5.

Bovet D, Bovet-Nitti F, Oliverio A. *Recent advances on learning and retention.* Accademia Nazionale Dei Lincei, 1968;109.

Cahill L, Vazdarjanova A, Setlow B. The basolateral amygdala complex is involved with, but is not necessary for, rapid acquisition of Pavlovian 'fear' conditioning. *Eur J Neurosci* 2000;12:3044–3050.

Canli T, Zhao Z, Brewer J, Gabrieli JDE, Cahill L. Event-related activation in the human amygdala associates with later memory for individual emotional experience *J Neurosci* 2000;20:RC99.

Cerletti U, Bini L. Electric shock treatment. *Boll Accad Med Roma* 1938;64:36.

Coons EE, Miller NE. Conflict versus consolidation of memory traces to explain "retrograde amnesia" produced by ECS. *J Comp Physiol Psychol* 1960;53:524–531.

Davis M. The role of the amygdala in conditioned and unconditioned fear and anxiety. In Aggleton JP, ed. *The amygdala: A functional analysis*, 2nd edition. New York: Oxford University Press, 2000;213–287.

Duncan CP. The retroactive effect of electroshock on learning. *J Comp Physiol Psychol* 1949;42:32–42.

Emptage NJ, Carew TJ. Long-term synaptic facilitation in the absence of short-term facilitation in *Aplysia* neurons. *Science* 1993;262:253–256.

Gardner EG. *Fundamentals of neurology*. Philadelphia: W.B. Saunders, 1947.

Gallagher M, Kapp BS, Musty RE, Driscoll PA. Memory formation: Evidence for a specific neurochemical system in the amygdala. *Science* 1977;198:423–425.

Gallagher M, Kapp BS, Pascoe JP, Rapp PR. A neuropharmacology of amygdaloid systems which contribute to learning and memory: In Ben-Ari Y, ed. *The amygdaloid complex*. Amsterdam: Elsevier/North Holland, 1981;343–354.

Gerard RW. The fixation of experience. In Delafresnaye JF, ed. *Brain Mechanisms and Learning*. Springfield, IL: Charles C Thomas Publishing, 1961;21–35.

Goddard GV. Amygdaloid stimulation and learning in the rat. *J Comp Physiol Psychol* 1964:58:23–30

Gold PE, Greenough WT. *Memory consolidation: Essays in honor of James L. McGaugh*. Washington, DC: American Psychological Association, 2001;1–402.

Gold PE, van Buskirk R. Facilitation of time-dependent memory processes with posttrial epinephrine injections. *Behav Biol* 1975;13:145–153.

Gold PE, van Buskirk R. Posttraining brain norepinephrine concentrations: Correlation with retention performance of avoidance training and with peripheral epinephrine modulatin of memory processing. *Behav Biol* 1978;25:509–520.

Hamann SB, Elt T, Grafton S, Kilts C. Amygdala activity related to enhanced memory for plesant and aversive stimuli. *Nature Neurosci* 1999;2:289–293.

Hebb DO. *The organization of behavior*. New York: John Wiley & Sons, 1949.

Hilgard ER. *Theories of learning*. New York: Appleton-Century-Crofts, 1948.

Izquierdo I, Barros DM, Mello e Souza T, de Souza MM, Izquierdo LA. Mechanisms for memory types differ. *Nature* 1998;393:635.

Jensen R. Neural pathways mediating the modulation of learning and memory by arousal. In Gold PE, Greenough WT, eds. *Memory consolidation: Essays in honor of James L. McGaugh*. Washington, DC: American Psychological Association, 2001;129–140.

Kety S. Brain catecholamines, affective states and memory. In McGaugh JL, ed. *The chemistry of mood, motivation and memory*. New York: Plenum Press, 1972; 65–80.

Lashley KS. The effect of strychnine and caffeine upon rate of learning. *Psychobiology* 1917;1:141–170.

LeDoux J. The amygdala and emotion: A view through fear. In Aggleton JP, ed. *The amygdala*. New York: Oxford University Press, 2000;289–310.

Lehmann H, Treit D, Parent MB. Amygdala lesions do not impair shock-probe avoidance retention performance. *Behav Neurosci* 2000;114:107–116.

Müller GE, Pilzecker A. Experimentelle Beitrage zur Lehre vom Gedächtniss. *Z Psychol* 1900;1:1–288.

Roozendaal B. Glucocorticoids and the regulation of memory consolidation. *Psychoneuroendocrinology* 2000;25:213–238.

Tolman EC. *Purposive behavior in animals and men.* New York: The Century Co., 1932.

Williams CL, Clayton EC. In Gold PE, Greenough WT, eds. *Memory consolidation: Essays in honor of James L. McGaugh.* Washington, DC: American Psychological Association, 2001;141–164.

Woodworth RS. *Experimental psychology.* New York: Henry Holt and Co., 1938.

Young MP. The organization of neural systems on the primate cerebral cortex. *Proc R Soc* 1993;252:13–18.

Randolf Menzel

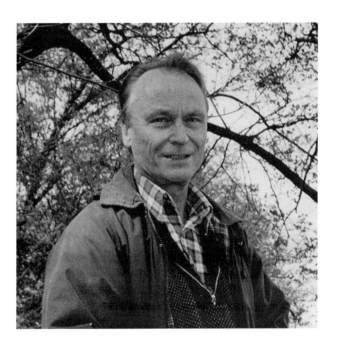

Randolf Menzel

BORN:

Marienbad, Czech Republic/Germany
June 7, 1940

EDUCATION:

University Frankfurt/Main, Ph.D.

APPOINTMENTS:

University Frankfurt/Main (1967)
Technical University Darmstadt (1969)
Australian National University Canberra (1973)
Technical University Darmstadt (1974)
Free University Berlin (1976)

HONORS AND AWARDS (SELECTED):

Hörlein Price of the German Biology Society (1960)
Fellow of the Academy of Arts and Sciences (1991)
Leibniz Award of the German Research Council (1991)
President of the International Society of Neuroethology
(1992)
Fellow of the Academy of Science, Berlin (1993)
Fellow of the Academy of Natural Sciences Leopoldina,
Halle (1996)
Fellow of the Royal Norwegian Academy of Sciences (2000)
Körber Award of European Sciences (2002)

Randolf Menzel pioneered the honeybee as a model system in neuroscience with respect to color vision, olfaction, learning, and memory. Combining levels of analysis from natural behavior to single neurons, he traced perceptual and cognitive capacities to their neural and cellular substrates. He established the first evidence for the role of the insect mushroom body in memory formation and characterized the cellular and neural correlates of different phases of memory.

Randolf Menzel

We carry our ancestors' genes within us; they define the surroundings in which body and spirit develop. The information genes contain is not directly available to us—not now, not in the foreseeable future—but certain genetic effects are reflected in our forefathers' life stories. Therefore, understanding ourselves implies remembering our ancestors' histories as well. We still don't know to what extent our ancestors' physical and mental characteristics are determined by the entirety of their genes, their life circumstances, and their experiences. We also know nothing about how combinations of genes from different lines of our ancestors, together with the particular experiences of these individuals, result in who they were, but occasionally, we discover surprising resemblances between their characters and life history and ours. This reminds us about the framework in which our physical and mental constitution develops.

Some of My Ancestors

This choice is, of course, not objective, because written history about many forefathers is so severely limited that it is impossible to describe them, and one naturally looks for similarities to one's own biography and picks out the favorable features.

My father's family came from a small village (Fulnek) in Moravia, on the Czech/Polish border. The village was one of those areas in eastern Europe where Germans, Poles, and Czechs lived together for centuries. His mother's family line (the Schindler family in Brünn) crosses with that of Gregor Mendel. Brünn is well known because it is the town near the monastery where Gregor Mendel did his famous cross-breeding experiments with peas.

The Germans in this multicultural border region were mainly members of the upper class: teachers, lawyers, factory owners, and clergy. My father's family (architect and brickyard owner) was well-to-do until the political upheavals resulting from World War I occurred (collapse of the old Austrian Habsburg monarchy). After 1924 the region was divided up into Polish and Czech territory, and the Germans had to decide to adopt either Polish or Czech citizenship. My father, who was studying languages and philosophy at the Charles University in Prague at the time, voted for Czech, while everyone else in his family voted for Polish citizenship. Many personal and social sore spots were created by the break up of German–Austrian culture in this area (as in many other multicultural areas in Czech, Polish, and Hungarian border regions); later (1939/1940), these wounds had devastating effects on political events.

After studies in philosophy, English and German philology in Prague and Vienna, my father completed his doctorate with a thesis on Heinrich von Kleist and worked as a secondary school teacher and director of a teacher-training college in Marienbad until 1944. The American army held him as a prisoner of war until 1948. Then he worked as a secondary school teacher in Gernsheim, a small town south of Frankfurt/Main, where the family had found a new home after being forced to leave western Sudetenland (the German settlement area of Behemian Lands: Bohemia and Moravia).

My mother's family line can be followed on the paternal side back over more than 10 generations to the early 16th century. They lived in the western Sudetenland; Marienbad, Plan, and Eger are the larger towns in this region. Her forefathers were farmers, millers, weavers, and other artisans. My mother's grandfather, Michl Urban, was a country doctor, local history buff, and poet. During his long life (1847–1936) he wrote numerous articles and pamphlets about rural medicine and the science of medicinal baths in the area around Marienbad and collected fairy tales, poems, folksy comedies, and historic studies about local towns, castles, and churches.

My mother's family line leads back to England and to the city of Graz in southern Austria. I want to dwell a bit on her grandfather, Robert von Lendenfeld (1858–1913), because he was a remarkable personality and the first scientist in the family tree.

He grew up in Graz and studied natural sciences at the university there. In 1881 he finished his doctorate on dragonfly flight under the supervision of F. E. Schultze, the zoologist who later headed the Zoological Institute and the Natural Sciences Museum of the Berlin University, and played a central role in developing evolutionary-biologically oriented animal taxonomy. For example, in 1936 Schultze edited the multivolume work *The Animal Kingdom* (*Das Tierreich*, published by Walter de Gruyter, Berlin).

R. von Lendenfeld left Europe immediately after receiving his doctorate (1881) and headed to Australia with his wife, whose dowry was important for this adventurous project. As a naturalist and mountaineer, he verified the glaciation of the Snowy Mountain area, determined the highest mountain in Australia, and gave his name to several mountain ridges in the Snowy Mountains. In the New Zealand Alps, several mountains were named by him or carry his name. For example, he was the first person to climb the second highest peak in New Zealand, the Hochstetter Dom. He wrote about his Australian and New Zealand expeditions in his book, *Australian Trip* (1892). This book is a gold mine of lively depictions of Australian flora and fauna, geology, landscape structures, and the way of life of the Australian settlers at the end of the 19th century. (My friend and colleague David Sandman, New South Wales University, Sydney, translated the book into English, but, unfortunately, it has not yet been published.) von Lendenfeld's own work was on primitive marine animals, predominantly Porifers und Coelenterates, but he was also interested in deep-sea fish (in particular, the histology of their light-producing organs). In 1886 R. von Lendenfeld went to London to work on Porifers and rhizostomatic Meduses as Ray Lancaster's assistant at the British Museum. Via the universities of Innsbruck and Czernowitz, he arrived at the Charles University in Prague and in 1897 was named Head of its Zoology Institute. For several years around 1910 he was rector of this famous university, founded by Charles the Fifth as the first university north of the Alps. With his group, he worked on the Porifers from the Challenger and the Valdivia expeditions and the catch from the "Albatross," an American research ship. R. von Lendenfeld's many and mostly quite long books are full of spectacular, often multi-colored lithographies, which show the sponges' habits, histology, and, most importantly, their needles. Drawing morphological structures, for publications and as wall diagrams for use in teaching, was an important activity in his institute, and my grandfather, Ferdinand Urban, also drew lots of teaching materials and illustrated publications for his doctoral supervisor, who later became his father-in-law. In order to be able to mass produce high-quality drawings, he ran his institute in Prague with military precision and included his family and his many children in his work. Both the drawings and the stories about them and how they were produced were passed on through the generations and made a deep and lasting impression on me.

R. von Lendenfeld's work is relevant to neuroscience at a core level, namely, in connection with the question of how the nervous system, in its simplest form, developed during the course of evolution. In his early publications, still in Australia, he joined Ernst Haeckel in his belief that the Porifers (Spongae) belong to the Coelenterates. He soon corrected this and acknowledged the completely different histological organization as a much simpler parachymatic arrangement of various cell types. As early as 1885 (von Lendenfeld, 1885a,b) he described neuron-type and sensory cell-type cells that exist alongside contracting muscle cells and the various types of epithelial cells, with or without flagellas. Using Cajal's reduced silver impregnation method and vital dyes, he found individual, randomly distributed cells that were not bound in a network, which he designated "nerve" and "sensory" cells (von Lendenfeld, 1887). He attributed to these cells a stimulus-transmitting and a coordinating function for the sponge's contractions, which are caused by mechanical and chemical stimuli (Lendenfeld, 1889). For decades, this view was held to be wrong; people believed that the obvious muscle cell contractions and changes in shape of the whole sponge or its parts as a reaction to mechanical and chemical stimuli were achieved only by direct effects, even though von Lendefeld had already demonstrated that even stimuli in remote regions of the sponge can trigger responses and that curare can block this action. The standard work on invertebrates,

Structure and Function in the Nervous Systems of Invertebrates, by Bullock und Horridge (1969) names von Lendenfeld as the discoverer of nerve and sensory cells in the porifers (p. 450 ff.). A French group gave lasting support to von Lendenfelds interpretations from 1952 on (Tuzet and Pavans, 1953). However, the neural function of these cells and their sensory and coordinating effect are still unclear, since it was not possible to measure neural excitation and conduction directly (Lawn, 1982). In 1977, Bullock wrote: "We conclude that Porifera lack a true nervous system," and this perception is still accepted today. A true nervous system certainly cannot exist, because their tissue systems are inherently unstable (Pavans de Ceccatty, 1974). Is the earliest physiological preliminary stage of the nervous system a loose connection of neuroid cells that transports signals (transmitters; biogenic amines, acetylcholine, and peptides have been identified) by wandering? How can neuroid cells identify their destinations, and how are they excited by the sensory cells? Is it conceivable that an integrative system similar to that possessed by the sponges was used by some remote ancestor of the Metazoa? Such a structure would lend itself to the emergence of a true nervous system, one comparable to that found in the Coelenterates (Lawn 1982; Cavalier-Smith et al., 1996). In his writings, von Lendenfeld follows this line of argumentation.

R. von Lendenfeld was a remarkable character. In his youth he was extremely strong and fit; in his later years he was a massive and imposing figure, which helped to reinforce his authority. For example, when he was rector of the Charles University, the German-language university, and Czech students attacked his office, he successfully rescued the university's centuries-old official seal. He gave his lectures in English and kept in contact with his colleagues all over the world with research trips to marine research stations, especially on the Mediterranean.

Ferdinand Urban (1879–1951), his assistant and, later, his son-in-law, was working on marine and freshwater biology and preparing to succeed von Lendenfeld. However, even though Urban was, like his father-in-law, a strong, short-tempered personality, it was difficult to exist in his shadow. So after finishing his doctorate (on a collection of Californian calcium sponges, which Professor Heath from Stanford University had sent), he left research and became a secondary school teacher. In addition to his teaching job, he carried on his research privately for many years, working on the calcium sponges collected on the Valdivia expedition and the "Gauss" South Pole expedition and those Agassiz found during the Albatross expedition. In his early teaching years around 1910, he possessed the largest collection of calcium sponges in the world and was considered their foremost expert. During stays at marine research stations, foremostly the Stazione Zoologica di Napoli, which Anton Dohrn founded in 1872 (see autobiography of Brian B. Boycott in this series: Vol. 3, p. 38, 2001), he focused on sponge development and degeneration, using physiological experiments. Unfortunately, these studies were never brought to an end and published because—severely overworked as he was—he began to lose sight in his left eye, his "microscope eye," and suffered from massive headaches. His lifelong relationship with zoology was full of longing, melancholy, and woe. His vast amount of material was given to the Naturkundemuseum in Berlin, where I was able to see it and read his notes. I have more to say about his books below.

My parents (Dr. Hans Menzel, 1903–1977; Dr. Helene Menzel, 1906–2002) were both philologists. My mother, whose strong influence on every living thing within reach was surely inherited from her father, stimulated and encouraged my early interests in identifying and observing flora and fauna. We made signs for the wild plants in our yard and caught insects, frogs, and reptiles to keep in a terrarium.

Memes

My early childhood years were during the final phase of World War II. My earliest memories were happy ones of a large family (I was the fourth child; later, two more were born) in a nice house with a large yard on a river, the Eger, in the town of Eger (now Cheb, a city north of Marienbad in the Czech Republic). I was born in Marienbad in 1940. However, these few pleasant childhood memories were soon replaced by alarming and ominous events. Our father became a soldier in 1944 and then disappeared. We fled from the attacks by the American army and went to Plan, the village where our great-grandparents (Michel und Anna Urban) lived. Their house, a splendid Gothic building with walls three feet thick and primitive sanitary facilities, had a wondrous yard, where my grandfather (Ferdinand Urban) introduced me to all the plants and animals. When American planes set the village on fire, we watched from the edge of the forest. We saw the flames devastating the houses and hoped that "our" house wouldn't be destroyed. In fact, it suffered only minor damage. These flash memories from those days are from the last year of the war, as the American army came in from the west, occupying towns and stopping just outside of Prague. My mother, who had been begging at a farm, trying to get some goat's milk for us kids (we were hiding in the forest nearby), was spotted by a small military plane and shot at. She ran in zigzags like a crazed rabbit, avoiding the machine guns, as we watched from our hiding place. A German tank blew up a bridge and sank in the mud. Endless streams of refugees filled the village and endangered our survival: scared people coming from the east, trying to flee from the Russians. The local American military authorities converted the basement of the town hall into a prison, and soon I discovered my father's face at a window there. He was a prisoner of war. My mother's brother was murdered by Czechs, and my father's brother was murdered by Poles. In the fall of 1946, the American army withdrew westward and, according to the Potsdam Agreement for carving up Europe among the Allies, turned over the area that became Czechoslovakia to the Russians. This meant that we had to flee westward immediately. My mother was able to get her four youngest children onto a cattle car in the last train leaving town. Our mother carried what little she could, and several days later, after an adventurous trip, we arrived in a refugees' camp near Nürnberg.

During this time something happened about which I heard only many years later and which instilled in me a deep appreciation for the international scientific community; I believe that this event had a decisive influence on my choice of work later in life.

Due to his poor health, my grandfather, Ferdinand Urban, would not have survived one of the customary mass transports during the Germans' expulsion from the Sudetenland. Furthermore, he was unable to leave behind his scientific library, a collection that he had inherited from his father-in-law, R. von Lendenfeld, and to which he had added countless volumes. My mother, who was working as a translator for the local American military administration, was able to make contact with a soldier who had studied marine biology in Berkeley and who was familiar with von Lendenfeld's and Urban's scientific publications. My grandfather's request was to give the books to Professor Heath in Palo Alto, the man who had given him the material for his doctoral project and after whom he had named the most beautiful calcium sponge in his collection. The military authorities, however, denied this request. So the soldier from Berkeley simply loaded the old man and his collection into a Jeep and drove him across the western border into safety, thus saving the old man's life and rescuing the library—thousands of reprints, zoological books from the final decades of the 19th century and the first half of the 20th century, and all of von Lendenfeld's and his own publications. In Urban's will, he stated that the library should be passed on to those descendants that studied biology. I inherited the collection many years later. I donated the materials to the library of the Senckenberg Museum in Frankfurt and was made a permanent member of this venerable museum—a great, unearned honor.

Amid the storms of the postwar period, survival was everything. We ended up living in a tiny hamlet in the Rhine region south of Frankfurt. I have memories of the incredible CARE packages from the United States and of my 14-year-old brother's black market dealings in all the surrounding towns in order to get such crucial items as matches, a bit of fuel for a cook stove, toothbrushes, and paper. My mother displayed unfailing strength, not only keeping us all alive, but making us inquisitive by keeping up a lively family life, having us perform plays, giving us religious instruction, and encouraging our imagination. All four of her sons later became scientists, and I attribute this to my mother's influence during these years. Schools were chaotic in the postwar era. I first went to a one-room school in which kids of all ages were taught by one teacher and then to a school quite far away (I had to walk, of course). I was in a class with 70 kids. Here the teacher spent the first hour of every day caning pupils. These school years left behind a deep mistrust of the importance of teaching curriculum and lesson plans. As I look back, I would say that the most valuable experience was my time in the one-room school, because the teacher radiated satisfaction with his work and he had enough imagination to adequately deal with the impossible situation he was in. My life became a bit more normal when I entered the Gymnasium (college-preparatory secondary school) when I was 10. My father had returned and was teaching at a Gymnasium; we moved to a little house in Gernsheim, a town on the Rhine. Here we had the signs on the plants and the terrariums that I mentioned earlier.

An event that was crucial for my career choice was when, at 15, I received my deceased grandfather's microscope, a brass model from Leitz built in 1900 and kept in a polished wooden box. Ferdinand Urban had bought this microscope for 400 guilders, money earned from private tutoring during his second semester in Prague. He needed the microscope for his marine biology course in Triest. In his memoirs, he wrote: "... my precious, beautiful microscope, that has accompanied me throughout my life as a dear, true comrade. It was an exquisite instrument ... it widened my horizon and influenced my entire relationship to science." That microscope may have had magic powers, since the same miracle happened to me 55 years later and brought me into biology.

A few weeks after my first experiments with the miraculous microscope, the pond that I had built began to turn red. I poured pond water through a fine net and found the microscopic wonders of my pond: red globules that dyed the water. I also found plankton plants and plankton animals. My enthusiasm was roused, and from that moment on my plankton net and I visited every pond in the Rhine plain. During my final years at secondary school, I did systematic studies of pond ecology throughout the four seasons; I determined and drew hundreds of plankton algae, rotifers, copepods, phylopods, and ciliates. I was interested in the interrelationships between the physical and chemical parameters in ponds, those of the plankton, and their changes during the day and throughout the years. My observations and drawings culminated in a 256-page work with over 100 illustrations, written in 1960, the year I finished secondary school, and which won the prize for the best student biology report in all of Germany (Hörlein Prize of the German Biology Society). Thus, my choice was made for biology as my university major subject and my professional field.

My affinity for freshwater biology brought me into contact for the first time with a famous scientist and a research lab. Franz Ruttner, the famous limnologist, who for many years was Head of the Research Station in Lunz am See in Austria, was a college friend of my grandfather's. I visited the station when I was still a secondary school student, participated as a young college student in various summer courses there, and met Professor Ruttner. I will always remember this distinguished senior scientist's eyes agleam with pride as he showed me "his" nanno-plankton (plankton organisms smaller than 5 μm) under the microscope and his readiness and generosity in giving a mere high school student a guided tour of his lab. This incident made a strong impression on me as to what the ideal scientist should be. I was an ardent admirer of the contemplative working atmosphere in the research station. Work out in the field, lab work, taxonomic and ecological studies, chemical-physical readings, and physiological experiments were combined with each other. Exhausting mountain hikes, taking samples from lakes and rivers, were compensated for with long nights at the microscope and in the library. Even as a first-year student, I got a pleasant glimpse of research work, and I met scholars who became my role models.

However, my course of studies at the University was a bit less attractive. I was studying biology, chemistry, and physics at the University of Frankfurt/Main. The zoology and botany courses consisted exclusively of making drawings. The lectures were mere obligatory rituals, and only a few of the excursions were at all interesting. However, physics and chemistry were different; there were enthralling lectures and interesting courses.

The situation in the Zoology Institute was especially adverse. The professor position was empty, and a retired professor, Professor Giersberg, gave lectures on classic zoological topics that were from prewar days. Almost no classes were offered in animal physiology. This was made worse by the fact that there was no real textbook for this field. It was only in 1963 that I read an animal physiology textbook: Prosser's *Comparative Animal Physiology* (1961). No classes were offered in ecology and behavioral biology, so I spent my first two college years studying physics, chemistry, and microbiology.

The course of studies in biology at a German university at this time was poorly structured. The only degrees offered were a doctorate or a secondary school teaching certificate. There were no directives about when one had to take which courses, and there were practically no exams during the course of studies. So we students put together our own degree programs; this gave us a great deal of academic freedom, but left us completely alone and often overwhelmed and a bit lost. Therefore, it was very fortunate for me, right away in first semester, to find friends with whom I have stayed in contact through the years, first as college pals and then as colleagues: Rüdiger Wehner and Günther Fleißner. We organized our own excursions (both Rüdiger and Günther are outstanding bird experts), attended the same lectures and courses, and had intense discussions about the topics covered in them.

Since five of the kids in my family were in college at the same time, I had to work during semester breaks. My skills in freshwater biology proved to be useful; I took a course at the University of Munich and became a qualified wastewater biologist. With this certification, I got a job with the Merck Pharmaceutical Company in my hometown, Gernsheim, where I did independent work in a small research lab on biological processes for the company's waste. The job had many good features: its research relevance, the freedom to be able to plan my work myself, good pay, and the fact that I could work during semester breaks. In fact, I was even able to continue my work on the Rhine Valley ponds; I published my first scientific article on this topic (Menzel, 1968b). Nevertheless, this taste of life in the commercial sector convinced me that I didn't want to pursue a career in industry: there was no open discussion (which I had grown to value in the Institute in Lunz and at the university); the staff was not thrilled with its work; all results had to remain secret; and, most importantly, the factory that I worked in polluted the Rhine to such an extent that I was in a major moral quandary, wondering whether I should bring this out into the open. My bosses forbade me to publicize the pollution, threatening me with legal action. It's surely understandable that I generalized about my experiences with big industry and that, with my leftist political leanings of the time, I characterized them as typical for the capitalist system. These semester breaks working in industrial surroundings even dimmed my interest in limnology, and I became unsure whether I wanted to pursue a career in freshwater biology or ecology.

The deficiencies in the animal physiology degree program at the University of Frankfurt motivated my friend Günther Fleißner and me to study at the University of Tübingen for one semester. As luck would have it, we were able to participate in a lab course held by Werner Loher (who later became a professor at the University of California, Berkeley). Furthermore, I attended lectures by Franz Huber (on color changes in the animal kingdom). Meeting Franz Huber was pivotal for finding my new field of interest. Unlike the other zoology lectures that I had endured, Huber's classes sparkled, full of verve and zeal. They linked together morphological, physiological, behavioral, and neurobiological aspects, creating a convincing overall picture. And he was available for his students. At the end of the semester, in summer 1963, I asked him what he thought of the idea of studying the physiology of learning processes in the microscopically small, transparent rotifers (e.g., in *Asplanchna*); after all, their nerve cells are directly visible, and they can be bred easily. Without my really having noticed, this question combined my two main motivating interests in biology: limnology and learning mechanisms. Huber encouraged me in my basic notion of studying something so complicated as learning in such well-suited model organisms. He recommended Prosser (1961) and Kenneth Roeder (1963) as suitable textbooks, and then lent me (but only over the weekend) a huge pile of proofs: Bullock and Horridge's book. Before he dismissed me with the proofs, he asked something very simple, which was, for me, incredibly enlightening: Why should these animals in fact learn, seeing as they swim around in an unstructured and unlimited ocean, and can neither avoid nor seek anything? This little question opened my eyes to ethological-behavioral argumentation.

All of this happened before 1964, when Tauc und Kandel published the first cellular analyses of synaptic plasticity in the nervous system of

Aplysia, when intracellular recording was still quite rare in neuroscience, and before the successful single-cell analysis of invertebrate nervous systems had started. But things were evolving at a fast pace. Franz Huber prepared us for these new developments by reporting on the exciting developments going on in labs all over the world and by telling us what he was working on: the attempt to ascribe behavior to the function of individual nerve cells or small neuronal networks. I got a vague idea of what direction I wanted to go, but how could I combine this direction with my interests in the mechanisms of learning processes? Huber didn't want to get involved with such a project; he recommended Martin Lindauer, who had taken up the professorship for zoology in Frankfurt. So I returned to Frankfurt and began my doctoral work on color learning in bees (Menzel, 1967).

Lindauer himself showed me how to train bees; he talked about his professor, Karl von Frisch, and then left me to work almost completely on my own for two years. Since my friend Rüdiger Wehner had also just started working with bee-training experiments, we were able to help each other. I built a complicated spectral apparatus with a strong Xenon bulb to train the bees to monochromatic light. In Germany, this kind of bee training is only possible from mid-July (when there is little nectar available) through the end of October (if it hasn't already gotten too cold). During this period, there are no free weekends, and if the apparatus breaks down, you repair it at night. Alongside our experimental work, we had time to read and have discussions. The role models I found in my readings were Karl von Frisch (1965), Thorpe (1963), Lashley (1950), Thorndike (1932), Pavlov (1927), von Holst (1935), Tolman (1932), and Köhler (1921), a colorful mixture, representing conflicting schools within behavioral biology. I could understand how important it was to use objective and quantifiable criteria to record behavior; my own experimental work was an intensive effort in this direction, but I was disappointed that behavioral biology did not refer to the brain. The American learning psychologists caught my eye, but they were also the most disappointing because they thoroughly dismissed any connection to brain mechanisms. Ethologists, on the other hand, disappointed me because they ignored learning processes and instead developed such rather strange concepts as "release mechanism modified by experience" as the only possible explanation for learning, even though learning quite obviously consists of acquiring totally new skills. Despite being enthralled with Karl von Frisch and having devoured his book with unflagging interest, I couldn't quite understand why he concentrated exclusively on sensory mechanisms when successful decision-making during nectar search, dance communication, navigation, social coordination, and more is clearly the result of brain mechanisms.

These questions were discussed with Rüdiger Wehner, but there was no great interest in discussions in the Zoology Institute; in particular, no one was familiar with Parlow or the American psychologists. Therefore, it was a great discovery to attend a seminar in the Psychology Institute which covered Hermann Ebbinghaus (reprinted 1964) and Müller and Pilzecker (1900). Vague perspectives appeared here: the correlation of behavioral tasks with neurological pathologies, comparative studies in animals and humans, and EEG recordings and retention measurements. A defining moment was when I read McGaugh's article on memory phases (1966). A new world opened up for me: so there were indeed possibilities to closely correlate strict behavioral events (retention) with mechanisms of brain function. After reading his article, and inspired by the early works by Agranoff, Davis, and Brink (1966), Flexner, Flexner, and Roberts (1966), and others, I knew what I wanted to do. I had a vague inkling that the task was to create a synthesis between the inconsistencies of the various behavioral biological schools of thought.

Finding My Own Way

Since in the meantime (having completed my doctorate in 1967) I had a thorough knowledge of my experimental animal, it was clear to me that I wanted to continue to work with bees. Bees learn very quickly and have a good, long-lasting memory (Martin Lindauer had just reported that even after 5 months bees can remember the characteristics of nectar source); enough animals are available year-round, the experimental animals are genetically closely related (daughters of one queen); and they demonstrate complex behavior. I, meanwhile, knew how to work with them in the open, in order to pose questions and quantify their behavior. However, whether they were suitable for laboratory experimentation and for neurophysiological studies was still unclear. I gathered some hope from the fact that intracellular recordings of retinula cells of the bee eye had been successfully carried out (Naka: 1961, Autrum and von Zwehl, 1964). Even though I had not yet prepared a bee brain and had no experience with neurophysiological methods, I wanted to study the neuronal foundations of their behavior, particularly, behavior that plays a role in learning and memory formation.

I'd like to make a comment about my supervisor Martin Lindauer and the state of behavioral/neurobiological research in Germany in the 1960s. Lindauer had been Karl von Frisch's most important pupil, and he carried on Frisch's work on orientation and communication in bees. His scientific skills came to fruition in his work with bees and in personal discussions about specific problems in bee research. He was not an especially brilliant lecturer or a great organizer. His teaching was not top notch. However, in everything he did he transmitted a sense of pleasure in his research work; ongoing curiosity about the wondrous accomplishments of his experimental animal, the bee; and an ability to immerse himself in bee biology. Strict discipline in experiments, dedication during difficult and long projects, and a critical view of one's own data were exemplary traits that we learned from him. In Germany at this time, the most influential zoologist was Hans-Jochen Autrum, Head of the Zoology Institute in Munich; Lindauer had worked there before going to Frankfurt. Autrum's pupils filled many professorships, broadening the influence and increasing the dominance of his field, sensory physiology. Lindauer was not part of this "inner circle," nor was Franz Huber. Although Lindauer himself never made the switch to neurophysiological studies, he prepared his pupils for them. For him, receptor and communication tasks in the bee were not exclusively carried out by receptors, but included brain processes. He began to think about learning and memory formation and, in doing so, distanced himself from two strong traditions which had been a firm basis for his previous work: sensory physiology from the behavioral-analytical point of view, and ethology (more in Tinbergen's sense than in Lorenz's). His discoveries in magnetic field orientation, communication, comb building, and bees' choice strategy got him thinking about the unknown processes in the bee brain that still needed to be investigated. His curiosity infected his pupils; many of his direct and indirect pupils became neuroscientists or spent at least part of their careers working in neurophysiology (Markl, Rathmayer, Wehner).

So the first thing I needed to do was to learn neurophysiology. Martin Lindauer helped me get a postdoc position and agreed that I should learn intracellular recording of retinula cells in the bee eye in Dietrich Burkhardt's lab; he was the second professor in the Institute. Back then (1967), capillary electrodes were pulled with homemade pullers and were filled by keeping them in water vapor for days. It was rare to get a successful recording. I began the journey down the thorny path of electrophysiology; in spite of many methodological improvements through the years, it is still a difficult discipline. Nowadays, we know that the bee brain is a difficult object for electrophysiologists, most likely because the neurons are especially thin, the mechanical stability of the brain is minimal, and the prepared brain is exceedingly sensitive to a lack of oxygen. Still, my fascination with these intracellular recordings has not faded, and to this day I spend time in the lab working on these recordings.

In the fall of 1967 I met Karl von Frisch. Martin Lindauer had a get together for his research group in Frisch's house on Lake Wolfgang in Austria, and von Frisch (who was then 81 years old) gave those of us who had just finished our doctorates an extra oral exam. I remember how startled I was by his question for me: Which bees move from blossom to blossom without ever flying? I first thought he was joking because I did not know very much about these strange little solitary bees that wait in flowers for big bees and clamp to their legs when they fly off to the next flower. So, I guess, Karl von Frisch did not get a good impression about my knowledge of general bee biology.

After the exam we told him about our experiments, and he encouraged us with tips that proved that he understood the underlying problem. I reported that bees learn violet spectral light especially quickly, and that this effect cannot be due to a sensory mechanism, but rather must be based on an evaluation process made by the central nervous system. von Frisch had worked on a similar query with his pupils at a time when little was known about color vision in bees, and his results could not be correlated with mine. The inconsistencies interested him the most. Since my attempts to explain things relied on many details from the psychophysics of color vision, I feared the discussion would become a bit sticky. Nothing of the kind: von Frisch was exceptionally well informed, wanted to learn from me, and gave me numerous tips for further experimentation. He didn't want to follow my core argumentation, however, which was the differentiation between peripheral and central mechanisms of estimating color.

Another topic of our conversation concerned color vision in bees, and this discussion was even more controversial. Let me dwell on this topic because it can serve as an illustration for the conceptual shift in sensory physiology at this time. von Hess (1913) had shown that bees act like color-blind animals in their phototactical behavior, whereas von Frisch (1914) proved that bees do differentiate colors when they learn food cues. von Frisch maintained that his finding proved von Hess' assumption wrong. However, this assumes that both phototaxis and learning color differences make use of the same central color vision system. My theory (speculative back then, but in the meantime experimentally proven, see Menzel und Greggers, 1985) was that this is not the case, but rather that the bee has various central chromatic integration systems that are assigned to various behaviors. This way of thinking was alien to von Frisch, which told me that he, following the tradition of sensory physiology from the first half of the 20th century, equated perception with peripheral (mostly receptor) performance. This mindset was surely remarkably successful and had led to great discoveries by Karl von Frisch and his students (i.e., seeing UV light, seeing polarized light, odor perception, and differentiation between acoustic and vibratory mechanosensory perception). The limitations of this way of thinking seemed obvious to me, but I could not satisfy von Frisch; he could not accept the existence of central evaluating mechanisms as a basis for an explanation. He was right with that, of course, as long as nothing is known about these hypothetical central mechanisms. I took this as a challenge to work on exactly this problem and to search for these central mechanisms.

In the fall of 1969, I took a position as an Assistant in the Zoology Institute of the Technical University of Darmstadt, where Hubert Markl had just taken over as Director. I was able to form my own research group. I wanted to work in parallel on two topics: the search for the neuronal basis of learning and memory and color vision in bees. The experimental approach for the former was greatly helped along by my visit to the Max-Planck-Institute for Behavioral Physiology in Seewiesen in 1970. There I met a doctoral student of Dietrich Schneider's, Ekkehard Vareschi, who was studying odor discrimination in the bee (Vareschi, 1971). He showed me the experiment that had been developed 20 years earlier by Masutaro Kuwabara (1957) in Karl von Frisch's lab: classical conditioning of the proboscis extension response (PER) in bees mounted in small tubes. I immediately saw that this was the experimental setup that I had been looking for. Even though I was familiar with Kuwabara's publications, I hadn't thought of using this paradigm for my studies. From that moment on, throughout my entire scientific life, this paradigm has accompanied me in my work and has made quintessential contributions to current knowledge of behavioral and neural mechanisms of appetitive olfactory learning and memory formation.

The PER paradigm has an interesting history. In the 1930s and 1940s Karl von Frisch's group studied bees' perception of food substances, especially sugar. He used Minnich's (1932) method; Minnich had noticed that hungry insects activate their mandibles when their tarsi or antennae are stimulated with sucrose solution. Hungry bees will extend their proboscis. One of von Frisch's students (Kantner) was determining the perceptual threshold for various sugars and believed that he had discovered an exceedingly high sensitivity; even a few sugar molecules per liter of water should be sufficient to release the response. von Frisch was skeptical and sent the student home (von Frisch, 1965, p. 533). In the 1950s, when Kuwabara joined his group, von Frisch told him about this peculiar experiment, and Kuwabara repeated the experiments. Kuwabara stimulated their antennae or front leg tarsi with a drop of sucrose solution. The bees' reflexes caused them to stick out their probosces. When he stimulated the sugar receptors on the tarsi, Kuwabara usually cut off the antennae, because that helped him achieve a more reliable reaction. But now, without antennae, the bees had lost their extremely high sensitivity to sugar. Kuwabara surmised that the bee perceives other stimuli (e.g., water vapor) simultaneously with the rewarding sugar stimulus and then associatively links the two. Kuwabara and Takeda (1956) then proceeded to prove that the antennae do indeed perceive the water vapor and that, after being repeatedly coupled with sugar stimulation, water vapor alone will trigger the PER. As a control, he stimulated the bees for the same number of trials with plain water. It was thus clearly a case of classical conditioning. Kuwabara was able to prove this quite convincingly when he used colored lights as the conditional stimulus and, after cutting off the antennae, stimulated only the sugar receptors on the tarsi (Kuwabara, 1957). Here he didn't use control groups, but he did test for color discriminatiation and at the end of the experiments carried out an extinction series. Conditioning to colored stimuli takes much longer than to water vapor or odors. It is noteworthy that Karl von Frisch (1965) cited work by Kuwabara and his colleagues only where it dealt with proofs of sensory capabilities and not regarding learning.

While my first two doctoral students (Jochen Erber und Thomas Masuhr) worked on learning and memory formation, I was searching for

ways to become acquainted with central vision physiology. My skills in intracellular recordings from photoreceptors in insect eyes were still limited, and
my attempts to get recordings from visual neurons failed. Adrian Horridge
invited me to spend a year at his institute at the Australian National University (ANU) in Canberra, where I learned electrophysiology from his doctoral
student Simon Laughlin. My goal was to study the role the primary visual
interneurons, the monopolar cells, in the bee lamina play in coding color
stimuli. This proved to be technically overwhelmingly difficult then, and it
still is (Menzel, 1974; de Souza et al., 1992), but in the intellectually stimulating atmosphere with Allan Snyder and Simon Laughlin I got a totally
new perspective on visual physiology and also did some intensive work on
photoreceptors in the bee eye. Allan Snyder, a brilliant theoretical physicist
and an expert on the theory of optical wave guides, was establishing the
new field of photoreceptor optics. In the shade of the eucalyptus trees on the
ANU campus, we carried out our intellectual flights of fancy, recognizing
the lateral filter principle in the fused rhadom, and searched for the receptor
mechanisms for analyzing the e-vector of light. In these studies I measured
the retinula cells' sensitivity to linear polarized light and found, to my great
surprise, that only a few of the UV-sensitive cells had sensitivity to polarized
light; all the other cells—even the UV-sensitive cells, which were seen more
often—had miniscule sensitivity. I was, of course, familiar with von Frisch's
explanation for the bees' ability to detect polarization patterns in daylight
(see von Frisch's star filter model, 1967). My data were diametrically opposite to his model, which assumes that all visual cells in the bee ommatidium
are sensitive to polarized light. How would von Frisch and how would my
revered former supervisor Lindauer react to these findings and my interpretation? Did I have any chance at all to publish these results, and would
I have any chance to do research in Germany in a situation like this? With
great trepidation, I submitted my manuscript to the *Journal of Comparative
Physiology*, and asked Autrum, the Editor, to pass it on to von Frisch for
evaluation. von Frisch was enthusiastically supportive, and the article was
immediately accepted for publication. A scientist's true greatness is shown
not only in his discoveries, but in his ability to correct his opinions when
faced with a new results.

In the pre-Internet era, with the erratic Australian postal service and
without phone contact, I tried to keep in touch with my group in Darmstadt
via a constant barrage of letters. At the same time I was substituting for
Horridge in administrative matters in his Institute, because he was off
in Oxford taking a sabbatical year. These multiple duties, ranging from
the various research topics represented in the Institute to the unavoidable
administrative tasks, added up to pose an enormous challenge. In addition,
at age 32, I was living in an English-speaking country for the first time and
had to rise to the challenge of communicating effectively in a foreign language. The defining event of my time in Australia was the zeal for theoretical

and experimental research that pervaded the group around Allan Snyder and Simon Laughlin. We came up with an experiment and did it the following day. If it didn't succeed, which happened often, of course, we looked for ways to simplify it. Theoretically picking apart a problem so tenaciously before setting up an experiment was a completely new experience for me.

I returned to Darmstadt as a professor in 1973. The German ambassador in Canberra swore me in as a professor, which was a good thing, because otherwise I would have ended up staying in Canberra (they had made me an offer). It wasn't very easy to adapt to the German zoology scene after my experience abroad. It was especially difficult for me, since my research work, especially on learning and memory formation, didn't fit into the narrow zoology curriculum taught at German universities. The ethologists didn't understand what I and many other young researchers were doing, and they decided who would get hired as behavioral biology professors in this small country. The neurophysiologists, under the powerful influence of Hans-Jochen Autrum, were exclusively sensory physiologists, and many professor positions had just been filled, directly or indirectly, with Autrum's pupils. During this phase, which was critical for my career, a new discipline was coming into existence, due to the initiative of Franz Huber, Ernst Florey, Hubert Markl, Werner Rathmayer, and Gerhardt Neuweiler; it aimed to study the neural basis of behavior, with emphasis on central mechanisms. The German Research Council (Deutsche Forschungsgemeinschaft) set up a nationally organized framework which provided intensive support to 20 research groups, with my small group included. For 15 years (1970–1985) the members of this program met regularly in stimulating sessions. Looking back, I have the impression that the most innovative neuroscience research in the zoological sector in Germany was carried out during this period. There was definitely a sense of making a fresh start. New methods in intracellular electrophysiology and new ways to dye neurons opened new perspectives. It was possible for the first time to correlate single-neuron analyses, foremostly in insects, with behavior. Our enthusiasm was boundless in 1970 when Zettler showed us an intracellularly marked neuron, one of the first intracellular markings worldwide. The unique neuron concept, the command neuron concept, and the identified neuron concept were all discussed intensively. Franz Huber was the central figure in this circle. His group at the Max-Planck-Institute for Behavioral Biology in Seewiesen set the standards, and he established the upbeat tone of our discussions. We were also quite sure that neuroscientists working on the insect nervous system were far ahead of those working on mammalian brains. Within the small brains of our insects, with their rich behavioral repertoire, we were able to point out individual neurons and describe their intracellularly recorded activity during almost normal behavior. Therefore, we thought, it should be possible to understand—from its individual elements—the function of natural neuronal networks in the context of biologically relevant sensory and motor processes. Each newly identified neuron was greeted with glee and seen as another stepping-stone along the way to achieving our goal. Today, many of us are still following this path, albeit with a more realistic attitude regarding our high hopes in those early years, but we are still convinced that neuronal networks can only be understood on the basis of neurons' individuality, their singular conformations and connectivities, their physiological attributes, and their specific forms of ontogenetic and experience-dependent plasticity.

Meanwhile, it was 1976, and I was busy establishing my group at the Free University of Berlin (FU). I was still blissfully unaware of the problems I would be facing in this enormous university (about 60,000 students during the 1980s and 1990s). I had decided to go to Berlin, and not to Princeton (where I would have succeeded Vincent Detier) or to the university in Hamburg. Perhaps my decision would have turned out differently if I had known that the FU students hardly ever came to lectures (and were encouraged in this behavior by other professors); that they were carrying out massive student strikes at the university, trying to get rid of exams; and that serious research on an international level was hard to find. During these years of turmoil on all levels of academic life at the FU, and violent encounters between political extremes, I fled every summer to the Marine Biological Laboratory (MBL) in Woods Hole, MA, to teach the course on "Neural Systems and Behavior" that had been founded by Alan Gelperin and Ron Hoy. The enthusiasm of the American students and the collegiality among the lecturers reminded me of a long-lost academic way of life, which was only reestablished at the FU in the mid-1980s.

In the rest of this autobiography I'll talk about some research projects that I've worked on over the years. First, however, I would like to comment on a central activity in Germany universities: teaching. The teaching load for professors at German universities is considerably higher than for our colleagues in the United States. Required teaching is normally 90–120 academic hours per semester, and if lab courses and seminars are involved, that number can be much higher. This workload, combined with numerous oral exams and supervisory duties for Diploma and Master's theses, is enormous and greatly reduces the time available for research during the semester. A crucial prerequisite for work at a university is therefore the willingness to teach ever-new generations of students. In my early years at the Technical University in Darmstadt, I taught general zoology, taxonomy, morphology, physiology, behavior, and ecology, with some of the disciplines being rather remote from my own areas of research. Later, in Berlin, I was able to concentrate my teaching on animal physiology and behavior. Satisfaction with teaching comes when the teacher is successful in conveying to the students the intellectual journey that he made while preparing the lecture, presenting valuable material such that it expands the insights and captures the interest of those listening to the finished product. The communicative process involved is hugely suspenseful and risky. When boredom and disinterest have taken over the lecture hall, everything is lost; I have bitter memories of this from some semesters in the late 1970s. Luckily, the student generation changed in the early 1980s, and university teaching returned to its normal, rewarding state.

Research

Color Vision

The first step in understanding color vision in any animal is to relate the spectral properties of the various receptor types in the eye with color perception. Bees were the first animals for which the spectral properties of receptors, as measured by intracellular recordings, allowed one to interpret basic characteristics of color perception (Autrum and von Zwehl, 1964; Daumer, 1956; von Helversen, 1972). My first contribution to this field was the proof that all three of the spectral receptor types are present in the ommatidium and play a role in the function of the fused rhabdom (Menzel and Blakers, 1975). This structure is designed to keep the narrow spectral sensitivity functions of each individual receptor, although it provides a high quantum yield (Menzel and Snyder, 1975). Assigning the functional receptor types to their respective morphological types led to the development of a wiring diagram of the peripheral visual neuropils of the bee brain, and this was, at least partially, verified with intracellular recordings of the primary visual interneurons. As is also the case in other color vision systems, further neuronal processing occurs in chromatically antagonistic neurons (Kien and Menzel, 1977; Hertel, 1980). Since it was extremely difficult to perform intracellular analysis on visual interneurons (and even to this day, there have been no further investigations of neuronal coding of color information in the bee brain either in our lab or elsewhere), we switched our emphasis to psychophysical studies, in which we took advantage of the possibility of easily training bees to color stimuli. Backhaus (Backhaus and Menzel, 1987) used these data as the basis for his model of color vision in the bee, which correlates very well with our neurophysiological findings and additional behavioral results (Menzel and Backhaus, 1991). Brandt and Vorobyev (1997) showed that Backhaus' model was one of a general class of models which psychophysical methods have shown all have identical levels of precision. At this time, Lars Chittka was also working on modeling color vision in our lab; he used data on color discrimination in various hymenoptera species. He developed a pragmatic, even though not completely coherent graphic model of color discrimination, the color hexagon. These three—Backhaus, Vorobyev, and Chittka—made fundamental advances in this discipline, but had mighty clashes of opinion among themselves. Our attempts at further experimentation—striving to reach a unified bee color vision model that could be accepted by all three of our experts—unfortunately did not succeed. Therefore, this problem was dropped, to be clarified by someone in another lab somewhere. There are serious problems involved: (1) too little data exist to resolve the problems caused by the non-linear relationship between color loci, as determined by a receptor-based model, and color discrimination; (2) the role of adaptation, especially its temporal dynamics, is still largely unknown; (3) spatial aspects of color vision have been briefly touched upon, but still require very thorough study (this is a topic currently active in my lab); and (4) higher order color vision phenomena (color constancy, color sensations, color evaluation, and meaning) are only understood at a basic level. My doctoral dissertation contributed something to the latter topic, namely, that color stimuli are evaluated independent of their receptor-related properties such as threshold and discriminability. For example, colors are discriminated equally well in the violet portion of the spectrum (around 400 nm) as they are in the blue-green portion (490 nm), but violet is learned much more quickly and at a higher level of performance than blue-green. After 30 years of research, we still do not have a clear explanation of this phenomenon. It makes lots of sense biologically, since blossoms that hymenopterans visit and pollinate (foremostly, the large hymenopterans [Menzel and Shmida, 1993]) are predominantly violet and blue in their blossom colors and blossom patterns. The co-evolutionary relationship between blossom color and color vision mentioned here is a subject that has interested me since my student days. It was a surprising discovery to find that this signal-receiver matching has no effect on the spectral characteristics of the photoreceptors in the pollinating insects' compound eyes, but does have an effect on their central nervous evaluation function. Rather, we found that the spectral characteristics of the receptors constitute an optimal peripheral filter system for all colors (in the spectral range from 300 to 650 nm [Vorobyev et al., 2001]).

The strength of the neuroethological approach, as used in our color vision studies, may be demonstrated by the following example: a blossom's shape and/or color pattern plays a decisive role in how a pollinating insect recognizes, lands on, and manipulates that blossom. Current explanations for pattern recognition in insects are at least incomplete or even faulty: do insects measure the pattern's flickering frequency as they fly over the flower (flicker frequency hypothesis), or do they see a pattern only when its image appears at exactly the same spot on the retina where it appeared when the animal first saw that pattern (retinotopic matching hypothesis), or do they simply measure the directions of all border lines and sum them up in three categories arranged 120° to each other (directional feature detector hypothesis) and sum these up in respective directional channels? In order to demonstrate the tasks involved in pattern recognition and the deficits of the explanations offered so far, we studied the bee's pattern generalization and abstraction capabilities (Giurfa, Eichmann, and Menzel, 1996). When bees learn different bilateral symmetrical (or asymmetrical) patterns, they transfer this ability to the discrimination of completely new symmetrical and asymmetrical patterns. All three hypotheses mentioned above and used so far to explain pattern recognition in insects can be dismissed by these results: the flicker frequencies do not differ between such patterns; the patterns cannot be matched to a retina-stable template, and the directional components of the contrast borders do not provide a specific feature of such patterns. The bees need not only discriminate between such patterns, but must extract a common feature (symmetry) and learn to associate this to reward. It turns out that bees are not only able to perform this generalization, but they can learn the reciprocal task much more quickly, thus demonstrating a certain capacity for abstraction. None of the existing models for pattern recognition can explain this performance. Therefore, we must assume that insects' ability to perceive chromatic and achromatic patterns is much more powerful and flexible than we had hitherto believed.

These experiments led us to question whether a brain as small as the bee brain is able to learn rules. To do so, we chose a matching-to-sample experiment (or matching-to-nonsample, respectively), and we demonstrated that such a task can indeed not only be solved, but that the bee transfers its response to new stimuli (Giurfa et al., 2001). The task that bees in our experiment had to carry out was to choose the blue target after seeing a blue signal (given a choice between blue and yellow) and choose the yellow target after seeing a yellow signal (given the same choice). Other bees had to solve the non-sample task (choose the blue target after seeing a yellow signal and the yellow target after seeing a blue signal). After the bees learned the task in the color domain, they were able to solve it without training in the pattern domain and even in the odor domain.

Ultimately, we need to explain such cognitive faculties and many others yet to be discovered in the bee on a neuronal basis. Demonstrating such faculties in a brain of 1 mm^3 with fewer than 1 million neurons, will hopefully help us search for and identify neural mechanisms at a reduced level of complexity. Whether insect scientists are able to contribute to such an enterprise is not at all clear, but we shall try, working together with our colleagues who work on "big brains" (Menzel and Giurfa, 2001).

Learning and Memory

After reading McGaugh's *Science* article (1966), I was eager to find out whether bees have short- and long-term memory (STM, LTM). Indeed, they do (Menzel, 1968a). The next step was to localize the consolidation of STM to LTM in the brain. We succeeded at this using the PER paradigm (see above) and found that robust learning can be observed after one-trial conditioning, even when the head capsule had been opened and the brain was made accessible to recording and manipulation. Using thin cold probes (200 μm in diameter), we were able to reversibly switch off small areas of the brain at different times after conditioning (Menzel et al., 1974). These experiments determined the particular importance of the bee brain's mushroom bodies in creating memory, even before studies on *Drosophila* came to similar conclusions (Heisenberg et al., 1985). It also became clear that memory is created not only in the mushroom bodies, but also in the primary sensory neuropil, the antennal lobe, an idea that we verified years later using other methods (Hammer and Menzel, 1998).

Back then, in 1975, experimental psychological procedures had not yet been systematically applied to study the PER paradigm. Since I was immersed in ethological tradition, with its rejection of experimental psychological concepts and techniques, I had no idea of the required testing procedures. I did, however, know from reading the literature that this knowledge was urgently needed. I got some preliminary impressions from a workshop held by Bitterman and Lolordo in Germany in 1976 (Bitterman et al., 1979). A subsequent collaboration with Jeff Bitterman during his stay in our lab in 1982 led to ongoing intensive behavioral-analytical studies of the PER paradigm in our group (Bitterman et al., 1983). Many paradigms were tested and found to lead to phenomena of conditioning similar to what are seen in laboratory mammals.

I'd like to dwell on one paradigm—the blocking phenomenon—because it led to controversial results that are still unresolved, even though the researchers involved (Bertram Gerber and Brian Smith) have been working cooperatively on clarifying it. In blocking, a novel stimulus is not learned if it occurs together with an already-learned stimulus. Brian Smith (Chandra and Smith, 1998), a former postdoc in my lab, demonstrated blocking, but Bertram Gerber, working on his doctorate in our lab, could not (Gerber and Ullrich, 1999). Both used rather similar conditioning procedures, but partially different odors, and one worked with German bees, while the other worked with American bees. If the nationality does not count, it is likely that unknown properties of the conditioned odor have a stronger impact on blocking than hitherto believed. I mention this to show that discrepancies in results need not necessarily lead to a breakdown in personal friendship and professional communication. This was, however, not always the case in connection with the PER paradigm. Jeff Bitterman, for example, was unsuccessful with PER conditioning in his lab (even though he had previously observed the experiments in our lab [Bitterman et al., 1983], and he then felt it necessary to include in his lectures his opinion that PER conditioning is a hoax. This gave me, during lectures in the United States, the opportunity to present a live conditioning trial, carried out on the overhead projector, and the bees erased all doubts with their convincing demonstration.

We still needed to prove the usefulness of the PER paradigm for physiological studies. One of my graduate students, Juliane Mauelshagen, succeeded here by using intracellular recording to show that a single identified neuron, the PE1 (a mushroom body-extrinsic neuron), selectively changes its response properties to odors when an animal learns (Mauelshagen, 1993). The next step was even more important. My graduate student Martin Hammer recorded from another single identified neuron, the VUM_{mx1}, (Hammer, 1993), and proved with elegant experiments that VUM_{mx1} excitation represents the reinforcing component during olfactory conditioning. He did this, after penetrating the neuron with an intracellular electrode, by substituting the sucrose reward in odor conditioning by current injection into this neuron. A forward pairing of odor and VUM excitation led to the same increase of conditioned responding in the animal as in normal conditioning when sucrose was used as a reward. A backward pairing of US and CS did not lead to learning in either experimental condition. This was a major breakthrough. The VUM's morphology was reconstructed, and it showed that the CS and US pathways anatomically converge at three locations (antennal lobe, mushroom body input site, and the lateral region of the brain) in both sides of the brain. This unique structure appears to be the substrate for the distributed memory trace (see above). The putative transmitter of VUM_{mx1} was identified with immunocytological methods (octopamine), and this led to the possibility of running a substitution experiment using local octopamine injection as the US (Hammer and Menzel, 1998). Meanwhile, we know that there are only 2 VUM neurons with the morphology of VUM_{mx1}, although the class of VUM neurons has 15 members. Thus, two neurons in the bee brain may be sufficient to represent the reward pathway in olfactory learning. It is most likely that no other VUM neuron is involved in visual learning, because no other VUM neuron converges with the visual neuropils in the bee brain.

Martin Hammer was an exceptional scientist, intellectually very strong and experimentally most skillful, and a gifted lecturer. He was also a true friend and extraordinary co-worker. Martin died in a car accident in 1997.

As mentioned above, intracellular electrophysiology is not an easy task when carried out within the bee brain, and neither are extracellular recordings. Somata of central neurons of insects are electrically disconnected from the integrating and conducting parts of the neurons. Thus, little current is available extracellularly. Against this background, it is rather impressive to see what graduate students and postdocs in the lab have learned about learning-related plasticity in the central nervous system (e.g., Grünewald, 1999; Mauelshagen 1993).

Nowadays, it has gotten quite a bit harder to attract a student to a research topic which requires high frustration tolerance, and the intracellular studies carrying the most risk are reserved for my own experimental work. The reason is not that students are less dedicated, but rather that new techniques are more attractive, particularly imaging techniques. Indeed, these new approaches have turned out to be most useful in studying both olfactory coding and neural plasticity related to olfactory learning (Faber, Joerges, and Menzel, 1999; Galizia and Menzel, 2000). The bee brain is well-suited for these studies, because selected areas can be exposed to the microscope under conditions when the whole animal learns and remembers an odor stimulus. The normal sensory inputs and motor outputs are intact, and under favorable conditions the animal may even be able to display motor responses. In my view we are on the verge of a new journey into a normally functioning nervous system using multiphoton-microscopy and intelligently designed sensing dyes. What the bee brain may be able to contribute in these new endeavors is an insight into neural mechanisms involved in accomplishing a cognitive task of midlevel complexity, e.g., natural forms of learning that transcend elementary associative processes, memory processing over many hours and days in a fully functional brain, configural and context-dependent learning and memory retrieval, attentional components in learning and memory, decision making under competing memory conditions, and the like. The question will be whether we can manage to handle and interpret the enormous amount of data from imaging a large number of neurons under such conditions, a task that can only be accomplished by intensive collaboration with colleagues from the theoretical disciplines.

A short note on how we started with the imaging experiments. In 1991 I received the prestigious Leibniz Prize from the DFG, the German Research Council, which came with $1.5 million. For the first time I had the chance to start new research projects without being forced to justify and document that I was qualified for the work. I decided to establish three new labs, each of them devoted to an experimental approach that I had never before been involved in and that had not yet been applied to the study of the bee brain: imaging, patch electrophysiology, and biochemistry. For the imaging project I recruited two graduate students (Jasdan Joerges and Armin Küttner) who, like me, had no experience whatsoever with optical measurements of neural or cellular functions. We only had our fantasies and no clear ideas about how to get optical signals from the bee brain. No research institution would have ever given us money for this undertaking. Back then, the digital cameras and the computers had to be programmed by the user—not an easy task for two biology students. The major problem was the preparation, and we worked hard for two years before we found a way to get the FM ester of Ca-green into the neurons and were able to measure signals from the dye and not from the moving brain.

The biochemistry lab was established by Uli Müller, who had been involved in protein chemistry with the *Drosophila* brain. Uli turned out to be a wonderful addition to the lab at a time when several people (Martin Hammer, Brian Smith, Frank Hellstern, and Bertram Gerber) had to test all the wonderful paradigms in the literature on associative learning (see above). He managed to measure kinase activities in single antennal lobes at very short intervals after single and multiple trial conditioning. The notion of STM and LTM in the bee brain, established by behavioral tests at the beginning of my scientific career, was successfully put to mechanistic scrutiny for the first time. I remember the excitement when we discussed his first set of data on PKA activity and the involvement of NO synthase on LTM, but not on STM induction (Müller, 1996). One might argue that it might not be necessary after all to test such basic concepts of the cellular correlates of STM and LTM, since *Aplysia, Drosophila*, and the many studies on LTP and LTD in mammals had already told us the story. I disagree wholeheartedly! General mechanisms in biological functions are discovered only through comparative studies. Furthermore, any species and any selected component of neural function has its own phylogenetic history and cannot be assumed at the outset to represent a general phenomenon. Specific adaptations of species to their ecological niches shape the functional components, and there is no way to distinguish between the specificities and the generalities. Take, for example, protein synthesis and LTM induction. When we found that 24-hr retention does not depend on protein synthesis in bees, we had a hard time getting the data published (Wittstock, Kaatz, and Menzel, 1993). Meanwhile, we know that bees are not as special as thought; they rely on translation-dependent early LTM and transcription-dependent late LTM as other animals do, but on a different time scale (Menzel, 1999).

The Bee in Its Environment: Choice Strategy, Navigation, Communication

Karl von Frisch said that observing a bee colony is an endless source of insight: that the longer one watches, the more one observes, and the more there is to be observed. Working with free-flying bees in their natural environment has been a constant throughout my research work. I repeatedly went back to just observing their behavior inside and outside the colony, and most of the questions that were followed up in laboratory studies stem from these observations. There has been additional motivation for me. Bees come in large numbers and look alike. When you have worked with a group of bees for a while you will identify individuals on the basis of their behavior; however, it is normally not possible to recognize an individual bee, a prerequisite for any careful study. In my view, Karl von Frisch was so successful with his research because, from the very beginning, he identified bees individually using dots of colored paint on their thoraces. He designed his experiments so that he knew exactly what each bee had been exposed to or had experienced before he tested it. I used von Frisch's colored dot method throughout my life, but we also developed all kinds of automatic recognition and testing devices to keep track of individuals, making the behavioral tests more objective; taking advantage of the large number of potential experimental animals; saving time, effort, and the risk of unpleasant experiences (watching bees at the hive entrance can lead to attacks and stings); and automating data collection.

One example might suffice. When we wanted to study bee choice strategy, my long-term co-worker Uwe Greggers, an excellent engineer, built computer-controlled feeders that detected an individual bee; provided a particular volume of sucrose solution according to a particular computer program (e.g., simulating a constant flow rate of sucrose solution), with a precision in the nanoliter range; and recorded the behavior (feeder handling, licking time, etc.). Four such feeders formed a patch in which bees performed hundreds of choices per bout, and each of the choices was recorded with its characteristic parameters (Greggers and Menzel, 1993). The huge amount of data and their computerized format allowed testing rather sophisticated models of choice performance (Greggers and Mauelshagen, 1997; Fülöp and Menzel, 2000).

Another topic studied over two decades is navigation. Whereas von Frisch and his co-workers, as well as current researchers (Thomas Collett, Rüdiger Wehner, and Mandyam Srinivasan), focused on the sensory and perceptual aspects of navigation (e.g., the role of the polarized light pattern, mechanisms of visual landmark recognition, time sense, and sequential views of landmarks), we were more interested in the cognitive structure of spatial orientation. Initially, I believed (as other researchers did) (Wehner and Menzel, 1990) that long-distance navigation is fully described by the assumption that bees establish vector memories from path integration and that such vector memories are associated with large-scale landmarks. When Gould (1986) came up with the proposal that bees might also refer to a geometric representation of experienced space, we performed a large number of experiments that dismissed this proposal. Although this dismissal is still correct, Gould's speculation is substantiated by new data. The problem with all studies on bee navigation is that only the initial flight path could be recorded after the bee was released at an unexpected site (vanishing bearings). During this initial flight phase, the bee follows the vector it would have taken if it had not been transferred to a new site. However, if the bee's full flight path is recorded using a radar tracing technique, we recently found (unpublished data) that the bee is able to return in direct flight from practically any location around the hive within a radius of approximately 500 m, indicating that bees refer to an allometric representation of space which allows them to localize themselves according to landmark constellations and to fly along the shortest route back to the intended goal. Such an intended goal is usually the hive, but can also be the feeding place.

von Frisch's famous discovery of the bee dance is supported by an overwhelming battery of impressive data (von Frisch, 1965), but a direct proof is lacking. A direct proof would be to trace the flight path of a bee recruited by a dancing bee and show that the recruited bee flies exactly according to the information gathered from the dancer. This proof is now available. Using the same radar technique, we documented a large number of flights by recruited bees and found that indeed bees perform a vector flight whose direction and distance were indicated by the dance.

Epilogue

"Bees are insects; their nervous centers are, as far as their anatomic evolvement goes, paltry, as compared to the human brain. Nevertheless, these creatures are able to tell their peers about a goal that is important for the entire colony." Karl von Frisch wrote that in 1965 at the end of his book on bee dance communication and orientation. von Frisch, Lindauer, and many other researchers devoted their entire professional lives to understanding the remarkable achievements of these small insects. My contributions are marginal when compared to the heroic deeds of my scholarly predecessors. Along with my co-workers, I was aiming for a paradigm change, from describing phenomena to analyzing neuronal mechanisms. I was inspired by the general "new beginning" in neurosciences in the early 1970s; by the enormous advances made in the methodology of measuring brain functions at this time; and by the example set by my older colleagues, Franz Huber, Ernst Florey, Werner Rathmayer, and Hubert Markl. However, I also had to free myself of some constraints which had been established by the strong German traditions in ethology and sensory physiology. In these zoological disciplines, experience-dependent adaptation by organisms is not held to be a subdiscipline; many influential zoologists even believe that this should not and cannot be considered a legitimate field of study.

When I ask myself what I have learned so far from my studies of how the nervous system works, I can suggest this answer. (1) We expect too little from small brains. One million neurons allow the bee to sense a huge sector of environmental energy distributions; to steer the body in elegant flight, even under rough weather conditions over long distances, and most effectively between a patchwork of potentially attractive food sources; to adapt the sensory and motor circuits such that effective behavioral control, well-timed expectations, and appropriate communication with its community occur; and to implement rules from sequences of learning. Little brains do not appear to produce more stereotyped behavioral patterns than big brains. There is also no indication that a small brain, by necessity, has a more limited memory capacity, at least within the boundaries of its cognitive faculties. Experience-dependent neural plasticity, and the memory trace resulting from it, is such a basic property of nervous systems that it does not require any particular level of network complexity or total number of neurons. The primary parameter for brain size is body size, and the additional function components with relatively increased brain size are very hard to uncover, indeed. (2) The intelligence of simple heuristics is underestimated, and cognitive tasks may require much less "cognition" than usually believed. The brain does not work in isolation, but is embedded in the functional properties of its sensors and actions. What these peripheral organs solve does not need to be solved by the brain. The complex polarization pattern of the sky, for example, is preanalyzed by the structure of the compound eye, and the brain receives not just generally useful information, but information selected for just one task, namely, to detect the great circle through the (unseen) sun such that the sun's azimuth can be calculated (Wehner, 1992). An astronomer would be unhappy with such a measuring device, but the pilot of a plane or the captain of a ship, facing the same problem as the bee (estimating the position of the sun from a patch of blue sky in an otherwise overcast sky), would find the combined hardware/software system immensely useful. The same argument applies to brain function. For example, the storage capacity and temporal dynamics of appetitive STM in bees appear to be adapted to their food sources (flowers), which are rather unreliable, provide very little food, and grow in patches (Menzel, 1999). Such heuristics are not exclusive to small brains; any brain, including the human one, takes advantage of them (Gigerenzer and Selten, 2000). (3) Rather similar environmental demands are made of small and big brains. Are different neural strategies implemented in small and big brains to solve similar problems? I do not believe so, and in particular, I do not consider small brains to be less flexible and less quick to adapt. Franz Huber asked me nearly 40 years ago why plankton rotiferas learns; he didn't ask "Why do you think such little nervous systems learn?" This is the key issue. If an animal species has an extended lifespan (in the case of the bee, the colony's lifespan is the deciding factor), and the individual animals are exposed to a changing environment, their nervous system will develop strategies to cope with these changes effectively, irrespective of the absolute size of its brain. This does not mean that the neural and cellular mechanisms are the same in small and big brains, but the mechanisms should be related to each other because of common phylogenetic histories.

For the reader who has never worked with bees, my opinion about the irrelevance of absolute brain size will sound strange and unconvincing. I can only recommend studying and watching these wonderful animals and getting caught up in their impressive behavior. It could become a lifelong commitment.

Selected Bibliography

Agranoff BW, Davis RE, Brink JJ. Chemical studies on memory fixation in the goldfish. *Brain Res* 1966;1:303–309.

Autrum HJ, von Zwehl V. Die spektrale Empfindlichkeit einzelner Sehzellen des Bienenauges. *Z Vergl Physiol* 1964;48:357–384.

Backhaus W, Menzel R. Color distance derived from a receptor model of color vision in the honeybee. *Biol Cybern* 1987;55:321–331.

Bitterman ME, Lolordo VM, Overmier JB, Rashotte ME. *Animal learning—Survey and analysis*. New York: Plenum Press, 1979;v-510.

Bitterman ME, Menzel R, Fietz A, Schäfer S. Classical conditioning of proboscis extension in honeybees (Apis mellifera). *J Comp Psychol* 1983;97:107–119.

Brandt R, Vorobyev MV. Metric analysis of threshold spectral sensitivity in the honeybee. *Vision Res* 1997;37:425–439.

Bullock T, Horridge GA. *Structure and function of the nervous system of invertebrates*. San Francisco: Freeman, 1969.

Cavalier-Smith T, Allsopp MTEP, Chao EE, Boury-Esnault N, Vacalet J. Sponge phylogeny, animal monophyly and the origin of the nervous system: 18S rRNA evidence. *Can J Zool* 1996;74:2031–2045.

Chandra S, Smith BH. An analysis of synthetic processing of odor mixtures in the honeybee. *J Exp Biol* 1998;201:3113–3121.

Daumer K. Reizmetrische Untersuchung des Farbensehens der Bienen. *Z Vergl Physiol* 1956;38:413–478.

de Souza J, Hertel H, Ventura DF, Menzel R. Response properties of stained monopolar cells in the honeybee lamina. *J Comp Physiol A* 1992;170:267–274.

Ebbinghaus H. *Memory. A contribution to experimental psychology*. Originally published in 1885. New York: Dover, 1964.

Faber T, Joerges J, Menzel R. Associative learning modifies neural representations of odors in the insect brain. *Nature Neurosci* 1999;2:74–78.

Flexner LB, Flexner JB, Roberts RB. Stages of memory in mice treated with ace-toxycyclohexamide before or immediately afer learning. *Proc Natl Acad Sci USA* 1966;56:730–735.

Fülöp A, Menzel R. Risk-indifferent foraging behaviour in honeybees. *Anim Behav* 2000;60:657–666.

Galizia CG, Menzel R. Odour perception in honeybees: Coding information in glomerular patterns. *Curr Opin Neurobiol* 2000;10:504–510.

Gerber B, Ullrich J. No evidence for olfactory blocking in honeybee classical conditioning. *J Exp Biol* 1999;202:1839–1854.

Gigerenzer G, Selten R. *Bounded rationality: the adaptive tool box*. Cambridge, MA: MIT Press, 2000a.

Giurfa M, Eichmann B, Menzel R. Symmetry perception in an insect. *Nature* 1996;382:458–461.

Giurfa M, Zhang S, Jenett A, Menzel R, Srinivasan MV. The concepts of 'sameness' and 'difference' in an insect. *Nature* 2001;410:930–933.

Gould JL. The locale map of honey bees: Do insects have cognitive maps? *Science* 1986;232:861–863.

Greggers U, Mauelshagen J. Matching behavior of honeybees in a multiple-choice situation: The differential effect of environmental stimuli on the choice process. *Anim Learn Behav* 1997;25:458–472.

Greggers U, Menzel R. Memory dynamics and foraging strategies of honeybees. *Behav Ecol Sociobiol* 1993;32:17–29.

Grünewald B. Physiological properties and response modulations of mushroom body feedback neurons during olfactory learning in the honeybee *Apis mellifera*. *J Comp Physiol A* 1999;185:565–576.

Hammer M. An identified neuron mediates the unconditioned stimulus in associative olfactory learning in honeybees. *Nature* 1993;366:59–63.

Hammer M, Menzel R. Multiple sites of associative odor learning as revealed by local brain microinjections of octopamine in honeybees. *Learn Mem* 1998;5:146–156.

Heisenberg M. Initiale Aktivität und Willkürverhalten bei Tieren. *Naturwiss* 1983;70:70–78.

Heisenberg M, Borst A, Wagner S, Byers D. *Drosophila* mushroom body mutants are deficient in olfactory learning. *J Neurogenet* 1985;2:1–30.

Hertel H. Chromatic properties of identified interneurons in the optic lobes of the bee. *J Comp Physiol* 1980;137:215–231.

Holst E von. Über den Prozess der zentralnervösen Koordination. *Pflügerg Arch Gesamte Physiol* 1935;236:149–158.

Kien J, Menzel R. Chromatic properties of interneurons in the optic lobes of the bee II. Narrow band and colour opponent neurons. *J Comp Physiol A* 1977;113:35–53.

Köhler W. *Intelligenzprüfung an Menschenaffen*. Berlin, 1921.

Kuwabara M. Bildung des bedingten Reflexes von Pavlovs Typus bei der Honigbiene, *Apis mellifica*. *J Fac Sci Hokkaido Univ Ser 6 Zool* 1957;13:458–464.

Kuwabara M, Takeda K. On the hygroreceptor of the honeybee, Apis mellifica. *Physiol Ecol* 1956;7:1–6.

Lashley KS. In search of the engram. *Symp Soc Exp Biol* 1950;4:454–482.

Lawn ID, Porifera. In Shelton GAB, ed. *Electrical conduction and behaviour in 'simple' invertebrates*. Oxford: Clarendon Press, 1982, 49–72.

Mauelshagen J. Neural correlates of olfactory learning in an identified neuron in the honey bee brain. *J Neurophysiol* 1993;69:609–625.

McGaugh JL. Time-dependent processes in memory storage. *Science* 1966;153:1351–1358.

Menzel R. Das Erlernen von Spektralfarben durch die Honigbiene (Apis mellifica). Doctoral thesis at the University of Frankfurt/Main, 1967.

Menzel R. Das Gedächtnis der Honigbiene für Spektralfarben. I. Kurzzeitiges und langzeitiges Behalten. *Z Vergl Physiol* 1968a;60:82–102.

Menzel R. Zur Ökologie eines Kolkes während der Sommerstagnation. *Arch Hydrobiol* 1968b;65:100–123.

Menzel R. Spectral sensitivity of monopolar cells in the bee lamina. *J Comp Physiol* 1974;93:337–346.

Menzel R. Memory dynamics in the honeybee. *J Comp Physiol A* 1999;185:323–340.

Menzel R, Backhaus W. Colour vision in insects. In Gouras P, ed. *Vision and visual dysfunction. The perception of colour*. London: MacMillan Press, 1991;262–288.

Menzel R, Blakers M. Functional organization of an insect ommatidium with fused rhabdom. *Cytobiologie* 1975;11:279–298.

Menzel R, Erber J, Masuhr T. Learning and memory in the honeybee. In Barton-Browne L, ed. *Experimental analysis of insect behaviour.* Berlin: Springer-Verlag, 1974;195–217.

Menzel R, Giurfa M. Cognitive architecture of a mini-brain: The honeybee. *Trends Cognitive Sci* 2001;5:62–71.

Menzel R, Greggers U. Natural phototaxis and its relationship to colour vision in honeybees. *J Comp Physiol* 1985;157:311–321.

Menzel R, Shmida A. The ecology of flower colours and the natural colour vision of insect pollinators: The Israeli flora as a study case. *Biol Rev* 1993;68:81–120.

Menzel R, Snyder AW. Introduction to photoreceptor optics—an overview. In Snyder AW, Menzel R, eds. *Photoreceptor optics.* Berlin-Heidelberg-New York: Springer-Verlag, 1975;1–13.

Minnich DE. The contact chemoreceptors of the honey bee Apis mellifera. *J Exp Zool* 1932;61:375–393.

Müller GE, Pilzecker A. Experimentelle Beiträge zur Lehre vom Gedächtnis. *Z Psychol* 1900;1:1–288.

Müller U. Inhibition of nitric oxide synthase impairs a distinct form of long-term memory in the honeybee, *Apis mellifera. Neuron* 1996;16:541–549.

Naka K. Recording of retinal action potentials from single cells in the insect compound eye. *J Gen Physiol* 1961;44:571–584.

Pavans de Ceccatty M. Coordination in sponges. The foundations of integration. *Am Zool* 1974;14:895–903.

Pavlov I. *Conditioned reflexes.* New York: Dover Publications, 1927.

Prosser CL. *Comparative animal physiology.* Philadelphia: Saunders, 1961;1–688.

Roeder KD. *Nerve cells and insect behavior.* Cambridge, MA: Harvard University Press, 1963.

Thorndike EL. *The fundamentals of learning.* New York: Columbia University Press, 1932.

Thorpe WH. *Learning and instinct in animals.* London: Methuen, 1963.

Tolman EC. *Purposive behavior in animals and men.* New York: Century, 1932.

Tuzet O, Pavans de Ceccatty M. Les cellules nerveuses de l'éponge calcaire homocoele *Leucandra johnstoni* Cart. *CR Acad Sci Paris* 1953;236:130–133.

Vareschi R. Duftunterscheidung bei der Honigbiene: Einzelzell-Ableitungen und Verhaltensreaktionen. *Z Vergl Physiol* 1971;75:143–173.

von Frisch K. Der Farbensinn und Formensinn der Biene. *Zool Jb Physiol* 1914;37:1–238

von Frisch K. *Tanzsprache und Orientierung der Bienen.* Heidelberg: Springer-Verlag, 1965.

von Helversen O. Zur spektralen Unterschiedsempfindlichkeit der Honigbiene. *J Comp Physiol* 1972;80:439–472.

von Hess C. Experimentelle Untersuchungen über den angeblichen Farbensinn von Bienen. *Zool Jb* 1913;34:81–106.

von Lendenfeld R. Das Nervensystem der Spongien. *Zool Anz* 1885a;8:47–50.

von Lendenfeld R. The histology and nervous system of the calcareous sponges. *Proc Linn Soc NS W* 1885b;9:977–983.

von Lendenfeld R. Synocils, Sinnesorgane der Spongien. *Zool Anz* 1887;10:142–145.

von Lendenfeld R. Experimentelle Untersuchungen über die Physiologie der Spongien. *Z Wiss Zool* 1889;48:406–700.

von Lendenfeld R. *Australische Reise*. Innsbruck: Verlag der Wagner'schen Universitäts-Buchhandlung, 1892;1–325.

Vorobyev MV, Brandt R, Peitsch D, Laughlin SB, Menzel R. Colour thresholds and receptor noise: Behaviour and physiology compared. *Vision Res* 2001;41: 639–653.

Wehner R. Arthropods. In Papi F, ed. *Animal homing*. London: Chapman & Hall, 1992;45–144.

Wehner R, Menzel R. Do insects have cognitive maps? *Annu Rev Neurosci* 1990;13:403–414.

Wittstock S, Kaatz H-H, Menzel R. Inhibition of brain protein synthesis by cycloheximide does not affect formation of long–term memory in honeybees after olfactory conditioning. *J Neurosci* 1993;13:1379–1386.

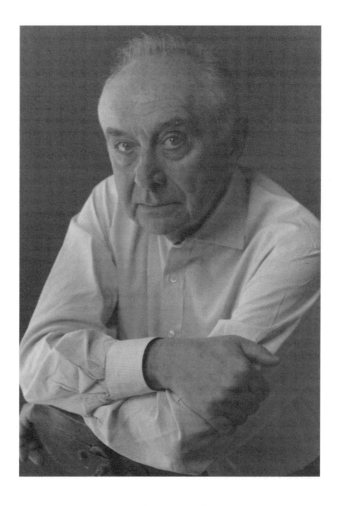

Mircea Steriade

BORN:

Bucharest (Romania)
August 20, 1924

EDUCATION:

Faculty of Medicine, Bucharest, M.D. (1945–1952)
Institute of Neurology, Romanian Academy of Sciences,
D.Sc. (1952–1955)
Université de Bruxelles, with F. Bremer (1957–1958)

APPOINTMENTS:

Head of Neurophysiology Laboratory, Institute of Neurology,
Bucharest (1958–1968)
Professor of Neuroscience, Laval University,
Québec (1968–present)

HONORS AND AWARDS (SELECTED):

Membre d'Honneur de la Société de Neurologie de Paris
(1957)
Médaille Claude Bernard de l'Université de Paris (1965)
Distinguished Scientist Award, Sleep Research Society (1989)
Scientific Prize of Québec (1991).
Member of the Academy of Sciences, Royal Society of Canada
(1994)
Award of the American Society for Clinical Neurophysiology
for Outstanding Achievements in Research (1998)
Presidential Lecture at the Society for Neuroscience Meeting
(1999)
Editor-in-Chief, *Thalamus & Related Systems* (2001, Elsevier)
Honor Member of the Romanian Academy of Medical
Sciences (2003)

*Mircea Steriade pioneered research that identified the network operations
and neuronal properties in corticothalamic systems, which are implicated
in the generation of normal brain rhythms during different states of
vigilance and different types of electrical seizures. He was the first to
demonstrate the role of GABAergic thalamic reticular neurons in the
production of sleep spindles. Using intracellular recordings in animals and
field potential recordings during human sleep, he also discovered a new
type of sleep rhythm, the slow oscillation, which is generated intracortically.*

Mircea Steriade

Initiation in Neurosciences

I was interested in neuroscience since my first year of medical studies in Bucharest (1945) when I was reading, aside from the usual textbooks, Lorente de Nô's chapter and other chapters on the cerebral cortex and thalamus in Fulton's 1938 book *Physiology of the Nervous System*. I remember being fascinated during those early years at the Faculty of Medicine by the hypothesis of Dusser de Barenne and McCulloch, who postulated the presence of connections from cortex to thalamus and back to different cortical areas. I tried to convey to some classmates my excitement by drawing esoteric arrows running from the motor cortex to basal ganglia and thalamus and back. These reciprocal projections that occurred to me right at the initiation in neuroscience anticipated the core of my entire research life, which is centered on the role of corticothalamic reciprocal loops in the generation of various (normal and paroxysmal) brain rhythms and their control by generalized modulatory systems. In 1950, an article by Hsiang-Tung Chang, then at Yale, presented convincing electrophysiological evidence in favor of reverberating circuits between cortex and thalamus. My inclination toward neuronal operations in these reciprocally connected networks explains why I was rather disappointed during the 1960s when Per Andersen and John Eccles discarded the influence of the cerebral cortex on thalamic spindles, a hallmark sleep rhythm. I first challenged their idea in 1972 by eliciting spindles from the contralateral cortex, through the callosal and corticothalamic pathways (to avoid backfiring of thalamocortical cells), and, more recently (1996), we demonstrated the crucial role played by corticothalamic projections in the spatiotemporal coherence of this oscillation.

I became actively involved in neuroanatomical work during the third year at the Faculty of Medicine when, as an Assistant in the Department of Anatomy, I sectioned brains of human embryos and stained monkey cerebral cortex with a modified Golgi technique in the histology laboratory of Professor I.T. Niculescu. (He repeatedly advised me to "be more patient and ally yourself with time." I respectfully disobeyed then as well as now.) I used to look through the microscope all day long, at the expense of some medical disciplines that I regarded as marginal and for which I remained a layman. I already knew that all my life would be spent with the brain and its operations.

After earning an M.D., I was offered in 1952 a position as a young research scientist working toward a D.Sc. (Ph.D.) at the Institute of Neurology of the Romanian Academy of Sciences. It is vivid in my memory how puzzled I was when, a few days after entering that institute, I was asked to deliver a talk on iron metabolism. I had been ignorant of the fact that heavy metals are present in the brain. Because the literature on this topic was mainly from German authors, I used my knowledge of German and the seminar appeared to go well, but I retained some resentment about the idea that unorthodox chemical elements were found in such a noble tissue.

The years of my doctorial studies, until 1955, were busy with experiments on cats and dogs, which led to a thesis on cerebello-cortical relationships. I also underwent training in neurology and neurosurgery. After seven years of clinic, I realized that what mainly interested me in patients was the site(s) of their lesion(s). I subsequently abandoned clinical work to be free for experiments. Nevertheless, those years (1952–1960) of clinical neurology and animal experiments contained the embryo of my future scientific life. In 1955, I became an independent researcher in the Laboratory of Neurophysiology of the Institute of Neurology.

Thus, in the clinic, I had the privilege to follow up an elderly woman who had had a hypersomnia for more than two years. I fed and nurtured that patient until her end, and, in histology, I found bilateral, butterfly-like lesions in thalamic intralaminar nuclei. We published in 1958 a paper in *Revue de Neurologie (Paris)* with those clinical-anatomical data, which were confirmed several years later by French neurologists at the Salpêtrière hospital in Paris. That report was my first important study, and it marked my first foray into research on brain stem activating systems relayed by thalamic intralaminar nuclei with widespread cortical projections. In a similar vein, I published two cases of akinetic mutism, one of them with a dorsolateral pontine tegmental lesion. In that case, there was an interruption of ascending projections, but no loss of effector pathways because the patient, a young boy, could answer complex questions by raising a finger or two. This was a case of pure *Antriebsmangel* (lack of incitement to action) due to interruption of ascending activating systems, a topic that occupied part of my research time with immunohistochemical/tracing studies and intracellular recordings during the 1980s and early 1990s.

The defense of my D.Sc. thesis in 1955 caused a bit of a stir. This was the first thesis defense to take place at the Romanian Academy of Sciences. (To give an idea of my enthusiasm when I had entered the fray three years before, I should say that when I heard, while fulfilling my obligation in the army, that a competition had been open for those wishing to pursue the D.Sc. degree, I obtained leave, immediately took the train, and, without changing from my soldier's uniform, went directly to the Academy of Sciences to register.) My thesis defense was attended by many people. One of them, who seemed to be viewed favorably by the regime, attacked the assumption implied by my title that cerebellar lesions influence neocortical electrical activity and conditioned reflexes. He bitterly questioned such a possibility, arguing that Ivan Pavlov had taught us that the cerebral cortex governs subcortical structures and not the other way around. If this man were aware of my present views according to which, indeed, the cortex exerts a powerful influence on the thalamus and other brain sites, he would have been satisfied. At that time, however, his point was simply political: how could the "rank-and-file" influence the "top?" My thesis became a monograph at Masson in Paris (1958), but it paled in comparison with the book on the cerebellum by Dow and Moruzzi published in the same year. Nonetheless, Wilder Penfield sent a congratulatory letter. I also remember that Alf Brodal asked me details about transneuronal degeneration in red nucleus neurons after cerebellar lesions, and, notably, Frédéric Bremer wrote me very nice words about the results of my experiments. Bremer remained highly vivid throughout my scientific life. In those early years, I also did my first experiments on epilepsy, succeeding to establish conditioned Jacksonian seizures in dogs by combining sound with electrical stimulation of the motor cortex.

The topics of brain stem-thalamic activating systems, relationships between the cerebral cortex and subcortical structures, and the neurophysiology of epileptic seizure, which I approached in the 1950s with global electrophysiological methods, morphological techniques, and clinical observation, have remained close to my heart during my entire career. These developments are discussed below.

Encountering Frédéric Bremer

When the proofs of my book on the cerebellum arrived in 1957, I finally obtained permission to go to the publishing house in Paris (after repeated failures to obtain an exit visa for the International Congress of Neurology in Brussels, 1957) and, then, to stay on as a postdoctoral fellow in Bremer's laboratory in Brussels. Bremer was well known as a world-leading neurophysiologist for his work on the spinal cord and cerebellum (this is why he accepted me in the laboratory after I sent him my D.Sc. thesis). Bremer was especially well known for the crucial discoveries made possible by the two types of brain stem transections he introduced during the 1930s: the *encéphale isolé* preparation (with a bulbo-spinal cut), whose brain fluctuates between electrical activity patterns of waking and sleep; and the *cerveau isolé* preparation (with an intercollicular cut), which is comatose and displays uninterrupted sequences of spindle waves, virtually identical to those that occur during natural sleep. These discoveries led a decade later (in 1949) to the experiments by Moruzzi and Magoun on a brain stem reticular substrate of arousal. The Moruzzi–Magoun concept of sleep as a consequence of fall in the activity of brain stem reticular ascending impulses had the flavor of Bremer's ideas about the *tonus cortical* maintained by specific afferents acting on brain stem structures. Giuseppe Moruzzi had worked in Bremer's laboratory during the late 1930s, before he went to work with Lord Adrian in Cambridge. Most investigators used to consider the idea of a non-specific brain stem reticular activating system as opposite to Bremer's concept that specific sensory systems are responsible for the maintenance of the waking state. However, these two views are not irreconcilable because sensory pathways, which have access to discrete thalamocortical projections, also lead (through cortico-brain stem projections) to more widespread activation. Thus, Bremer and Carlo Terzuolo showed that cortical actions of specific sensory and motor systems have a descending effect on the upper brain stem reticular core, with the consequence that widespread cortical activation results from this cortico-brain stem feedback. Terzuolo worked in the Brussels laboratory a few years before me, and technicians in that lab told me that we were equally impetuous (to use a euphemism).

Bremer explained to me, from the very beginning, that he did not have the means to provide the cats I needed for my own experiments. So I asked him if he would agree that, after the end of the experiments he conducted with Nicolas Stoupel, I could continue on the same *encéphale isolé* cat until the nighttime. He accepted my proposal and afterwards he called me *"l'infatigable monsieur Steriade."* In line with my previous work on cerebello-cortical relations, I stimulated the auditory cerebellar area (revealed in the 1940s to 1950s by Ray Snider) and recorded different types of evoked potentials in the auditory cortex. To substantiate the hypothesis that longer latency responses in the postero-inferior ectosylvian area (in contrast to the primary responses recorded from the antero-superior ectosylvian field) are transmitted to cortex through a relay in the brain stem core, I lesioned the brain stem reticular core and abolished long-latency responses. (The possibility that connections between the primary and secondary ectosylvian areas may account for differences in latency, which came to my mind later, was not tested.) Bremer was interested in my findings and spent many afternoons discussing the data with me. Yet, when I asked him to co-author my article (in collaboration with Stoupel, who showed me how to do the electrolytic lesions), he said that when you see one or two authors on a paper, you may be (almost) sure who did the experiments, but beyond two ... then, he declined. One day, Bremer asked for my opinion about his manuscript on cerebral and cerebellar potentials that would be published in 1958 in *Physiological Reviews*. I first thought that he was joking because I did not feel capable of giving any useful opinion, certainly not about Bremer's article. But he insisted, so I read and made some minor comments that, obviously, couldn't basically change his review.

When I remember now those experiments (Bremer with Stoupel, and my own work), which began in the morning and ended quite late, I cannot forget how we made the photographs of evoked potentials on large, thick, glass slides, as was done by professionals until recent times. I am often amused to compare this technique with the faster method used during the 1970s, when my technician spent the day developing hundreds of meters of 35-mm films, or with the method of today, when we no longer use such techniques and instead whole figures with numerous panels (as in Eccles' illustrations) are made on computers.

I could not return to Brussels until 1965 because I was prevented for seven years from obtaining a passport (because of many, many errors on my part ...). One of those errors was that I had already been able to go abroad when, generally, Romanians were not allowed (exceptions were made, for example, for the Director of my Institute who went to many different congresses and symposia, but used to ask me about the polarity of evoked potentials before lecturing in Western countries). The other "error" (the Romanian word in the *langue de bois* of that time was "weakness," generally used in the plural) was that I continued to publish in international journals, such as the *Journal of Neurophysiology*, *Brain*, or *The EEG Journal*, instead of publishing in Russian, Bulgarian, or other highly recommended journals in "brotherly" countries. When Hsiang-Tung Chang arrived from Shanghai to lecture in Bucharest in 1965, he asked to see me (as he knew and had cited my 1960 *Journal of Neurophysiology* paper with Demetrescu, showing brain stem reticular effects on light-evoked responses in the lateral geniculate nucleus). However, I was "very ill" according to his officially appointed guide. Chang insisted, and eventually, I met him. He organized my visit at his brain institute in Shanghai. I did numerous experiments on cats in Shanghai, one every day, performing (rather bad) impalements of visual cortex neurons, which oscillated when the lateral geniculate nucleus was stimulated (one of those recordings is in my 1968 *Brain Research* paper on flash-evoked after-discharges). Chang taught me how to enter the thalamus without a stereotaxic apparatus (!), as he didn't have the equipment at that time. "Look," he said, while taking an oblique position with his stimulating electrode in his hand, positioned as in a martial art exercise. In exchange, I taught him the *encéphale isolé* preparation that I had learned in Bremer's laboratory because I wished to avoid the barbiturate anesthesia that Chang usually employed. But Chang was an immensely capable physiologist (his chapter on evoked potentials in the 1959 *Handbook of Physiology* is a gem), and I was a child compared to him and his knowledge. I met him for the last time in Pisa in 1980 at a symposium in honor of Moruzzi.

After so many years, things apparently changed a little (not very much) in Romania, and I was able to return to see Bremer in 1965. It was an afternoon, sometime in the spring, about 3:00 or 4:00 PM, when we had our rendezvous in his Brussels laboratory. I knocked at the door, and he opened, embraced me effusively, and, just a minute later, asked (after six or seven years of absence): "Tell me, Steriade, do you think there is an active inhibition in the cerebral cortex?" I don't know if my young colleagues know what was believed in the early 1960s, but at that time Bremer accepted inhibition in the spinal cord, while still thinking that there was no consistent evidence for active inhibitory processes in forebrain structures. I must say that the poor quality of some intracellular recordings in the 1960s might well have inspired Bremer's earlier skepticism about active inhibition in the thalamus and cortex. Nevertheless, I was amazed. I reminded him of his question later, in the 1970s, during a meeting in Bruges, and he laughed. Not only had he become aware of the presence of IPSPs in thalamic and cortical neurons, but he also assumed that inhibitory processes from the preoptic area to the upper brain stem reticular core may be operational in the process of falling asleep. He was among the first to conceive of this circuit. It was later that excitement developed about the hypnogenic properties that preoptic neurons might exert by inhibiting activating systems.

It must be clear by now what role Bremer played in my life: he was the only mentor that I highly admired and continue to love. In fact, I succeeded to impart this feeling to some of my former students, certainly to Diego Contreras. I remember the thrill while, on a tramway in Bucharest in 1961, I opened Moruzzi's *Archives Italiennes de Biologie* and found the (for me) astonishing sentence of Bremer's 1960 paper in which he confirmed my results with the brain stem reticular facilitation of photically evoked responses in the visual thalamus. I don't know if I cried, but, if not, I was not far from it. Generally, French investigators, among them some of my friends in Paris, do not much like Bremer because, they say, he was harsh in his public comments about some speakers (possibly themselves).

The place of Bremer in neuroscience is not assured by his place in the Medline or Citation Index because, as it sadly happens, our field is for today and possibly tomorrow, and (with some exceptions) the young researchers do not bother with papers published before yesterday. But Bremer's contributions are not limited to his crucial discoveries about the role played by brain stem structures in states of vigilance, which opened the path to modern investigations. He was the first, well before the 1990s work on gamma oscillations (the magical "40-Hz" rhythm), to report an *"accélération synchronisatrice"* of cortical electrical activity in response to arousing brain stem reticular stimulation (see the legend of Fig. 5 in his 1960 *Archives Italiennes de Biologie* paper [Bremer, Stoupel, and Van Reeth, 1960]). This expression sounded unorthodox at that time and for most investigators today, in view of the fact that Moruzzi's epigones describe this response as a "desynchronizing" reaction. Bremer's paper preceded by more than three decades the description of spontaneously occurring, synchronized gamma rhythms during brain-alert states, as demonstrated with multisite, extra- and intracellular recordings from cortical and thalamic neurons in my laboratory, as well as with magnetoencephalographic recordings in humans by Llinás and Ribary. Also, Bremer should be credited for his concept of autonomous neuronal activity (1949) that evolved into what is now known as *intrinsic* neuronal activity, a concept that has been added to the purely

reflexologic (input-output) view of brain operations. Intrinsic neuronal properties have been intensely studied since the early 1980s by Rodolfo Llinás and
many younger fellows working in brain slices maintained *in vitro*. Lately, I
have had to fight the simplistic assumptions of some colleagues who are not
shy to jump from a 0.4-mm-thick slice to global states of behavior; but this
occurred during the most recent (hopefully not last) period of my scientific
life and is discussed toward the end of this chapter.

Out of Romania

I left Romania in 1968. I intended to settle abroad because of the lack of
resources for science in that country and difficulties in maintaining normal relations with my colleagues in Western countries. This was indeed an
adventure for a man in his mid-40s. My first daughter, Donca, advised me to
follow regular procedures and ask for a legal passport to emigrate. It was difficult to follow such advice. Those who did so were first forced to leave their
job and then waited for long years, long enough to forget their earlier scientific training. Instead, I left Bucharest in May 1968 with a passport valid for
three months. Pierre Buser had invited me to deliver a lecture at the University of Paris, but the students were busy with the May "revolution" and
had better things to do than attend lectures. My French colleagues, Buser
and Yves Galifret, have been very friendly and generous with me; even my
first visit at the Institut Marey in 1966 could not have been possible without
the kind invitation of Denise Albe-Fessard, whom I had met in Warszaw in
1961, when both of us had been asked by Jerzy Konorski to give alternating
lectures during one week.

Turmoil reigned in Paris in May 1968, but that period is still favorably
colored for me by several encounters with Emil Cioran, a philosopher and
moralist of Romanian origin who is now appreciated as one of the most
accomplished stylists in French literature, a kind of improved Chamfort.
I tried first to talk with Cioran in Romanian, but he answered in French
"because I'm not yet perfect in this language" (he had been in France since
1938). We walked through the *Jardin du Luxembourg* (he lived next door at
the top floor of a building in an apartment like a monastery with a patio that
had a *vue imprenable sur le Théâtre de l'Odéon*), and we walked in the garden
of the *Palais Royal*, talking about Mao and minor dictators, such as the man
governing Romania at that time. While Cioran is known for his sharp mind,
he surprised me by saying "the truth is with you, with science." I laughed and
explained to him the ephemeral nature of scientific "truth," but I am sure
he stood by his convictions. I never could explain the style of Cioran, who
wrote with joy, delight, and roguishness about the inconvenience of being
born, the black despair of decomposition, and the syllogisms of bitterness.
He seemingly liked suffering those states of the soul or, more probably,
regarded ours with an Olympian eye.

As Paris was busy, I went to Marseille where Jean Massion, a distinguished investigator of motor control, asked me to meet Jean-Pierre Cordeau, who was a visiting professor from Montréal spending his sabbatical in Marseille. I had lunch with Cordeau. He knew me from some papers and, like that, without introduction, asked if I would accept a position of visiting professor at the Université de Montréal. I didn't think too much before saying yes. Back in Paris, I called the Director of my Institute in Bucharest to ask for permission to remain abroad for a longer period. He summoned me back immediately, but the Secretary of the Academy of Science, Professor Ştefan Milcu, wrote a very kind letter that permitted to stay. Cordeau asked when I would like to go (he paid for my flight ticket, for I was as poor as Job). I thought that August 20th (my birthday) would be a good start for a new life, and I left Paris with mixed hope and anguish.

Working in Canada: The Beginnings

I arrived in Montréal on the day Russians invaded Prague. My wife at the time sent me word from Bucharest, through a painter friend, to remain and try to bring our daughter, Donca, to Canada. My attempt to do this continued until 1973, when the Romanian ambassador invited me for lunch in Ottawa and asked me for my fondest wish. When I asked why I deserved the honor of this question, he answered candidly that I was known in circles of scientists and that I had never complained publicly about the regime. I simply said: my daughter. This took place on a Friday. The following Monday, two strapping fellows arrived at the University in Bucharest where my daughter was a student in classical philology, took her out of the amphitheater, and told her to pack her luggage immediately, as she would be leaving for Canada. Donca was not so ready to leave and certainly not on these terms. It was another year before I obtained a tourist passport for her, which was not the same as a definitive emigration. This passport has had the same destiny as mine: she arrived (greeted me with "hello" at the airport as if we had seen each other the day before), began studying linguistics, and received a Master's degree from Laval University. She then moved to Yale and MIT and is now a full Professor of Phonology at MIT (I don't know if she kept that 3-month 1974 passport). Those six years, from 1968 to 1974, until my daughter came, and the fear of what might happen to her and my wife at that time, cost me much sleep. This is not, however, the reason why I was, and continue to be, working on the topic of sleep for I do not deal with practical issues such as insomnia (and those who deal with such issues cannot influence the politics of bizarre governments or bosses who make life and sleep difficult).

I began working at the Université de Montréal, in collaboration with J.P. Cordeau, on brain stem reticular influences on auditory cortical responses, a topic we were both interested in. We had both published a series of papers on state-dependent changes in thalamic and cortical responses that are evoked by electrical stimuli applied to central pathways (see Steriade, 1970). At the first seminar I delivered, on fluctuations of cortical and thalamic responses evoked by central volleys during states of vigilance, Herbert Jasper asked me if we receive electrical stimuli during normal life and wondered why I did not use light flashes instead. Results with flash-evoked responses were also presented in my talk, but I preferred to answer that stroboscopic flashes are as abnormal as electrical stimuli applied to central pathways, with the disadvantage that there are additional synapses in the retina that may further complicate the data. Cordeau was delighted and told me after the seminar that my reply was the only way to deal with the great man if one did not want to be crushed. In any case, Jasper was extremely favorable to me throughout my Canadian career.

I never trusted Jasper's concept of a "centrencephalic system" that has no anatomical reality. Nor do I think that 3-Hz stimulation of the medial thalamus induced spike-wave complexes similar to those in absence (petit-mal) epilepsy, as he claimed in his 1949 paper with Drooglever-Fortuyn. This paper is a favorite citation for those who have read only the title and the abstract, without looking at the figure showing *responses* but no self-sustained activity, as should be the case in a seizure. Curiously, despite his preference for the idea that spike-wave seizures are generated by some deep-lying brain structures, Jasper was probably the first to show, in his 1938 paper with Hawkes, that EEG local epileptic activities may shift from one cortical region to another. Later, topographical analyses of spike-wave complexes in humans, carried out by others, showed that the "spike" component can propagate from one hemisphere to another with time lags as short as 15 ms, too quickly to be estimated by visual inspection. All these data are incompatible with the conventional notion of "suddenly generalized, bilaterally synchronous" spike-wave seizures due to a pacemaking "centrencephalic system." Since the 1970s, I have claimed that spike-wave seizures are cortical in origin, a conclusion based on experiments in behaving monkeys. In the 1990s, we strengthened this hypothesis with multisite, extra- and intracellular recordings from various cortical fields and thalamic nuclei. I fully disagreed with Jasper on this issue, and we publicly expressed our contradictory views in Marseille in 1974, when Henri Gastaut invited both of us to lecture in the same morning on the origin and mechanisms of spike-wave seizures.

In any case, I have always believed that Jasper's contribution to neuroscience was invaluable, and I am sure that some of his lapidary statements had a great influence on thinking in neuroscience, certainly on me. For example, Jasper's idea (1958) that activation processes are not entirely ascribable to a globally energizing process and that sculpturing inhibition should be included in the activated response was fully confirmed experimentally with extra- and intracellular recordings. Some very good investigators had reported during the 1960s and 1970s that a global disinhibition occurs in the thalamus as a consequence of brain stem reticular activating impulses (we learned later that this might have been due to the hyperpolarization of thalamic GABAergic reticular neurons). However, studies in several laboratories (mine and others, including the laboratory of Livingstone and Hubel) showed that prolonged and rhythmic inhibitory processes are blocked upon brain stem reticular stimulation or natural awakening, but that short-lasting inhibition is preserved, the specificity of the response in thalamic as well as neocortical neurons is enhanced, and irrelevant responses are eliminated. These findings made sense for a response that occurs during the waking state, at a time when sculpturing inhibition and discrimination processes would seem important. With my students Denis Paré and Roberto Curró Dossi, we showed that the earliest IPSP in thalamocortical neurons is enhanced during reticular-induced arousal (see below), in full confirmation of Jasper's idea that inhibition is included in the activation process. In the late 1950s, Jasper also asked rhetorically: "Can the melody of the mind be played on a (brain) keyboard ... with *rigidly determined functional characteristics?*" (italics mine), and he considered the role of widely distributed neuronal networks as well as the behavioral state of vigilance as determined by the effects of generalized activating systems. This simple question anticipated my view that the mechanisms underlying global states of behavior cannot be investigated in extremely simplified preparations that are fashionable nowadays and which were at the basis of research performed *in vivo* in my laboratory during the past decade. Moreover, the above question by Jasper anticipated our intracellular data obtained in the late 1990s, which showed that the firing patterns due to intrinsic properties of single neurons are not inflexible because they can be overwhelmed and drastically changed by synaptic activities in complex neuronal networks and by shifts in behavioral states of vigilance (see below).

In My Québec Laboratory during the 1970s and 1980s

After my arrival in Montréal, I was invited to lecture at many Canadian universities, including McGill where I always had friendly relations with Krnjević, and I received various proposals for a position as professor and researcher in neurosciences. Eventually, I accepted an offer for a permanent position at the Faculty of Medicine of Laval University in Québec, because there was no neuroscientist in that University and I thought it would be exciting to create a team. Québec, about 240 km northeast of Montréal (I mention this because many of my colleagues still ask me: "How is it in Montréal?"), is a small city, a provincial capital, and a university town. You can visit the old city, for which many tourists come to see "Europe," in about 1 hr. Otherwise, the city is a monastery for work in the lab, dinner with family, and sleep (with some recitals and chamber music, more and more rare because the public has come increasingly to prefer other types of entertainment).

I arrived in December 1968 and gave a lecture. The Head of the Physiology Department took me to his home and between the car and the house asked me if I would accept the salary he proposed. I thought I was becoming scandalously rich. Later on, he asked me why I did not bargain; I did not have any bargaining technique, and, to this day, I prefer to have none. (I have always thought that the salaries of researchers like me are too high. To avoid the entrance of undesirable people into the temple, one should give them less and see if they still express a passion for science. Otherwise, they may begin immediately to think about tenure and, not so long afterwards, to dream about retirement.) I immediately accepted, and we went for dinner in the old city. The rector (Rector Magnificus, a bishop, Monseigneur Parent, as it was a Catholic university at that time) sent me a long letter, containing the memorable words: *"Monsieur, vous êtes professeur à vie."* I wish it were as simple as that for my younger colleagues.

The initial space provided for my research was minuscule, but it progressively increased. As first pieces of equipment, I had some amplifiers, an oscilloscope, and one stimulator (not significantly more sophisticated than in Bucharest), but the laboratory continuously evolved into what it has now become. These days (especially when I arrive, about 6:00 AM), I go into the labs alone, look at them, and I do not believe my eyes. The Medical Research Council of Canada accepted my first grant application, and, since 1969, I have been continuously funded by this federal agency to the point that I received an award for maintaining uninterrupted grants during these 33 years. This is not the place to acknowledge the financial support for my research, but without it (from different Canadian federal agencies, the Human Frontier Science Program, and an RO1 from the U.S. National Institutes of Health), our research would not have been possible.

During 1969 I did experiments alone, recording along the cerebello-thalamo-cortical pathway. Thereafter, I accepted Ph.D. students. As I mentioned above, initially, I had few experimental facilities to offer my students. Improved facilities came later, during the luxurious 1980s and 1990s. This is why I decided to share a chronically implanted macaque monkey, making the left hemisphere available to one team for cortical recordings and the other hemisphere available to another group from my laboratory. One morning, they all came in my office and asked to have one animal for each team. (Don't forget that I came from Romania, where such an action would have caused trouble for the petitioners.) I had to make a quick decision: either I remain alone or I agree. I did the reasonable thing. During the 1970s my most gifted student was Martin Deschênes, who left his training in psychology to do experiments with me on neuronal activity in the motor cortex of cats and monkeys. The reason he left psychology, he explained to me, was that he had read my book on the physiology of visual pathways, which was published again at Masson in Paris (Steriade, 1969) and dealt mainly with my experiments.

Several findings came out of the work with Deschênes, and these were published as two companion papers in the *Journal of Neurophysiology* (Steriade and Deschênes, 1974). First, we dissociated the arousal-related firing rates of fast-conducting pyramidal cells from those of slow-conducting cells that were identified antidromically, and we characterized the discharge features of presumed local interneurons during sleep and waking. Interestingly, fast-conducting pyramidal cells stopped firing for about 10 sec upon natural arousal, but their antidromic responses were enhanced and the break between the initial segment and somadendritic components of action potentials disappeared. This observation suggested that the arrest in spontaneously occurring discharges does not reflect inhibition but disfacilitation, a hypothesis later confirmed by Oshima and his colleagues in Japan. Second, testing feedback and feedforward inhibitory processes in pyramidal neurons of monkey precentral gyrus during natural states of vigilance showed that well-pronounced (but short-lasting) inhibition during wakefulness provides a mechanism for accurately analyzing excitatory signals and for following rapidly recurring messages. Currently, we are doing experiments on the same topic using intracellular recordings in chronically implanted cats. Last, but not least, after Deschênes left for a postdoctoral term with Mike Bennett at the Albert Einstein School of Medicine in the Bronx, I was left to analyze the data, and, in addition to the sleep–waking findings, I discovered on tapes what subsequently became one of my favorite topics: the occurrence of seizures with spike-wave complexes during states of drowsiness or light sleep. This was an accidental finding. While the tape showed that the monkey was sleepy, the EEG potentials suddenly became so ample that the pen of the ink-writing machine started jumbling. I thought these were artifacts, but I fortunately diminished the gain and what I saw were beautiful, typical, spike-wave complexes in a seizure lasting about 12–15 sec that recurred in the same form several times. Simultaneously, there was an increased firing of neurons in the monkey's motor cortex during the EEG "spike" component, which was rhythmically interrupted by long pauses of the "wave" component. Focal field potentials recorded from the cortical depth, together with action potentials, displayed typical spike-wave complexes at 3 Hz (though the surface EEG did not always reflect the drama that was occurring in the cortical depth). Notably, at the beginning and end of these seizures the monkey had tonic eye movements, as in the absence epilepsy of children and adolescents. I wrote a paper, and this was the beginning of my current claim that spike-wave seizures originate in local neuronal pools of the cerebral cortex, only to spread later to other pools and, eventually, to the thalamus. Those 1974 data were at the origin of all our efforts in this direction during the late 1990s.

During the 1980s, our experiments multiplied in several directions. One set of studies dissected the electrophysiological basis of neuronal steps in the brain stem activating reticular system. With Lloyd Glenn, a postdoctoral fellow who did his Ph.D. with William Dement at Stanford, we identified in 1982 "beyond hypothesis the final corticopetal link in the anatomical substratum of the phenomenon of diffuse cortical arousal," as Nauta and Kuypers wrote in 1958, describing it as a topic for future experiments. In other words, we demonstrated monosynaptic excitation from midbrain reticular neurons to thalamocortical cells in intralaminar nuclei, which could be antidromically activated from different cortical areas. This bisynaptic, brain stem-thalamic-cortical link, which explained the prolonged somnolence of my 1958 patient with bilateral thalamic intralaminar lesions (see above), proved also to be the basis of PET activation in the midbrain reticular core and intralaminar thalamus during complex tasks in humans, as shown in 1996 by Roland's group in Stockholm. The widespread cortical projections of thalamic intralaminar nuclei, first shown anatomically by E.G. (Ted) Jones, explain the importance of this nuclear complex in the maintenance of alertness. With Glenn, we also investigated the firing patterns and excitability of thalamic intralaminar neurons during the whole waking–sleep cycle of cats. Another line of research during the 1980s was the combination of retrograde tracing techniques with immunohistochemistry to demonstrate the projections of mesopontine cholinergic neurons to thalamic relay, associational, intralaminar, and reticular nuclei in cats and monkeys.

The most important achievements of my laboratory during the 1980s have been the disclosure of the pacemaker role played by thalamic reticular GABAergic neurons in the generation of sleep spindles and the analysis of the low-threshold spike (LTS) response of thalamocortical neurons *in vivo*. To start with the LTS, Deschênes and I published this phenomenon in the early 1980s (a short paper in 1982 and a full-length paper in 1984). During the very same two years, Llinás and Jahnsen revealed this current and its ionic nature in thalamic slices maintained *in vitro*. It is fair to state, however, that Llinás discovered the LTS in an earlier paper on the inferior olive, published with Yosi Yarom in 1981, in which he suggested that similar events may take place in the thalamus (possibly, this guess may have been emboldened by some experiments on thalamic cells that were already in place). Of course, the transient Ca^{2+} current (I_T) that gives rise to the LTS was revealed *in vitro*, because the *in vitro* condition allows manipulations that can disclose ionic conductances (this is the *raison d'être* of slice work). We then decided to move *in vivo* and see how the LTS looks in the intact-brain animal. Actually, the animal was not so intact, as we worked intracellularly in the thalamus with a partially removed cortex to allow for the safe penetration of micropipettes. This technique is what we still use, although it is possible that completely intact corticothalamic as well as other synaptic projections may influence the intrinsic properties of thalamic cells.

In fact, more recently, Igor Timofeev, a postdoctoral fellow, and I have shown that the LTS is greatly modified by afferent synaptic activities arising in prethalamic relays such as the cerebellum (Timofeev and Steriade, 1997). The Ca^{2+}-mediated LTS, which is de-inactivated (uncovered) by membrane hyperpolarization, is probably the best example of similarity between the results obtained *in vitro* and *in vivo*. The LTS of thalamocortical neurons gives rise to a high-frequency burst of fast Na^+ action potentials (the postinhibitory rebound) that reach cortex. Therefore, this intrinsic neuronal property accounts for the transfer of thalamically generated sleep spindles to the cerebral cortex and their expression at the macroscopic level of the EEG. Nevertheless, the dissimilarities between data from slices and from intact-brain structures exceed the similarities. This is what we realized beginning in the mid-1980s and especially during the 1990s and is discussed below. To anticipate, the LTSs of thalamic anterior neurons are similar to those of other thalamocortical neurons, but, at least in cat, anterior nuclei do not receive synaptic connections from the pacemaker spindle generator (the thalamic reticular nucleus), and therefore, the anterior nuclei as well as their projection areas in the anterior cingulate gyrus do not display this sleep oscillation. Thus, intrinsic properties alone cannot generally account for the generation of oscillation. The only exception is the clock-delta rhythm of thalamocortical neurons, but that oscillation is also under the influence of corticothalamic and brain stem-thalamic synaptic activity (see below).

The description of LTSs in thalamic neurons and their role in spindle oscillations during sleep have been the topics of two symposia I organized in 1984 at The Neurosciences Institute of the Neuroscience Research Program, when it was at the Rockefeller University in Manhattan. The first symposium dealt mainly with the structure of thalamocortical systems, and the second symposium dealt with their functional properties. These two symposia have initiated a fruitful collaboration with Rodolfo Llinás and Ted Jones, which led to our 1990 monograph on the thalamus (Steriade, Jones, and Llinás, 1990).

Coming to sleep spindles, the neuronal mechanisms of this major brain rhythm have been elucidated intracellularly, first in my laboratory working *in vivo* since the 1980s (but also more recently) and, subsequently, in other laboratories working on thalamic slices during the 1990s. However, with the exception of hypotheses that have been tested in my laboratory very recently, showing that rhythmic sequences of spindle oscillations (or their experimental model, augmenting responses) may strengthen synaptic responses, the functional significance of these waxing-and-waning brain waves is not yet completely elucidated.

Despite the uncertainty as to their functional role, spindles have become quite fashionable due to numerous *in vitro* and *in computo* studies that followed our *in vivo* experiments. The slice work was done by David McCormick and his team at Yale. At a University of California at Los Angeles (UCLA) symposium on the thalamic reticular nucleus, organized by Arne Scheibel during the early 1990s, the speakers were asked to give publicly a brief explanation of what pushed them into research on the thalamus. McCormick kindly acknowledged that it was my 1984 review with Deschênes that opened his eyes and persuaded him to work on the thalamus. This statement has touched me, especially because I appreciated McCormick's experiments done with David Prince at Stanford and the collection of papers he produced with Prince on neurotransmitter actions on thalamic neurons. McCormick's work on spindle activity analyzed this rhythmic activity in lateral geniculate slices, as did Alain Destexhe's computational models, done first with Terry Sejnowski at the Salk Institute and later with me in Québec. One of the discrepancies between David's experimental results in slices and our data *in vivo* mainly concerned the absence of spindles in the isolated thalamic reticular nucleus in slices. *In vivo*, spindles are abolished in thalamocortical systems after lesions of thalamic reticular neurons, whereas this oscillation is preserved in the deafferented thalamic reticular nucleus. We agreed to explain the difference between our results in our 1993 long article in *Science* by a lack of intact collections of reticular neurons *in vitro*. The slicing procedure cuts the very long dendrites of these neurons (which are crucial in the generation of spindles) and thus mutilates the equipment required for this oscillation. Numerous modeling studies, reviewed in the recent monograph by Destexhe and Sejnowski (2001), predict the occurrence of spindles in the isolated GABAergic reticular nucleus. Other divergent results between *in vivo* and *in vitro* studies in the thalamus came later and are discussed in the next section.

The Last Decade Was the Most Exciting, in the Company of Gifted Students Who Taught and Tolerated Me

Throughout my career, I had a large number of excellent Ph.D. students and postdoctoral fellows, which reached a climax in the late 1980s and during the 1990s when I worked with (in chronological order) Denis Paré, Roberto Curró Dossi, Angel Nuñez, Florin Amzica, Diego Contreras, Igor Timofeev, Dag Neckelmann, and François Grenier, some of them Ph.D. students, some postdoctoral fellows, but all technically gifted and intellectually creative. The work was impressive: the experiments were done by a team in a room with the main electrophysiological setup, and the analysis of data was done the next day in another room with a similar setup while a second team took the experimental room. Note that before Denis left for Rutgers in December 2001, I had just one experimental room; in the past few months, I organized a second laboratory (the first for intracellular recordings in chronic animals, the second for acute experiments). People who visited me were amazed that, with a single setup, my young colleagues were able to produce the amount of data that came out of our laboratory. The man in charge of the electronic part of the work was, and is, responsible for the technical achievements; without Pierre Giguère, I don't think we would have been so happy.

Now, what did we do? The main topics are still (1) brain oscillations during states of vigilance and neuronal plasticity related to these rhythms; (2) the influences exerted by modulatory systems on thalamic and cortical responsiveness; and (3) the neuronal mechanisms of different types of electrical seizures, a project that has marked my scientific life since its beginnings. These three facets of my activity are closely interrelated. Thus, brain rhythms in the cerebral cortex and the thalamus are under the control of brain stem and forebrain modulatory systems, and the types of seizures we investigate occur with much greater propensity during slow-wave sleep than during waking or REM sleep. Although I have not changed radically the focus of my research, in that what we do currently reflects my early years in neuroscience, the techniques have greatly improved during the past seven or eight years. This apparently minor matter (minor only for those who do not rely on the electrical activity of neurons) has been essential in changing concepts in our field. Thus, dual intracellular recordings *in vivo*, which was science fiction a decade ago, have been accomplished by Florin Amzica in the neocortex and by Diego Contreras in cortex, as well as in related cortical and thalamic neurons (even triple such recordings are now feasible in Igor Timofeev's cortical slabs *in vivo*). Florin's analyses revealed unexpected temporal relations among neurons recorded from multiple sites; Diego demonstrated that thalamic oscillations are under the control of neocortex; and Igor succeeded in obtaining intracellular recordings in naturally sleeping and awake cats, which opens new windows in our research. All these studies, related to global behavioral states, require intact-brain preparations: for me, this is probably the most important notion I acquired during these recent years. This notion does not mean that we are inattentive to the host of ionic conductances in the neurons that we are recording. In fact, I think that each laboratory also needs an *in vitro* setup if the researcher wants to put his/her finger on the ionic nature of channels, the different subtypes of receptors, and so forth. But I am allergic to the use of great words, such as "sleep," "waking," "absence epilepsy," and even "consciousness," when referring to a 0.4-mm-thick brain tissue. In sum, we continue to work *in vivo* because this is the reality of the brain. Not long ago, we were regarded as the last of the Mohicans. However, this was illusion, or wishful thinking, as we (the Mohicans) are alive and well and some of the best *in vitro* investigators recently discovered the brain in its entirety and now perform nice experiments this way.

The 1990s began with a series of papers on neuronal activity recorded from mesopontine cholinergic neurons during the natural waking–sleep cycle and done with my Ph.D. students Denis Paré and Roberto Curró Dossi and other fellows. During transition from slow-wave sleep to either waking or REM sleep, we showed increases in firing rates in those neurons, in advance of the most precocious changes in global electrical activity of the forebrain. This finding suggests that a cardinal role is played by brain stem cholinergic neurons in these shifts from disconnected to activated states. Also, we described five types of neurons that fire or cease firing in conjunction with ponto-geniculo-occipital (PGO) potentials during REM sleep, while only one type had been known before. This led us to propose a plausible circuitry for the genesis of these potentials, "the stuff dreams are made of."

The very friendly relations between Denis and Roberto have been beneficial for the laboratory as they collaborated on a series of experiments. One of the most important of these led to the 1991 disclosure of a new type of IPSP in thalamocortical neurons, occurring before the well-known, biphasic $GABA_{A-B}$ components. The earliest, shortest, small-amplitude IPSP is Cl^- dependent (like the $GABA_A$-receptor-mediated one), and we postulated, on physiological and morphological grounds, that it is generated by presynaptic dendrites of local interneurons in glomeruli. The other series of experiments revealed that this IPSP, called $GABA_a$, which was confirmed one year later by Soltesz and Crunelli in another thalamic nucleus, is not obliterated by brain stem reticular arousing volleys and may even be enhanced. I cherished this finding in view of my earlier extracellular experiments at the cortical and thalamic level, which demonstrated that some inhibitory processes *must* be included in the process of brain activation (see above). The actions of brain stem cholinergic neurons on thalamocortical cells are not confined to simple depolarization and increased input resistance, as these actions lead to prolonged potentiation of synaptic responses in thalamic anterior (limbic) neurons. In papers and a book chapter published with Paré, we showed the muscarinic nature of this prolonged facilitation of synaptic responses that is induced by stimulating brain stem cholinergic nuclei, and we suggested that the cholinergic system could provide a way to regulate the flow of information along the mammillothalamic axis and modify the strength of the functional relationship between the hippocampal formation and cortical memory storage sites (see also Squire and Alvarez, 1995).

Other projects, with Curró Dossi and Nuñez, explored the relationships between oscillatory events generated by interplay between the ionic currents of thalamocortical cells and network (potentiating and suppressing) influences on these intrinsic properties. *In vitro* studies by McCormick and Pape, as well as by Leresche, Crunelli, and their colleagues in the early 1990s, have applied DiFrancesco's description of a pacemaker current (I_H) in cardiac cells to the level of thalamic neurons, which happen to oscillate, due to the interplay between I_H and I_T, within the frequency range of 1–4 Hz. We investigated intracellularly this oscillation *in vivo* and proposed that it represents the thalamic component of sleep delta waves. More importantly, we demonstrated that, despite the fact that this is an intrinsic oscillation of single cells, pools of thalamic neurons can be synchronized by corticothalamic inputs, which drive thalamic reticular GABAergic neurons and thus set thalamocortical neurons at a hyperpolarized membrane potential that is required for delta generation. Then, singly oscillating thalamic neurons can be synchronized by synaptic activity in corticothalamic networks, and this coherent activity is then reflected at the macroscopic EEG level. By contrast, data in the same 1991 paper showed that depolarization of thalamocortical cells by ascending activating cholinergic impulses results in obliteration of sleep delta potentials, as is indeed the case upon awakening. Our work had such an impact that many people in the EEG field took it for granted that *all* delta waves are generated in the thalamus, despite my cautionary note that this is just one component of delta waves, with the other being cortical in nature.

Looking for generators of delta activity (1–4 Hz) in visual thalamic reticular neurons, we did not find convincing evidence in this sector of the nucleus or in more rostral sectors. However, to our surprise, Curró Dossi and Contreras recorded a *slow* oscillation of intracellularly recorded thalamic reticular cells, with a frequency of less than 1 Hz. Where could such an oscillation possibly arise, which has the typical features of a synaptically generated rhythm and which has never been described before? Then, I decided to ask Nuñez and Amzica to look at the neocortical level, knowing that the most potent drive for GABAergic thalamic reticular neurons is the corticothalamic projection. We recorded neocortical neurons, and, indeed, in the first experiment in the summer of 1991, the *slow* oscillation appeared in its entire splendor, generally between 0.3 and 1 Hz. The disclosure of a novel brain rhythm in virtually all neocortical neurons (both pyramidal and local-circuit inhibitory cells, as subsequently identified by Contreras using intracellular staining) was surprising because of previous intensive investigations of cortical neurons. Probably, this sleep oscillation was ignored (like other slow or very slow rhythms) because low frequencies of EEG activity are so often filtered out. On the other hand, small cortical regions *in vitro* may exhibit synchronous activity, but such limited circuits are not adequate to support oscillations for prolonged periods of time unless the bathing milieu contains an abnormally high K^+ or other ionic manipulations that set cortical or thalamic neurons into action. The slow sleep brain oscillation gradually became so fashionable after our 1993 papers that it came to occupy researchers at many levels, ourselves *in vivo* in the beginning, but also EEG and MEG researchers of human sleep, and believe it or not, even *in vitro* investigators.

Francis Crick once asked me: "Why so many oscillations?" There are indeed at least three major types of brain rhythms during slow-wave sleep (spindle, delta, and slow oscillations). Their variations in frequency, patterns, origins, and underlying cellular mechanisms are due to the different electrophysiological and connectivity features of thalamocortical, thalamic reticular, and neocortical neurons that generate these brain rhythms. Nonetheless, to answer now Crick's reasonable question, the cortically generated slow oscillation, which we revealed in a series of three papers in one 1993 issue of *Journal of Neuroscience*, has the virtue of including other sleep rhythms generated in cortex and thalamus within complex wave sequences that contain both the slow oscillation and spindles as well as delta waves. This is due to the powerful impact of corticocortical and corticothalamic projections. Thus, *the variations in oscillation frequency are less important than the unified picture of sleep oscillations* that was detected by performing intracellular recordings from cortex or cortex and thalamus in collaboration with Nuñez, Amzica, Contreras, and Timofeev. In other words, the apparently "many oscillations" can be simplified into one complex oscillatory type. A recent paper on human sleep by other investigators (Mölle et al., 2002) supports this view. The cortical nature of the slow oscillation (it survives thalamectomy and brain stem transection) was recently confirmed in cortical slices by Mavi Sanchez and McCormick, and the impact of cortical inputs on metabotropic receptors of thalamic neurons was nicely demonstrated in thalamic slices by Crunelli and his group (Hughes et al., 2002). Still, the combination of slow and spindle oscillations within complex sequences can be seen only in intact corticothalamic networks. This combination gives rise to K-complexes, known for a long time in clinical EEG but only recently investigated intracellularly in our laboratory.

The slow sleep oscillation was studied in our laboratory during the past decade because it provided the best example of a unified corticothalamic network. At this point, let me confess that I am less interested in sleep per se than in the miraculous arrangement of long- and short-axoned neurons in the cortex and thalamus and in the control exerted by brain stem and basal forebrain modulatory systems upon them. We do not know why we sleep. One can speculate, but one can also approach the problem experimentally. We have tested our hypothesis that some sleep oscillations (in particular, spindles) contribute to plasticity and consolidation of memory traces acquired during wakefulness. These experiments were done in our laboratory, and computational models of experimental data were elaborated in collaboration with Maxim Bazhenov and Terry Sejnowski from The Salk Institute. First (1997) we demonstrated that short-term plasticity occurs in thalamic neurons of decorticated animals. This progressively increased synaptic responsiveness occurs in two forms: low-threshold and high-threshold augmentation. Second, in intact thalamocortical networks, we showed (1998) that cortical augmentation of responses is dependent on spike bursts fired by thalamic relay neurons, but cortical neurons oscillate in a self-sustained manner within the same frequency range as the evoked responses during the prior period of stimulation, whereas thalamic neurons simultaneously remain under the hyperpolarizing pressure from the GABAergic thalamic reticular neurons. If prolonged, the self-sustained cortical activity may reach dramatic intensity, and, ultimately, it becomes paroxysmal. Thus, the cortical neuronal equipment is itself capable of displaying normal as well as paroxysmal forms of plasticity, even in the absence of the thalamus.

Sleep and waking are reproducible behaviors that change the internal states of, and linkages among, all these neurons, thus teaching us how the brain operates on time scales from milliseconds to hours. This is why we (1) analyzed the effects of brain stem cholinergic and monoaminergic systems on cortical slow oscillations; (2) determined the ionic nature of the rhythmic, hyperpolarizing phase of the slow oscillation in acutely prepared and chronically implanted animals and demonstrated that this phase is not (as expected) inhibitory, i.e., it is not produced by local-circuit GABAergic actions, but is due to disfacilitation and some K^+ currents; (3) tested the responsiveness of cortical and thalamic neurons during different components of the slow oscillation; and (4) above all, realized that the slow sleep oscillation progressively develops, without discontinuity, into spike-wave seizures or the pattern of the Lennox-Gastaut syndrome that is a more severe epileptic disease than absence epilepsy. Needless to say, what we have studied in the past seven years is the neuronal basis of an electrographic pattern, strikingly resembling that seen in humans, and not the disease itself. This is why I never use the term *epilepsy*, but, instead, I refer to electrical seizures of one type or another, and I am always bemused when I read about "absence epilepsy" in some studies conducted on thalamic slices.

The studies on neuronal substrates of seizures strengthened the views expressed in my 1974 paper on behaving monkeys, namely, that spike-wave seizures originate in neocortex. I remember the summer of 1993, when I realized with Diego, using dual intracellular recordings from cortex and thalamus, that, during tempestuous activity in neocortical neurons, thalamic reticular neurons faithfully follow the paroxysmal depolarizing shifts in cortex, but thalamocortical neurons (targets of thalamic reticular GABAergic neurons) are steadily hyperpolarized and display phasic IPSPs that are closely related to each spike burst of cortical and thalamic reticular cells. The finding of thalamic reticular paroxysmal excitation, which contrasts with the sustained inhibition of thalamocortical cells (without rebound bursts), may be astonishing, but only for those who think that thalamic relay cells are actively implicated in the generation of spike-wave seizures. We published these findings in a 1995 *Journal of Neuroscience* paper, and they are now fully confirmed in genetic strains of rats that develop spike-wave seizures. Indeed, Crunelli's group showed, on the one hand, paroxysmal excitation of thalamic reticular neurons (Slaght et al., 2002) and, on the other hand, sustained hyperpolarization and phasic IPSPs in thalamocortical neurons during cortical spike-wave seizures in a strain of rats with inherited absence epilepsy (Pinault et al., 1998). The contrasting effects of corticothalamic paroxysmal volleys on thalamic reticular GABAergic neurons and on thalamocortical neurons have recently been explained by Ted Jones' team. They showed that the numbers of glutamate receptor subunit GluR4 are 3.7 times higher at corticothalamic synapses in thalamic reticular neurons, compared to thalamocortical neurons, and that the mean peak amplitude of corticothalamic excitatory postsynaptic currents (EPSCs) is about 2.5 times higher in thalamic reticular neurons than in thalamocortical neurons (Golshani, Liu, and Jones, 2001). In a series of four papers published in a 1998 issue of *Journal of Neurophysiology*, we showed that spike-wave seizures occur initially in the neocortex and spread only later to the thalamus.

If asked what have been the main achievements during the past decade, I would of course enumerate the above, but my personal focus was also to shed light on the innumerable differences between the results obtained by us and a few other colleagues working *in vivo* and those coming from extremely simplified preparations. Data from my laboratory, mentioned above, justify my assumption that topics dealing with complex behavioral states, from sensory experiences to motor control, states of vigilance, memory, and paroxysmal discharges, can only be approached in the intact brain. This may seem a trivial statement. Still, "those studying the intact brain are often asked to justify findings that diverge from those obtained *in vitro*." This sentence, from a book review (*Neuroscience*, 2003) of my 2001 MIT monograph by a distinguished *in vitro* researcher, Alex Thomson, working at the University College in London, seemed to her "humorous if it were not so dangerous." I remember, for example, that the depolarizing envelope of spike bursts fired by thalamic reticular neurons during spindles *in vivo* contrasted with a hyperpolarizing envelope found *in vitro*. Although everyone knows now that thalamic reticular neurons fire during spindles over a depolarizing envelope, the inference of the *in vitro* investigators was that the membrane *should be* deteriorated in experiments performed *in vivo*; later on, however, they realized by examining their own data that the depolarizing envelope is the reality at the level of membrane potential usually seen *in vivo*. Another example, from very recent intracellular recordings in behaving animals, involved my challenge of the idea that intrinsically bursting patterns of some pyramidal neurons are inflexible. One of the two reviewers (most probably an *in vitro* researcher who never did chronic experiments) asked that we provide morphological evidence using intracellular staining (note: in a chronically implanted animal who is studied for many long weeks!) that we were indeed recording from a pyramidal cell, as if this were the issue, rather than the change in firing pattern with shift in behavioral state. These are technical matters for most readers, but they indicate the climate of this kind of work.

Thus, in view of what we have learned since the 1980s, throughout the 1990s, and during the first years of this millennium, we continue to work *in vivo*, and my students who left the laboratory to become professors elsewhere have taken the same main path in their own research.

A Few Words on Some Subtle Issues: Circumscribed Neuronal Circuits, Neuronal Types, and Consciousness

I expressed my view on the tantalizing issue of the role played by specific neuronal types or circuits in consciousness in my book *The Intact and Sliced Brain* (Steriade, 2001b). This question excites nowadays many distinguished minds, especially theoreticians, as very few active neuroscientists devote more than a few brief sentences on this topic at the end of their papers, if they do so at all. This does *not* mean that consciousness, as a whole, is generated outside the brain, nor does it imply that some elementary components cannot be studied at the single neuron level. Indeed, different forms of memory have been investigated using neuronal recordings, attentive behavior has been studied in the cortex and thalamus, the brain stem circuitry that gives rise to thalamocortical processes that are implicated in dreaming mentation has been identified, and the sites of brain stem and thalamic lesions that produce loss of wakeful conscious states in humans have been described. These relations between neuronal activities and behavioral states merely refer to some *fragments* of activity that build up states of consciousness, but none of those studies (so numerous that is difficult to cite them here) were aimed at revealing the role of specific neuronal types or brain circuits in the generation of the global state of consciousness, which includes, of necessity, subjective experience. The crucial issue is that even the basic elements of first-order consciousness, namely, perceptual experience, imply subjective states, but the mechanisms behind the emergence of subjectivity are hidden.

Knowing that recordings of identified neuronal types cannot be made systematically in humans, and knowing that animals can perform behavioral tasks but do not possess the virtue of expressing their subjective states, how can consciousness be studied at the neuronal level? This is the major obstacle in understanding how action potentials can give rise to a subjective sensory experience—which is just a first step in consciousness.

Some authors have suggested that there are special sets of awareness neurons somewhere in cortical layer V, that these are bursting cells, and that it is only a matter of time before specific molecular markers are found in those neuronal elements of consciousness (Crick and Koch, 1998; Koch, 1998). It remains difficult to understand why layer V is important and not also layers III–IV or other layers; why only bursting and not also regular-spiking neurons are important; and what role fast-spiking inhibitory interneurons may have, which play a cardinal role in focusing attention on relevant messages by ignoring non-relevant signals during conscious states. The issue is that the firing patterns of cortical neuronal types are not inflexible, but change with the level of membrane potential and during epochs rich in synaptic activity, as is the case for wakeful consciousness. One of the most striking examples is the transformation of bursting cortical neurons into regular-spiking neurons, which occurs during transition from slow-wave sleep to brain-activated states, such as REM sleep or wakefulness (Steriade, Timofeev, and Grenier, 2001). Moreover, we showed in the same article that intrinsically bursting cells represent fewer than 5% of the cortical neuronal population, because their firing patterns transform into regular spiking during the waking state when consciousness arises. Thus, it is difficult to speculate about the role in consciousness of specific neuronal types having distinct firing patterns, because the intrinsic properties of neurons are overwhelmed by synaptic activities when shifts occur in the state of vigilance.

Confronted with these difficulties in relating consciousness to specific neuronal types, which are located in distinct cortical layers or neuronal circuits, thereby leaving aside many other brain systems, and confronted with the impossibility of having simultaneous access to electrophysiologically identified neurons belonging to all structures that organize conscious processes in a concerted way, those interested in subtle mental states may continue to read Flaubert, Dostoyevsky, Proust, and Joyce, among others, and to devote their research time to topics that can be defined more precisely and successfully attacked.

How Did My Life Arise and Develop?

These final lines remind me of those who created a privileged environment for my development.

My mother was not easygoing, and I am sure that my drive and working ability come from her. Her memory is always present, and I often think that she played a critical role in my career. She gave me professors for French and piano lessons beginning at age 5 and for German and English beginning at age 10 or 11. I stopped studying German when I entered the Faculty of Medicine. As for English, I tried to learn it again alone, much later, when I started writing papers. All these lessons beyond the usual schoolwork, especially the piano and French, completely filled my days. My mother used to come at 10:00 AM to the high school to bring me a sandwich (which she could have given me in the morning). But the point was not the sandwich. She wanted to know what grade I got on the math quiz or in natural sciences or history. If it was 9 or 10 out of 10, did someone else have the same or a better grade? The gap between my grades and those of other students was never satisfactory for her. She never spent the afternoon going out, as her friends did; all her time was devoted to me. Having quit school before the 10th grade, she could not always monitor efficiently my work in physics or other such subjects. For this reason, I had to learn the lessons in all their details to convince her that the job had been done. In her 90s, a decade ago, she often asked me on telephone (I was in Canada and she in Bucharest) if I was productive enough that year, "because, you know, you never worked very much." All in all, the relationship was not always peaceful, but she remained for me an example of how work could be done well and on time. My father, who completed only four years of elementary school classes but had intellectual inclinations (he wrote poems), was an admirable man whom I also loved. The only regret is that I did not spend enough time telling him about my work when I became a researcher.

I was blessed with two families, both of which I adore. I was first married to Fana, who gave me Donca in 1951. The family was close knit and we had extended, friendly debates around the dinner table, but at that time I was not very smart, as I often wanted to go out with my wife instead of being with my daughter at home. Since high school Donca grew very well, read the great novels of the Russian and French literature of the 19th century, and began publishing papers in literary periodicals. Now that she has become a well-known Professor of Phonology at UCLA and recently at MIT, those beginnings do not mean a lot for her, but they do for me. I suspect that she is more attracted to so-called hard science than to soft science, and this might explain why she lately moved closer to phonetics. Yet to me, the general rules of linguistics and the underlying brain mechanisms seem more exciting than the peripheral aspects. In any case, she was and continues to be a very close friend with whom I consult on every crucial occasion. There was a time when I used to call her my moral conscience, an expression that some of my friends strongly disapproved of. Besides my former wife, who remained a close friend, Donca is the only person with whom I use my native language. Our only opportunity to speak Romanian is during phone conversations and, more rarely, when we go together to Paris or elsewhere.

My second wife is French-Canadian. Jacqueline gave me the second daughter, Claude, in 1989, when I was 65. This was indeed a gift at my age, especially because being wiser I spend my evenings with her. We spend more time together on her piano and less at her schoolwork: she no longer needs supervision. My wife tells me that I am too demanding and that her gift for piano was acquired through tears (no longer now), but after all I am my mother's son. As with Fana and Donca, every evening is spent around the dinner table with Jacqueline and Claude discussing North American, France or Middle East politics, listening to classical music, and having fun. Claude is the best in her class and very good also at the Music Conservatory. We never leave her alone and do all our traveling in Europe with her. Donca is a very good advisor to Claude for readings of great literature and recommended *War and Peace* to her as well as other novels. I suggested that she read Flaubert, and Claude is now a great reader of French, Russian, and English literature. More recently, Donca suggested Plato's *Apology of Socrates*. To be sure that this would fit Claude, I took Plato's book on one of my travels and read and annotated it, identifying the passages I thought essential. Claude is now reading what seems to me was beyond my abilities when I was her age or even older. I do not know if her taste for classical music, literature, and good painting accounts for the closer relations she has with us, her parents, than with her peers, but I am not dissatisfied when it comes to the development of her inclination toward art and literature. When asked what will she do, she answers (of course) neurophysiology, but she may change her mind.

I spend all day at the laboratory, from very early in the morning, 6:00 AM or so, until late afternoon. I was the Head of the Department for a few years, but when asked if I would consider renewing my candidacy for the position, I declined because I dislike the administrative work. To me, the only activity that seems worth spending time on is the research. I am fully active, have grants for many years (possibly beyond my biological limit), and my country is wise enough not to ask for mandatory retirement of those who still want to work. Am I satisfied with what I have done? Yes and no. I am sure that some of our data have created paths for research and that what we are doing right now holds some promise toward an understanding of the functional significance of brain rhythms. Some of my former students and postdoctoral fellows continue to explore the thalamic and neocortical world with passion and with exciting results. But I am not so happy with my mathematical and physical background (despite my mother's supervision!). This is partially due to the fact that, since my arrival in Canada, I have always been in a hurry to produce and to produce, to prove to myself that I did not come for reasons other than research. Besides my laboratory and my family, I am also blessed with my love for music. However, knowing what really playing piano well means, I do feel pain when I sit and play. I also take a different approach from other non-professional pianists who, as a rule, go through the piece as best they can and take pleasure in it. I cannot play this way and instead work on a few lines at a time until I am satisfied, but I often get no further than some short parts of a sonata movement. Then, I decide to put on a CD and listen to Argerich, Benedetti Michelangeli, or Solomon or Sokolov or Perahia, and I get depressed. But afterward, I am able to show Claude how to play a few bars in a piece!

Everything is fine. Let's work.

Selected Bibliography

Achermann P, Borbély A. Low-frequency (<1 Hz) oscillations in the human sleep EEG. *Neuroscience* 1997;81:213–222.

Amzica F, Steriade M. Disconnection of intracortical synaptic linkages disrupts synchronization of a slow oscillation. *J Neurosci* 1995a;15:4658–4677.

Amzica F, Steriade M. Short- and long-range neuronal synchronization of the slow (<1 Hz) cortical oscillation. *J Neurophysiol* 1995b;75:20–38.

Amzica F, Steriade M. The K-complex: Its slow (<1 Hz) rhythmicity and relation to delta waves. *Neurology* 1997;49:952–959.

Amzica F, Steriade M. Neuronal and glial membrane potentials during sleep and paroxysmal oscillations in the cortex. *J Neurosci* 2000;20:6648–6665.

Andersen P, Andersson SA. *Physiological basis of the alpha rhythm.* New York: Appleton-Century-Crofts, 1968.

Bazhenov M, Timofeev I, Steriade M, Sejnowski TJ. Self-sustained rhythmic activity in the thalamic reticular nucleus mediated by depolarizing $GABA_A$ receptor potentials. *Nat Neurosci* 1999;2:168–174.

Bremer F. Cerveau "isolé" et physiologie du sommeil. *CR Soc Biol (Paris)* 1935;118:1235–1241.

Bremer F. Considérations sur l'origine et la nature des "ondes" cérébrales. *Electroencephalogr Clin Neurophysiol* 1949;1:177–193.

Bremer F. Cerebral and cerebellar potentials. *Physiol Rev* 1958;38:357–388.

Bremer F. The isolated brain and its aftermath. In Worden FG, Swazey JP, Adelman G, eds. *The neurosciences: paths of discovery.* Cambridge, MA: MIT Press, 1975;267–274.

Bremer F, Stoupel N, Van Reeth PC. Nouvelles recherches sur la facilitation et l'inhibition des potentiels évoqués corticaux dans l'éveil réticulaire. *Arch Ital Biol* 1960;98:229–247.

Bremer F, Terzuolo C. Contribution à l'étude des mécanismes physiologiques du maintien de l'activité vigile du cerveau. Interaction de la formation réticulée et de l'écorce cérébrale dans le processes du réveil. *Arch Int Physiol* 1954;62:157–178.

Chang H-T. The repetitive discharges of cortico-thalamic reverberating circuits. *J Neurophysiol* 1950;134:235–258.

Contreras D, Destexhe A, Sejnowski TJ, Steriade M. Control of spatiotemporal coherence of a thalamic oscillation by corticothalamic feedback. *Science* 1996;274:771–774.

Contreras D, Destexhe A, Sejnowski TJ, Steriade M. Spatiotemporal patterns of spindle oscillations in cortex and thalamus. *J Neurosci* 1997;17:1179–1196.

Contreras D, Steriade M. Cellular basis of EEG slow rhythms: A study of dynamic corticothalamic relationships. *J Neurosci* 1995;15:604–622.

Contreras D, Steriade M. Spindle oscillation: The role of corticothalamic feedback in a thalamically generated rhythm. *J Physiol (Lond)* 1996;490:159–179.

Crick F, Koch C. Consciousness and neuroscience. *Cereb Cortex* 1998;8:97–107.

Curró Dossi R, Nuñez A, Steriade M. Electrophysiology of a slow (0.5–4 Hz) intrinsic oscillation of cat thalamocortical neurones *in vivo. J Physiol (Lond)* 1992;447:215–234.

Curró Dossi R, Paré D, Steriade M. Short-lasting nicotinic and long-lasting muscarinic depolarizing responses of thalamocortical neurons to stimulation of mesopontine cholinergic nuclei. *J Neurophysiol* 1991;65:393–406.

Curró Dossi R, Paré D, Steriade M. Various types of inhibitory postsynaptic potentials in anterior thalamic cells are differentially altered by stimulation of laterodorsal tegmental cholinergic nucleus. *Neuroscience* 1992;47:279–289.

Deschênes M, Paradis M, Roy JP, Steriade M. Electrophysiology of neurons of lateral thalamic nuclei in cat: Resting properties and burst discharges. *J Neurophysiol* 1984;51:1196–1219.

Destexhe A, Contreras D, Steriade M. Spatiotemporal analysis of local field potentials and unit discharges in cat cerebral cortex during natural wake and sleep states. *J Neurosci* 1999;19:4595–4608.

Destexhe A, Sejnowski TJ. *Thalamocortical assembly.* Oxford: Oxford University Press, 2001.

Façon E, Steriade M, Wertheimer N. Hypersomnie prolongée engendrée par des lésions bilatérales du système activateur médial: Le syndrome thrombotique de la bifurcation du tronc basilaire. *Rev Neurol (Paris)* 1958;98:117–133.

Glenn LL, Steriade M. Discharge rate and excitability of cortically projecting intralaminar thalamic neurons during waking and sleep states. *J Neurosci* 1982; 2:1287–1404.

Golshani P, Liu XB, Jones EG. Differences in quantal amplitude reflect GluR4-subunit number at corticothalamic synapses on two populations of thalamic neurons. *Proc Natl Acad Sci USA* 2001;98:4172–4177.

Hughes SW, Cope DW, Blethlyn KL, Crunelli V. Cellular mechanisms of the slow ($<1\,Hz$) oscillation in thalamocortical neurons in vitro. *Neuron* 2002;33: 947–958.

Inubushi S, Kobayashi T, Oshima T, Torii S. An intracellular analysis of EEG arousal in cat motor cortex. *Jpn J Physiol* 1978;28:689–708.

Jahnsen H, Llinás R. Electrophysiological properties of guinea-pig thalamic neurones: An *in vitro* study. *J Physiol (Lond)* 1984a;349:205–226.

Jahnsen H, Llinás R. Ionic basis for electroresponsiveness and oscillatory properties of guinea-pig thalamic neurones *in vitro*. *J Physiol (Lond)* 1984b;349:227–247.

Jasper HH. Recent advances in our understanding of the ascending activities of the reticular system. In Jasper HH, Proctor LD, Knighton RS, Noshay WC, Costello RT, eds. *Reticular formation of the brain*. Boston: Little Brown, 1958;319–331.

Jasper HH. Problems of relating cellular and modular specificity to cognitive functions: Importance of state-dependent reactions. In Schmitt FO, Worden FG, Adelman G, Dennis SG, eds. *The organization of the cerebral cortex*. Cambridge, MA: MIT Press, 1981;375–393.

Jasper HH, Droogleever-Fortuyn J. Experimental studies on the functional anatomy of petit-mal epilepsy. *Res Publ Assoc Res Nerv Ment Dis* 1949;26:272–298.

Jasper HH, Hawkes WA. Electroencephalography. IV. Localization of seizure waves in epilepsy. *Arch Neurol (Chicago)* 1938;39:885–901.

Jones EG. *The thalamus*. New York: Plenum, 1985.

Kinomura S, Larsson J, Gulyás B, Roland P. Activation by attention of the human reticular formation and thalamic intralaminar nuclei. *Science* 1996;271:512–515.

Koch C. The neuroanatomy of visual consciousness. In Jasper HH, Descarries L, Castelucci VF, Rossignol S, eds. *Consciousness: At the frontiers of neuroscience*. *Adv Neurol* Philadelphia: Lippincott-Raven, 1998;77:229–241.

Leresche N, Lightowler S, Soltesz I, Jassik-Gerschenfeld D, Crunelli V. Low-frequency oscillatory activities intrinsic to rat and cat thalamocortical cells. *J Physiol (Lond)* 1991;441:155–174.

Livingstone MS, Hubel DH. Effects of sleep and arousal on the processing of visual information in the cat. *Nature* 1981;291:554–561.

Llinás RR. The intrinsic electrophysiological properties of mammalian neurons: Insights into central nervous system function. *Science* 1988;242:1654–1664.

Llinás RR, Paré, D. Of dreaming and wakefulness. *Neuroscience* 1991;44:521–535.

Llinás RR, Ribary U. Coherent 40-Hz oscillation characterizes dream state in humans. *Proc Natl Acad Sci USA* 1993;90:2078–2081.

Llinás RR, Yarom Y. Electrophysiology of mammalian inferior olivary neurones *in vitro*. Different types of voltage-dependent ionic conductances. *J Physiol (Lond)* 1981;315:549–567.

McCormick DA. Neurotransmitter actions in the thalamus and cerebral cortex and their role in neuromodulation of thalamocortical activity. *Progr Neurobiol* 1992;39:337–388.

McCormick DA, Pape HC. Properties of a hyperpolarization-activated cation current and its role in rhythmic oscillation in thalamic relay neurones. *J Physiol (Lond)* 1990;431:291–318.

Mölle M, Marshall L, Gais S, Born J. Grouping of spindle activity during slow oscillations in human non-REM sleep. *J Neurosci* 2002;12:10941–10947.

Moruzzi G. The sleep-waking cycle. *Ergeb Physiol* 1972;64:1–165.

Moruzzi G, Magoun HW. Brain stem reticular formation and activation of the EEG. *Electroencephalogr Clin Neurophysiol* 1949;1:455–473.

Nauta WJH, Kuypers HGJM. Some ascending pathways in the brain stem reticular formation. In Jasper HH, Proctor LD, Knighton RS, Noshay WC, Costello RT, eds. *Reticular formation of the brain*. Boston: Little Brown, 1958;3–30.

Neckelmann D, Amzica F, Steriade M. Spike-wave complexes and fast components of cortically generated seizures. III. Synchronizing mechanisms. *J Neurophysiol* 1998;80:1480–1494.

Paré D, Curró Dossi R, Steriade M. Three types of inhibitory postsynaptic potentials generated by interneurons in the anterior thalamic complex of cat. *J Neurophysiol* 1991;66:1190–1204.

Paré D, Steriade M. Control of mamillothalamic axis by brain stem cholinergic laterodorsal tegmental afferents: Possible involvement in mnemonic processes. In Steriade M, Biesold D, eds. *Brain cholinergic systems*. Oxford: Oxford University Press, 1990;337–354.

Paré D, Steriade M, Deschênes M, Oakson G. Physiological properties of anterior thalamic nuclei, a group devoid of inputs from the reticular thalamic nucleus. *J Neurophysiol* 1987;57:1669–1685.

Paré D, Steriade M, Deschênes M, Bouhassira D. Prolonged enhancement of anterior thalamic synaptic responsiveness by stimulation of a brain stem cholinergic group. *J Neurosci* 1990;10:20–33.

Pinault D, Leresche N, Charpier S, Deniau JM, Marescaux C, Vergnes M, Crunelli V. Intracellular recordings in thalamic neurones during spontaneous spike and wave discharges in rats with absence epilepsy. *J Physiol (Lond)* 1998;509:449–456.

Sanchez-Vives MV, McCormick DA. Cellular and network mechanisms of rhythmic recurrent activity in neocortex. *Nat Neurosci* 2000;3:1027–1034.

Simon NR, Mandshanden I, Lopes da Silva FH. A MEG study of sleep. *Brain Res* 2000;860:64–76.

Slaght SJ, Leresche N, Deniau JM, Crunelli V, and Charpier S. Activity of thalamic reticular neurons during spontaneous genetically determined spike and wave discharges. *J Neurosci* 2002;22:2323–2334.

Soltesz I, Crunelli V. $GABA_A$ and pre- and post-synaptic $GABA_B$ receptor-mediated responses in the lateral geniculate nucleus. *Progr Brain Res* 1992;90: 151–169.

Squire LR, Alvarez P. Retrograde amnesia and memory consolidation: A neurobiological perspective. *Curr Opin Neurobiol* 1995;5:169–177.

Steriade M. Development of evoked responses into self-sustained activity within amygdalo-hippocampal circuits. *Electroencephalogr Clin Neurophysiol* 1964;16: 221–236.

Steriade M. The flash-evoked after discharge. *Brain Res* 1968;9:169–212.

Steriade M. *Physiologie des Voies et Centres Visuels*. Paris: Masson, 1969.

Steriade M. Ascending control of thalamic and cortical responsiveness. *Int Rev Neurobiol* 1970;12:87–144.

Steriade M. Interneuronal epileptic discharges related to spike-and-wave cortical seizures in behaving monkeys. *Electroencephalogr Clin Neurophysiol* 1974;37: 247–263.

Steriade M. Cortical long-axoned cells and putative interneurons during the sleep-waking cycle. *Behav Brain Sci* 1978;3:465–514.

Steriade M. The excitatory-inhibitory sequence in thalamic and neocortical cells: State-related changes and regulatory systems. In Edelman GM, Gall WE, Cowan WM, eds. *Dynamic aspects of neocortical function*. New York: Wiley, 1984; 107–157.

Steriade M. Alertness, quiet sleep, dreaming. In Peters A, Jones EG, eds. *Cerebral cortex: Normal and altered states of function*, vol. 9. New York: Plenum, 1991; 279–357.

Steriade M. Synchronized activities of coupled oscillators in the cerebral cortex and thalamus at different levels of vigilance. *Cereb Cortex* 1997;7:583–604.

Steriade M. Coherent oscillations and short-term plasticity in corticothalamic networks. *Trends Neurosci* 1999;22:337–345.

Steriade M. Corticothalamic resonance, states of vigilance, and mentation. *Neuroscience* 2000;101:243–276.

Steriade M. Impact of network activities on neuronal properties in corticothalamic network. *J Neurophysiol* 2001a;86:1–39.

Steriade M. *The intact and sliced brain*. Cambridge, MA: MIT Press, 2001b.

Steriade M. *Neuronal substrates of sleep and epilepsy*. Cambridge: Cambridge University Press, 2003.

Steriade M, Amzica F, Contreras D. Synchronization of fast (30–40 Hz) spontaneous cortical rhythms during brain activation. *J Neurosci* 1996;16:392–417.

Steriade M, Amzica F, Neckelmann D, Timofeev I. Spike-wave complexes and fast runs of cortically generated seizures. II. Extra- and intracellular patterns. *J Neurophysiol* 1998;80:1456–1479.

Steriade M, Amzica F, Nuñez A. Cholinergic and noradrenergic modulation of the slow (~0.3 Hz) oscillation in neocortical cells. *J Neurophysiol* 1993;70:1384–1400.

Steriade M, Botez MI, Petrovici I. On certain dissociations of consciousness levels within the syndrome of akynetic mutism. *Psychiatr Neurol (Basel)* 1961;141: 38–58.

Steriade M, Contreras D. Relations between cortical and thalamic cellular events during transition from sleep pattern to paroxysmal activity. *J Neurosci* 1995;15: 623–642.

Steriade M, Contreras D, Amzica F, Timofeev I. Synchronization of fast (30–40 Hz) spontaneous oscillations in intrathalamic and thalamocortical networks. *J Neurosci* 1996;16:2788–2808.

Steriade M, Contreras D, Curró Dossi R, Nuñez A. The slow (<1 Hz) oscillation in reticular thalamic and thalamocortical neurons: Scenario of sleep rhythm generation in interacting thalamic and neocortical networks. *J Neurosci* 1993;13:3284–3299.

Steriade M, Curró Dossi R, Nuñez A. Network modulation of a slow intrinsic oscillation of cat thalamocortical neurons implicated in sleep delta waves: Cortical potentiation and brain stem cholinergic suppression. *J Neurosci* 1991;11: 3200–3217.

Steriade M, Datta S, Paré, D, Oakson G, Curró Dossi R. Neuronal activities in brain stem cholinergic nuclei related to tonic activation processes in thalamocortical systems. *J Neurosci* 1990;10:2541–2559.

Steriade M, Demetrescu M. Unspecific systems of inhibition and facilitation of potentials evoked by intermittent light. *J Neurophysiol* 1960;23:602–617.

Steriade M, Deschênes M. Inhibitory processes and interneuronal apparatus in motor cortex during sleep and waking. II. Recurrent and afferent inhibition of pyramidal tract neurons. *J Neurophysiol* 1974;37:1093–1113.

Steriade M, Deschênes M. The thalamus as a neuronal oscillator. *Brain Res Rev* 1984;8:1–63.

Steriade M, Deschênes M, Oakson G. Inhibitory processes and interneuronal apparatus in motor cortex during sleep and waking. I. Background firing and synaptic responsiveness of pyramidal tract neurons and interneurons. *J Neurophysiol* 1974;37:1065–1092.

Steriade M, Deschênes M, Domich L, Mulle C. Abolition of spindle oscillations in thalamic neurons disconnected from nucleus reticularis thalami. *J Neurophysiol* 1985;54:1473–1497.

Steriade M, Domich L, Oakson G, Deschênes M. The deafferented reticularis thalami nucleus generates spindle rhythmicity. *J Neurophysiol* 1987;57:260–273.

Steriade M, Glenn LL. Neocortical and caudate projections of intralaminar thalamic neurons and their synaptic excitation from the midbrain reticular core. *J Neurophysiol* 1982;48:352–371.

Steriade M, Hobson JA. Neuronal activity during the sleep-waking cycle. *Progr Neurobiol* 1976;6:165–376.

Steriade M, Jones EG, Llinás RR. *Thalamic oscillations and signaling.* New York: Wiley-Interscience, 1990.

Steriade M, Jones EG, McCormick DA. *Thalamus: Organisation and function* Vol. 1, Oxford: Elsevier, 1997.

Steriade M, Llinás RR. The functional states of the thalamus and the associated neuronal interplay. *Physiol Rev* 1988;68:649–742.

Steriade M, McCarley RW. *Brain stem control of wakefulness and sleep.* New York: Plenum, 1990.

Steriade M, McCormick DA, Sejnowski TJ. Thalamocortical oscillation in the sleeping and aroused brain. *Science* 1993;262:679–685.

Steriade M, Nuñez A, Amzica F. A novel slow (<1 Hz) oscillation of neocortical neurons *in vivo*: Depolarizing and hyperpolarizing components. *J Neurosci* 1993a;13: 3252–3265.

Steriade M, Nuñez A, Amzica F. Intracellular analysis of relations between the slow (<1 Hz) neocortical oscillation and other sleep rhythms. *J Neurosci* 1993b;13:3266–3283.

Steriade M, Paré, D, Datta S, Oakson G, Curró Dossi R. Different cellular types in mesopontine cholinergic nuclei related to ponto-geniculo-occipital waves. *J Neurosci* 1990;10:2560–2579.

Steriade M, Paré, D, Hu B, Deschênes M. *The visual thalamocortical system and its modulation from the brain stem core.* Berlin: Springer-Verlag, 1990.

Steriade M, Paré, D, Parent A, Smith Y. Projections of cholinergic and non-cholinergic neurons of the brain stem core to relay and associational thalamic nuclei in the cat and macaque monkey. *Neuroscience* 1988;25:47–67.

Steriade M, Parent A, Hada J. Thalamic projections of nucleus reticularis thalami: A study using retrograde transport of horseradish peroxidase and double fluorescent tracers. *J Comp Neurol* 1984;229:531–547.

Steriade M, Timofeev I. Neuronal plasticity in thalamocortical networks during sleep and waking oscillations. *Neuron* 2003;37:563–576.

Steriade M, Timofeev I, Dürmüller N, Grenier F. Dynamic properties of corticothalamic neurons and local cortical interneurons generating fast rhythmic (30–40 Hz) spike bursts. *J Neurophysiol* 1998;79:483–490.

Steriade M, Timofeev I, and Grenier F. Natural waking and sleep states: A view from inside neocortical neurons. *J Neurophysiol* 2001;85:1969–1985.

Steriade M, Timofeev I, Grenier F, Dürmüller N. Role of thalamic and cortical neurons in augmenting responses: Dual intracellular recordings *in vivo*. *J Neurosci* 1998;18:6425–6443.

Timofeev I, Bazhenov M, Sejnowski TJ, Steriade M. Contribution of intrinsic and synaptic factors in the desynchronization of thalamic oscillatory activity. *Thal Relat Syst* 2001;1:53–69.

Timofeev I, Grenier F, Bazhenov M, Sejnowski TJ, Steriade M. Origin of slow oscillations in deafferented cortical slabs. *Cereb Cortex* 2000;10:1185–1199.

Timofeev I, Grenier F, Steriade M. Disfacilitation and active inhibition in the neocortex during the natural sleep-wake cycle. *Proc Natl Acad Sci USA* 2001;98:1924–1929.

Timofeev I, Steriade M. Fast (mainly 30–100 Hz) oscillations in the cat cerebellothalamic pathway and their synchronization with cortical potentials. *J Physiol (Lond)* 1997;504:153–168.

Richard F. Thompson

Judith R. Thompson

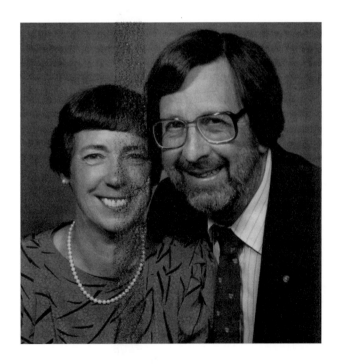

Richard F. Thompson

BORN:
Portland, Oregon
September 6, 1930

EDUCATION:
Reed College, B.A. (Psychology, 1952)
University of Wisconsin, M.S. (Psychology, 1953)
University of Wisconsin, Ph.D. (Psychology, 1956)
University of Wisconsin, Postdoctoral Fellow
(Neurophysiology, 1956–1959)

APPOINTMENTS:
University of Oregon Medial School (1959)
University of California, Irvine (1967)
Harvard University (1973)
Stanford University (1980)
University of Southern California (1987)

HONORS AND AWARDS (SELECTED):
Councilor, Society for Neuroscience (1972–1976)
Society of Experimental Psychologists (1973)
Warren Medal, Society of Experimental Psychologists (1989)
President, Division 6, American Psychological Association (1972)
Distinguished Scientific Contribution Award,
American Psychological Association (1977)
National Academy of Sciences, USA (1977)
American Academy of Arts and Sciences (1989)
William James Fellow, American Psychological Society (1989)
President, American Psychological Society (1995–1996)
President, Western Psychological Association (1994–1995)
John P. McGovern Award (1999)
American Philosophical Society (1999)

Richard F. Thompson pioneered the use of simplified neural and behavioral systems in mammals to study basic processes of learning and memory. With William Alden Spencer, he showed that spinal flexion reflexes exhibited the properties of behavioral habituation and sensitization and analyzed putative mechanisms. Using classical conditioning of discrete responses (e.g., eyeblink) in mammals, he and his associates identified the cerebellum and its associated circuitry as the essential neural system for this form of learning; identified the CS, US, and CR pathways; localized the "basic" memory trace to the interpositus nucleus; and elucidated the role of the cerebellar cortex.

Richard F. Thompson

I was born September 6, 1930, in Portland, OR. My father, Frederick Albert Thompson, Jr., worked for the International Harvester Co., initially in Southern California. He was transferred to the Portland branch of the company in 1928 as office manager and later as branch manager. My mother, Margaret St. Claire Marr, and he were married in 1922 in San Francisco and lived initially in Southern California. Although they tried for years to have children, I was the only issue.

A few words about my family history. My father's father, Frederick Albert Thompson, was a career army man, a captain, and was for a time stationed in the Philippines, where my father spent part of his childhood. My grandfather apparently played a role in the development of Army Camp Kearney in Southern California. My father returned to the Oakland, CA, area for high school and then attended the University of California at Berkeley for one year; he then enlisted in the army at the U.S. entry into World War I. He was a lieutenant and sharp shooter instructor and did not serve overseas. After the war he farmed for a while, and then after marriage became an accountant, eventually with the Harvestor Co. (My mother, having grown up on a farm, gave him the choice of marrying her or farming.) My father was a very good and gentle man.

My mother had a remarkable career for a woman of that era. She was the youngest of nine children born and raised on a farm in New Brunswick, Canada. Her family name was Marr—the family came originally from Scotland before the revolution and settled in the colonies. Apparently, they were loyalists because they moved to New Brunswick before the revolution. An ancestor Marr fought on the British side in the revolution. It is likely that a Thompson of the time fought on the U.S. side.

My mother attended normal school to train as a teacher and taught school in New Brunswick. She saved enough money to train as a nurse at the Peter Bent Brigham Hospital in Boston, MA. When World War I began, she enlisted in the British army nurses corps, spent time in the front line hospitals in France, and was awarded a citation by King George V. She returned to Boston and when the United States entered the war, she joined the U.S. army nurses corps and went to France again. She kept a diary of her experiences in France, which I treasure.

The Early Years

In retrospect, growing up in Portland before World War II was about as idyllic as one could hope, although I of course did not realize it at the time. We lived in a modest house near Grant High School, which had a large public playground, swimming pools, and tennis courts. In my early years my mother and I would go there every day in the summer if the weather was nice. I learned to swim there at an early age.

There was a street car stop only a few blocks from our house, and my friends and I (grade school age) would take it downtown regularly on weekends and in the summer. Portland seemed a very safe place then. The stop where I got on and off was at Thompson Street. The conductor got to know us, and when we came to my stop he would call out "Thompson street for Dick Thompson!" Growing up, I had several very close friends in the neighborhood.

In grade school we were thoroughly drilled in the basics, although I somehow never mastered penmanship. One remarkable teacher stands out in my memory: Miss Crawford. She was an Irish lady who wore dark wool suits and button top shoes. She taught natural history and a good deal about life and morality. She kept us enthralled with her stories of how the British would mow down innocent Irish people. But more important, she taught us literature, an episode at a time. I think it took her at least a semester to read us the full novel *Les Miserables*.

I had learned to read before I entered first grade (no kindergarten in those days) and early on read voraciously everything from Peter Rabbit to Viking legends. Perhaps it was Miss Crawford who introduced me to good literature. Later and into the high school years, I would take the street car downtown to Portland's main library on 10th Avenue and check out a pile of books each week. I started at the A's in novels and read all the way to the Z's.

During the years from about 10 to 15, I developed interests in chemistry and electricity. Early on I had a chemistry set that I expanded. I began with color change assays, but found this rather dull and branched out. In those days in Portland kids could buy almost any chemical, including very dangerous ones. We discovered sodium. We could buy a pound of the metal for about a dollar. Sodium, of course, catches fire and explodes when it comes in contact with water, which led to all sorts of possibilities. Our greatest achievement was a sodium cannon—an iron pipe with an inside diameter a little larger than a marble and sealed at one end. We filled it half full of water and dropped in some sodium and a marble. We set it up in my backyard and aimed it at our garage wall. Our first trial was our last. There was an incredible explosion that blew the marble entirely through the garage wall. Several neighbors came running, thinking our furnace had exploded.

My fascination with electricity stemmed, in part, from a biography of Nikola Tesla. A friend and I constructed a Tesla coil to generate very high frequency, high voltage in my room. We made a spark gap out of two nails; our condenser was a milk bottle half full of salt water and wrapped in tinfoil; the power source was a 15,000-V transformer we obtained from a neon sign shop. I gave "shows" for my long-suffering parents and their friends. Holding a metal rod, I would draw a large continuous spark from the coil, and it would light up a light bulb I held in my other hand. (I also put on magic shows, but I fear my talents did not lie in that direction.)

When activated, our Tesla coil system broadcast a wide band electrical signal that caused very loud static in radios in a several mile radius. My friend had a Tesla setup as well, and we would send signals to each other via radios. Of course, everyone in that part of town also received our loud static signals on their radios. Given that this occurred in the war years, it is surprising no authorities ever investigated us.

I was also generally very interested in science and the "big" questions— the nature of the universe and the mind. It wasn't until I was in Grant High School that I realized education had anything at all to do with my interests. I took all the math and science courses, Latin, and extra literature. The most remarkable teacher I had was Miss Curie (no relation to the Nobel Laureate), who taught physics. She had worked as a graduate student with the physicist Robert Milliken and told us many stories. For extra credit, I made heavy water, only to have the janitor dump it down the drain.

Reed College, 1948–1952

I entered Reed College in 1948 with the intention of majoring in theoretical physics. Reed was (and is) remarkable—the course work was intense, and we read several full volumes a week in the humanities course. For the first time I really had to work at my studies. In my sophomore year in physics, I attempted to repeat Milliken's measurement of the charge on the electron and failed. More important, several of my classmates had an intuitive grasp of math and physics that I did not. I was good at math, enjoyed it and could work through the problems, but with no intuition. I began to have second thoughts about my major.

I became very interested in philosophy and read widely, particularly in epistemology. Writers such as Bertrand Russell, Ludwig Wittgenstein, and others convinced me, at least, that science, as imperfect as it is, was the only way to learn about "reality." At about that time I took Introductory Psychology from Monty Griffith, a Welshman who was an early admirer of John Watson and behaviorism. He was a realist, some would say cynic, and cut through much of the mystique in the field. He was also intellectually brilliant and entertaining. The other key faculty member in the Psychology

Department was Fred Courts, an excellent behavioral scientist who had done research on human factors. Thanks in part to Monty and Fred, I changed my major to psychology.

At Reed, all seniors had to complete a comprehensive thesis. I attempted to solve the continuity–non-continuity controversy—do we learn to see new perceptions by building on details (continuity) or do so *de novo* (non-continuity) as gestalts? Karl Lashley argued the latter. I built a Lashley jumping stand: rats had to jump from a platform against one of two cards. The correct card would fall back and the rat could enter and obtain food. The incorrect card would not move and the rat would fall onto a hammock. I had planned the experiment carefully, but had not counted on the rats. No self-respecting rat would jump against a wall; instead, if they jumped at all, most jumped all the way down to the floor. I did manage to get some data, but my results were inconclusive. However, I learned a good bit about rat psychology.

University of Wisconsin—Graduate and Postdoctoral Years, 1952–1959

In any event, I became greatly interested in brain bases of behavior, particularly learning and memory. I applied to several graduate schools and received good offers from W.J. Brogden at the University of Wisconsin in Madison and Kenneth Spence at the University of Iowa. Fred Courts advised me to go with Brogden, who had done classic work with Culler and Gantt on brain substrates of learning. However, when I arrived in Madison, I discovered that Brogden had changed his interests to human learning and performance. So I completed several studies of target pursuit learning and learning of "mental mazes" with fellow graduate students George Briggs and James Voss. Although at the time I was unhappy about this, in retrospect it was very good experience. Brogden was a very rigorous behavioral scientist with the highest standards. I learned scientific writing by his tearing apart my drafts over and over again.

The Psychology Department at the University of Wisconsin at that time was extraordinary. A number of leading behavioral scientists were at their most productive periods—Wulf Brogden, Jack Gilchrist, David Grant, Harry Harlow, Hershel Liebowitz, Fred Mote, Donald Meyer (a visiting Professor) and Will Thurlow. Clinton Woolsey's neurophysiology laboratory at the medical school (all on the same campus) was deeply involved in brain-behavior research and encouraged psychology graduate students to participate.

The Wisconsin psychology faculty had a strong empirical orientation; it was sometimes referred to by more theoretically oriented psychology departments as the "dust bowl of empiricism." (Harry Harlow had a chamber pot so labeled in his office.) But the Wisconsin faculty were broadly interested in the issues of psychology at that time. Looking back, we, the graduate students, felt that the 1950s were the golden years of the Department. My fellow students of that era included Norman Anderson, William Battig, Lyle Bourne, George Briggs, Gilbert French, Isidore Gormezano, Leslie Hicks, William Prokasy, Allan Schrier, Joseph Sidowski, and James Voss. The graduate program then was Darwinian. I believe more than 30 began in my graduate class and 6 received their Ph.D.

As was true of many others, my interests in brain substrates of memory were greatly stimulated by Donald Hebb's remarkable book *The Organization of Behavior* (1949). Hebb tried to reconcile Lashley's "mass action" with neuronal connectivity. Hebb's book revitalized this field, which had been somewhat dormant since Lashley's 1929 monograph. When it came to details, Hebb was rather lacking, particularly about synaptic processes. But in all fairness, John Eccles discovered synaptic inhibition only about the same time as Hebb's book.

Because of my interests, Brogden agreed to set up an animal training laboratory and Woolsey graciously allowed us to do so in his facilities. I completed several studies of *sensory preconditioning* using shock avoidance with cats. Brogden had discovered this phenomenon much earlier working in Gantt's laboratory at Johns Hopkins. I also began a series of studies on stimulus generalization and lesion studies on the role of the auditory cortex in frequency discrimination (cats) (Thompson, 1960). I obtained a three-year NIH postdoctoral fellowship to work with Woolsey.

Woolsey's laboratory was a most exciting environment. Much of the work focused on the organization of the motor cortex in a series of primates, including chimpanzees, using electrical stimulation and on the organization of sensory cortical areas using surface-evoked potentials. P.W. Davies visited the lab and described the new extracellular microelectrode technique he and Jerzy Rose had developed at Johns Hopkins. During that time (Davies taught us a seminar), I read the Hodgkin–Huxley papers with great admiration. Jerzy Rose visited one summer, and using the Davies–Rose electrode, we completed the first single-unit recording study of the tonotopic organization of the primary auditory cortex (in cat) (see Hind et al., 1960).

During my time (and of course, earlier and later, as well) there were extraordinarily talented scientists in the laboratory. Konrad Akert provided solid expertise in neuroanatomy; Joseph Hind was expert in the auditory system and all matters acoustic; and W.I. Welker and Robert Benjamin were young scientists at the height of their productivity. There were many others as well. Woolsey was a very tolerant laboratory chief. If the work we did was to some degree relevant to cortical organization and functions and was carefully done, we were free to follow our own interests. Personally, Woolsey was a gentle man. I never saw him lose his temper. He was an ideal role model in that he was totally focused on the work (and his family), was objective, and never engaged in *ad hominem*. However, if you took a particular position on cortical organization, you had better be prepared to defend it. He had very high standards and expected the same of everyone. Morale in Woolsey's laboratory was extremely high.

Woolsey was a superb but infrequent lecturer, often teaching by demonstration. At that time, textbooks stated that complete removal of the neocortex in monkeys caused virtual paralysis. In the medical student physiology course, Woolsey once demonstrated a fully decorticate rhesus monkey, which he held on a stick chain while the monkey chased him around the lectern trying to bite him. This finding was, of course, much more than simply a demonstration. Travis and Woolsey showed that after bilateral removal of all neocortex in stages, monkeys could show considerable recovery of motor function and became capable of locomotion if given adequate postoperative physical therapy. Recovery of function following brain injury was of deep interest to Woolsey. I assisted Woolsey in preparation of two of the decorticate macaques (we did them in two stages) and in their postoperative care. Woolsey had developed a method of subpial surgical aspiration of cortex that made it possible to remove localized regions without damage to adjacent regions or of an entire hemisphere of cortex with minimal bleeding. He was a superb experimental neurosurgeon; my skill in this area is due to his teaching.

In Woolsey's lab, Ron Sindberg and I began mapping auditory and association areas of the neocortex in cat using chloralose anesthetic, which provided very responsive cortical tissue. At that time, several scientists in France, particularly Pierre Buser and Madam Albe-Fessard, had reported separate sensory responsive areas in association areas of the cortex. In this initial work, Ron and I looked at association areas (see Thompson and Sindberg, 1960) and at auditory responses in a region of ventral auditory cortex that we discovered. We used the difficult technique that Woolsey and Walzl had developed of electrically stimulating different regions of auditory nerve fibers in the exposed cochlea to determine tonotopic organization. In addition, I studied neuroanatomy with Konrad Akert and collaborated with Joseph Hind, W.I. Welker, Robert Benjamin, William Cox, Jean Hirsch, and others on various research projects.

The University of Oregon Medical School, 1959–1967

In 1959 I accepted an appointment as an Assistant Professor at the University of Oregon Medical School, initially in the Psychiatry Department under George Saslow as Chairman and subsequently in the Department of Medical Psychology when it formed as a separate department under Joseph D. Matarazzo as Chairman. My responsibilities were to do research and to teach a little to medical and graduate students. I was indebted to John Brookhart, Chairman of the Physiology Department, for providing much encouragement and advice and also my first laboratory—a small room in the basement that quickly became both overcrowded and immensely stimulating. Ron Sindberg spent a brief time in my laboratory in Portland, and we completed our study of the ventral auditory cortex (Sindberg and Thompson, 1962).

The move back to Portland was exactly what I had wished for. Indeed, I was thrilled when Woolsey told me of the job and offered to write a letter, as did Wulf Brogden, Harry Harlow, and others. So I returned home. My mother had died when I was in Wisconsin, and I moved into my father's house. We lived very happily—he was a great cook and I know he enjoyed having someone in the house—he had been alone since my mother died. I was single, had a great place to live, had a great job, owned an Austin-Healy sports car, and really felt on top of the world. But I stress that my world was mostly science.

There were other reasons why the move back to Portland was important to me. Growing up, my closest friend was Michael Baird. We went to grade school, high school, and college together. When I went to Wisconsin he entered the University of Oregon Medical School, and when I returned he was just completing a residency in internal medicine. His father, David Baird, was Dean of the Medical School, and I knew the family well. Michael and I had become good friends with William Alden Spencer at Reed College. Indeed, Michael later married Alden's sister Jane. Alden also went to the University of Oregon Medical School and did elegant research with John Brookhart. After a rotating internship, Alden joined the NIH for the research equivalent of a residency in Wade Marshall's laboratory, where he and Eric Kandel did their pioneering work on hippocampal physiology. Alden later return to the University of Oregon Medical School in the Physiology Department in 1961. Alden and I developed a joint research program which I will describe later.

While working with medical students and my superb technician, Hilton Smith, I made the first discovery that was entirely my own. In the course of carefully mapping the sensory responsive regions in associative areas (cat), à la Woolsey, I realized that the responses were not sensory specific, but rather polymodal. The French scientists had always described them as sensory specific, but they were not—the areas of activation were identical for all three modalities of stimulation (auditory, visual, tactile) and the responses showed the same refractory periods both within and across modalities. I was very excited by this discovery and submitted an abstract to the XXII International Congress of Physiological Sciences in Holland in 1962, my first solo presentation at an international meeting.

When I stood up to give my talk, Madam Albe-Fessard came to the front of the room, stood directly in front of me with her arms crossed, and glowered at me throughout my presentation. At the end she accused me in no uncertain terms of stealing her ideas. I was devasted; it was my first real encounter with the dark side of science. Vernon Mountcastle was in the audience and has told this story more than once. The bottom line, however, is that I appeared to be correct (see Thompson et al., 1963a,b).

In the summer of 1959 I met my wife-to-be, Judith Pedersen, at the Psychiatry Department picnic at Merwin Dam in Washington. At that time, Judith and I were both very strong swimmers. Together, we swam way out to a log border in the lake and got to know each other. Judith was born and grew up in Denmark, and spent part of her life during the Nazi occupation. At 18 she came to the United States on a scholarship to the University of Oregon in Eugene. She was very good in science, particularly chemistry, biology, and math, and would have gone to medical school except at that time medical schools were only admitting one or two women a year. Consequently, Judith majored in pre-nursing and obtained her B.S. and R.N. in the joint program between the University and the Medical School in Portland. At the time I met Judith, she was on the staff in the Psychiatry Department. Because office space was tight, my office was actually, on the ward, so I got to know Judith and the other nurses and aides and many of the patients. It was my first real experience with psychosis—our ward was experimental and our typical patients were very bright, young adult schizophrenics.

Judith and I were married in May 1960 and moved into an apartment near the Medical School. At Christmas time we went to visit her family in Denmark and also traveled through France and Italy. We joined Alden Spencer and his wife Diane for a week in Pisa—Alden was doing a postdoctorate in Moruzzi's lab. During this week Alden and I developed our joint research plans—he had already accepted his appointment in the Physiology Department at the University of Oregon Medical School. We decided to focus on mechanisms of behavioral and synaptic plasticity in the spinal cord, where neurophysiological analysis was possible (see below).

Judith entered the graduate school of nursing in 1961 to obtain a Masters degree in psychiatric nursing, supported by a Public Health Fellowship. We discovered she was pregnant about Christmas time of 1961, and so that year we bought a house in Beaverton, a mixed blessing. It had an unheated swimming pool, usable about one month in Portland (although we did ice skate on it one winter), a septic tank that backed up, and a large overgrown backyard. Our first child, Kathryn, was born in August 1962, and I abandoned my family to attend the aforementioned International Congress in September. Judith and our newborn baby moved in with a nursing friend while I was gone. Then, in November, we lived through the "Columbus Day" storm. It blew down many of the trees at the end of our yard and took quite a few shingles from the roof. We were without power for about a week and sterilized the baby bottles on the barbeque.

Meanwhile, Judith had finished all her course work before Kathryn was born and was able to concentrate on her thesis. She received her Masters degree in the summer of 1963. She was appointed an Instructor at the University of Oregon School of Nursing. Our second daughter, Elizabeth, was born in 1964. (Our third daughter, Virginia, was born in Newport Beach in 1968). Judith interrupted her own career to devote more time to the children. In later years, Judith joined me in the laboratory, and we have now worked together for many years. Judith became a superb neuroanatomist, completing a number of pathway tracing studies. She, along with a graduate student, Jo Anne Tracy, received the D.G. Marquis Behavioral Neuroscience Award in 1999 (American Psychological Association) for the most outstanding research paper of the year (Tracy et al., 1998).

When I joined the medical school in Portland, I obtained an NIH grant, which I held for many years. I have been most fortunate in having adequate grant support over the years from the NIH, NIMH, NSF, ONR, and other sources. Indeed, I have had continuous federal research grant support since 1959 and am currently supported through 2007. In 1962 I received a Career Development Award from NIMH which permitted me to devote even more time to research.

Our small Department of Medical Psychology at the medical school developed a Ph.D. program in "biopsychology." A critical factor was the hiring of Judson Brown, a distinguished behavioral scientist from the University of Iowa. Thanks to Jud, I gained a better appreciation of the importance of behavioral analysis at both empirical and theoretical levels. Jud came out of the Hull-Spence tradition and was a leading theorist in the field of motivation. He and I discussed and argued at length about the value of neuronal analysis of behavior and attempts to interrelate neural and behavioral phenomena. My paper on stimulus generalization (Thompson, 1965) illustrates this approach; indeed, it was much influenced by discussions with Jud. I felt this was my most important "theoretical" contribution to that time. Unfortunately, it was published as a chapter in a book. Judging from responses from colleagues, perhaps five people read it.

As a result of teaching courses in neurophysiology and behavior to our small but very capable group of graduate students in our Ph.D. program in Portland, I felt the need for a modern text in physiological psychology. My goal was to "explain" neurophysiology to psychology students and attempt, as far as possible, to analyze behavioral phenomena in neuronal terms. The result was my first (and best) text, *Foundations of Physiological Psychology*, written during the period 1964–1967 (Thompson, 1967). Our small graduate program, incidentally, produced a number of excellent scientists, e.g., Joel Davis, Mary Meikle, Timothy Teyler, and Richard Vardaris (Joel and Mary were my students).[1] David S. Phillips, my first postdoc, joined me

---

[1] I list in the footnotes the graduate students, postdocs, visiting professors, and others who worked in my laboratories at several institutions. If I have omitted anyone I apologize. Students in my laboratory at the University of Oregon Medical School (including MD-MS students) 1959–1967: Lew Bettinger, David Bliss, Joel Davis, Linda Fitzgerald, Richard Johnson, Robert Kramer, Mary Meikle, David Phillips, Robert Sack, Jon Shaw, Hilton Smith, and Ellen Zucker.

in 1962; Dave is now and for many years has been a full Professor at the medical school. The Department of Medical Psychology evolved into the current Department of Behavioral Neuroscience, a basic science department at the medical school. In October 2001, I had the great pleasure of being one of the speakers to dedicate this new version of our old department and graduate program in the medical school at the now Oregon Health Sciences University.

Alden Spencer and I began our collaboration in 1962. Alden had a basement lab adjoining mine. We had opted for the study of processes of behavioral plasticity in the acute spinal preparation. Thanks, in part, to the work of Eccles and his many associates, more was known at that time about the synaptic physiology of the spinal cord than other neural systems. Our goal was to develop spinal reflex models of behavioral processes of learning and memory so we could analyze synaptic mechanisms—in short, to develop simplified neuronal *models* of complex behavioral phenomena. I believe this was the first explicit attempt to develop the model system approach for analysis of the neuronal mechanisms of learning and memory. At least we thought so. In a broad context our approach was not, of course, entirely new; Pavlov had a somewhat analogous approach, using the conditioned reflex to study "psychic" processes.

We selected habituation of the hindlimb flexion reflex of the acute spinal cat as our model system. Flexion reflex habituation was a very robust and repeatable phenomenon. We first showed that habituation of this model system had all the properties of behavioral habituation in intact organisms (Thompson and Spencer, 1966). In the course of this work, we discovered that dishabituation was actually a superimposed process of sensitization, both in our preparation and in intact vertebrate behavior.

At the same time, we analyzed sites and mechanisms of plasticity underlying short-term habituation and sensitization (e.g., Spencer, Thompson, and Neilson, 1966). For habituation, we ruled out muscle fatigue, sensory adaptation, and changes in motor neurons and in primary afferent fibers. Our results were consistent with a process of synaptic depression in interneurons, although we could not prove it. Later, Kandel and associates demonstrated this to be the case in a monosynaptic system in *Aplysia*, and we did so in a monosynaptic pathway in the isolated frog spinal cord (e.g., Farel and Thompson, 1976). At the University of California, Irvine, Philip Groves, a graduate student, and I elaborated all these findings and results from our spinal interneuron recordings into the "dual-process" theory of habituation (Groves and Thompson, 1970). The Thompson and Spencer 1966 paper on the parametric properties of habituation (later a citation classic) and the dual-process theory had a significant impact on the field and indeed are still cited to this day.

In 1966 I took a six-month sabbatical in the neurophysiology laboratory of Anders Lundberg at the Salgrenska in Göteborg, Sweden. At that time,

Lundberg was perhaps the leading scientist in spinal neurophysiology. During the time I was there, I was fortunate to work on a project with Anders, Charles Phillips from England, and others on the patterns of monosynaptic Ia connections to hindlimb motor nuclei in the baboon (see Hongo et al., 1984; yes the data were collected in 1966, but not published until 1984). I learned a great deal more about intracellular recording in this project. Because baboons are, of course, very valuable and the experiments were acute, the work was intensive, with each preparation (and all the experimenters) going for 36 hr or more. Judith and our daughters spent much of this time with relatives in Denmark.

University of California, Irvine, 1967–1973

In 1967 I accepted a professorship in the Department of Psychobiology at the University of California, Irvine, at that time chaired by James L. McGaugh. When I moved to Irvine, I was awarded a Research Scientist Career Award from NIMH, which I held until I left Irvine in 1973. The period at Irvine was very productive, both in terms of research and scholarship and in terms of the growth and increasing importance of the Department of Psychobiology. I had an outstanding group of graduate students and postdoctoral fellows during this period.[2] Indeed, the graduate program we developed was one of the first and most successful programs in the broad field of behavioral neuroscience. While at Irvine I continued research on the neurobiology of habituation and on the organization and functions of cerebral cortex and developed a research program on neuronal mechanisms of associative learning, using the somewhat controversial spinal conditioning preparation (e.g., Pattersen, Cegavske, and Thompson, 1973). We actually began this work in Oregon (Fitzgerald and Thompson, 1967). We did indeed demonstrate an associatively induced increase in the amplitude of the flexor reflex (acute spinal cat); however, unlike associative learning in intact organisms, there was no change in response latency with learning. As with habituation, we were able to rule out changes in motor neurons and sensory afferent terminals, but could go no further.

During the time at Irvine, I collaborated and interacted with a number of colleagues: Carl Cotman, Gary Lynch, James McGaugh, Marcel Verzeano, Norman Weinberger, Richard Whalen, and others. I particularly valued, and still do, my discussions with McGaugh, Lynch, and Weinberger and my collaborations with Verzeano. Intellectually, it was an exciting time as we

[2]Graduate students and postdoctoral fellows at the University of California, Irvine, 1967–1973: Lew Bettinger and Joel Davis moved with us; Herman Birch, Craig Cegavske, Ray Demarco, Paul Farel, Michael Gabriel, Fay Glanzman, Dennis Glanzman, Philip Groves, Dexter Irvine, Kathleen Mayers, Michael Patterson, Richard Robertson, Richard Roemer, Edwin Rubel, Timothy Teyler, Knut Wester, and William Wheeler.

developed the graduate program and our own research programs. During the time at Irvine, I collaborated with Harry Harlow and James McGaugh in writing an introductory psychology text that emphasized the biological point of view (Harlow, McGaugh, and Thompson, 1971). I also began editing a series of volumes on methods in physiological psychology and, in collaboration with James Voss, edited a book on learning and performance dedicated to W.J. Brogden and written by Brogden's students (Thompson and Voss, 1972). We were able to present a typescript copy of the book to Wulf Brogden at a Psychonomic Society meeting in St. Louis before he died. Although in poor health, Wulf, in typical fashion, wrote a critique of each chapter for each author. But we could tell he was very pleased. I know how he must have felt. Just this past year many of my former students and colleagues wrote and published a book dedicated to me (Steinmetz, Gluck, and Solomon, 2001). My students also wrote articles for a full issue of the journal *Neurobiology of Learning and Memory* (2001, 76, pp. 225–461).

At Irvine and later at Harvard, I collaborated with Gardner Lindzey and Calvin Hall in writing yet another introductory text in psychology (Lindzey, Hall, and Thompson, 1975). I had gotten to know Gardner via committees; he was then at the University of Texas, and he played a key role in convincing me to accept the position at Harvard, where he had agreed to serve as Chair of the Department. Gardner was extremely knowledgeable and influential in psychology and very stimulating. Calvin Hall was also a most impressive intellect. I greatly enjoyed my interactions with these more senior individuals.

It was also during this period at Irvine that I became involved in editorial activities, beginning as Editor-in-chief of the journal *Physiological Psychology* published by the Psychonomic Society. In this context I got to know Cliff Morgan well; he was an extraordinary person. I became one of the Associate Editors of the *Annual Review of Neuroscience* in 1981; I enjoyed my interactions with Max Cowan and the other Associate Editors. In 1981 I agreed to become Editor of the *Journal of Comparative and Physiological Psychology (JCPP)* (1981–1982) published by the American Psychological Association, but with a condition. At that time there was serious strife between comparative and physiological psychologists; their methods, approaches, and interests had become quite divergent and the *JCPP* was suffering. The *JCPP* had a long history as *the* psychological journal in the field. My condition was to separate it into two journals, *The Journal of Comparative Psychology* and *Behavioral Neuroscience*. I was thus the "founding" Editor of *Behavioral Neuroscience* (1983–1990). Several senior people in the field were rather outraged by this change in title, but the separation worked. *Behavioral Neuroscience* is now the leading journal in the field.

During this period at Irvine, I was not satisfied with spinal conditioning as a model for analysis of mechanisms of associative learning and memory in intact mammals and cast about for other approaches. At that time, Michael

Patterson, a postdoc in the lab, argued persuasively for eyeblink conditioning (actually nictitating membrane conditioning) in rabbit, with the preparation developed by his Ph.D. mentor, Isidore (Dore) Gormezano. I was, of course, familiar with his work and a great admirer of it; Dore and I had been fellow graduate students at Wisconsin. Mike set up the instrumentation, and we trained a few rabbits. I was enormously impressed with the very robust and reliable learned behavior and the possibilities for neurobiological analysis.

Harvard University, 1973–1975

In 1973 I moved to the Department of Psychology and Social Relations at Harvard University, where I held the professorship previously held by Karl Lashley—a very special honor, since Lashley had been a particular hero from undergraduate days. Harvard provided me with superb laboratory facilities and support, and I found, as expected, that the intellectual atmosphere, students, and colleagues at Harvard were truly outstanding.

While at Harvard we discovered the massive engagement of hippocampal neurons in eyeblink conditioning (Berger, Alger, and Thompson, 1976). We characterized this result at length: the increase in neuronal activity had all the properties of a memory trace except that, as we knew from the earlier literature, the standard delay eyeblink conditioned response (CR) was neither prevented nor abolished by removal of the hippocampus. This seeming paradox bedeviled us for years (see Berger, Berry, and Thompson, 1986; Thompson et al., 1976). Theodore Berger was and is an extraordinarily talented scientist.

Actually, we set out to map the entire rabbit brain in 1-mm steps in well-trained animals using unit cluster recordings. Since the amplitude-time course of the behavioral eyeblink CR forms the envelope of the unit cluster response in the motor nuclei, and this motor CR response has to be driven from higher systems, we looked for similar patterns in unit cluster recordings throughout the brain. We did not, of course, look randomly, but brain structure/system by system. The hippocampus was the first structure we mapped. But in the end, we mapped all the major brain systems. Other than the hippocampus and, of course, brain stem motor nuclei, the cerebellum showed the most prominent neuronal model of the CR, both in areas of cerebellar cortex and in the nuclei (see, e.g., McCormick, Lavond, and Thompson, 1983). This mapping led us to the cerebellar memory system (see below).

Timothy Teyler played a key role in our research program at Harvard. Tim had been a postdoc in my lab at Irvine. He then took a further postdoc in Per Andersen's laboratory in Oslo, Norway, where he learned the hippocampal explant (slice) preparation and long-term potentiation (LTP). I was able to hire Tim as an Assistant Professor at Harvard. He set up a hippocampal slice lab in the floating room built initially for von Bekesy in my laboratories.

During that time, Gary Lynch visited our lab and learned the slice technology from Tim. I believe that Tim's lab at Harvard and Philip Schwartzkroin's lab at the University of Washington (he had also done a postdoc in Oslo) were the first two hippocampal slice labs devoted to physiology and synaptic plasticity in the United States. At Harvard I had outstanding facilities and a large number of spectacular undergraduates, outstanding graduate students, and postdocs, and we mounted a number of different research projects.[3] When I left Harvard I held a dinner party at the faculty club for my people; I believe there were about 50 in attendance.

Although my wife and I liked Harvard very much, and indeed, Judith began working with me in the lab there, neither we nor our daughters liked living in the Boston area at all so we returned to the University of California, Irvine and to Newport Beach in 1975. In 1977 I was elected to the National Academy of Sciences, the honor that pleased me the most in my career.

University of California, Irvine, 1975–1980

At Irvine we continued work on hippocampal substrates of eyeblink conditioning (Theodore Berger came with me to Irvine to complete his thesis and stayed on as a postdoc). Yet again, I had superb graduate students and postdocs in the lab.[4] Steve Berry discovered a key relationship between hippocampal EEG frequency and learning (eyeblink conditioning) (Berry and Thompson, 1978). Ron Kettner made what I have always thought to be a major discovery, namely, that at absolute acoustic detection threshold (rabbit eyeblink CR) neurons in auditory nuclei detected the signal equally on behavioral detection and non-detection trials (thus ruling out auditory nuclei as a site of memory trace formation), whereas hippocampal neurons (and cerebellar neurons) only responded on detection trials (Kettner and Thompson, 1982, 1985). Paul Solomon (a visiting professor) and Don Weisz (a postdoc) made a key discovery we had been waiting for: hippocampal lesions markedly impaired learning of the trace (but not delay) eyeblink CR (Solomon et al., 1986; although not published until 1986, the initial lesion

---

[3] I had undergraduates, graduate students, and postdocs at Harvard University, 1973–1975: Craig Cegavske, Fay and Dennis Glanzman, Richard Roemer, and William Wheeler moved with us; Timothy Teyler rejoined us as an Assistant Professor; Bradley Alger, Theodore Berger, Theresa Harrison, William Levy, Patricia Mensah, Jacqueline Metzler, Sheryl Spinweber, and Richard Young.

[4] I had graduate students and postdocs at the University of California, Irvine, 1975–1980: Theodore Berger, Fay and Dennis Glanzman, and Patricia Mensah moved with us; Steve Berry, Gregory Clark, Steve Coates, Fred Hoehler, Ronald Kettner, Brenda Lonsbury-Martin, Laura Mamounas, Glen Martin, Russell Richardson, Patricia Rinaldi, Robert Shannon, Paul Solomon, Donald Weisz, and Bo Yi Yang.

work was done at Irvine). The role of the hippocampus in trace conditioning in animals and humans has developed into a field, thanks in part to a
subsequent study by Jeansok Kim and Robert Clark in my lab at the University of Southern California (USC) (Kim, Clark, and Thompson, 1995) and
to work by John Disterhoft, Larry Squire, Robert Clark, and others. It may
provide a simple approach to the study of awareness.

In 1978–1979 we spent a year at the Center for Advanced Study in the
Behavioral Sciences at Stanford. Gardner Lindzey was now Director of the
Center and encouraged me to come. We developed a special interest group in
learning and memory. During this year at the center, Leslie Hicks and I, with
the long-distance help of V.B. Shvyrkov, wrote up the proceedings of a joint
Soviet–U.S. symposium on brain substrates of learning and memory I had
hosted at the University of California Irvine in 1978 (see Thompson, Hicks,
and Shvyrkov, 1980). This symposium was preceded by a rather difficult visit
to Moscow Judith and I made as a part of a delegation from the U.S. National
Academy of Sciences to the Soviet Academy of Sciences to arrange a series of
such joint symposia. Arranging the meeting at Irvine was extremely difficult.
We (U.S. side) had insisted that Evgeny Sokolov, their most distinguished
scientist in this field, be included, but in the end the Soviet authorities
refused. (Evgeny tells me that now he is free to travel as he pleases, but
no longer has adequate funds from the Russian government to do so.) Over
the years, I made several trips to the Soviet Union and more recently to
Russia. Although events during visits in the Soviet days could be complex,
even mysterious, I have always enjoyed my Russian colleagues and my visits
there.

Stanford University, 1980–1987

Judith and I and our daughters very much liked living at Stanford and, of
course, Stanford University. I accepted a position at Stanford University in
1980 as Bing Professor of Human Biology with a primary appointment in
the Psychology Department. I had developed some interest in administration
and chaired the Human Biology program (a popular undergraduate major)
for five years. Although the program was successful during my reign—the
number of majors virtually doubled and many of the students were great—I
felt it took far too much time away from my research. Of course, the Psychology Department at Stanford was and is outstanding, and I greatly enjoyed
my colleagues there and in the university-wide neuroscience Ph.D. program.
(I served as acting Chair for a semester.)

It was at Stanford that we discovered the essential involvement of the
cerebellum in standard delay eyeblink conditioning (McCormick et al., 1981).
I will never forget the day Dave McCormick showed me the polygraph
record from the first successful cerebellar lesion. The conditioned eyeblink
response was completely gone, even on CS (tone) alone test trials and the

reflex eyeblink response to the corneal airpuff US was unchanged. We had hints from recording studies by McCormick (see above) and by Kettner and lesion work by David Lavond that the cerebellum was involved in eyeblink conditioning, but the cerebellar lesion data were decisive. Key players in our cerebellar work at Stanford also included Paul Chapman, Gregory Clark, Nelson Donegan, Michael Foy, Mark Gluck, Barbara Knowlton, Christine Logan, Michael Mauk, Laura Mamounas, Ronald Skelton, Joseph Steinmetz, and Diana Woodruff-Pak.

I make special mention of several of my associates in the cerebellar work at Stanford. Mark Gluck introduced me to computational modeling and developed several useful connectionist level computational models of the cerebellar learning circuitry, models that made specific, verifiable (and verified!) predictions about the circuit (Gluck, Reifsnider, and Thompson, 1990; Gluck et al., 2001). David Lavond showed that kainic acid lesions in the correct place in the interpositus nucleus not much larger than 1 mm^3 abolished the eyeblink CR, thus ruling out fibers of passage and demonstrating extreme localization (Lavond, Hembree, and Thompson, 1985). Michael Mauk showed that high decerebrate animals could retain the CR and provided key evidence re the US pathway (Mauk, Steinmetz, and Thompson, 1986). David McCormick was the key player in the initial recording and lesion studies identifying the essential cerebellar circuit (McCormick and Thompson, 1984). Joe Steinmetz, more than anyone else, was the key player to identify the CS pathway and, with David McCormick and Michael Mauk, the US pathway and showed that electrical stimulation of mossy fibers as a CS and climbing fibers as a US resulted in normal behavioral learning (Steinmetz, Lavond, and Thompson, 1989). Diana Woodruff-Pak argued persuasively and demonstrated empirically that eyeblink conditioning in rabbits and humans provided an extremely useful model for studying the neurobiological effects of aging on learning and memory (Woodruff-Pak and Thompson, 1988). Laura Mamounas demonstrated the key role of GABA in cerebellar memory processes (Mamounas et al., 1987). Most of these scientists continue to work on the neuronal substrates of basic associative learning and memory in their current research programs.

Our cerebellar discoveries were not met with unanimous acclaim. Indeed, several cerebellar physiologists, among others, not only did not believe our findings, but attacked us in every conceivable way, both legitimate and otherwise—another lesson in the dark side of science. However, we or at least data from our lab and subsequently from other labs as well (e.g., Yeo et al., 1985) prevailed. A fact that often gets lost because of the emphasis on eyeblink conditioning is that our cerebellar findings apply to classical conditioning of *all* discrete responses learned with aversive events, e.g., limb flexion, head turn, etc. The studies by Theodore Voneida at the Northeastern Ohio Medical School on cerebellar substrates of forelimb flexion conditioning in the cat are an elegant example (e.g., Voneida, 1999, 2000; Voneida et al., 1990).

Yet again, I was able to assemble an outstanding group of undergraduates, graduate students, postdocs, and visiting professors at Stanford.[5] During the eight years we were at Stanford, we identified the entire essential circuitry for delay eyeblink conditioning, ran a number of control studies ruling out various alternative hypothesis, and completed some computational models of the cerebellar circuitry. Much of the work during this period is summarized in Gluck, Reifsnider, and Thompson, 1990; Steinmetz and Thompson, 1991; Thompson, 1986, 1990; and Woodruff-Pak and Thompson, 1988.

There was considerable interest some years ago in electrical stimulation of cerebral cortex as a CS. Robert Doty reported several such studies using limb flexion conditioning. At the time, it was thought that the memory trace was formed in the cerebral cortex, but definitive evidence was lacking. For her thesis at Stanford, Barbara Knowlton used electrical stimulation of the auditory cortex of the rabbit as a CS in eyeblink conditioning. She was able to show that, as with peripheral stimuli, the critical structure was the cerebellum, and, with Judith, she identified the CS pathway: from auditory cortex to a region of the pontine nuclei and to the cerebellum as mossy fibers (Knowlton and Thompson, 1992; Knowlton, Thompson, and Thompson, 1993). It was very satisfying to bring this earlier unresolved literature to closure.

The issue of the role of the cerebellar cortex in eyeblink conditioning was tackled in detail by Christine Logan for her thesis at Stanford University using rabbit eyeblink. She obtained the first really decisive data showing that very large cortical lesions including the anterior lobe result in a dramatic decrease in CR latency in addition to impairing learning (Logan, 1991). We had earlier seen a suggestion of this, but not so clearly (McCormick and Thompson, 1984). These general results—impairment in acquisition and amplitude of CR and a decreased latency with very large cerebellar cortical lesions—have been replicated in many other studies. On the other hand, the only lesion that consistently and completely abolishes the behavioral CR is a lesion of the interpositus nucleus.

While at Stanford I developed a collaborative research program with my colleague in the Psychiatry Department, Seymore (Gig) Levine. Gig was (and is) a world authority in the field of stress. Michael Foy had joined my lab as a postdoc after receiving his Ph.D. with Tim Teyler at Northeastern Ohio

----

[5]I had an outstanding group of undergraduates, graduate students, postdocs, and visiting professors at Stanford University, 1980–1987: Gregory Clark, Ronald Kettner, Laura Mamounas, Russell Richardson, and Bo Yi Yang moved with us; Paul Chapman, Nelson Donegan, Michael Foy, Mark Gluck, Deborah Haley, Lee Holt, Barbara Knowlton, David Lavond, Christine Logan, John Madden, Michael Mauk, David McCormick, Merle Prim, Ronald Skelton, Mark Stanton, Joseph Steinmetz, and Diana Woodruff-Pak.

Medical School, where he mastered the hippocampal slice and LTP. Mike had the idea that behavioral stress might be important in LTP, perhaps accounting for the variable results across laboratories in the degree of LTP reported at that time. Together with another postdoc, Mark Stanton, we completed a study where we first acutely stressed rats (immobilization and tail shock) and then prepared hippocampal slices and induced LTP (Foy et al., 1987). The results were striking; prior behavioral stress completely prevented the subsequent induction of LTP in the slice (CA1).

When I moved to USC (see below), Mike Foy accepted a position in the Psychology Department at Loyola-Marymount University in Los Angeles, where he is now a full Professor. He continues to work with us on hippocampal plasticity. By the time I moved to USC, we were joined by a superb postdoc, Tracey Shors, who also worked on the project.

University of Southern California, 1987–present

In 1987 I was given an offer I "could not refuse" from USC. They were in the process of developing a neuroscience program and had raised the money to build a research building. In addition to the usual setup funds, my offer included a substantial permanent research fund, a position for Judith, and other forms of support. I was appointed Keck Professor of Psychology and Biological Science, with a light teaching load. We had rented out our house in Newport Beach when we moved to Stanford, so we moved back yet again to Newport Beach. This time, however, there was a formidable commute.

Development of the Neuroscience Program at USC was due to the vision of a remarkable man, William Wagner, then Dean of Natural Sciences and a physicist by training. He labeled the program NIBS—Neural, Informational and Behavioral Sciences—with a strong focus on cognitive and computational aspects of neuroscience. I agreed to become Director of the program in 1989 and set about hiring. I had a budget of over one million dollars that was designed to self-destruct. Each time we hired someone for the NIBS program, that person had to have a primary appointment in a department and the first year of his/her salary came as a permanent reduction in the NIBS budget, thereafter to be picked up by the University. So NIBS and the home departments had to agree on the appointments. It was also the case that setup funds for each new appointee would come from my budget and then be replaced in my budget the following year.

In the first several years, I hired or facilitated hiring of an outstanding group of scientists: Michel Baudry, Theodore Berger, Irving Biederman, Roberta Brinton, Mary Ellen MacDonald, Mark Seidenberg, Larry Swanson, and Alan Watts. Together with Michael Arbib and Christoff von der Malsburg, already in the program, we were well on our way to becoming an outstanding neuroscience program with foci on synaptic plasticity and learning and memory and with a strong emphasis on cognitive and computation approaches.

Although it took some time and effort, I was finally able to establish a university-wide Ph.D. program in neuroscience in 1996. This has proved to be the glue that holds the neuroscience program together, at least until now. From the beginning there was a fundamental structural problem in the NIBS/neuroscience program. The initial budget for the program, including the Hedco Neuroscience research building (due in large part to a gift from the Hedco Foundation), came entirely from the School of Letters, Arts and Sciences (LAS), but the program was university-wide. The revenue sharing system at USC pits school against school, so problems were inevitable.

The NIBS program was strongly supported in the early days by then Dean of LAS, William Spitzer. However, he retired and support for the NIBS program declined rapidly under a succession of LAS deans who cut the budget, changed the rules on setup funds, and were generally not supportive. I was not able to make any more hires in the program, and we basically stalled. It was most unfortunate.

In 1999 our neuroscience program received an external review by an outstanding group (Leon Cooper, Fred Gage, and Larry Squire). Their report was very supportive of our program and its goals and very critical of the University for its lack of support. There was no response from LAS. Eventually, however, the Provost (with university-wide authority) intervened and provided much needed support in terms of graduate student stipends and operational costs. I stepped down as Director in 2001 to be replaced by Larry Swanson.

Although I enjoyed many aspects of administering the neuroscience program, it did interfere substantially with my research program. But, yet again, I was able to assemble an outstanding group in my laboratory.[6] In 1991 I was appointed a "corresponding" member of the Center for the Neurobiology of Learning and Memory at the University of California, Irvine. I have greatly enjoyed my continuing interactions with my many friends and colleagues at Irvine.

I will note here just a few high points of our research at USC. First, I must acknowledge my debt to two colleagues at USC: Michel Baudry and Caleb (Tuck) Finch. Michel is a superb neurochemist/physiologist and a long-time

---

[6]I had an outstanding group in my laboratory at the University of Southern California, 1987–present: Paul Chapman, Barbara Knowlton, David Lavond, and Christine Logan moved with us (we continued long-distance collaborations with several colleagues: e.g., Mark Gluck, Joseph Steinmetz, and Diana Woodruff-Pak); Gabor Bartha, Shaowen Bao, Gil Case, Chong Chen, Lu Chen, Kimberly Christian, Robert Clark, Michael Foy, Rene Garcia, David Gellerman, Hiroshi Gomi, Jeffrey Grethe, Stephanie Hauge, Richard Hinchliffe, Dragana Ivkovich, Tsugio Kaneko, Jeansok Kim, Jon Lockard, Yi Chun (Ingrid) Liu, Steve Maren, Matti Mintz, Shahriar Mojtahedian, Nancy Nichols, Alan Nordholm, Gorica Petrovich, Andrew Poulos, Xiaoxi Qiao, Oscar Ramirez, Karla Robleto, Andrea Scicli, Paul Shinkman, Tracey Shors, Steve Standley, William Sun, Rodney Swain, Georges Tocco, Jo Anne Tracy, Benjamin Tran, Noriaki Uenishi, Rosemarie Vouimba, Craig Weiss, Martha Weninger (ne Berg), and Kenji Yoshimi.

friend and collaborator who has done his best to educate me in molecular matters. Tuck is a leading scientist in the neurobiology of aging and a greatly valued friend and collaborator. At USC we continued to characterize the essential circuitry for delay classical conditioning of eyeblink and other discrete responses. I had decided at Stanford that a way to approach the issue of localizing the memory trace in the circuit was by reversible inactivation. A visiting professor in my lab at Stanford tried to develop a reversible cooling system, but without success. David Lavond became interested in this approach; he had moved with us to USC, where he was a Research Assistant Professor in my laboratory. (He is now a full Professor in the Psychology Department.) He successfully developed a cryoprobe using freon, based on a system initially developed at the University of California at Los Angeles (UCLA).

Meanwhile, a superb graduate student in my laboratory, David Krupa, developed a complementary approach by infusion of muscimol, a competitive $GABA_A$ agonist, an approach initially suggested to me at Stanford by Eric Knudsen. Muscimol hyperpolarizes and thus inactivates all neurons with $GABA_A$ receptors for a period of several hours, followed by complete recovery. Alan Nordholm, another excellent graduate student, utilized lidocaine for reversible inactivation (Nordholm et al., 1993). Judith worked with Krupa and with Nordholm on these projects. Using all these methods, we were able to localize the memory trace to the cerebellum.

More specifically, inactivation of the motor nuclei or the red nucleus during training did not prevent learning at all, even though performance of the response (CR for red nucleus CR and UR for motor nuclei) was completely prevented. Similarly, inactivation of the superior cerebellar peduncle, all the output from the interpositus (now using tetrodotoxin), does not prevent learning at all, even though performance of the CR is prevented during training. In marked contrast, muscimol inactivation limited to the interpositus nucleus completely prevented learning. Subsequent postinactivation learning occurred with no savings at all compared to an appropriate control group, even though all projections to the cerebellar cortex were completely functional (except, of course, for projections from the interpositus) (Krupa and Thompson, 1995, 1997; Krupa, Thompson, and Thompson, 1993; Krupa, Weng, and Thompson, 1996).

Paul Shinkman, a Professor in the Psychology Department at the University of North Carolina and an old friend, joined me for a number of summers and a sabbatical year to work on a most interesting project following up on a study my Wisconsin Professor, Wulf Brogden, published with W. Horsley Gantt in 1945. In brief, they reported that movements elicited by electrical stimulation of cerebellar white matter (e.g., limb flexion, eyeblink, etc.) could be conditioned to a neutral tone or light CS (dogs). With Rodney Swain, a graduate student, we replicated and extended these observations in rabbit (Swain et al., 1992). The responses elicited by cerebellar stimulation relayed through the interpositus nucleus rather than by antidromic activation via the inferior olive or pontine nuclei and the effective stimulus appeared due to activation of climbing fibers. Indeed, we were able to condition the movements elicited by stimulating white matter (US) directly under an oval surface electrode stimulating parallel fibers as a CS, thus creating what we hope is an extremely localized memory trace (see Shinkman, Swain, and Thompson, 1996; Swain et al., 1992; Thompson et al., 2000).

An extraordinary group in my lab, Jeansok Kim (postdoc), Lu Chen, and Shaowen Bao (graduate students), established procedures for eyeblink conditioning in the freely moving mouse. We based this on earlier work by two former postdocs in the lab, Ron Skelton and Mark Stanton, who had initially developed procedures for eyeblink conditioning in the rat, infant rat, and mouse. Because of the large number of mutant and transgenic mouse strains available, a number of issues concerning possible mechanisms of learning and memory can be analyzed. In particular, the issue of cerebellar cortex versus interpositus nucleus (as the site of memory storage) could be addressed by use of the Purkinje cell degeneration (pcd) mouse. This mutant, with no functional cerebellar cortex at all, learns eyeblink conditioning, albeit more slowly, to a lesser degree and with shorter CR latencies (Chen et al., 1996), just as with large cerebellar cortical lesions or inactivation. But lesion of the interpositus nucleus in the pcd mouse completely prevents learning.

Lu and Shaowen, together with Xiaoxi Qiao and others, completed an important series of studies on the Stargazer mouse (e.g., Chen et al., 1999). This mouse, incidentally, was discovered by Xiaoxi Qiao and Ray Nobilis at the Jackson lab. It lacks BDNF in cerebellar cortical granule cells; these cells have no functional AMPA receptors and eyeblink conditioning is much impaired. We collaborated with Susumu Tonegawa, Shigeyoshi Itohara, Hiroshi Gomi, and others in studies of transgenic mice (see Kim et al., 1996).

In our cerebellar projects in the rabbit, Jeansok Kim and David Krupa were able to show that the behavioral phenomenon of "blocking" in eyeblink conditioning was mediated by the GABAergic projection from the interpositus to the inferior olive (Kim, Krupa, and Thompson, 1998). Jeansok was also much interested in hippocampal functions in eyeblink conditioning. As a graduate student with Michael Fanselow at UCLA, they showed that lesions of the hippocampus in fear conditioning (rats) abolished freezing to context, but only if made soon after training. In my lab, Jeansok, together with Robert Clark, obtained similar results for trace eyeblink conditioning in rabbits: large bilateral lesions of hippocampus immediately after training abolished trace (but not delay) conditioning. The same lesions made a month after training had no effect (Kim, Clark, and Thompson, 1995). Shaowen Bao, Lu Chen, and Jeansok Kim completed an extraordinary study using both mouse interpositus slice and intact trained rabbit and provided very strong evidence that in standard eyeblink conditioning the basic memory trace is established in the interpositus nucleus (Bao et al., 2002). Currently, I have an outstanding group of graduate students focusing on cerebellar substrates of conditioning: Kimberly Christian, Ka Hung Lee, Shahriar Mojtahedian, Andrew Poulos, and Karla Robleto.

In our ongoing project on stress and hippocampal LTP, Tracey Shors completed a lovely study showing that stress impairment of LTP is truly "psychological." Animals were given shock escape training—they learned rapidly—and yoked animals were given identical shocks, but could do nothing about it. The escape animals showed little subsequent impairment of LTP (hippocampal slice), but the yoked animals, who could not control the situation, showed marked impairment of LTP (Shors et al., 1989). More recently, Jeansok Kim and Mike Foy showed that behavioral stress enhanced subsequent LTD (hippocampal slice) and that both stress impairment of LTP and enhancement of LTD required NMDA receptor activation (Kim et al., 1996). In current work with Mike Foy and in collaboration with our colleague Michel Baudry, we discovered that acute application of physiological levels of estrogen to the bath enhanced LTP, prevented stress impairment of LTP, and prevented stress enhancement of LTD (Bi et al., 2001; Foy et al., 1999, 2000; Vouimba et al., 2000).

Conditioned fear has always been of interest to me. We collaborated with our superb colleague in the School of Pharmacy at USC, Jean Shih, in showing that MAOA KO mice exhibited markedly enhanced conditioned fear, but no change in eyeblink conditioning (Kim et al., 1997). With our colleagues, Larry Swanson, Gorica Petrovich, and Andrea Scicli, we characterized enkephalin mRNA levels in the amygdala (Petrovich et al., 2000). In current work, Ingrid Liu is exploring the role of BDNF in conditioned fear.

In this essay I have focused on the "voyages of discovery" I have been so fortunate to make with my many students and associates. There is no intellectual thrill greater than discovering something entirely new that has never been known before. However, in the long run, I feel the most important thing to me is family—my wife, children, and now grandchildren (we have seven). In looking back, I so wish I had spent more time with my daughters as they were growing up. For many years I was too much involved in professional activities—committees of the National Science Foundation, the National Institute of Mental Health, the American Psychological Association, the National Academy of Sciences, the National Research Council, the Society for Neuroscience, and others. Such activities may be useful, but in my case they took far too much time away from my family.

I have been very gratified by the many honors and awards I have received. But in the end, I and most other scientists will be forgotten. The discoveries we have made will be listed in the textbooks as facts not associated with names, and this is as it should be. Unlike other approaches to knowledge, scientific knowledge is cumulative

Selected Bibliography

Bao S, Chen L, Kim J, Thompson RF. Cerebellar cortical inhibition and classical eyeblink conditioning. *Proc Natl Acad Sci USA* 2002;99:1592–1597.

Benjamin RM, Thompson RF. Differential effects of cortical lesions in infant and adult cats on roughness discrimination. *Exp Neurol* 1959;1:305–321.

Berger TW, Alger BE, Thompson RF. Neuronal substrate of classical conditioning in the hippocampus. *Science* 1976;192:483–485.

Berger TW, Berry SD, Thompson RF. Role of the hippocampus in classical conditioning of aversive and appetitive behaviors. In Isaacson RL, Pribram KH, eds. *The hippocampus, vols. III and IV*, New York: Plenum Press, 1986;203–239.

Berger TW, Rinaldi PC, Weisz DJ, Thompson RF. Single unit analysis of different hippocampal cell types during classical conditioning of the rabbit nictitating membrane response. *J Neurophysiol* 1983;50(5):1197–1219.

Berger TW, Thompson RF. Limbic system interrelations: Functional division among hippocampal-septal connections. *Science* 1977;197:587–589.

Berger TW, Thompson RF. Identification of pyramidal cells as the critical elements in hippocampal neuronal plasticity during learning. *Proc Natl Acad Sci USA* 1978a;75(3):1572–1576.

Berger TW, Thompson RF. Neuronal plasticity in the limbic system during classical conditioning of the rabbit nictitating membrane response. I. The hippocampus. *Brain Res* 1978b;145(2):323–346.

Berger TW, Thompson RF. Neuronal plasticity in the limbic system during classical conditioning of the rabbit nictitating membrane response. II: Septum and mammillary bodies. *Brain Res* 1978c;156:293–314.

Berry SD, Rinaldi PC, Thompson RF, Verseano M. Analysis of temporal relations among units and slow waves in rabbit hippocampus. *Brain Res Bull* 1978;3: 509–518.

Berry SD, Thompson RF. Prediction of learning rate from the hippocampal EEG. *Science* 1978;200:1298–3000.

Berry SD, Thompson RF. Medial septal lesions retard classical conditioning of the nictitating membrane response in rabbits. *Science* 1979;205:209–211.

Bi R, Foy MR, Vouimba R-M, Thompson RF, Baudry M. Cyclic changes in estradiol regulate synaptic plasticity through the MAP kinase pathway. *Proc Natl Acad Sci USA* 2001;98:13391–13395.

Cegavske CF, Patterson MM, Thompson RF. Neuronal unit activity in the abducens nucleus during classical conditioning of the nictitating membrane response in the rabbit. Oryctolaqus cuniculus. *J Comp Physiol Psychol* 1979;93:595–609.

Cegavske CF, Thompson RF, Patterson MM, Gormezano I. Mechanisms of efferent neuronal control of the reflex nictitating membrane response in the rabbit *(Oryctolagus cuniculus). J Comp Physiol Psychol* 1976;90:411–423.

Chen L, Bao S, Lockard JM, Kim JJ, Thompson RF. Impaired classical eyeblink conditioning in cerebellar lesioned and Purkinje cell degeneration (pcd) mutant mice. *J Neurosci* 1996;16:2829–2838.

Chen L, Bao S, Qiao X, Thompson RF. Impaired cerebellar synapse maturation in *waggler*, a mutant mouse with a disrupted neuronal calcium channel γ subunit. *Proc Natl Acad Sci USA* 1999;96:12132–12137.

Chen L, Bao S, Thompson RF. Bilateral lesions of the interpositus nucleus completely prevent eyeblink conditioning in Purkinje cell degeneration mutant mice. *Behav Neurosci* 1999;113:204–210.

Chen C, Kano M, Abeliovich A, Chen L, Bao S, Kim JJ, Hashimoto K, Thompson RF, Tonegawa S. Impaired motor coordination correlates with persistant multiple climbing fiber innervation in PKCγ mutant mice. *Cell* 1995;83:1233–1242.

Chen C, Kim JJ, Thompson RF, Tonegawa S. Hippocampal lesions impair contextual fear conditioning in two strains of mice. *Behav Neurosci* 1996;110:1177–1180.

Chen C, Thompson RF. Temporal specificity of long-term depression in parallel fiber-Purkinje synapses in rat cerebellar slice. *Learn Mem* 1995;2:185–198.

Clark GA, McCormick DA, Lavond DG, Thompson RF. Effects of lesions of cerebellar nuclei on conditioned behavioral and hippocampal neuronal responses. *Brain Res* 1984;291:125–136.

Davis RT, Leary RW, Stevens DA, Thompson RF. Learning and perception of oddity problems by lemurs and seven species of monkey. *Primates* 1967;8:311–322.

Farel PB, Glanzman DL, Thompson RF. Habituation of a monosynaptic response in the vertebrate central nervous system: Lateral column-motoneuron pathway in isolated frog spinal cord. *J Neurophysiol* 1973;36:1117–1130.

Farel PB, Thompson RF. Habituation of a monosynaptic response in frog spinal cord: Evidence for a presynaptic mechanism. *J Neurophysiol* 1976;39:661–666.

Fitzgerald LA, Thompson RF. Classical conditioning of the hindlimb flexion reflex in the acute spinal cat. *Psychonomic Sci* 1967;8:213–214.

Foy MR, Henderson VW, Berger TW, Thompson RF. Estrogen and neural plasticity. *Curr Directions Psycholog Sci* 2000;9:148–152.

Foy MR, Stanton ME, Levine S, Thompson RF. Behavioral stress impairs long-term potentiation in rodent hippocampus. *Behav Neural Biol* 1987;48:138–149.

Foy MR, Xu J, Xie X, Brinton RD, Thompson RF, Berger, TW. 17β-Estradiol enhances NMDA receptor-mediated EPSPs and long-term potentiation. *J Neurophysiol* 1999;81:925–929.

Garcia R, Vouimba R-M, Baudry M, Thompson RF. The amygdala modulates prefrontal cortex activity relative to conditioned fear. *Nature* 1999;402:294–296.

Gluck MA, Allen MT, Myers CE, Thompson RF. Cerebellar substrates for error-correction in motor conditioning. *Neurobiol Learn Mem* 2001;76:314–341.

Gluck MA, Reifsnider ES, Thompson RF. Adaptive signal processing and the cerebellum: Models of classical conditioning and VOR adaptation. In Gluckand MA, Rumelhart DE, eds. *Neuroscience and connectionist models*. Hillsdale, NJ: Lawrence Erlbaum Associates, 1990;131–185.

Gluck MA, Thompson RF. Modeling the neural substrates of associative learning and memory: A computational approach. *Psycholog Rev* 1987;94:176–191.

Groves PM, Thompson RF. Habituation: A dual-process theory. *Psycholog Rev* 1970;77:419–450.

Harlow HF, McGaugh JL, Thompson RF. *Psychology*. San Francisco: Albion, 1971.

Hebb DO. *The organization of behavior*. New York: John Wiley & Sons, 1949.

Hind JE, Rose JE, Davies PW, Woolsey CN, Benjamin RM, Welker WI, Thompson RF. Unit activity in the auditory cortex. In Rasmussen GL, Windle WF, eds. *Neural mechanisms of the auditory and vestibular systems*. Springfield, IL: Charles C Thomas, 1960;201–210.

Hongo T, Lundberg A, Phillips CG, Thompson RF. The pattern of monosynaptic Ia-connections to hindlimb motor nuclei in the baboon: A comparison with the cat. *Proc R Soc Lond* 1984;221:261–289.

Ivkovich D, Lockard JM, Thompson RF. Interpositus lesion abolition of the eyeblink CR is not due to effects on performance. *Behav Neurosci* 1993;107:530–532.

Kettner RE, Thompson RF. Auditory signal detection and decision processes in the nervous system. *J Comp Physiol Psychol* 1982;96(2):328–331.

Kettner RE, Thompson RF. Cochlear nucleus, inferior colliculus, and medial geniculate responses during the behavioral detection of threshold–level auditory stimuli in the rabbit. *J Acoust Soc Am* 1985;77(6):2111–2127.

Kim JJ, Chen L, Bao S, Sun W, Thompson RF. Genetic dissections of the cerebellar circuitry involved in classical eyeblink conditioning. In Nakanishi S, Silva AJ, Aizawa S, Katsuki M, eds. *Gene targeting and new developments in neurobiology*. Tokyo: Japan Scientific Societies Press, 1996;3–15.

Kim JJ, Clark RE, Thompson RF. Hippocampectomy impairs the memory of recently, but not remotely, acquired trace eyeblink conditioned responses. *Behav Neurosci* 1995;109:195–203.

Kim JJ, Foy MR, Thompson RF. Behavioral stress modifies hippocampal plasticity through N-methyl-D-aspartate (NMDA) receptor activation. *Proc Natl Acad Sci USA* 1996;93:4750–4753.

Kim JJ., Krupa DJ, Thompson RF. Inhibitory cerebello-olivary projections mediate the "blocking" effect in classical conditioning. *Science* 1998;279:570–573.

Kim JJ, Shih JC, Chen K, Chen L, Bao S, Shin MJ, Maren SA, Anagnostaras SG, Fanselow MS, Maeyer ED, Seif I, Thompson RF. Selective enhancement of emotional, but not motor, learning in monoamine oxidase A-deficient transgenic mice. *Proc Natl Acad Sci USA* 1997;94:5929–5933.

Knowlton BJ, Thompson RF. Conditioning using a cerebral cortical CS is dependent on the cerebellum and brainstem circuitry. *Behav Neurosci* 1992;106:509–517.

Knowlton BJ, Thompson JK, Thompson RF. Projection from the auditory cortex to the pontine nuclei in the rabbit. *Behav Brain Res* 1993;56:21–30.

Krupa DJ, Thompson RF. Inactivation of the superior cerebellar peduncle blocks expression but not acquisition of the rabbit's classically conditioned eyeblink response. *Proc Natl Acad Sci USA* 1995;92:5097–5101.

Krupa DJ, Thompson RF. Reversible inactivation of the cerebellar interpositus nucleus completely prevents acquisition of the classically conditioned eyeblink response. *Learn Mem* 1997;3:545–556.

Krupa DJ, Thompson JK, Thompson RF. Localization of a memory trace in the mammalian brain. *Science* 1993;260:989–991.

Krupa DJ, Weng J, Thompson RF. Inactivation of brainstem motor nuclei blocks expression but not acquisition of the rabbit's classically conditioned eyeblink response. *Behav Neurosci* 1996;110:219–227.

Lavond DG, Hembree TL, Thompson RF. Effect of kainic acid lesions of the cerebellar interpositus nucleus on eyelid conditioning in the rabbit. *Brain Res* 1985;326:179–183.

Lindzey G, Hall C, Thompson RF. *Psychology.* New York: Worth Publishers, 1975.

Logan CG. Cerebellar cortical involvement in excitatory and inhibitory classical classical conditioning. *Doctoral Dissertation*, Stanford University, 1991.

Mamounas LA, Thompson RF, Lynch GA, Baudry M. Classical conditioning of the rabbit eyelid response increases glutamate receptor binding in hippocampal synaptic membranes. *Proc Natl Acad Sci USA* 1984;81(8):2548–2552.

Mamounas LA, Thompson RF, Madden J, IV. Cerebellar GABAergic processes: Evidence for critical involvement in a form of simple associative learning in the rabbit. *Proc Natl Acad Sci USA* 1987;84:2101–2105.

Maren S, Tocco G, Standley S, Baudry M, Thompson RF. Postsynaptic factors in the expression of long-term potentiation (LTP): Increased glutamate receptor binding following LTP induction *in vivo. Proc Natl Acad Sci USA* 1993;90: 9654–9658.

Mauk MD, Steinmetz JE, Thompson RF. Classical conditioning using stimulation of the inferior olive as the unconditioned stimulus. *Proc Natl Acad Sci USA* 1986;83:5349–5353.

McCormick DA, Lavond DG, Clark GA, Kettner RE, Rising CE, Thompson RF. The engram found? Role of the cerebellum in classical conditioning of nictitating membrane and eyelid responses. *Bull Psychonomic Soc* 1981;18(3):103–105.

McCormick DA, Lavond DG, Thompson RF. Concomitant classical conditioning of the rabbit nictitating membrane and eyelid responses: Correlations and implications. *Physiol Behav* 1982;28:769–775.

McCormick DA, Lavond DG, Thompson RF. Neuronal responses of the rabbit brainstem during performance of the classically conditioned nictitating membrane (NM/eyelid response). *Brain Res* 1983;271:73–88.

McCormick DA, Steinmetz JE, Thompson RF. Lesions of the inferior olivary complex cause extinction of the classically conditioned eyeblink response. *Brain Res* 1985;359:120–130.

McCormick DA, Thompson RF. Cerebellum: Essential involvement in the classically conditioned eyelid response. *Science* 1984a;223:296–299.

McCormick DA, Thompson RF. Neuronal responses of the rabbit cerebellum during acquisition and performance of a classically conditioned nictitating membrane-eyelid response. *J Neurosci* 1984b;4(11):2811–2822.

Mintz M, Lavond DG, Zhang AA, Yun Y, Thompson RF. Unilateral inferior olive NMDA lesion leads to unilateral deficit in acquisition and retention of eyelid classical conditioning. *Behav Neural Biol* 1994;61:218–224.

Nordholm A, Thompson JK, Dersarkissian C, Thompson RF. Lidocaine infusion in a critical region of cerebellum completely prevents learning of the conditioned eyeblink response. *Behav Neurosci* 1993;107:882–886.

Patterson MM, Cegavske CF, Thompson RF. Effects of classical conditioning paradigm on hindlimb flexor nerve response in immobilized spinal cat. *J Comp Physiol Psychol* 1973;84:88–97.

Petrovich GD, Scicli AP, Thompson RF, Swanson LW. Associative fear conditioning of enkephalin mRNA levels in central amygdalar neurons. *Behav Neurosci* 2000;114:681–686.

Phillips DS, Denney DD, Robertson RT, Hicks LH, Thompson RF. Cortical projections of ascending nonspecific systems. *Physiol Behav* 1972;8:269–277.

Qiao X, Chen L, Gao H, Bao S, Hefti F, Thompson R, Knusel B. Cerebellar brain-derived neurotrophic factor-TrkB defect associated with impairment of eyeblink conditioning in *stargazer* mutant mice. *J Neurosci* 1998;18:6990–6999.

Robertson RT, Mayers KS, Teyler TJ, Bettinger LA, Birch H, Davis JL, Phillips DS, Thompson RF. Unit activity in posterior association cortex of cat. *J Neurophysiol* 1975;38:780–794.

Schreiber SS, Tocco G, Najm I, Thompson RF, Baudry M. Cycloheximide prevents kainate-induced neuronal death and c-fos expression in adult rat brain. *J Mol Neurosci* 1993;4:149–159.

Shibuki K, Gomi H, Chen L, Bao S, Kim JJ, Wakatsuki H, Fujisaki T, Fujimoto K, Ikeda T, Chen C, Thompson RF, Itohara S. Deficient cerebellar long-term depression, impaired eyeblink conditioning and normal motor coordination in GFAP mutant mice. *Neuron* 1996;16:587–599.

Shinkman PG, Swain RA, Thompson RF. Classical conditioning with electrical stimulation of cerebellum as both conditioned and unconditioned stimulus. *Behav Neurosci* 1996;110:914–921.

Shors TJ, Seib TB, Levine S, Thompson RF. Inescapable versus escapable shock modulates long-term potentiation in the rat hippocampus. *Science* 1989;244: 224–226.

Shors TJ, Weiss C, Thompson RF. Stress-induced facilitation of classical conditioning. *Science* 1992;257:537–539.

Sindberg RM, Thompson RF. Auditory response fields in ventral temporal and insular cortex of cat. *J Neurophysiol* 1962;2:21–28.

Solomon PR, Vander Schaaf ER, Thompson RF, Weisz DJ. Hippocampus and trace conditioning of the rabbit's classically conditioned nictitating membrane response. *Behav Neurosci* 1986;100(5):729–744.

Spencer WA, Thompson RF, Neilson DR Jr. Decrement of ventral root electronic and intracellularly recorded PSPs produced by iterated cutaneous afferent volleys. *J Neurophysiol* 1966;29:253–274.

Steinmetz JE, Gluck MA, Soloman PR. *Model systems and the neurobiology of associative learning*. Mahwah, NJ: Lawrence Erlbaum, 2001.

Steinmetz JE, Lavond DG, Ivkovich D, Logan CG, Thompson RF. Disruption of classical eyelid conditioning after cerebellar lesions: Damage to a memory trace system or a simple performance deficit? *J Neurosci* 1992;12:4403–4426.

Steinmetz JE, Lavond DG, Thompson RF. Classical conditioning in rabbits using pontine nucleus stimulation as a conditioned stimulus and inferior olive stimulation as an unconditioned stimulus. *Synapse* 1989;3(3):225–232.

Steinmetz JE, Logan CG, Rosen DJ, Thompson JK, Lavond DG, Thompson RF. Initial localization of the acoustic conditioned stimulus projection system to the cerebellum essential for classical eyelid conditioning. *Proc Natl Acad Sci USA* 1987;84:3531–3535.

Steinmetz JE, Thompson RF. Brain substrates of aversive classical conditioning. In Madden J IV, ed. *Neurobiology of learning, emotion and affect.* New York: Raven Press, 1991;97–120.

Swain RS, Shinkman PG, Nordholm AF, Thompson RF. Cerebellar stimulation as an unconditioned stimulus in classical conditioning. *Behav Neurosci* 1992;106: 739–750.

Teyler TJ, Shaw C, Thompson RF. Unit responses to moving visual stimuli in motor cortex of cat. *Science* 1972;176:811–813.

Thompson RF. The effect of training procedure upon auditory frequency discrimination in the cat. *J Comp Physiol Psychol* 1959a;52:186–190.

Thompson RF. Effect of acquisition level upon the magnitude of stimulus generalization across sensory modality. *J Comp Physiol Psychol* 1959b;52:183–185.

Thompson RF. Function of auditory cortex of cat in frequency discrimination. *J Neurophysiol* 1960;23:321–334.

Thompson RF. Role of the cerebral cortex in stimulus generalization. *J Comp Physiol Psychol* 1962;55:279–287.

Thompson RF. Role of cortical association fields in auditory frequency discrimination. *J Comp Physiol Psychol* 1964;57:335–339.

Thompson RF. The neural basis of stimulus generalization, In Mostofsky D, ed. *Stimulus generalization.* Stanford, CA: Stanford University Press, 1965; chap. 12, pp. 154–178.

Thompson RF. *Foundations of physiological psychology.* New York: Harper & Row, 1967.

Thompson RF. The neurobiology of learning and memory. *Science* 1986;233:941–947.

Thompson RF. Neural mechanisms of classical conditioning in mammals. *Philos Trans R Soc Lond B* 1990;329:161–170.

Thompson RF, Berger TW, Cegavske CF, Patterson MM, Roemer RA, Teyler TJ, Young RA. The search for the engram. *Am Psychol* 1976;31:209–227.

Thompson RF, Hicks TW, Shvyrkov VB, Eds. *Neural mechanisms of goal directed behavior and learning.* New York: Academic Press, 1980.

Thompson RF, Johnson RH, Hoopes JJ. Organization of auditory, somatic sensory, and visual projection to association fields of cerebral cortex in the cat. *J Neurophysiol* 1963;26:343–364.

Thompson RF, Krupa DJ. Organization of memory traces in the mammalian brain. *Annu Rev Neurosci* 1994;17:519–549.

Thompson RF, Mayers KS, Robertson RT, Patterson CJ. Number coding in association cortex of cat. *Science* 1970;168:271–273.

Thompson RF, Patterson MM, Teyler TJ. Neurophysiology of learning. *Annu Rev Psychol* 1972;23:73–104.

Thompson RF, Sindberg RM. Auditory response fields in association and motor cortex of cat. *J Neurophysiol* 1960;23:87–105.

Thompson RF, Smith HE, Bliss D. Auditory, somatic sensory, and visual response interactions and interrelations in association and primary cortical fields of cat. *J Neurophysiol* 1963;26:365–378.

Thompson RF, Spencer WA. Habituation: A model phenomenon for the study of neuronal substrates of behavior. *Psycholog Rev* 1966;173:16–43.

Thompson RF Swain R, Clark R, Shinkman PS. Intracerebellar conditioning— Brogden and Gantt revisited. *Behav Brain Res* 2000;110:3–11.

Thompson RF, Voss JF, Eds. *Topics in learning and performance.* New York: Academic Press, 1972.

Thompson RF, Welker WI. Role of auditory cortex in reflex head orientation by cats in auditory stimuli. *J Comp Physiol Psychol* 1963;56:996–1002.

Tocco G, Devgan KK, Hauge SA, Weiss C, Baudry M, Thompson RF. Classical conditioning selectively increases AMPA/quisqualate receptor binding in rabbit hippocampus. *Brain Res* 1991;559:331–336.

Tracy J, Thompson JK, Krupa DJ, Thompson RF. Evidence of plasticity in the ponto-cerebellar CS pathway during classical conditioning of the eyeblink response in the rabbit. *Behav Neurosci* 1998;112:267–285.

Voneida TJ. The effect of rubrospinal tractotomy on a conditioned limb response in the cat. *Behav Brain Res* 1999;105:151–162.

Voneida TJ. The effect of brachium conjunctivum transection on a conditioned limb response in the cat. *Behav Brain Res* 2000;109:167–175.

Voneida TJ, Christie D, Bogdanski R, Chopko B. Changes in instrumentally and classically conditioned limb-flexion responses following inferior olivary lesions and olivocerebellar tractotomy in the cat. *J Neurosci* 1990;10:3583–3593.

Vouimba R-M, Garcia R, Baudry M, Thompson RF. Potentiation of conditioned freezing following dorsomedial prefrontal cortex lesions does not interfere with fear reduction in mice. *Behav Neurosci* 2000;114:720–724.

Weisz DJ, Clark GA, Yang BY, Solomon PR, Berger TW, Thompson RF. Activity of dentate gyrus during NM conditioning in rabbit. In Woody CD, ed. *Conditioning: Representation of involved neural functions.* New York: Plenum Press, 1982;131–145.

Wester K, Irvine DRF, Thompson RF. Acoustic tuning of single cells in middle suprasylvian cortex of cat. *Brain Res* 1974;76:493–502.

Woodruff-Pak DS, Thompson RF. Cerebellar correlates of classical conditioning across the life span. In Baltes PB, Featherman DL, Lerner RM, eds. *Life span development and behavior, vol. 9.* Hillsdale, NJ: Lawrence Erlbaum Associates, 1988:1–37.

Yeo CH, Hardiman MJ, Glickstein M. Classical conditioning of the nictitating membrane response of the rabbit. I. Lesions of the cerebellar nuclei. *Exp Brain Res* 1985;60:87–98.

Young RA, Cegavske CF, Thompson RF. Tone-induced charges in excitability of abducens motoneurons and the reflex path of the rabbit nictitating membrane response. *J Comp Physiol Psychol* 1976;90:424–434.

Index of Names